Nanoparticles in Cancer Theranostics

This book comprehensively reviews the application of nanoparticles in cancer diagnosis and treatment. The introductory section provides a fundamental understanding of cancer biology, its global incidence and prevalence, and the intricate nano–bio interactions at the cellular level. The subsequent section discusses the pivotal role of nanoparticles in precise cancer detection, enhancing cancer imaging and serving as contrast agents for accurate diagnosis. It also presents cutting-edge nanotechnology-based methods for detecting HTLV-1 retroviruses. The following section covers the utilization of lipid-based nanoparticles, monoclonal antibodies, and advanced nanotherapeutics for targeted cancer treatments. This book is a useful resource for researchers, clinicians, and students in the fields of oncology and nanotechnology.

Nanoparticles in Cancer Theranostics

Current Progress in Cancer Management

Editor
Dr. Prudhvi Lal Bhukya
Scientist B, Preclinical Vaccine Testing Laboratory, Rodent Experimentation Facility, ICMR–National Animal Resource Facility for Biomedical Research, Department of Health Research, Ministry of Health and Family Welfare, Government of India, Genome Valley, Shamirpet, Hyderabad, Telangana 500078, India

Corresponding Editor
Dr. Neelam Thakur, Assistant Professor, Department of Zoology
Sardar Patel University, (a State Govt. University), Vallabh Government College Campus, Paddal, Kartarpur, Mandi 175001, Himachal Pradesh, India

CRC Press
Taylor & Francis Group
Boca Raton London New York

CRC Press is an imprint of the
Taylor & Francis Group, an **informa** business

First edition published 2025
by CRC Press
2385 NW Executive Center Drive, Suite 320, Boca Raton FL 33431

and by CRC Press
4 Park Square, Milton Park, Abingdon, Oxon, OX14 4RN

CRC Press is an imprint of Taylor & Francis Group, LLC

ISBN: 978-1-032-73228-2 (hbk)
ISBN: 978-1-032-73229-9 (pbk)
ISBN: 978-1-003-46319-1 (ebk)

DOI: 10.1201/9781003463191

Typeset in Times LT Std
by Apex CoVantage, LLC

This book is dedicated to our families, teachers, friends, and all well-wishers.

Contents

PART III Nanoparticles in Cancer Therapy

Preface

Cancer is a collective term for a number of the deadliest and frequently diagnosed pathophysiological conditions in the world. Although it has captured the interest of researchers for many years, there are still many unanswered questions regarding the intricate cellular and molecular pathology of cancer. The diseased state is usually characterized by uncontrolled-fashion cell division and dysfunctional pathways of replicative senescence.

As per the recent fact sheet data of the World Health Organization, cancer is the leading cause of death in 112 nations, out of 183 countries. Cancer death ranks third or fourth in the remaining 23 countries, and fifth to eighth in 48. Changes in lifestyle brought on by socioeconomic development, population growth, and the incidence and distribution of cancer risk factors are all being blamed for the rise in cancer-related mortality.

Diagnosis of cancer usually starts with identifying the symptoms associated with the disease, and it plays a pivotal role in understanding the history and mechanism behind the causes and timely management of the disease so as to prevent loss of life. It is the type and location of the tumors that determine the diagnostic methods used for detection and help in early treatment of the disease. For optimal cancer treatment, the most important steps are early detection of cancer cells and drug applications with reduced systemic toxicities. Conventional cancer diagnostics and therapeutics are not sufficient to find cancer cells at early stages and to reduce the drug toxicities, so other strategies, including nanotechnology, are being used nowadays to ameliorate diagnosis and alleviate the severity of disease. The conventional treatments of cancers include the therapies which are used worldwide, like surgery, radiotherapy, and chemotherapy. However, the conventional methods of diagnosis and treatment have their own pros and cons which need to be addressed for better diagnosis and treatment in the future.

The current research and development in nanotechnology offers a novel approach in enhancing the standards of diagnostics and treatments of many communicable and non-communicable diseases. The use of nanotechnology in cancer therapeutics has improved the pharmacokinetics and reduced the systemic toxicities of chemotherapies by selectively targeting and delivering anticancer drugs to tumor tissues in both viral oncogenesis and non-viral oncogenesis.

Nanoparticles in Cancer Theranostics: Current Progress in Cancer Management covers the application of nanotechnology in the field of cancer diagnosis and therapy. Nanotechnology has emerged as a groundbreaking field with immense potential in the diagnosis and treatment of cancer. As such, a comprehensive book on this subject is timely and needed to disseminate knowledge and insights to researchers. It is relevant to healthcare practitioners, researchers, pharmaceutical, and medical device industry professionals.

The book covers a wide range of topics, from introducing the concepts of nanotechnology to the types of nanoparticles and nano–bio interactions at the cellular level and their applications at clinical interphase.

The book is organized into three parts offering comprehensive updates on recent emerging developments in nanotechnology. Part I explicates the basic concepts of cancer, national and international cancer incidences, and gives a glimpse of recent advancements in nanotechnology. This section throws a light on mechanism and challenges in shaping the nanomaterials for wide biomedical applications.

Part II gives in detail insights on the use of nanoparticles in cancer diagnosis and their advantage in comparison with the conventional methods of cancer diagnosis. Nanoparticles, nanodevices, and nano-based imaging methods are highlighted with updated information. This section also especially focuses on nanotechnology-based diagnosis of oncogenic viral diseases like retro and herpes infections.

Meanwhile, Part III throws light on the types of nanoparticles and their application in treating cancers. This section highlights in detail lipid-based nanoparticles, monoclonal-based nanoparticles, and nanoparticles in immunotherapy.

Overall, this book is a valuable guide covering the most recent scientific progress in the field of nanotechnology for cancer management and will serve as the best resource for undergraduates, graduates, medical professionals, researchers, public health physicians, and national and international health authorities. The information in this book can help apply their expertise to more advanced study that could have positive societal and economic effects.

Altogether, the present editorial work provides an in-depth understanding of nanotechnology and its applications in cancer-causing infectious and non-infectious agents. Our authors have explored all the current advancements in nanoparticles for the treatment and diagnosis of cancers.

It is our immense pleasure to present this comprehensive summary to the scientific community for the benefit of health care and society at large.

Dr. Prudhvi Lal Bhukya
Scientist B, Preclinical Vaccine Testing Laboratory, Rodent Experimentation Facility
ICMR–National Animal Resource Facility for Biomedical Research,
Genome Valley, Shamirpet, Hyderabad–Telangana 500101, India

Dr. Neelam Thakur (Corresponding Editor)
Assistant Professor, Department of Zoology
Sardar Patel University (a State Govt. University)
Vallabh Government College Campus, Paddal, Kartarpur, Mandi 175001,
Himachal Pradesh, India

About the Editors

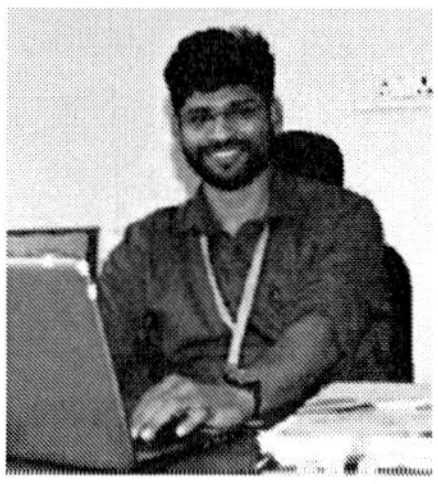

Dr. Prudhvi Lal Bhukya is a virologist currently serving the ICMR–National Animal Resource Facility for Biomedical Research (NARFBR), Hyderabad, as a scientist. Presently, he is associated with the preclinical vaccine testing laboratory at NARFBR. His area of working includes preclinical vaccinology studies, host–virus interactions studies of emerging human viral infections, and prevention and control of diseases and development of tools to prevent outbreaks. He has done his PhD in ICMR–National Institute of Virology, Pune, on human hepatitis B virus. He proved his credentials by working on HBV and HEV with his publication record. He has presented his work in numerous national and international conferences. He has proved his accolades with several publications in international journals, like the *Journal of General Virology*, *Journal of Virology*, *Journal of Travel Medicine*, *Indian Journal of Medical Microbiology*, and *Science of Total Environment*. He is a well-experienced manuscript writer and has contributed to several book chapters for publication bodies like Springer Nature, CRC Press, IntechOpen, and IGI Global Publications. Dr. Prudhvi also edited a book with Springer Nature titled *Emerging Human Viral Disease*, in two volumes. His contributions to these books as an editor will act as catalysts, as his comments are really critical and an achievement for the books.

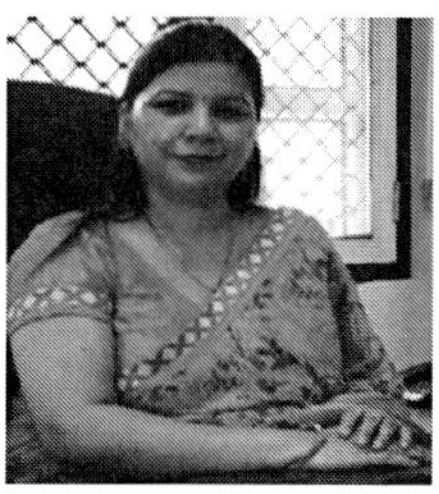

Dr. Neelam Thakur has worked as an assistant professor in the Department of Zoology, Sardar Patel University (a state government university), Mandi, Himachal Pradesh, since 2022. Before joining this university, she worked as an associate professor in the Department of Biosciences at Chandigarh University, Punjab. She obtained her PhD in genetics from Himachal Pradesh University in 2012. After her PhD, she joined as a research associate in the immunology lab of CSIR–Imtech, Chandigarh, in 2012. Her research interests are early diagnosis of tuberculosis and cancer, nanotechnology for cancer diagnostics and therapy, cytogenetic analysis of intellectually disabled individuals, and microbiome studies. She has supervised many master's students and is currently guiding PhD students as well. She has published 18 research papers in journals with good impact factor, like *Cellular Signalling*. Her patent titled "Antigenic Composition and Method of Expression Thereof" has also been published. She has received two Young Researchers Awards and one Eminent Researchers Award from government-registered societies/organizations for her contributions in research.

Contributors

Sujata Adhana
Department of Biomedical Sciences
Bhaskaracharya College of Applied Sciences, University of Delhi
India

Ishant Arora
Public Health
London School of Hygiene and Tropical Medicine
Keppel St., London

Arundhati
Department of Civil Engineering
Chandigarh University
Gharuan, Mohali, Punjab, India

Asvin Suresh Babu
King's College London
Stamford St., London

Vidushi Bahl
London School of Hygiene and Tropical Medicine
Keppel St., London

Divya Dhawal Bhandari
University Institute of Pharmaceutical Sciences
Panjab University
Chandigarh, India

Prudhvi Lal Bhukya
ICMR–National Animal Resource Facility for Biomedical Research
Genome Valley, Shamirpet, Hyderabad, India

Priyanka Chambial
Department of Biosciences
Chandigarh University
Gharuan, Mohali, Punjab, India

Jyoti Chaudhary
Department of Biotechnology, School of Engineering
Noida International University
India

Hitesh Chopra
Saveetha School of Engineering
Saveetha Institute of Medical and Technical Sciences
Chennai, Tamil Nadu, India

Anuradha Derashri
Gahlot Institute of Pharmacy
Navi Mumbai, Maharashtra, India

Akanksha Dwivedi
Acropolis Institute of Pharmaceutical Education and Research
Indore, Madhya Pradesh, India

Jyoti
Centralized Core Research Facility
All India Institute of Medical Sciences
New Delhi, India

Nitin Kolhe
Gahlot Institute of Pharmacy
Navi Mumbai, Maharashtra, India

Anil Kumar Mavi
Department of Botany and Life Sciences
Sri Aurobindo College, University of Delhi
India

L. Preethi
London School of Hygiene and Tropical Medicine
Keppel St., London

Sunita Saklani
Sidharth Govt. College Nadaun
Hamirpur, Himachal Pradesh, India

Akash Tripathi Satsangi
Hindustan College of Science and Technology
India

Akriti Sharma
Department of Civil Engineering
Chandigarh University
Gharuan, Mohali, Punjab, India

Bhagwati Prashad Sharma
Sidharth Govt. College Nadaun
Hamirpur, Himachal Pradesh, India

Anju Singh
Department of Chemistry
Chandigarh University
Gharuan, Mohali, Punjab, India

Gagandeep Singh
Department of Biosciences
Chandigarh University
Gharuan, Mohali, Punjab, India

Arshiya Sood
Department of Zoology
Sardar Patel University
Mandi, Himachal Pradesh, India

Kamal Kishor Thakur
Department of Chemistry
Chandigarh University
Gharuan, Mohali, Punjab, India

Neelam Thakur
Department of Zoology
Sardar Patel University
Mandi, Himachal Pradesh, India

Samjeet Singh Thakur
NSCBM Govt. College Hamirpur
Himachal Pradesh, India

Christy Thomas
London School of Hygiene and Tropical Medicine
Keppel St., London

Soumya Upadhyay
Bundelkhand University
India

Rhea Vas
London School of Hygiene and Tropical Medicine
Keppel St., London

Part I

Introduction

1 An Introduction to Fundamentals of Cancer Cell Biology

Neelam Thakur and Prudhvi Lal Bhukya

ABBREVIATIONS

Acronym	**Full Form**
ABL	Abelson
Arf	ADP ribosylation factor
AJ	adherens junction
BCR	breakpoint cluster region
CAFs	cancer-associated fibroblasts
CCL2	chemokine ligand 2
CDH	cadherin
CDK	cyclin-dependent kinase
CeRNA	competing endogenous RNA
CIP	CDK interacting protein
CKI	cyclin-dependent kinase inhibitors
CML	chronic myelogenous leukemia
CpG	cytosine-phosphate-guanine dinucleotides
CSC	cancer stem cell
CSCP	cancer stem cell plasticity
CSFs	colony-stimulating factors
CKs	cytokeratins
CRC	colorectal cancer
DMP1	dentin matrix acidic phosphoprotein 1
DNA	deoxyribonucleic acid
DS	desmosome
E2F	a group of genes that code for transcription factor
E2F-DP	E2F dimerization partner
EBV	Epstein–Barr virus
ECM	extracellular matrix
EGF	epidermal growth factor
EMT	epithelial–mesenchymal transition
EMTF	epithelial–mesenchymal transition factor
ErbB2	erythroblastic oncogene B
FOXM1C	forkhead box protein M
FOXO	forkhead box transcription factors
GTP	guanosine triphosphate
HATs	histone acetyltransferases
HCC	hepatocellular carcinoma
HDAC	histone deacetylase

DOI: 10.1201/9781003463191-2

HDS	hemidesmosome
HER2	human epidermal growth factor
HGF	hepatocyte growth factor
HOXD-AS1	HOXD cluster anti-sense RNA 1
INK	inhibitor of CDK (cyclin-dependent kinase inhibitor)
ISWI	imitation SWI
JUN	Ju-nana (proto-oncogene)
k-ras	Kirsten rat sarcoma viral oncogene homolog
KD	knock down
KIP	kinase inhibitory protein
KSHV	Kaposi's sarcoma–associated herpesvirus
lncRNAs	long noncoding RNAs
LC	lung cancer
MALAT1	metastasis-associated lung adenocarcinoma transcript 1
MBD2	methyl-CpG binding domain protein 2
MeCP	methyl-CpG binding protein
MET	mesenchymal–epithelial transition
MiRNA	microRNA
MMPs	matrix metallopeptidase/proteinases
MYC	myelocytomatosis (proto-oncogene)
NF1	neurofibromin 1
NFR1	nuclear respiratory factor 1
NK	natural killer
OC	ovarian cancer
PCa	pancreatic cancer
PDGF	platelet-derived growth factor
pRb	retinoblastoma protein
PTAR	pro-transition associated RNA
Pten	phosphatase and tensin homolog (deleted on chromosome 10)
Ras	a family of proteins (GPTases) responsible for cell proliferation
RNA	ribonucleic acid
SASP	senescence-associated secretory phenotype
SNAIL/SLUG	snail family transcriptional repressor
SOX4	SRY-related HMG-box 4
STAT3	signal transducer and activator of transcription 3
TCGA	The Cancer Genome Atlas
TGF-β	transforming growth factor beta
TJ	tight junction
TK	tyrosine kinase
TME	tumor microenvironment
TNF-α	tumor necrosis factor α
TSG	tumor suppressor genes
ZEB1	zinc finger E-box

1.1 INTRODUCTION

Despite being a prevalent disease globally, cancer is a life-threatening illness, owing to its molecular pathologies involved, which is characterized by a broad range of biological aggression that is really difficult to control. The past century has seen an astounding advancement in our knowledge of the biology of cancer (Hanahan and Weinberg 2011; Hickey et al. 2013). This progress has been especially accelerated in the last few decades by conceptual and technological developments in different fields, comprising large-scale next-generation sequencing, flow cytometry, the addition of "omic" sciences, high-resolution microscopy, individual cell sequencing and analysis, novel cell culture techniques, animal models development, etc. However, still a lot of unanswered questions and issues are there with this illness that needs to be resolved. Thus, it is necessary to view oncological research as essential.

According to reports from etiologic studies, there are a variety of potential causative agents for cancer. These include genetic mutations (such as somatic mutations, inherited mutations, and inevitable DNA replication errors), epimutations (such as hypomethylation of cancer-causing gene, that is, oncogene; hypermethylation of tumor suppressor genes; and chromatin remodeling), oncogenic viral infections (e.g., hepatitis B [HBV]and C [HCV] and human papillomavirus [HPV]), exposure to aflatoxin B, and so forth (Moore and Chang 2010). But lifestyle choices and/or exogenous risk factors may also contribute to an early development of some malignancies (De Flora and La Maestra 2015; Cai and Yuan 2017).

Carcinogenesis, also referred to as *tumorigenesis* or *oncogenesis*, is a process that involves interactions between an organism's genes and environment. These multistep, multifactorial molecular events are responsible for causing cancer. The known process is a multistep process, resulting in dysregulated hedonic homeostasis and unregulated cell proliferation. It involves successive mutations and/or epimutations (Hong 2018). Cancer-causing changes gradually alter the metabolism and behavior of cells. They modify the control over their multiplication, provide them with an endless lifespan, change how they communicate with nearby cells, and finally, give them the capacity to evade the immune system. In summary, despite any genetic and/or epigenetically caused harm, they are still capable of self-proliferation and division (Puneet et al. 2018).

Even while multicellular organisms undergo differentiation, which results in widespread cellular variety, cells share basic mechanisms for carrying out essential functions that control cell division and proliferation. The intracellular organization required for homeostasis in a multicellular organism is controlled by regulations that cancer cells fail to abide by. Cancer cells, therefore, put up a lot of effort to adapt, proliferate, and exploit their invasive aggression to defeat the immune system to invade surrounding tissues. The intricate complexity of cellular alterations frequently observed in cancerous cells was attempted to be shown by Hanahan and Weinberg in 2000 as what they named cancer hallmarks (Hanahan and Weinberg 2011). The permanent activation of the proliferative signal, resistance to apoptosis, evasion of growth suppressors, repeated replication, induction of angiogenesis, invasion, metastasis, dysregulation of cellular metabolism, dominant immune attack, genomic instability/mutations, tumor-promoting inflammation, and immune evasion are a few of these (Moses et al. 2018; Böttcher et al. 2020). Since then, the idea has continued to develop and has given cancer biologists new motivation. Thus, molecular and cellular processes comprise the basis of cancer etiology. In fact, improper management of the cell cycle drives the mechanisms that permanently activate carcinogenesis.

1.2 CELL CYCLE

A. Howard and S. Pelc conducted autoradiographic investigations in 1953 to report that the synthesis of DNA takes place at a specific moment throughout the process of cell division (Howard and Pelc 1953). The current understanding of the eukaryotic cell cycle stages was laid by this key experiment. The term "cell cycle" describes all the biological processes encompassed in the initiation, growth, and division of cells. It includes the interphase stages (resting phase: gap 1, DNA synthesis, and gap 2) and the mitotic stages (dividing phase: pro-, meta-, ana-, and telophases). Strict precision in the replication of DNA and equal distribution of genetic material in cells that follow one another are the ultimate goals of the cell cycle. DNA replication (during S phase), chromatin condensation, spindle formation, nuclear membrane degradation, and cytoskeleton remodeling are the outcomes of this process (Øvrebø, Ma, and Edgar 2022).

Regulatory checkpoints monitor the molecular and structural occurrences that occur with regard to the optimal cell cycle frame and regulate their consistency, conformity, and adherence throughout the process. At the checkpoints, anomalies are identified and initiate pathways that lead to different outcomes, such as necroptosis, apoptosis, cell arrest (senescence), and repair processes (DNA repair) (Elledge 1996). In unicellular species, the failure of a multiplying cell to activate either of these mechanisms results in a reduction of the reproductive capacity; in multicellular organisms, it causes unchecked cell division that may lead to cancer. The cell cycle is governed by two main categories of control mechanisms: internal mechanisms that are housed inside checkpoints' control, and extracellular routes for signals, that is, signaling pathways (Kastan and Bartek 2004; Lukas, Lukas, and Bartek 2004; Barnum and O'Connell 2014.

1.2.1 The Clinical Importance of Cell Cycle Control and Deregulation

In 1953, A. Howard and Pelc performed autoradiographic studies to describe, for the first time, that DNA synthesis occurs in a precise period during the cell division process (Howard and Pelc 1953). This milestone experiment set the groundwork for defining the eukaryotic cell cycle phases as we know them today. Mammals rely on complex regulatory systems that mainly control the cell cycle to ensure appropriate cell division (Figure 1.1). This regulation involves both intracellular and extracellular regulatory mechanisms. Extracellular signaling is necessary for a cell to cross the restriction point (R-point) and enter the G1 phase (Moore and Chang 2010). Following external signaling, the cell finally goes through the G2 phase, S phase, and mitosis, but only with the help of intracellular regulators. Genetic instructions essentially and independently govern the latter control

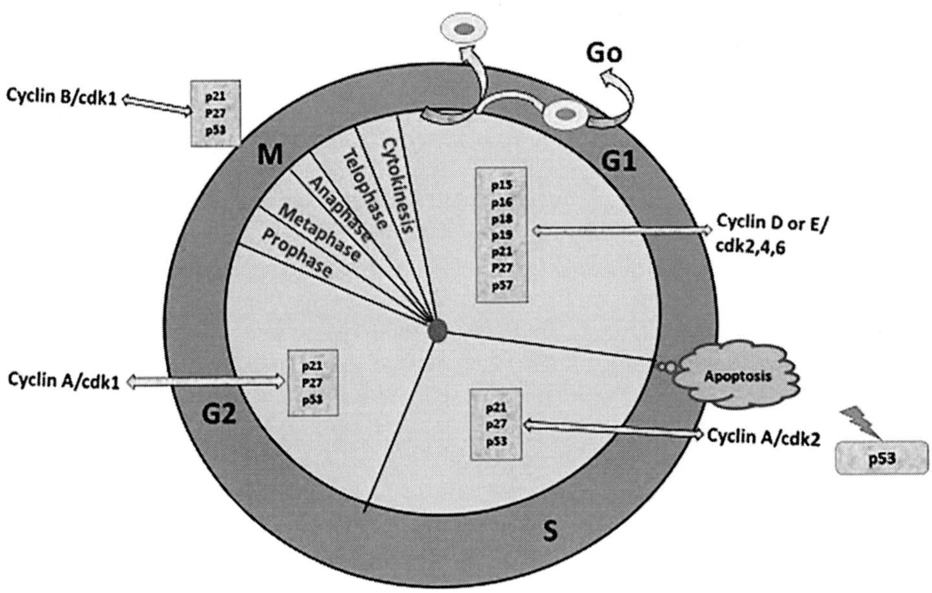

FIGURE 1.1 Diagram showing how the cell cycle progresses. The cell cycle phases of eukaryotes are governed by cell cycle regulators: G1 (gap1), S (DNA synthesis), G2 (gap2), and M (mitosis). During the G1 phase, the interphasic cells are diploids (2n). During the S phase, the cell duplicates its genetic material, or DNA, in order to get ready for a future division. The cell thus has doubled DNA (4n) in the latter S phase and G2 phase. As seen in the image, the mitotic division proceeds from prophase to telophase. There are two daughter cells formed at the end of mitosis. G0 represents a dormant state that cells may eventually pass through. The cyclin-dependent kinases depicted in the picture represent cell cycle checkpoints, each of which has the potential to ultimately dictate the fate of the cell in relation to the existence or dearth of growth factors and mitogens.

systems, known as checkpoints. The aforementioned checkpoints evaluate the integrity and fidelity of DNA replication as well as the cell's final passage through G2 and mitosis (Hanahan and Weinberg 2011). Enzymes and proteins, referred to as effector and regulator, play an indispensable part in the progression of the cell cycle. These catalytic enzymes and regulatory proteins can be identified as cyclin-dependent kinases (CDKs) and cyclins (A, B, D, E, and H) (Cai and Yuan 2017; Puneet et al. 2018). Cyclins serve as a regulatory component for cyclin-dependent kinases (Johnson and Walker 1999; Hydbring, Malumbres, and Sicinski 2016). Vertebrates possess four different kinds of CDKs, with the quantity of each type changing as the cell cycle progresses through different phases. Therefore, cyclins can be classified as G1 phase, G1/Sphase, Sphase, or Mphase.

To propel the cell through the subsequent phase, every single one of these cyclins combines with cyclin-dependent kinases. The quantity of cyclin-dependent kinases does not change throughout the cycle, even while the cell synthesizes and/or destroys cyclins (Morgan 1995). This is due to the fact that cyclin-dependent kinases come to be increasingly inactive when a given concentration of cyclins decreases (Ekholm and Reed 2000). On the other hand, an increase in cyclin concentration corresponds directly to the triggering of the corresponding phase's cyclin-dependent kinases (Vermeulen, Van Bockstaele, and Berneman 2003; Hydbring, Malumbres, and Sicinski 2016; Bertoni 2018).

Some cyclin-dependent kinases exhibit an ability to bind to numerous cyclins, while others do not share multiple cyclin binding. For example, CDK1 has a greater affinity for cyclin B but may possibly bind to other cyclins, like A, B, D, and E as well. Although CDK2 can also bind to cyclin B and D, it has a stronger affinity for cyclin A and E. While CDK7 binds to cyclin H, CDK4, CDK6, and CDK7 have a strong affinity for cyclin D. As their name suggests, phosphorylation and dephosphorylation, as well as protein interaction, also regulate the catalytic action of CDKs, besides to phase-specific cyclin production and degradation. The latter group of proteins are known as CKIs, or cyclin-dependent kinase inhibitors. They may belong to the INK4 family (cyclin-dependent kinase inhibitors), which includes proteins (p15, p16, p18, and p19) that are exclusive to CDK4, or they may be CIP (CDK interacting protein) (p21) and KIP (kinase inhibitory protein) (p27, p57), which are effective inhibitors of all CDKs (Harper et al. 1995; Denicourt and Dowdy 2004; Quereda et al. 2015; Corbet 2017).

In the G1 phase, the progress through the restriction point (R-point) is mediated by CDK–cyclin complexes, which phosphorylate the retinoblastoma protein family members, p107, p130, and Rb. Histone deacetylase (HDAC) combines with Rb and E2F in early to mid G. CDK–cyclins' phosphorylation of Rb facilitates the production of gene products required for the cell cycle's progression and promotes the release of E2F-DP transcription factors (Schulze et al. 1995; Ren et al. 2002; Morgunova et al. 2015; Thwaites et al. 2017).

Together, the parts of the cell cycle's regulatory apparatus provide the perfect environment for the cell cycle to progress in the right direction. The most well-studied cell cycle regulators that have roles other than merely acting as cell cycle checkpoints are the E2F family proteins, cyclins, CDKs, CIP, and CKI (Blanchet et al. 2011). These regulators could function independently from one another or together as complexes, as is the case with the cell cycle's regulation. Together, the parts of the cell cycle's regulatory apparatus provide the perfect environment for the cell cycle to progress in the right direction. In addition to their usual regulatory function in the cell cycle, several regulating checkpoints have extra responsibilities that could be assigned to different compartments of the cell. Examples of these non-ministerial functions in regulation are as follows: (1) cyclin E1 acting in tandem with CDK2 for the activation of MYC, transcription factor which inhibits senescence of cell; (2) CDK2 and CDK4, which act in tandem using cyclin D1, cyclin E1, and cyclin A2, leading to the activation of transcription factor FOXM1C, which acts to either repress cellular senescence or endorse the cycle promotion; (3) CDK4 and its partner cyclin D1, which impede transcription factor NFR1, thus inhibiting the functions of mitochondria; (4) cyclin D1, acting as a repressor to FOXO1, O3 transcription factor, so inhibiting anoikis; (5) CDK6, which activates the JUN transcription factor, acting as the stimulator of angiogenesis; and (6) E2F, which controls oxidative metabolism, and cyclin D2, which suppresses DMP1 (transcription factor), which modifies the pathway of p53 (Hydbring, Malumbres, and Sicinski 2016). In conclusion, non-canonical roles for regulatory machinery components are documented in different biological processes of cells, such as cellular differentiation, senescence, death, immune response, metabolism, mitochondrial activity, fission, apoptosis, and mitochondrial biogenesis. Underlying the intricate activities of the cell cycle is a critical need for energy commitments made by the mitochondria via a suitable adaptive metabolism. As a result, the mitochondria and the cell cycle's regulatory apparatus support a functional dynamism that propels cell division, growth, survival, and senescence (Wang et al. 2014; Bendris, Lemmers, and Blanchard 2015; Lopez-Mejia and Fajas 2015).

The pathognomonic trait, which is the result of a dysregulated cell cycle that leads to uncoordinated cell growth, is what makes all neoplastic diseases distinct. Expressional dysregulation and/or functional mutations of the genes coding the regulators of cell cycle have been shown to cause carcinogenic events. Because of this, it has become crucial to pay more attention to, and get in-depth knowledge of, the molecular mechanisms behind the cell cycle regulation. The dysregulated gene expression and erratic functional activity have been connected to numerous malignancies. Normal cell proliferation continues unabated even when some of these regulating proteins cease to function. Some malignant neoplasms have been shown to overexpress certain genes, though, and nowadays, this phenomenon has been utilized as a biomarker for diagnostic and prognostic applications (Musgrove et al. 2011). Tumor suppressor genes and oncogenes are the two categories of genes that regulate the cell cycle as a consequence. Additionally, scientists are trying to take note of the abnormalities in gene expression patterns and/or regulator functional activities observed in cancer cells, with the aim to develop targeted therapeutics (Asghar et al. 2015; Otto and Sicinski 2017).

1.3 CELLULAR MODELS OF CANCER CAUSE

Mammalian animals are made up of mosaic cell types, such as differentiated cells, which differ in shape, chemistry, and mitotic capability. We are more concerned about the mitotic competence in this case. Three types of cells might be identified using these criteria: cells that would never divide again, cells that cycle actively, and cells (stem cells, resting cells) that proliferate in response to stimuli. Stem cells are those that divide asymmetrically during mitosis in order to produce new cells that undergo differentiation processes and ultimately carry out a specific role, in addition to dividing to renew their own type. It is evident that the cell cycle regulators' dysregulated gene expression and/or subsequent abnormal functionality in the corresponding pre-cited cell types have different clinical implications. Actually, only a few different kinds of cells possess the capacity to multiply and ultimately cause a tumor to develop. Similar to the mosaicism of healthy cells of organisms cells, intratumoral heterogeneity is a feature of malignancies (Marjanovic, Weinberg, and Chaffer 2013). To put it another way, this means that the morphology, chemistry, and malignant potential of tumor cells vary greatly. In actuality, there are three widely accepted hypotheses that explain the mosaicity of cancerous cells: the clonal evolution model, phenotypic plasticity/plastic cancer stem cells model, and the cancer stem cell (CSC) model, as shown in Figure 1.2. Scientific publications that clarify the similarities and differences between these models and their respective advantageous clinical implications have been backed by these models. The growing corpus of knowledge arising from research on these models contributes to developing more understanding of cancer and facilitates the creation of more potent remedies and preventative measures (Jayachandran, Dhungel, and Steel 2016).

1.3.1 Cancer Stem Cell (CSC) Hypothesis

According to the hypothesis behind cancer stem cells (CSC), a small proportion of cancerous cells have traits of stem cells; they are accountable for the start, spread, metastasis, and ultimate cancer recurrence after treatment. The unique capacity of CSCs is to divide irregularly to produce descendants that ultimately and permanently differentiate, forming the hierarchical structure of the cancerous tissue in equivalence to normal, as well as regularly for self-renewing,

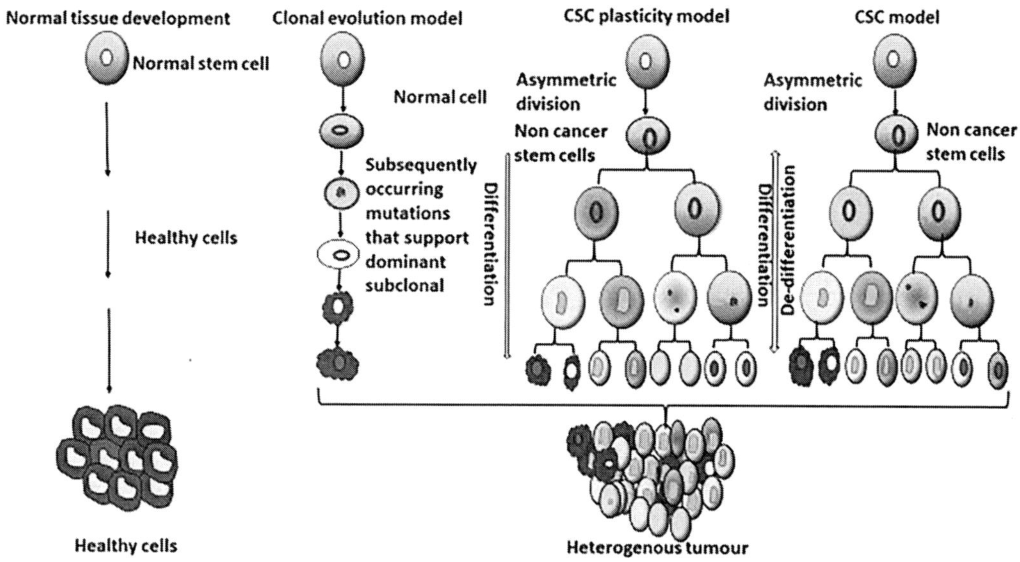

FIGURE 1.2 Intratumoral heterogeneity models. According to the clonal evolution concept, dominant subclonal cells benefit from subsequent mutational changes that lead to intratumoral heterogeneity. By cell differentiation, intratumoral heterogeneity arises, as per the cancer stem cell paradigm. The dedifferentiation process of cancerous cells may be the source of intratumoral heterogeneity, in accordance with the cancer stem cell plasticity paradigm.

to confirm the longevity of undifferentiated cancer stem cells (Jayachandran, Dhungel, and Steel 2016; Abou-Antoun et al. 2017). The cancer-initiating cells are also formed from precursor cells that were going to attain cancerous alterations (mutation or epimutation), which lends support to this scenario. This hypothesis proposes that cancer is a disease of stem cell. One of the main differences between malignant and healthy stem cells is that the former have dysregulated stemness pathways, whereas the latter have consistent genetic and epigenetic profiles and adhere to homeostatic stemness processes.

Additionally, these cells have quiescent characteristics, which could account for the spread of the disease as well as the late relapses that indicate the resistance of cancer to chemotherapy and/or radiation therapy. Conventional cancer treatments, such as radiation and chemotherapy, target pathogenetically growing cells in a broad, non-discriminatory manner. The sensitivity of non-tumorigenic cells and cancer stem cells to treatment varies. The ability of cancer stem cells to withstand therapeutic attack is high. This may be partly because of the high concentration of free radical scavengers, which allows to gradually repair DNA damage after DNA-targeting treatment (Batlle and Clevers 2017). Therefore, isolating cancer stem cells and researching the molecular mechanisms by which therapeutic resistance arises in them would probably further our understanding of the tumor recurrence mechanisms and ultimately inform the development of targeted therapies that target these mechanisms, particular to cancerous stem cells. The intricate heterogeneity of cancer in relation to therapeutic challenges, however, shapes the cancer stem cell model's nonuniversal applicability. This draws into uncertainty the epithelial–mesenchymal transition, the genesis of clonal cancer, and the therapeutic relevance of the cancer microenvironment (Pattabiraman and Weinberg 2014; Yoshida and Saya 2016; Qureshi-Baig et al. 2017; Bahmad et al. 2020).

1.4 TUMOR MICROENVIRONMENT (TME)

Solid tumors can be distinguished from other tumors like leukemia and lymphomas, which develop in connective tissues like blood and lymph, respectively. *Solid tumors* are defined as a growing cell mass in a particular tissue that is confined, in their early stages. In solid tumors, the malignant cells are encircled by TME and encased by the basement membrane (Albini et al. 2015; Butturini et al. 2019). The constituents of the TME are a range of inhabitant and invading host cells, extracellular matrix (ECM) components, and secreted factors, in addition to cancer cells (Figure 1.3). TME is a complex web of interconnected elements that controls the onset, spread, and metastasis of tumors and has a significant effect on the effectiveness of treatments (Klemm and Joyce 2015; Butturini et al. 2019). This is comparable to the structure of healthy tissues. The stroma of lymphomas and leukemias are made up of lymph and blood, respectively. There is scientific evidence that these structures develop in tandem and are interdependent during the whole course of cancer (Balkwill, Capasso, and Hagemann 2012). The basement membrane, stromal cells—genetically stable cells—and the extracellular matrix (ECM), a non-cellular matrix, make up the tumor stroma. The multistage pattern of carcinogenesis begins with an environmental attack, or initiation, and progresses to promotion events. Localized in their niches—privileged anatomical sites—cancer stem cells engage in crucial bidirectional communication with the surrounding microenvironment to ascertain the advancement or metastasis of primary tumors and the latency or proliferative status of malignant stem cells that have metastasized. Tumoral cells produce different biomolecules, such as growth factors, cytokines, proteases, etc., to cause changes in the local microenvironment that affect the physicochemical features of the host tissue (Mbeunkui and Johann 2009). It has been proposed that corrective modification of the tumor microenvironment might normalize the tumoral cells, preventing their ablation by only re-educating the stromal cells. Among the cells of tumor stroma are adipocytes, cancer-associated fibroblasts (CAFs), myeloid-derived suppressor cells, natural killer cells (NKs), neuroendocrine cells, regulatory T cells (Tregs), perivascular cells, and other cells, such as mast cells. A diverse mixture of macromolecules with a range of biochemical and biomechanical characteristics makes up the ECM. The ECM is made up of proteins, polysaccharides,

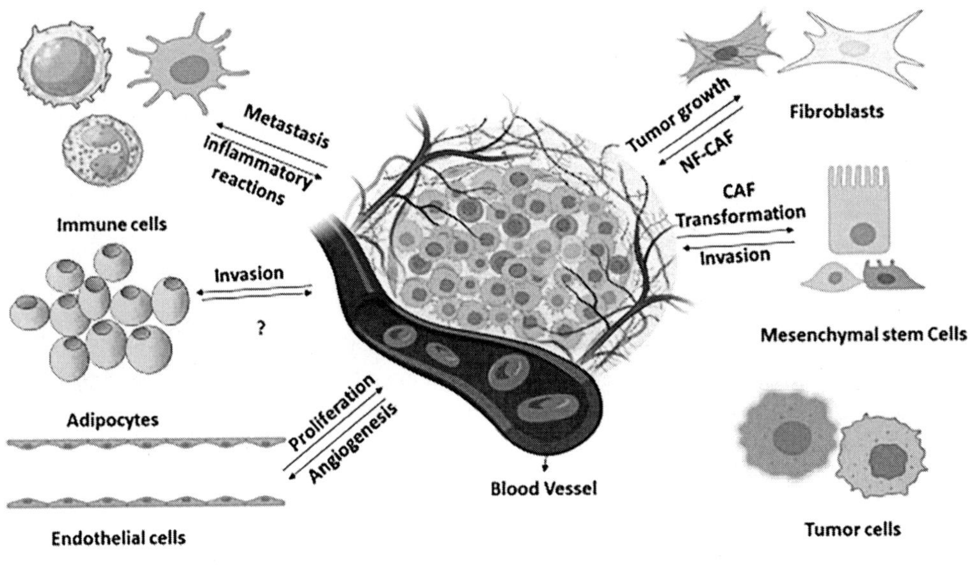

FIGURE 1.3 Tumor microenvironment. TME is formed of ECM, hematological (immune) cells, and mesenchymal (adipocytes, fibroblast, and endothelial) cells. The development of cancer depends on the interaction of the tumor and its microenvironment. Angiogenesis is encouraged by tumor cells, which also trigger an inflammatory response and cause mesenchymal stem cells and normal fibroblasts (NFs) to differentiate into CAFs. Conversely, endothelial cells stimulate tumor cell proliferation, mesenchymal stem cells and immune cells govern and promote tumor metastasis or dormancy, and adipocytes are essential for tumor cell invasion.

Source: Biorender.com.

glycoproteins, and proteoglycans. Although the ECM is strictly regulated throughout embryonic and organ homeostasis, neoplastic diseases frequently cause dysregulation of this matrix, which promotes anarchic cell proliferation and metastasis (Plaks, Kong, and Werb 2015).

In summary, the process would begin with the exudation of cytokines and growth factors by the CSCs that are released into the tissue microenvironment of the host. For example, in breast cancer, stem cells release platelet-derived growth factors (PDGF) to stimulate the formation of cancer-associated fibroblasts (Andrade et al. 2017). The fibroblasts linked to cancer are then stimulated by cancer stem cells, and this leads to the production of collagen I and II, which are the components of connective tissue, and extracellular matrix, or stroma, indicates solid tumor features. Blood arteries that irrigate the so-formed tumor stroma supply oxygen and nutrients and remove waste from the tumor cells. TGF-β is secreted and released by cancer cells to stimulate cancer-associated fibroblasts, which, in turn, alter the stroma over time. Collagen fibers, which comprise connective tissue, are broken down by metalloproteases (MMPs) released by activated cancer-associated fibroblasts. Eventually, HGF produced by CAFs would also cause tumor cells to proliferate and invade (Andrade et al. 2017; Tugues et al. 2019).

1.5 THE HETEROGENEITY OF CANCER CELLS AND THE CLONAL EVOLUTION THEORY

The "clonal evolution" model of cancerous cells proposed by Nowell in 1970s served as the inspiration for the present evolutionary biology of carcinogenesis. In this concept, cancer starts with a single mutant cell that multiplies and experiences successive further changes to form subpopulations of cells. These subpopulations' biology and clinical outcomes are dictated by natural selection and the fitness that the cells accumulate over time. One way to conceptualize the clonal evolution paradigm would be a lineage of malignant cell clones. Every new clone arises through the acquisition of novel mutations that give a selective advantage; the intratumoral heterogeneity is based on the clonal variety that results (Makohon-Moore et al. 2017).

The idea behind the clonal evolution model of malignancies clarifies how carcinogenesis is driven by mutations and/or epimutations of tumor suppressor and oncogenes. Nevertheless, any of these models could be applied to every type of cancer. The hierarchical architecture of tumor cells, which is the sine qua non of the "cancer stem cell" hypothesis, is the general forewarning to the "clonal evolution" model. Therefore, the best paradigm to treat this tumor would be clonal evolution, when the heterogeneity within the tumor arises from mutational and epimutational processes. To explain their inhomogeneity, certain tumors would need to use both models, while others would only need one or the other. The clonal evolution model could be the next step in the early phases of carcinogenesis, which could commence with the cancer stem cancer model (B. Zhao, Hemann, and Lauffenburger 2016; Makohon-Moore et al. 2017). Actually, depending on the point at which an environmental insult causes selected phenotypic and/or useful mutation(s)/epimutation(s) into a developing tumor, the intratumoral heterogeneity's model result would vary. Cancer stem cell models are required to address the following scenarios: (1) if the changes only affect cancer stem cells, in which case they will ultimately cause intratumoral heterogeneity among cancer stem cells; (2) if the changes affect non-tumorigenic cells, in which case they will not spread, as long as the tumorigenic status stays the same; and (3) if the changes impact tumorigenic cells that differentiate, in which case clonal evolution models and cancer stem cell models will then be essential to address the resulting intratumoral heterogeneity (Diori Karidio and Sanlier 2021)

1.6 EPITHELIAL–MESENCHYMAL TRANSITION (EMT) AND MESENCHYMAL–EPITHELIAL TRANSITION (MET)

The biological process by which epithelial cells lose their properties and acquire mesenchymal traits is known as the epithelial–mesenchymal transition (EMT). EMT is the crucial phase of embryonic physiology initially delineated in 1980s by Betty Hay, an American scientist of developmental biology. Epithelial cells gain mesenchymal markers, spindle cell shape, cell motility, and apical-basal polarity during EMT, while losing cell–cell connections and epithelial markers (Lai et al. 2020). Throughout this process, the immotile polarized epithelial cells gradually lose some of their innate qualities as they acquire those of mesenchymal cells, or as they transform into motile cancer metastases, according to biochemical and epigenetic processes. EMTs are therefore categorized separated into three subtypes: EMT types I, II, and III. Type III EMT is evident in invasive potentiated stromal cells; type II EMT is seen in fibrosis, tissue regeneration, and wound healing, and EMT I is shown during the development of embryos and organs (Kalluri 2009; Kalluri and Weinberg 2009; Zeisberg and Neilson 2009). Nevertheless, the intrinsic plasticity of mesenchymal cells remains unaltered while transitioning from epithelial cells. Because of this, epithelial and mesenchymal cells are both pluripotent (Hay 2008; Kiefer, Nieto, and Thiery 2008). Mesenchymal-to-epithelial transition (MET), the contrary of EMT, is likewise a physiologically observable process. The term "metamorphic plasticity events" describes the process by which nonpolarized, motile, and possibly mesenchymal cells that invade dedifferentiate into polarized, nonmotile epithelial cells connected to each other and packed on the basement membrane. EMT and MET are physiological processes that are strictly regulated and are detected in disease states like fibrosis, inflammation, and metastases of cancer.

1.6.1 Cancer's Epithelial–Mesenchymal Transition: Molecular Mechanisms

While the three biological subtypes of EMTs each has unique mechanistic characteristics, the molecular mechanisms driving EMTs share highly conserved hallmarks. Cells undergoing epithelial–mesenchymal transitions (EMTs) are typically exposed to genetic, epigenetic, and pharmacological processes that alter their phenotype and gene expression (Kalluri and Weinberg 2009; Nieto 2009). The process of cancer has only been fully explained in carcinomas, or the most common types of cancer that are diagnosed. The process can be divided into three main stages: (1) polarity loss and detachment of recruited epithelial cells for EMT; (2) basement membrane digestion, intravasation, and extravasation through the blood or lymph; and (3) invasion of tissue and dormancy (Nieto 2009; Nisticò, Bissell, and Radisky 2012). The process involves both cell-surrounding events and intracellular remodeling (Figure 1.4).

EMT enhances morphogenesis and stem cell plasticity during embryogenesis, supports tissue regeneration during wound healing, and causes metastasis—the final stage of cancer—in physiopathological conditions like cancer. Therefore, EMT is comparable to a nexus of homeostatic, pathophysiological processes in the life of human beings that ultimately react to external stimuli (i.e., growth factors, immunological response) and intrinsic stimuli (i.e., mutation, epimutation) (Son et al. 2016). Tumor cells exhibit cohesive adhesion with each other and the surrounding microenvironment prior to metastasis. This is because the cells release colony-stimulating factors (CSFs) to attract stromal cells and macrophages. Tumor cells release more CSF as a result of the macrophages' response, which involves the release of a positive feedback loop, that is, epithelial growth factors (EGFs). The main characteristics of EMT are then produced by the release of cathepsin B by macrophages (Radisky 2005; Zhang et al. 2015; Campos-da-Paz et al. 2018).

The loss of cytokeratins (CK8, CK18, CK19), desmoplakin, E-cadherin, mucin 1, and occludin is one of the main characteristics of EMT. The transmembrane protein N-cadherin (CDH) is coded by the CDH1 gene, which is also a tumor suppressor gene and has additional functions related to cell motility, polarization, differentiation, and stemness (Radisky 2005). Neighboring cells' extracellular E-cadherin segments link together, while alpha-catenin helps their intracellular tails attach to actin filaments. As cancer spreads and metastasizes, CDH1 experiences functional mutations or epimutations, which are transcriptional amplification of the repression factor, or hypermethylation of the gene's promoter. Consequently, basal-apical polarity and cell–cell adhesion are lost locally by epithelial cells. Because of this, they are permitted to separate and move towards the surrounding

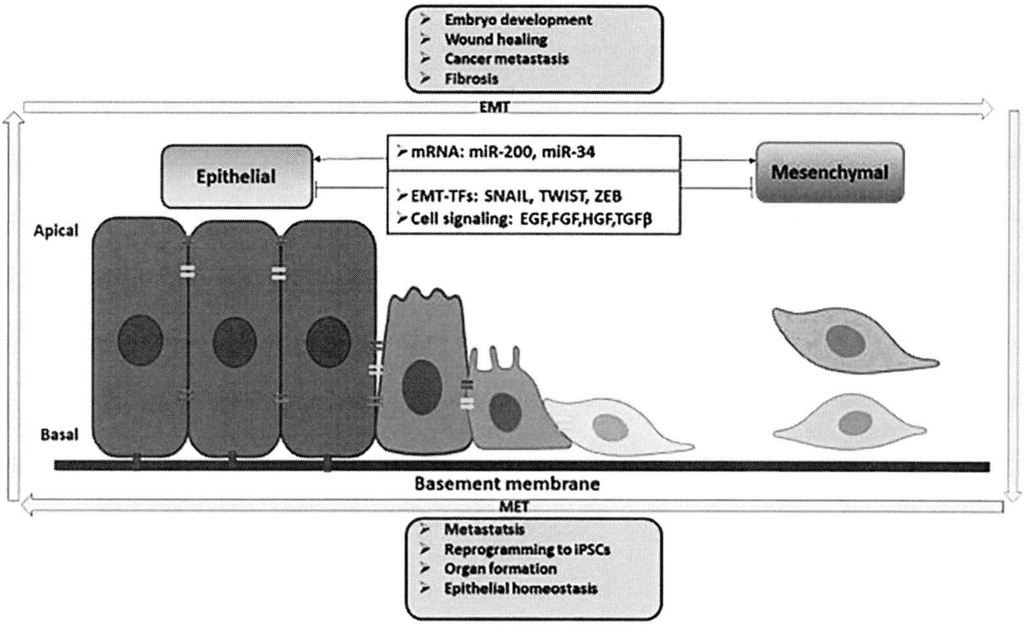

FIGURE 1.4 A brief glance at MET and EMT. Both EMT and its inverse process, MET, exhibit spectral characteristics and arise throughout physiological and pathological advancements. Epithelial cells lost their connections to the basement membrane and apical-basal polarity during EMT. Numerous factors, including transcription factors, cell signaling, and epigenetic modification, govern epigenetic modification (EMT). Note: *HDS* is hemidesmosome; *DS* is desmosome; *AJ* is adherens junction; and *TJ* is tight junction.

Source: Biorender.com.

tissue, while the cells in close proximity go through morphogenic rearrangement to close the space. Matrix metalloproteases (MMPs) are released by stromal cells in order to break down the basement membrane. This process creates a chemical gradient, which, in turn, causes the chemoattractant—that is, hepatocyte growth factors—to reorganize the cytoskeletal actin via Ras-like GTPases (Jerrell, Leih, and Parekh 2020). Actin fibers in the cytoskeleton reorganize to create stress fibers, which in turn produce lamellipodia, filopodia, and invadopodia (Machesky 2008). These structures are particularly important for the spread of cancer. Actin filaments shaped like wheels, called lamellipodia, mediate the motility of the cell. Spiky membrane projections, called filopodia, are used by cells to sense their surroundings. To break down the extracellular matrix, invasive polypodia create proteases that include vesicles (Revach and Geiger 2014; Weber et al. 2018).

Tumor necrosis factor α (TNFα) is produced by macrophages in conjunction with EGFs during the ongoing process. TNFα inhibits the epithelial E-cadherin synthesis by upregulating its repressors of transcription, also known as EMT-TFs, such as SLUG, SNAIL, ZEB1, ZEB2/SIP1, and increases the production of N-cadherin of mesenchyma. From then on, mesenchymal genes gradually "switch on" and epithelial genes gradually "switch down," enabling the change in phenotype from epithelial to mesenchymal and the corresponding traits. In the end, they develop resistance to apoptosis and senescence in addition to invasive powers (Kiesslich, Pichler, and Neureiter 2013; Tsai and Yang 2013; Lamouille, Xu, and Derynck 2014; Oral et al. 2016; Serrano-Gomez, Maziveyi, and Alahari 2016).

Consequently, intravasation is how those cells reach the circulatory system. They are attached to platelets as they travel through the circulatory system to shield them from immune system assaults. At the end of their voyage, they relocate the residence to the metastatic position after extravasation from the blood vascular system. It is thought that the metastatic cells go through MET before they colonize the secondary site. There are two probable outcomes for the metastatic site: the metastatic cells either (1) effectively inhabit the secondary location and develop into a secondary tumor following a dormant phase, known as tumor dormancy, which could linger for many years, or (2) transform back into normal epithelial cells (Tsai and Yang 2013; Serrano-Gomez, Maziveyi, and Alahari 2016; Gomis and Gawrzak 2017; Fares et al. 2020).

1.7 CANCER STEM CELL (CSC) PLASTICITY

The CSC plasticity concept links EMT, which systematically facilitates vigorous and bidirectional population of the CSC group and fundamentally shows the hierarchical-morphological, phenotypic, and functional heterogeneity of tumors, which is known as tumorigenicity. This reminds that the CSC model postulates that certain CSCs differentiate into tumor cells, which leads to the hierarchical organization of the tumor and the heterogeneity of tumors. However, clonal evolution suggests that cells pick up mutations that are transmissible through evolution as part of the sequential process of carcinogenesis, which leads to the emergence of tumor heterogeneity. The essential characteristics of the clonal evolution models and CSC are somehow combined in the CSCs' plasticity model through the use of EMT/MET. The CSC model's fundamental hierarchical structure is combined with a final vigorous interconversion of CSCs to non-CSCs bidirectionally to achieve this. From this angle, EMT functions as a switch for three alarming consequences of carcinogenesis: metastasis, non-CSC to CSC (restoration of the CSC group after chemotherapy), and interconversion of CSC to non-CSC in both directions (establishing the hierarchical structure of tumor cells). Additionally, according to the clonal evolution hypothesis, EMT deliberates non-genetic plasticity that facilitates a tumor's metastatic potential (Garg 2017)

The EMT-undergoing portion of a tumor's clonal evolution model would contain stemness characteristics that come from dedifferentiation in the end. Interestingly, the range of tumor cells' flexibility extends well beyond that of CSCs, which only reflect a small portion of cancer cells' plasticity. It is thought that after an aggressive therapy, more aggressive CSC may arise from the epimutation(s). Furthermore, CSC, non-CSC, EMT-CSC, and MET-CSC subpopulations would all be present in a tumor with history EMT (Heikenwalder and Lorentzen 2019)

1.8 MITOTIC CATASTROPHE

The term "mitotic catastrophe" is not universally agreed upon. Historically, the fundamental standards for characterizing mitotic catastrophe were established by the 1984 McIntosh study on "microtubule catastrophe" and the 1986 Russell and Nurse report on temperature-dependent deadly aberrant chromosomal segregation in *Schizosaccharomyces pombe* (Castedo et al. 2004; Vakifahmetoglu, Olsson, and Zhivotovsky 2008). A series of events known as a mitotic catastrophe is indicative of a type of cell death brought on by exposure to radiation, chemotherapy, or extreme heat. Although the precise mechanism causing mitotic catastrophe is unknown, it is assumed to be the result of aberrant, or early, mitosis, which is characterized by partial disintegration of anaphase nuclei (Castedo et al. 2004). This process of eradicating incompetent mitotic cells differs from apoptosis in that mitotic catastrophe happens in cells lacking p53 and having functionally defective apoptotic pathways (Orth et al. 2012). It is possible that cells that suffer fatal injuries from cytotoxic and radiation medications during their interphase will never undergo mitosis. Consequently, apoptosis is typically responsible for swift cell death. If not, injured cells that go through mitosis end up with irregular mitosis during either metaphase or anaphase. Because irregular mitosis incorrectly divides chromosomes, it results in the formation of a non-viable cell with two or more nuclei that are moderately or entirely parted from each another (Uetake and Sluder 2010; Hayashi et al. 2012).

The mitotic catastrophe's therapeutic significance accounts for much of its significance. As part of their mechanisms of action, a number of well-researched anticancer medications are recognized to cause mitotic catastrophe in cancerous cells. These medications include bleomycin, cisplatin, doxorubicin, etoposide, and taxol (Maskey et al. 2013). Anticancer medications that cause a metastatic event are significant for various reasons, including the following: because cells with defective apoptotic mechanisms experience mitotic catastrophe, (1) they are effective against apoptosis-resistant cancer cells, and (ii) they require lower doses than those that induce apoptosis. Furthermore, mitotic catastrophe may only affect cancer cells because it can happen to p53-deficient or G2/M checkpoint–weakened cells (Burns et al. 2003). Cells undergo either apoptosis or necroptosis after the mitotic catastrophe. In summary, mitotic catastrophe can be understood as a process wherein cells recognize genetic instability that may be harmful and react by inducing oncosuppressive events that result in necrosis/necroptosis or apoptosis. Consequently, the development of anticancer therapies will greatly benefit from a deeper comprehension of the underlying patterns of mitotic catastrophe (Woods et al. 1995; Fujie et al. 2005; Vitale et al. 2011; Trybus, Trybus, and Król 2022).

1.9 SENESCENCE

Senescence is defined by biochemical and morphological changes brought on either prematurely by external factors, such as medicine and oxidative stress destroying DNA, or by physiological processes of the cell, such as the shortening of telomeres after the cell cycle. As people age, cellular senescence happens more frequently and at a faster rate (Deursen and Jan 2014; Childs et al. 2015; Tominaga 2015; Lidzbarsky et al. 2018). Senescence is frequently thought of as a tumor-suppressive process. Scientific studies corroborate the idea that this is happening to stop a tumor suppressor gene from operating too suppressively or too aggressively. The oncogene-induced oncogenic stress triggers a hyperreplicative mechanism that leads to oxidative DNA damage by producing unsustainable oxidative damage (Buhl et al. 2019). An innate reaction involving the Arf/p53/p21, p16/pRb, and DNA damage response pathways is triggered by this. The deletion of Pten and NF1 in human and mouse cells serves as a case of how the loss of tumor suppressor genes can cause senescence. Senescence causation mechanism, however, is still poorly understood. There are certain contradictory results to the commonly recognized characteristics of senescent cells.

It is thought that senescent cells may function as a pro-inflammatory or fail-safe mechanism by suppressing tumor growth if it quickly advances to apoptosis, or they may have a pro-oncogenic effect due to the senescence-associated secretory phenotype (SASP)(Lee and Schmitt 2019).

1.10 INVASION AND METASTASIS

Metastasis, or *metastases* in plural, is derived from the Greek words "meta" (which means "change") and "histanai" (which means "to place, or cause to stand"). In other words, *metastasis* literally means "changing place." In the medical context, "metastasis" refers to the intricate and multistep process by which cells detach from the main tumor and move to colonize a specific microenvironment through the bloodstream or lymphatic system and initiate malignant growth (Beauchesne 2011). Metastases, not the original cancer, are the main cause of the high morbidity and death rates associated with cancer. Metastasis accounts for around 90% of cancer-related mortality (Lambert, Pattabiraman, and Weinberg 2017). Early-stage diagnoses of localized primary cancer are extremely rare. If detected early enough, localized solid cancer might theoretically be treated with surgery and local radiotherapy. On the other hand, most diagnosed patients have cancer that has already spread or is still spreading (Jiang et al. 2015; Thiam et al. 2016).

Metastasis is apparently the perfect and desired target of therapies for cancer control and restorative therapy since it is the main factor determining a patient's cancer's malignancy, diagnosis, and course of treatment. "All metastasized neoplasms are incontrovertibly malignant, but not all neoplasms are necessarily metastatic" is the basic rule. In actuality, the likelihood that a cancer may spread depends on its specific form. For example, the likelihood of skin squamous cell carcinoma spreading is modest, whereas lung squamous cell carcinoma frequently metastasizes. In gliomas, metastasis is also infrequently seen. Gliomas and squamous cell carcinoma are aggressive, locally invasive cancers that sporadically spread (Undabeitia et al. 2015; Li et al. 2015; Thompson et al. 2016; Sun et al. 2017; W. Wu et al. 2017).

When cancer spreads to other parts of the body, it usually colonizes the lymph nodes, brain, liver, bones, and lungs. Cancer may also spread, albeit less frequently, to the abdominal cavity, pleural space, and other organs, such as the skin, muscles, etc. Depending on the original cancer, metastasizing cells may spread throughout the body, although they typically target particular organs: usually, the adrenal glands, bones, brain, chest wall, liver, and lungs are colonized by metastatic breast cancer; lung cancer metastasizes to these locations; colonic cancer frequently metastasizes to the liver and lungs; and prostate cancer often metastasizes to the bones (Riihimäki et al. 2014; Strilic and Offermanns 2017; Prasanna et al. 2018).

A tumor's local invasion of surrounding tissues is the first step of the metastasis process, which also includes the intravasation of tumor cells into circulatory system. One or more micrometastatic lesions may develop as a result of neoplastic cells spreading from the original tumor to far locations. These lesions eventually enlarge to the point that they are clinically evident. The epithelial–mesenchymal transition (EMT), or the partial loss of epithelial characteristics and the development of mesenchymal qualities, is the process by which the cells that are able acquire migratory features (Pastushenko and Blanpain 2019). Cancer cells can move from their original tissue and enter surrounding blood arteries by going through a series of stages that result in the loss of their cuboidal epithelial-like phenotype and the development of a spindle-shaped mesenchymal morphology, which facilitates metastasis and invasiveness (Thwaites et al. 2017; Ribatti, Tamma, and Annese 2020) (Figure 1.5). Epithelial cells are

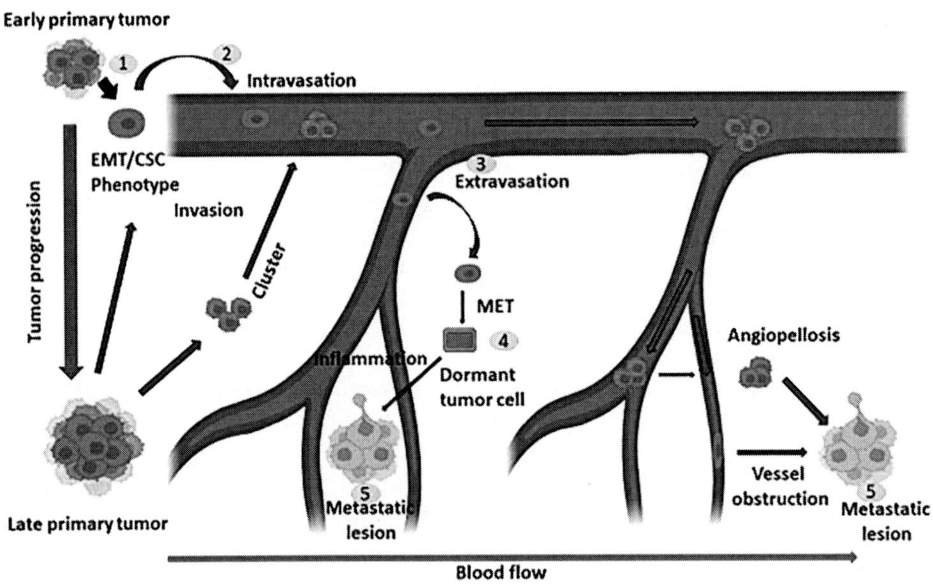

FIGURE 1.5 The cascade of invasion and metastasis. Both invasion and metastasis can happen early or late in the development of a tumor. In either scenario, (1) stem-like cells (cancer stem cells) that undergo the epithelial–mesenchymal transition (EMT) are what propel invasion into neighboring tissues. (2) Tumor cells enter the bloodstream either singly or in groups once they get close to blood vessels. (3) Extravasation occurs when cancer cells in the blood cling to the endothelium. Alternative pathways to extravasation may exist, such as angiopelosis, wherein the endothelium internalizes clusters of tumor cells. Moreover, tumor cells have the ability to block microvasculature at specific locations, which can immediately cause a metastatic lesion. (4) A tumor cell that has just stopped circulating may enter a metastasis in order to go dormant. (5) Quasi-slumbering metastatic cells can be roused by inflammatory signals, multiply, and produce a clinically discernible lesion.

Source: Biorender.com.

allowed to maintain their phenotype by the use of various markers of cell surface and cytoskeleton, for example, adherens junction–specific epithelial cadherin (E-cadherin) and tight junction–specific claudin, occludin, and zonula occludens. Additionally, they preserve the hemidesmosomes' cytokeratin filaments, which cling to the basement membrane and preserve the apical-basal polarity of epithelial cells (Gloushankova, Rubtsova, and Zhitnyak 2017; Fu et al. 2022).

Alongside epithelial markers such as E-cadherin, mesenchymal markers such as mesenchymal neural cadherin (N-cadherin), vimentin, integrins (α2β1, α5β1), type (I) and (II) collagens, fibronectin, and matrix metalloproteinases (MMPs 1, 3 and 9) start to be expressed or function less in cancer cells during the EMT process (Lamouille, Xu, and Derynck 2014; Lambert and Weinberg 2021). An intermediary filament protein called vimentin interacts to encourage cellular motility motor proteins that help move cellular organelles by pointing mesenchymal proteins in the direction of membranes (Mendez, Kojima, and Goldman 2010). N-cadherin stabilizes RTKs by means of its linkages with the cytoskeleton through α-, β-, and p120 catenin, which, in turn, improves their signaling and initiates EMT. Integrin α2β1 interacts with type (I) collagen in the ECM through ECM remodeling MMPs, facilitating translocation of the transcription factor β-catenin through nuclear membrane and E-cadherin dissociation. Integrin α5β1 stimulates cellular adhesion towards the extracellular matrix protein fibronectin, hence inducing cell migration. Different signaling pathways, comprising Notch, RTK, TGFβ, Wnt/β-catenin, and Hedgehog, are implicated in EMT (Brabletz et al. 2021; Imodoye et al. 2021). In the stimulation of mesenchymal genes and the repression of epithelial ones, various TFs have been integrated through these signaling pathways. Examples of these include zinc-finger E-box-binding (ZEB), ZEB1/2 and basic helix–loop–helix (TWIST1/2), and the Snail family, SNAIL1 and SLUG (also known as SNAIL2) (Wang et al. 2010; Lin and Wu 2020).

LncRNA, a type of transcript known as long noncoding RNA has more than 200 nucleotides and either no coding or very little coding capacity. Despite the fact that certain lncRNAs have been identified for decades, the human genome's full-length cDNA library sequencing project just recently revealed the tremendous diversity of lncRNAs. More than 16,000 lncRNA genes are estimated to be present in the human genome by the GENCODE project (Lagarde et al. 2017; Mattick et al. 2023). Because of their incredibly varied modes of action, lncRNAs influence the majority, if not all, of biotic processes. It has been discovered that lncRNAs' altered expression may be a contributing constituent in the development of numerous disorders, including cancer. According to a number of studies, lncRNAs (long noncoding RNAs)largely control EMT and migration/invasion processes to affect the spread of cancer (Table 1.1) (Ahmad et al. 2023).

TABLE 1.1
Examples of LncRNAs Linked to Metastasis

S. No.	LncRNA	Cancer Type	Function	Action Mechanism	Reference
1	HOTAIR	Non–small cell lung cancer	Induces metastasis	Col-1 activates HOTAIR transcription	Zhuang et al. (2013)
2	Gm26809	Melanoma	Causes migration and proliferation	Normal fibroblasts are reprogrammed to become CAFs	Zhuang et al. (2013); Thwaites et al. (2017)
3	H19	Different types	Causes the spread of metastases	Expression increased by TGF-β leads to an increase in SLUG	Matouk et al. (2014)
4	H19	Prostate cancer	Prevents migration	Suppresses TGF-βI by way of miR-675 that it derives	Zhu et al. (2014)

(Continued)

TABLE 1.1 ***(Continued)***
Examples of LncRNAs Linked to Metastasis

S. No.	LncRNA	Cancer Type	Function	Action Mechanism	Reference
5	LINC00092	Oral cancer	Induces metastasis	Interacts with PFKFB2 to promote persistent CAF characteristics and enhanced glycolysis	Zhao et al. (2017)
6	N-BLR	Colorectal cancer	Encourages invasion and migration	miR-200c-3p and miR-141–3p are the targets	Rigoutsos et al. (2017)
		Gastric cancer	Stimulates invasion and migration	Targets miR-200c-3p, causing N-cadherin, SNAIL, and ZEB1 to be upregulated	Youn et al. (2019)
7	HOXD-AS1	Hepatocellular carcinoma	Promotes invasion and migration	Suppresses miR-130a-3p, which causes SOX4 to be upregulated and EZH2 and MMP2 to be expressed concurrently	Wang et al. (2017); Terashima et al. (2018)
8	PTAR	Oral cancer	Increases metastasis and EMT	Suppresses miR-101–3p, which causes ZEB1 to be overexpressed	Liang et al. (2018)
9	MEG8	Lung cancer and prostate cancer	Causes EMT	Represses the miRNA-34a and miRNA-203 genes by interaction with EZH2, which causes SNAIL1/2 overexpression	Terashima et al. (2018)
10	CRYBG3	Lung cancer	Prevents invasion, migration, and proliferation	Prevents G-actin from polymerizing into F-actin by interacting with it	Pei et al. (2018)
11	ATB	Breast cancer	Enhances the spread of metastasis	Reduces miR-200 family expression, which raises ZEB1 and TWIST1	R.-H. Li et al. (2018)
12	MEG8	Lung cancer and prostate cancer	Causes EMT	Represses the miRNA-34a and miRNA-203 genes by interaction with EZH2, which causes SNAIL1/2 overexpression	Terashima et al. (2018)
13	MALAT1	Lung cancer	Causes metastasis and proliferation	Increases ZEB1 expression LC via suppressing miR-200a	Feng et al. (2019); Grimm et al. (2020)
14	DANCR	Hepatocellular carcinoma	Promotes metastasis	Suppresses miR-27a-3p, which causes LIMK1 to be upregulated	Guo et al. (2019)
15	H19	Hepatocellular carcinoma	Causes invasion, migration, and proliferation	Suppresses miR-15b, which causes Cdc42 to be upregulated	Zhou et al. (2019)
16	LCAT1	Lung cancer	Causes the spread of metastases	Suppresses miR-4715–5p, which causes Rac1 to be upregulated	Juze Yang et al. (2019); Chen et al. (2022)

TABLE 1.1 *(Continued)*
Examples of LncRNAs Linked to Metastasis

S. No.	LncRNA	Cancer Type	Function	Action Mechanism	Reference
17	LINC00452	Oral cancer	Encourages invasion and migration	Suppresses miR-501–3p, which causes ROCK1 to be upregulated	Yang, Wang, and Zhang (2020)
18	ZFAS1	Pancreatic adenocarcinoma	Induces metastasis	Suppresses miR-3924, which causes ROCK2 to be upregulated	Liu, Zhu, and Ge (2020)
19	NAS1	Breast cancer	Induces DTC dormancy	Interacts with NRF2 mRNA-5'UTR, causing NRF2 to be upregulated and ΔNp63 to be downregulated	Liu et al. (2021)
20	LINC00857	Prostate cancer	Promotes metastasis and proliferation	Suppresses miR-103b, which causes RhoA to be upregulated	Chen et al. (2022)

Source: Ahmad et al. (2023).

Mesenchymal ovarian cancer (OC) was identified by bioinformatic investigation of the ceRNA (competing endogenous RNA) network to recognize lncRNApro-transition associated RNA (PTAR). The Cancer Genome Atlas (TCGA) OC data sets showed that mesenchymal subtypes have PTAR-related elevation of ZEB1 EMT-associated TF in comparison to epithelial subtypes. Furthermore, whereas PTAR knockdown (KD) reduced OC tumorigenicity and metastasis in vivo, PTAR overexpression boosted OC EMT and metastasis in vitro. Functional analysis revealed the mechanism by which PTAR regulates ZEB1 levels. ZEB1 mRNA is directly targeted by PTAR, which functions as ceRNA for miR-101–3p; PTAR overexpression subsequently raises ZEB1 levels (Liang et al. 2018).

It has been discovered that lncRNA H19, irrespective of the underlying tumor origin, is highly expressed in many metastatic tissues. In a positive feedback loop, TGF-β-induced production of H19 causes the overexpression of SLUG TF, which, in turn, causes an increase in H19 expression. Multiple cancer cell types experience metastasis as a result of the ensuing suppression of E-cadherin (Matouk et al. 2014).

Maternally expressed RNA 8 (MEG8) is associated with TGF-β-mediated epithelial–mesenchymal transition (EMT) in cell lines of pancreatic cancer (PCa) and lung cancer (LC). MEG8 recruits EZH2, a PRC2-repressive complex component, to the promoter regions of the miRNA-34a and miRNA-203 genes. The consequent suppression of these miRNAs' expression leads to the overexpression of SNAIL1/2, the repression of E-cadherin, and the promotion of EMT (Terashima et al. 2018).

In vitro, hepatocellular carcinoma (HCC) cell metastasis in vitro, distant lung metastases, and poor prognosis have all been associated with lncRNA HOXD-AS1 (HOXD cluster anti- sense RNA 1) overexpression. It was demonstrated that SRY-related HMG-box 4 (SOX4) is induced by HOXD-AS1 overexpression mediated by STAT3 (signal transducer and activator of transcription 3). By competitively binding miR-130a-3p, HOXD-AS1 inhibits the degradation of SOX4 miRNA-mediated processes (Wang et al. 2017; Terashima et al. 2018). SOX4 has been linked to TGF-β-mediated EMT and metastasis, and it has been increased in different malignancies (Feng et al. 2019; Grimm et al. 2020).

TGF-β-activated (ATB) lncRNA is substantially expressed in patients with breast cancer (BC) and associated with a greater risk of metastasis and a lesser total survival rate. It was discovered that lncRNA ATB functions as ceRNA for a number of miRNAs belonging to the miR-200 family, including miR-141, miR-429, and miR-200a/b/c. Through these connections, ATB can raise the expression of TWIST1 and ZEB1, which, in response, promote the production of vimentin and the migration and invasion of BC cells (R.-H. Li et al. 2018).

When comparing gastric cancerous tissue of stomach to normal tissue, lncRNA N-BLR (pyknon-containing, primate-specific lncRNA) is highly expressed in GC tissue. The ability of GC cells to migrate and invade was diminished by the downregulation of lncRNA N-BLR. Mechanistic characterization revealed that miR-200c-3p was the target of N-BLR, which caused EMT. By suppressing SNAIL, ZEB1 TF, and N-cadherin, miR-200c-3p has anti-EMT features (Youn et al. 2019). In addition, by blocking the anti-metastatic miRNAs miR-200c-3p and miR-141–3p, N-BLR controls the metastasis of colorectal cancer (CRC), and its knockdown (KD) prevents the migration and invasion of CRC cells (Rigoutsos et al. 2017).

Additionally, by serving as a ceRNA (competing endogenous RNAs) for anti-metastatic miR-200a and triggering ZEB1 TF expression, the lncRNA metastasis-associated lung adenocarcinoma transcript 1 (MALAT1), which is increased in a variety of cancer types (Guo et al. 2021), encourages LC proliferation and metastasis.

It is intriguing to observe that ATB, N-BLR, and MALAT1 lncRNAs all influence EMT via the similar mechanism, which involves ceRNA connections with miRNAs belonging to the mir-200 family. The miRNA family has a wide range of functions in EMT, ECM remodeling during metastasis, and generally functions as leading regulators in the majority of processes connected to metastasis (Guo et al. 2021). Therefore, in this context, lncRNAs appear to function as a specific and effective instrument to regulate the action of miRNAs in a post-transcriptional way, contributing to the intricacy required to tune gene expression.

Many of the problems related to this process remain unresolved, despite the fact that several of the constituent parts are now understood. For example, in vivo, it is currently not feasible to track the exact moment at which it occurs (Thwaites et al. 2017); the precise point in tumor evolution at which a single cell or a group of cells starts to transfer to distant locations is also unidentified, as are the primary tumor's microenvironmental components that support such a transition. Intra- and intertumoral heterogeneity (Espinoza-Sánchez et al. 2017) offers a wide range of choices; therefore, it is challenging to suggest a general strategy that could resolve this problem.

Contrary to the popular idea that metastasis can only occur in the latter phases of tumor growth, previous research indicates that EMT and metastasis can begin early in the progression of the illness, for example, cells going through the epithelial–mesenchymal transition (EMT) can colonize the liver and form metastatic lesions in the initial stages of pancreatic cancer (Zhou et al. 2009; Rhim et al. 2012). Compared to individual tumor cells, metastatic cell clusters in peripheral blood (PB) have a higher propensity to develop a metastatic location (Aceto et al. 2014; Thwaites et al. 2017). In this field, novel approaches to lessen the development of EMT are being studied, such as the use of micro-RNAs (Tanabe et al. 2020). It should be highlighted, nonetheless, that the metastatic process appears to have other, less-frequent pathways, making it even more intricate than the EMT (Fischer et al. 2015; Zheng et al. 2015).

One of the most important stages in metastasis process is the intravasation of tumor cells—individually or in groups—into the lymphatic and/or bloodstream (Zavyalova et al. 2019). Furthermore, a lot of research is being done on these pathways since blocking them can allow the original tumor to stop spreading. Tumor cells travel to distant areas inside the peripheral blood circulation (PB), with the intention of becoming a metastasis. During their travels, these cells must withstand blood flow pressure and keep away from natural killer (NK) cells (Zavyalova et al. 2019; Luo et al. 2023). Tumor cells often envelop themselves in thrombocytes to avoid them, in addition to generating chemicals such as VEGF (vascular endothelial growth factor), CCL2 (chemokine ligand 2), angiopoietin-2, and angiopoietin-4, which are implicated in the increase of vascular permeability (Lambert, Pattabiraman, and Weinberg 2017; Foss et al. 2020). Moreover, neutrophils contribute to metastasis of lung in the bloodstream by the extravasation of tumor cells and the secretion of IL-1β and metalloproteases (Spiegel et al. 2016).

The following stage of metastasis is called extravasation, and it is here that tumor cells might use a range of tactics, either individually or in groups. One such tactic is angiopellosis that comprises rearranging the endothelium barrier to permit one or more cells to enter a tissue (Allen et al. 2019). Our understanding of the mechanism behind leukocyte extravasation has progressed to the point that several recommended treatments to prevent extravasation now include integrin inhibitors, which are molecules necessary for tumor cell attachment, rolling, and extravasation (Vadillo et al. 2018; Allen et al. 2019; Sökeland and Schumacher 2019). As a therapeutic strategy, antibodies that support vascular integrity can be utilized to prevent tumor cells from migrating through endothelial cells and aid in their elimination in peripheral circulation (Sökeland and Schumacher 2019; Khan and Kerbel 2020).

After extravasation, tumor cells can go quiescent for several years, a process called the mesenchymal–epithelial transition, during which they return to an epithelial phenotype. They achieve this by vying for certain niches that transmit signals via the Notch and Wnt pathways, such as those found in the brain, intestinal mucosa, and bone marrow (Oskarsson, Batlle, and Massagué 2014). Tumor cells adopt a sluggish state of the cell cycle through the Wnt pathway, and they release chemicals that prevent natural killer cells (NK cells) from destroying other cells (Malladi et al. 2016). Two characteristics of quiescent extravasated tumor cells are common to all stem cells: they must be able to self-renew and produce all the cells that make up the secondary tumor.

The metastatic process raises a number of unresolved questions. The significance of EMT for metastasis or chemoresistance is still up for debate (Fischer et al. 2015; Zheng et al. 2015). It is imperative to determine whether there is a pattern in the development of cells that can carry out EMT in each tumor. Controlling metastasis requires an understanding of the intrinsic mechanisms affecting this transformation and the causes of the migratory phenotypic development. Furthermore, it is vital to comprehend if this process is caused by the variety of epigenetic changes or mutations associated with the original tumor (Lambert, Pattabiraman, and Weinberg 2017). It is obvious that, depending on the type of original tumor, metastatic cells favor some tissues over others (see seed and soil hypothesis). Because of the various soluble substances released by the tumor and the immune system's recruitment of those areas, premetastatic niches may also be conditioned at a distance in addition to the location and route of the bloodstream or lymphatic fluid (Massagué and Obenauf 2016; Lambert, Pattabiraman, and Weinberg 2017). All the components that are involved in this process still need to be identified and described.

1.11 CANCER GENES

Irregular cell proliferation and resistance to apoptosis, or programmed cell death, are features of cancer. Three things happen: faulty tumor suppressor genes (TSGs), ineffective or inadequate DNA repair genes, and actively expressed oncogene(s), which could be used, at the gene level, to describe any cancer. These distinctive occurrences may interact with one another or work alone to give rise to malignant characteristics in a healthy cell. Three main categories can be used to classify functional mutations: mutational inactivation, mutational gain of function, and mutational activation.

Tumor suppressor genes typically experience mutational inactivation, which can manifest as either amorphic, hypomorphic, or antimorphic. One example of how genes might become activated by mutation is the activation of oncogenes through hypermorphic mutation. Finally, a mutation is referred to as neomorphic when it confers a novel function or functions on a gene (Strilic and Offermanns 2017)

1.11.1 Oncogenes and Proto-Oncogenes

In 1969, George Toddaro and Robert Heubner coined the oncogene term, which is derived from the Greek terms *onkos*, which means "mass/bulk," and gignere/genui, which means "beget/give birth."

Any gene that has the capacity to promote disordered cell development is referred to as an oncogene. Through experimental techniques, a normal cell with an activated tumorigenic phenotype could develop into a tumor in the naked mice, for example, by transfecting normal cells or nude mice with activated oncogenes in vitro or in vivo. Nevertheless, it takes more than one oncogene to produce cancerous cell characteristics in healthy cells. The oncoprotein that emerges from the oncogene's expression would eventually need additional environmental cues, for example, viral infection, or synergistic activation of another oncogene or faulty tumor suppressor gene. In reality, aggressive carcinogenesis requires oncogene collaboration. Consequently, the concepts of clonal evolution and cancer stem cells are compatible with oncogene cooperation (Afrikanova et al. 2002; Shields et al. 2011; Ashton et al. 2012; Wichmann et al. 2014; Fang et al. 2016; Caswell and Swanton 2017).

Hence, oncogenes explore the functional sides of genes that, if aberrantly overexpressed or acquire constitutive expression, would ultimately aid in the development of tumors. In healthy cells, proto-oncogenes mediate cell proliferation. They resemble oncogene precursor genes in certain ways. On the other hand, they are frequently and abusively called oncogenes. Proto-oncogenes would eventually become oncogenes after undergoing oncomutation(s). The four primary mechanisms by which oncogenic activation occurs are gene amplification (e.g., ErbB2/HER2; Myc), specific point mutations in the gene sequence (e.g., H-ras, K-ras, N-ras; EGFR), oncoviruses infection (Hobbs, Der, and Rossman 2016; Naab et al. 2018), and DNA translocation to more transcriptionally active chromosomal sites, or the emergence of a novel fusion gene that codes a protein with higher biological activity (e.g., CML, chronic myelogenous leukemia) (D. Hanahan 2023)(Figure 1.6). Human cancer frequently involves chromosomal translocations, especially in hematopoietic and lymphoid cancers. They contribute in the development of certain cancers, albeit the precise process is unclear. These translocations might give some stem or progenitor cells a discerning growth benefit or increase the likelihood of later mutations, which might then start the progression of some malignant tumors. Gene rearrangements may alter the initial positions of proto-oncogenes in oncogenic chromosomal translocations, leading to the evident impact on phenotype through two main pathways (Fröhling and Döhner 2008; Nambiar, Kari, and Raghavan 2008). Making oncogenic fusion proteins is one of them. The most notable example is the translocation of the Philadelphia (Ph) chromosome [t(9;22)], which occurs in chronic myeloid leukemia (CML) and causes the translocation of the proto-oncogene ABL (Abelson) at 9q34 to BCR (breakpoint cluster region) on chromosome 22. Tyrosine kinase (TK) aberrant activity is linked to the development of BCR-ABL oncoprotein and is linked to the carcinogenesis of acute lymphoblastic leukemia and CML (Pui, Relling, and Downing 2004). Another method involves the interaction of the novel cis-regulatory elements with proto-oncogenes. The proto-oncogene c-MYC is overexpressed in Burkitt lymphoma

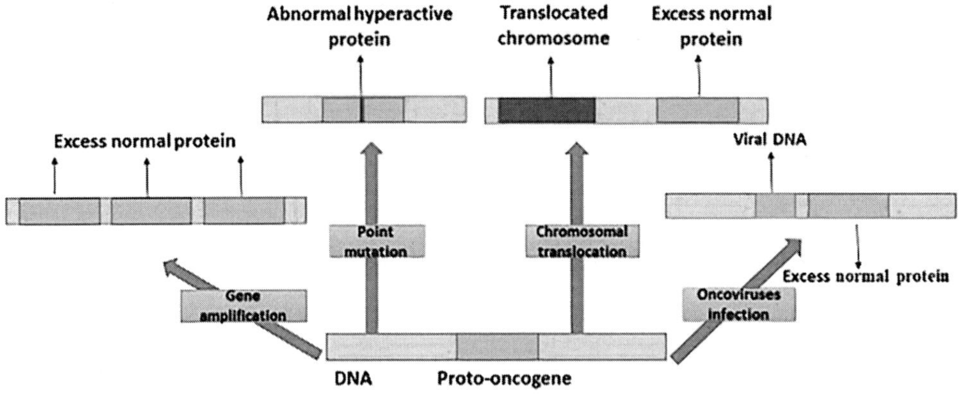

FIGURE 1.6 Oncogene activation mechanisms: gene amplification, point mutation, chromosomal translocation, and oncoviruses infection.

as a result of t(8;14), which causes c-MYC to be in opposition to heavy chain (IGH) regulatory elements of immunoglobulin. This is a classic case (J. Zheng 2013). In vivo chromosomal translocations are a complicated biological process that requires two prerequisite steps to be fulfilled. First, there are synchronous DNA double-strand breaks (DSBs) at the two loci. Second, DSB ends are illegally connected together and must approach one another. Beyond these fundamental processes, mounting data indicates that a number of additional factors, including activation-induced deaminase (AID)–mediated V(D)J recombination, nuclear architecture, gene expression, and additional unidentified mechanisms, also affect the formation of chromosomal translocations (Aplan 2006; Raghavan and Lieber 2006; Hakim et al. 2012).

It is essential to highlight that RNA viruses, or retroviruses, are the original source of oncogenes. Since then, it has been established that numerous RNA viruses are linked to cancer in both people and animals. Even while oncogenes are not present in many retroviruses, those that do have them are extremely carcinogenic when they infect both humans and animals. Retroviruses incorporate a corresponding DNA (cDNA) copy of their genome haphazardly into the DNA of their host cells. The virus occasionally inserts itself adjacent to a proto-oncogene in the cell. This has two potential mechanisms to increase the proto-oncogene's transcription. Enhancer insertion occurs when a nearby proto-oncogene's transcription is stimulated by the enhancer found in the lengthy terminal repeats of the inserted retrovirus. This technique functions even if the virus is introduced in a distance that is greater than 10,000 base pairs, since enhancers can act over such distances (Meisenberg and Simmons 2012).

The retroviral cDNA inserts itself immediately upstream of the proto-oncogene during promoter insertion. This may result in the abnormally high rate of transcription of the proto-oncogene from the promoter in the virus's downstream long terminal repeat without the presence of the typical negative controls. Among the well-known oncogenic viruses are the Merkel cell polyomavirus, hepatitis B and C viruses, Epstein–Barr virus (EBV), Kaposi's sarcoma–associated herpesvirus (KSHV), and T-lymphotropic virus. Numerous oncogenes associated with human malignancies have been identified since the 1970s. Their prevalence in different cancer subtypes ranges from one to the other. As an illustration of how k-ras on computation functions, a mutation in the gene sequence is common in lung adenocarcinoma and non–small cell lung carcinomas, but uncommon in small cell lung carcinomas. Additional example is the overexpression of the myc gene; however, this time it manifests as the overexpression of an oncogene. Both small cell and non–small cell lung carcinomas exhibit this (Chaturvedi et al. 2011; Chen et al. 2015; Yuan et al. 2017; Cao and Li 2018; Hussein et al. 2018; Yeo-Teh, Ito, and Jha 2018).

1.11.2 Tumor Suppressor Genes (TSGs)

TSGs are the genes that support in vivo homeostatic cell growth, differentiation, and motility prospects. When necessary, they function directly or indirectly to encourage DNA repair, inhibit cell division, and support apoptosis. Any type of mutation that ultimately modifies the function of these genes would put the cell on the route to cancer. One of four general pathways can lead to defective tumor suppressor genes: (1) direct mutation that leads to gene silencing, (2) gene deletion, (3) loss of heterozygosity, and (4) hypermethylation of promoter (Figure 1.7) (Roa et al. 2015; Dunford et al. 2016; Luchini et al. 2016; Gao et al. 2017; L. Li et al. 2018).

1.12 MOLECULAR UNDERPINNINGS OF EPIGENETIC CONTROL IN CANCER

The field of epigenetics studies how to alter gene expression without any change in DNA sequence. Conard Waddington originated the term in 1942; it is Greek in origin and means "above or over the genome" (Waddington 2012). Three chemical processes, including DNA methylation, RNA methylation, and chromatin remodeling patterns, are involved in the epigenetics process. These changes alter the structure of nucleic acids and histones, resulting in a distinct structure of chromatin

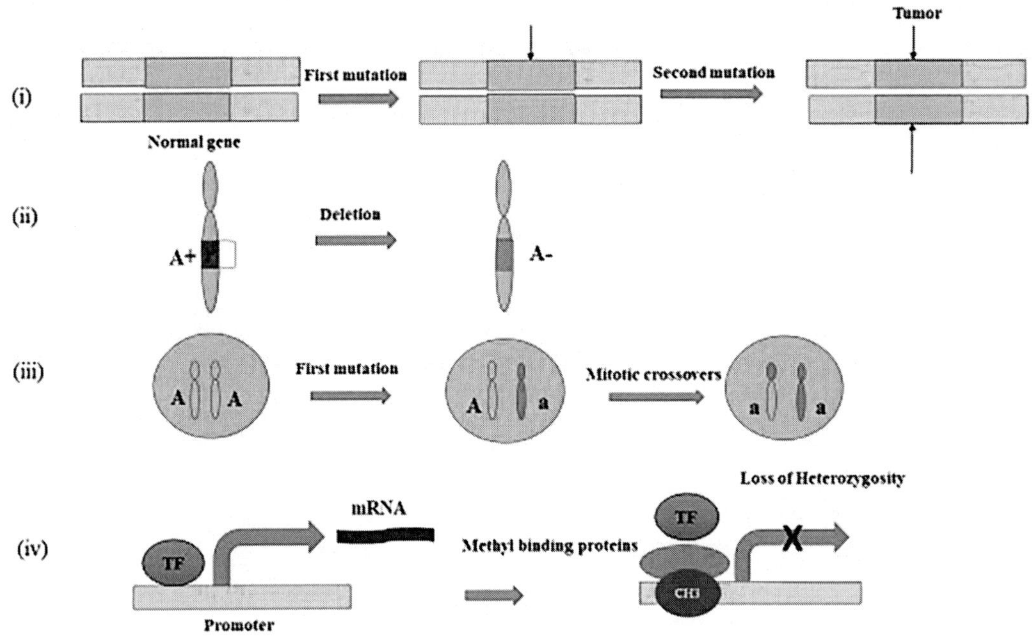

FIGURE 1.7 Loss of the function of tumor suppressor gene in cancer: (1) direct mutation that leads to gene silencing, (2) gene deletion, (3) loss of heterozygosity, and (4) hypermethylation of promoter.

(Ganesan et al. 2019). Several chemical changes are involved in these epigenetic alterations, and they are produced by a class of enzymes known as epigenetic tools. Enzymes involved in biochemical addition to DNA or histones are called "writers," while those involved in chemical tag removal are called "erasers." A distinct class of enzymes known as "readers" interprets all these alterations (Biswas and Rao 2018). Epigenetics regulates a number of activities, including DNA repair, replication, transcription, translation, post-transcriptional regulation, and translation (Dawson and Kouzarides 2012). Accordingly, abnormal epigenomic changes may cause dysregulation, which, in turn, may result in malignancies (Lu et al. 2020).

The main focus of epigenetics is on the molecular mechanisms that cause and/or sustain heritable, but reversible, changes in gene regulation due to environmental cues, independent of the DNA sequence (which is one of the causes it is most frequently linked to CSC). "Epimutations" refers to the epigenetic modifications. After their initial signal has vanished, they may either persist for a considerable amount of time (sometimes indefinitely) or vanish (reverting to their previous state). DNA methylation, polycomb group of proteins, noncoding RNAs (miRNA and others), chromatin remodeling, histone modification patterns, and chromatin remodeling are examples of epimutations. Epigenetic dysregulation may facilitate the development and spread of cancer. In one form or another, every one of the aforementioned epimutations has been documented as clinically relevant in relation to the genesis, diagnosis, and/or prognosis of cancer (Flavahan, Gaskell, and Bernstein 2017; Poli, Fagnocchi, and Zippo 2018).

1.12.1 Epigenetic Modulators, Modifiers, and Mediators

Three main types of genes—epigenetic mediators, modifiers, and modulators—are responsible for epigenetic modifications. Peptides and proteins known as epigenetic mediators are in charge of the stemness, pliability, and subsequent intratumoral heterogeneity of malignant tissues in cancer cells. They have interactions with HDAC (histone deacetylases), HAT (histone acetyltransferases), and HMT (histone methyltransferases) epigenetic modifiers. Through chromatin modulation, histone modification, DNA methylation, and other methods, the latter class lays the groundwork for epimutation. As they direct the progressions of cell and tissue differentiation, the third and final class of proteins, known as epigenetic modulators, is specific to particular tissues and is essential to normal cellular functions. They provide the epigenetic modifiers with environmental cues (Feinberg, Koldobskiy, and Göndör 2016); (Singh Nanda, Kumar, and Raghava 2016) (Figure 1.8).

1.12.1.1 DNA and RNA Methylation

Among the epigenetic modifications, methylation of DNA is among the most extensively researched and exemplary. In order to complete the process, a methyl group must be transferred to position 5′ of cytosine of 5′-CpG-3′-rich DNA sections known as CpG islands. These regions are made up of a palindromic collection of dinucleotides that are located in the promoter and in other genomic regions as well. When methylation occurs on the cytosine residues of one or both strands of DNA, the latter may be either hemi- or homoimethylated, respectively. Additionally, methylation on the cytosine of 5′-CT-3′ or 5′-CA-3′ residues may happen, but to a lesser degree. *DNA methylation* refers to the ability of methylating enzymes known as DNA methyltransferases to separate DNA from transcription factors, which is essential for activity. Certain repressor proteins, such as MeCP2 (methyl-CpG-binding protein 2), MBD2 (methyl-CpG-binding domain protein 1), MBD3 (methyl-CpG-binding domain protein 3), and others, are attracted to DNA methylation. Thus, a cell's transcriptional plasticity is regulated by DNA methylation. There have been reports linking various DNA methylation variations to the etiology of cancer and/or metastasis. These include aberrant hypermethylation (silencing of TSG), abnormal DNA hypomethylation (overexpression of carcinogenic proteins; lack of imprinting), and genomic imprinting (where the expression of specific genes is dependent on the parent of origin) (Jones and Laird 1999; Wainwright and Scaffidi 2017; Perduca et al. 2018) (Figure 1.8).

RNA methylation is a less well-studied epigenetic mechanism. It is almost seven times higher than the methylation of DNA. Transcript degradation and mRNA localization are the outcomes of these changes (Zaccara, Ries, and Jaffrey 2019). It is now clear that methyl alterations at the mRNA level may have an impact on the cellular processes leading to human diseases, due to the discovery of next-generation sequencing and the identification of RNA methylation–related proteins. Currently, more than 150 distinct RNA modifications have been identified; the most prevalent is N6-methyladenosine (m6A) modification, which is recognized by RNA-binding proteins and influences numerous aspects of mRNA function (Schwartz et al. 2014; Linder et al. 2015). Changes in RNA can impact the epigenetic regulation of gene expression (Tulsyan et al. 2022) (Figure 1.8).

1.12.1.2 Histone Modifications

Histones are the main (gene) regulatory proteins that encircle DNA in eukaryotes. The structural components of a nucleosome are two twists, or 146 base pairs (bp) of DNA wound around two H2A, H2B, H3, and H4 histones. H1 histone, an anchor used to stabilize some nucleosomes, is the histone linker H1. DNA is packaged within the nucleus, and gene expression is regulated by the position and direction of DNA packaging, which also determines the state of euchromatin and heterochromatin. The core canonical histones' N-terminal tails extend beyond the nucleosomes and are occasionally modified by covalent post-translational processes. At the aminoterminal tail of these histones, ADP-ribosylation, acetylation, methylation, phosphorylation, or ubiquitination are the processes that modify the histones. It is known that a number of enzymes catalyze the aforementioned processes. Histone kinases, histone methyltransferases, and histone acetyltransferases add acetyl, methyl, phosphate groups, and other functional groups to the histone aminoterminal tail. Known as writers, these epigenetic markers function as co-activators of transcription. Conversely, by the removal of these groups from the histone end, erasers—histone deacetylases (HDACs), histone demethylases (HDMs), and phosphatases—act as co-repressors of transcription (Li et al. 2020). The concurrent opening and closing of the chromatin structure, which is required for gene expression, is carried out by all these enzymes (Figure 1.8). Variations in these enzymes could result in changed post-transcriptional processes and gene transcription. These alteration patterns are collectively known as "histone code," which is one of the chromatin structure–altering regulatory mechanisms for gene expression. The alterations stop DNA from being accessed by the transcriptional machinery. The majority of the time, they are found on particular amino acids, such as arginine, leucine, lysine, serine, etc. (Lund and van Lohuizen 2004). Oncohistones, or aberrant histone modifications, have been linked to a number of cancer types.

1.12.1.3 Chromatin Remodeling Related to Cancer

As explained earlier, nuclear DNA in eukaryotic cells is tightly wound and wrapped around histones to form nucleosomes, which are repeating units of chromatin structure. The latter procedure involves packing meters of DNA efficiently in an active and inactive state of chromatin within a nuclear cell compartment, as well as regulating gene expression at the primary level (limiting access to gene promoter and enhancer regions). Epigenetic fingerprints on DNA and histones distinguish heterochromatin and euchromatin and enable their structural arrangement (Flavahan, Gaskell, and Bernstein 2017). The transcriptionally active and loosely packed genomic areas are known as euchromatin, whereas the densely packed and transcriptionally silent genomic regions are known as heterochromatin (facultative and constitutive). Compactly coiled genes in chromatin are not available to RNA polymerase or transcriptional factors, which are necessary for the genes' eventual expression. To provide admittance for the machinery of transcription (RNA polymerase, transcription factors, etc.), the chromatin "opens," deviating from its typical state in eukaryotic cells and exposing certain genes for expression. The dynamic, complex process known as "chromatin remodeling" modifies chromatin's structure to make genomic DNA visible. It is necessary for eukaryotic cells to function in balance. The process uses a range of multiportion complexes called chromatin remodelers, which employ ATP hydrolysis to mobilize and restructure nucleosomes. Remodelers are therefore essential for uncovering DNA to transcription, chromatin structure, DNA repair mechanisms, and other processes. Admittance to nucleosomal DNA is frequently made feasible by two basic types of multiprotein complexes: (1) covalent histone-modifying complexes (HATs, HDACs, etc.) and (2) ATP-dependent chromatin remodeling complexes for nucleosome mobility, ejection, and reformation (Feinberg, Koldobskiy, and Göndör 2016; Kang et al. 2020). CRCs relate to the four families of eukaryotes—SWI/SNF, ISWI, CHD, and INO80—that are different both physically and functionally. Histone modifications may promote chromatin "opening," which allows a specific region of DNA to become accessible and attract RNA polymerase II. Chromatin activation has been linked to a number of different histone modifications (Dawson and Kouzarides 2012; Feinberg, Koldobskiy, and Göndör 2016) (Figure 1.8).

1.13 MICROBIOTA, NUTRITION, BIOACTIVE DIETARY COMPONENTS, EPIGENETIC MODIFICATIONS, AND CANCER

It can be difficult to define cancer in terms of its genesis, diagnosis, prognosis, and/or treatment, and this might vary depending on the approach(s) taken. For example, cancer can be classified as a cellular, genetic, metabolic, chronic inflammatory, epigenetic (nutritional or not), dysbiosis, or hereditary disease. Numerous scientific studies proposed—supported by compelling data—that the gut microbiota's interaction with dietary components (nutrients and bioactive substances) may influence the pathways involved in gene expression through epigenetic modifications. Expanding the fields of study that aim to understand these mechanisms would be a significant step forward in the direction of new therapeutic methods in the treatment of cancer. Food ingredients and nutrients may alter their metabolic pathways and occasionally change the structure of the epigenome. To mediate an organism's phenotypic plasticity, they may employ epigenetic processes mentioned before. Thus, it is possible to argue that nutrients and other food ingredients are crucial for the etiology, development, management, and prevention of cancer. Among the most researched one-carbon nutrients are

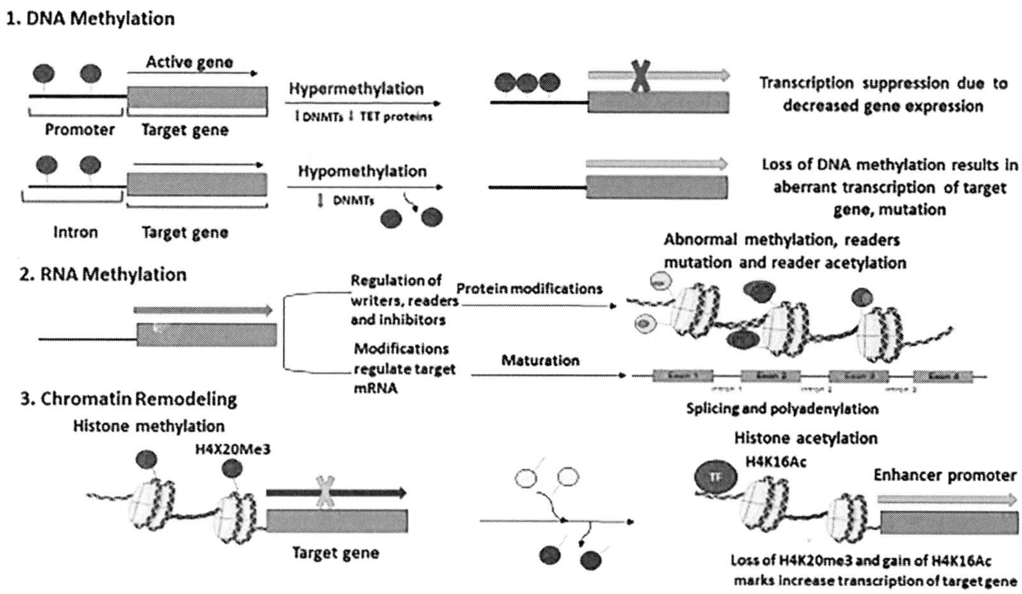

FIGURE 1.8 An illustration of epigenetic pathways. (1) DNA methylation: Gene promoter regions get an addition of methyl group by DNA methyltransferases (DNMTs). Conversely, DNA hypomethylation, which impacts the intronic and intergenic sections of the DNA and causes an overall reduction in methylation levels relative to normal cells, causes chromosomal instability and a rise in mutation occurrences. (2) RNA methylation: Deadenylation, or the removal of an mRNA's 3′ poly(A) tail, is brought on by miRNA's indirect translational repression, which increases mRNA breakdown. There are various ways in which the miRNA–mRNA interaction might result in direct translational inhibition removed, leading to augmented mRNA degradation. The miRNA–mRNA interaction can lead to several modes of direct translational repression. (3) histone modification (H4K20Me3): These methyl groups are eliminated by histone demethylases (HDM) and lysine demethylases (KDM6/4). It is connected to both silencing and gene expression. Histone acetylation is the process by which the histone acetylase (HAT) enzyme adds an acetyl group to histone H3K9Ac (lysine 9 in the enhancer/promoter region). To undo the alterations, transcriptional repressor (TR) and histone deacetylase (HDAC) interact.

folate (B9), choline, betaine, and vitamin B12. These nutrients supply the methyl group S-adenosyl homocysteine, which is then transformed into the universal methyl donor S-adenosylmethionine. The latter impedes the activity of methyltransferases, which methylate histone tails and DNA. In order to maintain the heredity of gene expression patterns, the over-, normo-, or undernutrition of one carbon donor can affect gene expression (by epimutations) as well as the creation of epigenetic fingerprints. As a result, it has a close relationship with the patterns of gene expression in pathological diseases such as cancer and developmental physiology. These micronutrients are necessary for the highly proliferating cancer cells to fuel their methylations, redox metabolisms, and DNA synthesis (Newman and Maddocks 2017; Rosenzweig, Blenis, and Gomes 2018; Zhao et al. 2018).

HATs/HDACs are essential for the transfer of an acetoxy group—from donor to acceptor in both plants and animals. Acetylation often takes place on the amino group of histone tail lysine residues, causing them to locally separate from their nucleosomes and allowing transcriptional machinery to access DNA, which in turn enhances gene expression. In contrast, deacetylation strengthens the interactions between histone tails and nucleosomal proteins, which protect nearby DNA from transcription. Animals need responses for a variety of physiological processes, from histone modifications to detoxifying foreign substances to regulating gene expression. HATs expression and activity in cancer and normal cells differ in an exciting way. There have been reports linking the overexpression and increased activity of HATs (P300/CBP) with certain oncogenes' expression during carcinogenesis and metastasis. On the other hand, increased HDAC expression and activity (which typically couple with decreased HAT expression and activity) would suppress tumor suppressors' expression and accelerate the development of tumors and metastases (Barnes, English, and Cowley 2019; Feron 2019; Narita, Weinert, and Choudhary 2019).

Evidences from research reports suggest that specific dietary constituents—such as those in fruits, whole grains, cruciferous plants, dietary fibers, etc.—have the capacity to modify histones. Acetylation would be encouraged by a large nuclear pool of acetate. Histone modifications begin early in embryogenesis and dynamically continue/reshape throughout life, similar to other epigenetic modification mechanisms. As a result, in addition to environmental stressors, maternal nutrition may have an impact early in pregnancy and reversibly continue (Bassett and Barnett 2014; Campit et al. 2020; Zhang et al. 2021)

The term "microbiota" describes populations of commensal bacteria (~2 kg) that inhabit the gastrointestinal tracts of mammals. According to reports, the interactions between the quantitative and qualitative components of the microbial flora and their host are crucial for maintaining homeostasis. Eubiosis is the process by which a significant balance of the anticipated microbial community has been established, and it is predicted or documented that this condition is linked to many medical disorders. On the other hand, dysbiosis, or an uneven distribution of desired versus undesired community members, has been linked to a number of illnesses. Food-related factors affect the microbial community's diversity and function, affecting the mucus's thickness and shielding the intestines from harm. Thick mucus typically indicates eubiosis, but thin mucus typically indicates dysbiosis (Ho and Dashwood 2010; Delage and Dashwood 2008; Ho and Dashwood 2010). The dietary composition and richness, in conjunction with the energy balance, determine the availability of specific nutrients that function as cofactors to enzymes engaged in epigenetic activities. To put it another way, they generated metabolites that might interact with or serve as substrates for processes like histone methylation/demethylation, methyltransferase (DNA), HATs/HDACs (histone acetylation/deacetylation), etc. According to Diori Karidio and Sanlier (*Journal of the Egyptian National Cancer Institute* 2021), different bacterial species that are part of the gut microbiota have been shown to produce oncometabolites, immunomodulatory, "onco-repressive," or oncolytic metabolites, which in turn facilitate pervasive epigenetic mechanisms (De Almeida et al. 2019; Lee 2019; Miro-Blanch and Yanes 2019; El-Sayed, Aleya, and Kamel 2021; Guz et al. 2021).

1.14 CONCLUSION AND FUTURE PROSPECTS

A thorough understanding of cancer from the outset, a multidisciplinary approach would be necessary to eventually identify the molecular etiology of metastasis and establish foundations to prevent its molecular disease. Advances in cancer research facilitate the dismantling of barriers across numerous scientific fields, resulting in an enormous corpus of multidisciplinary methods that combine the biological sciences for a deeper comprehension of the preservation of the desired organismal harmonic states and their various disturbances that could exacerbate carcinogenesis. According to molecular genetics, hereditary defects on genes involved in cell cycle checkpoints have the potential to progressively magnify unchecked cell proliferation. Conversely, the models of CSC and CSCP demolished the misconception of evolutionary carcinogenesis by explicating hypothetical mechanisms that were previously unknown. Research has indicated a correlation between low clinical outcome and cancer metastasis when it comes to the expression of lncRNAs. Similar to other characteristics of cancer, long noncoding RNAs (lncRNAs) control the metastasis of cancer cells via various signaling pathways. They also function as guide for chromatin-modifying complexes or as ceRNA for anti-metastatic microRNAs, which has an impact on the transcriptional and post-transcriptional levels of metastasis-associated genes. Additionally, cancer cell epigenetic pathways are linked to food and energy balance, which maintain the gut microbiota population and metabolism, producing anti-oxidants, anti-cancer, oncometabolites, and onco-suppressive metabolites.

Knowledge of these many aspects of the molecular pathophysiology and genesis of cancer would be more beneficial for drug discovery. Problems such as treatment resistance, target identification, biological system analysis, and variations between individuals will be minimized, with additional studies being carried out on the mechanisms. Future immunotherapy methods will offer cancer patients with a treatment choice with the lowest side effect rate and a high immune response rate.

In order to give patients successful cancer therapy, it becomes more and more important to develop and accurately evaluate molecular tumor profiles as new genetic and molecular drugs become available. Nonetheless, the notable developments in molecular techniques and the precision of the information that these tools offer are noteworthy. It is essential to go through clinical scenarios and the molecular analysis results to translate these molecular profiles into clinically useful information.

REFERENCES

Abou-Antoun, Tamara J., James S. Hale, Justin D. Lathia, and Stephen M. Dombrowski. 2017. "Brain Cancer Stem Cells in Adults and Children: Cell Biology and Therapeutic Implications." *Neurotherapeutics: The Journal of the American Society for Experimental NeuroTherapeutics* 14 (2): 372–84.

Aceto, N., A. Bardia, D. T. Miyamoto, M. C. Donaldson, B. S. Wittner, J. A. Spencer, M. Yu, et al. 2014. "Circulating Tumor Cell Clusters Are Oligoclonal Precursors of Breast Cancer Metastasis." *Cell* 158 (5). https://doi.org/10.1016/j.cell.2014.07.013.

Afrikanova, Iva, Ellen Yeh, David Bartos, Stephanie S. Watowich, and Gregory D. Longmore. 2002. "Oncogene Cooperativity in Friend Erythroleukemia: Erythropoietin Receptor Activation by the Env Gene of SFFV Leads to Transcriptional Upregulation of PU.1, Independent of SFFV Proviral Insertion." *Oncogene* 21 (8): 1272–84.

Ahmad, Mohammad, Louis-Bastien Weiswald, Laurent Poulain, Christophe Denoyelle, and Matthieu Meryet-Figuiere. 2023. "Involvement of lncRNAs in Cancer Cells Migration, Invasion and Metastasis: Cytoskeleton and ECM Crosstalk." *Journal of Experimental & Clinical Cancer Research: CR* 42 (1): 1–14.

Albini, Adriana, Antonino Bruno, Cristina Gallo, Giorgio Pajardi, Douglas M. Noonan, and Katiuscia Dallaglio. 2015. "Cancer Stem Cells and the Tumor Microenvironment: Interplay in Tumor Heterogeneity." *Connective Tissue Research* 56 (5): 414–25.

Allen, Tyler A., Dana Asad, Emmanuel Amu, M. Taylor Hensley, Jhon Cores, Adam Vandergriff, Junnan Tang, et al. 2019. "Circulating Tumor Cells Exit Circulation While Maintaining Multicellularity, Augmenting Metastatic Potential." *Journal of Cell Science* 132 (17). https://doi.org/10.1242/jcs.231563.

Andrade, Sheila Siqueira, Joana Tomomi Sumikawa, Eloísa Dognani Castro, Fabricio Pereira Batista, Edgar Paredes-Gamero, Lilian Carolina Oliveira, Izabel Monastério Guerra, et al. 2017. "Interface Between Breast Cancer Cells and the Tumor Microenvironment Using Platelet-Rich Plasma to Promote Tumor Angiogenesis—Influence of Platelets and Fibrin Bundles on the Behavior of Breast Tumor Cells." *Oncotarget* 8 (10): 16851–74.

Aplan, P. D. 2006. "Causes of Oncogenic Chromosomal Translocation." *Trends in Genetics: TIG* 22 (1). https://doi.org/10.1016/j.tig.2005.10.002.

Asghar, Uzma, Agnieszka K. Witkiewicz, Nicholas C. Turner, and Erik S. Knudsen. 2015. "The History and Future of Targeting Cyclin-Dependent Kinases in Cancer Therapy." *Nature Reviews. Drug Discovery* 14 (2): 130–46.

Ashton, John M., Marlene Balys, Sarah J. Neering, Duane C. Hassane, Glenn Cowley, David E. Root, Peter G. Miller, et al. 2012. "Gene Sets Identified With Oncogene Cooperativity Analysis Regulate In Vivo Growth and Survival of Leukemia Stem Cells." *Cell Stem Cell* 11 (3): 359–72.

Bahmad, Hisham F., Mohamad K. Elajami, Talal El Zarif, Jolie Bou-Gharios, Tamara Abou-Antoun, and Wassim Abou-Kheir. 2020. "Drug Repurposing Towards Targeting Cancer Stem Cells in Pediatric Brain Tumors." *Cancer Metastasis Reviews* 39 (1): 127–48.

Balkwill, Frances R., Melania Capasso, and Thorsten Hagemann. 2012. "The Tumor Microenvironment at a Glance." *Journal of Cell Science* 125 (23): 5591–6.

Barnes, C. E., D. M. English, and S. M. Cowley. 2019. "Acetylation & Co: An Expanding Repertoire of Histone Acylations Regulates Chromatin and Transcription." *Essays in Biochemistry* 63 (1). https://doi.org/10.1042/EBC20180061.

Barnum, Kevin J., and Matthew J. O'Connell. 2014. "Cell Cycle Regulation by Checkpoints." *Methods in Molecular Biology* 1170: 29–40.

Bassett, S. A., and M. P. Barnett. 2014. "The Role of Dietary Histone Deacetylases (HDACs) Inhibitors in Health and Disease." *Nutrients* 6 (10). https://doi.org/10.3390/nu6104273.

Batlle, Eduard, and Hans Clevers. 2017. "Cancer Stem Cells Revisited." *Nature Medicine* 23 (10): 1124–34.

Beauchesne, Patrick. 2011. "Extra-Neural Metastases of Malignant Gliomas: Myth or Reality?" *Cancers* 3 (1): 461.

Bendris, Nawal, Bénédicte Lemmers, and Jean Marie Blanchard. 2015. "Cell Cycle, Cytoskeleton Dynamics and Beyond: The Many Functions of Cyclins and CDK Inhibitors." *Cell Cycle*, June. https://doi.org/10.1080/15384101.2014.998085.

Bertoni, Gregory. 2018. "Cell Cycle Regulation by Chlamydomonas Cyclin-Dependent Protein Kinases." *The Plant Cell* 30 (2): 271.

Biswas, S., and C. M. Rao. 2018. "Epigenetic Tools (The Writers, The Readers and The Erasers) and Their Implications in Cancer Therapy." *European Journal of Pharmacology* 837 (October). https://doi.org/10.1016/j.ejphar.2018.08.021.

Blanchet, Emilie, Jean-Sébastien Annicotte, Sylviane Lagarrigue, Victor Aguilar, Cyrielle Clapé, Carine Chavey, Vanessa Fritz, et al. 2011. "E2F Transcription Factor-1 Regulates Oxidative Metabolism." *Nature Cell Biology* 13 (9): 1146–52.

Böttcher, Martin, Rebecca Baur, Andrej Stoll, Andreas Mackensen, and Dimitrios Mougiakakos. 2020. "Linking Immunoevasion and Metabolic Reprogramming in B-Cell-Derived Lymphomas." *Frontiers in Oncology* 10 (November): 594782.

Brabletz, S., H. Schuhwerk, T. Brabletz, and M. P. Stemmler. 2021. "Dynamic EMT: A Multi-Tool for Tumor Progression." *The EMBO Journal* 40 (18). https://doi.org/10.15252/embj.2021108647.

Buhl, Juliane L., Florian Selt, Thomas Hielscher, Romain Guiho, Jonas Ecker, Felix Sahm, Johannes Ridinger, et al. 2019. "The Senescence-Associated Secretory Phenotype Mediates Oncogene-Induced Senescence in Pediatric Pilocytic Astrocytoma." *Clinical Cancer Research: An Official Journal of the American Association for Cancer Research* 25 (6): 1851–66.

Burns, Timothy F., Peiwen Fei, Kimberly A. Scata, David T. Dicker, and Wafik S. El-Deiry. 2003. "Silencing of the Novel p53 Target Gene Snk/Plk2 Leads to Mitotic Catastrophe in Paclitaxel (taxol)-Exposed Cells." *Molecular and Cellular Biology* 23 (16): 5556–71.

Butturini, Elena, Alessandra Carcereri de Prati, Diana Boriero, and Sofia Mariotto. 2019. "Tumor Dormancy and Interplay With Hypoxic Tumor Microenvironment." *International Journal of Molecular Sciences* 20 (17). https://doi.org/10.3390/ijms20174305.

Cai, Qiliang, and Zhenghong Yuan. 2017. "Overview of Infectious Causes of Human Cancers." *Infectious Agents Associated Cancers: Epidemiology and Molecular Biology* 1–9.

Campit, S. E., A. Meliki, N. A. Youngson, and S. Chandrasekaran. 2020. "Nutrient Sensing by Histone Marks: Reading the Metabolic Histone Code Using Tracing, Omics, and Modeling." *BioEssays: News and Reviews in Molecular, Cellular and Developmental Biology* 42 (9). https://doi.org/10.1002/bies.202000083.

Campos-da-Paz, Mariana, José Garrofe Dórea, Alexsandro Sobreira Galdino, Zulmira Guerrero Marques Lacava, and Maria de Fatima Menezes Almeida Santos. 2018. "Carcinoembryonic Antigen (CEA) and Hepatic Metastasis in Colorectal Cancer: Update on Biomarker for Clinical and Biotechnological Approaches." *Recent Patents on Biotechnology* 12 (4): 269–79.

Cao, J., and D. Li. 2018. "Searching for Human Oncoviruses: Histories, Challenges, and Opportunities." *Journal of Cellular Biochemistry* 119 (6). https://doi.org/10.1002/jcb.26717.

Castedo, Maria, Jean-Luc Perfettini, Thomas Roumier, Karine Andreau, Rene Medema, and Guido Kroemer. 2004. "Cell Death by Mitotic Catastrophe: A Molecular Definition." *Oncogene* 23 (16): 2825–37.

Caswell, Deborah R., and Charles Swanton. 2017. "The Role of Tumour Heterogeneity and Clonal Cooperativity in Metastasis, Immune Evasion and Clinical Outcome." *BMC Medicine* 15 (1): 1–9.

Chaturvedi, A. K., E. A. Engels, R. M. Pfeiffer, B. Y. Hernandez, W. Xiao, E. Kim, B. Jiang, et al. 2011. "Human Papillomavirus and Rising Oropharyngeal Cancer Incidence in the United States." *Journal of Clinical Oncology: Official Journal of the American Society of Clinical Oncology* 29 (32). https://doi.org/10.1200/JCO.2011.36.4596.

Chen, Hongda, Xin-Zu Chen, Tim Waterboer, Felipe Andres Castro, and Hermann Brenner. 2015. "Viral Infections and Colorectal Cancer: A Systematic Review of Epidemiological Studies." *International Journal of Cancer* 137 (1): 12–24.

Chen, Peng, Zhirui Zeng, Jie Wang, Wenpeng Cao, Chunzhuo Song, Shan Lei, Yichuan Li, and Zhangxia Ren. 2022. "Long Noncoding RNA LINC00857 Promotes Pancreatic Cancer Proliferation and Metastasis by Regulating the miR-130b/RHOA Axis." *Cell Death Discovery* 8 (1): 198.

Childs, Bennett G., Matej Durik, Darren J. Baker, and Jan M. van Deursen. 2015. "Cellular Senescence in Aging and Age-Related Disease: From Mechanisms to Therapy." *Nature Medicine* 21 (12): 1424–35.

Corbet, Cyril. 2017. "Stem Cell Metabolism in Cancer and Healthy Tissues: Pyruvate in the Limelight." *Frontiers in Pharmacology* 8: 958.

Dawson, M. A., and T. Kouzarides. 2012. "Cancer Epigenetics: From Mechanism to Therapy." *Cell* 150 (1). https://doi.org/10.1016/j.cell.2012.06.013.

De Almeida, Carolina Vieira, Marcela Rodrigues de Camargo, Edda Russo, and Amedeo Amedei. 2019. "Role of Diet and Gut Microbiota on Colorectal Cancer Immunomodulation." *World Journal of Gastroenterology: WJG* 25 (2): 151–62.

De Flora, S., and S. La Maestra. 2015. "Epidemiology of Cancers of Infectious Origin and Prevention Strategies." *Journal of Preventive Medicine and Hygiene* 56 (1): E15–20.

Delage, B., and R. H. Dashwood. 2008. "Dietary Manipulation of Histone Structure and Function." *Annual Review of Nutrition* 28. https://doi.org/10.1146/annurev.nutr.28.061807.155354.

Denicourt, Catherine, and Steven F. Dowdy. 2004. "Cip/Kip Proteins: More Than Just CDKs Inhibitors." *Genes & Development* 18 (8): 851–55.

Deursen, Van, and M. Jan. 2014. "The Role of Senescent Cells in Ageing." *Nature* 509 (7501): 439–46.

Diori Karidio, Ibrahim, and Senay Hamarat Sanlier. 2021. "Reviewing Cancer's Biology: An Eclectic Approach." *Journal of the Egyptian National Cancer Institute* 33 (1): 32.

Dunford, Andrew, David M. Weinstock, Virginia Savova, Steven E. Schumacher, John P. Cleary, Akinori Yoda, Timothy J. Sullivan, et al. 2016. "Tumor-Suppressor Genes That Escape From X-Inactivation Contribute to Cancer Sex Bias." *Nature Genetics* 49 (1): 10–16.

Ekholm, S. V., and S. I. Reed. 2000. "Regulation of G(1) Cyclin-Dependent Kinases in the Mammalian Cell Cycle." *Current Opinion in Cell Biology* 12 (6): 676–84.

Elledge, Stephen J. 1996. "Cell Cycle Checkpoints: Preventing an Identity Crisis." *Science*, December. https://doi.org/10.1126/science.274.5293.1664.

El-Sayed, Amr, Lotfi Aleya, and Mohamed Kamel. 2021. "Microbiota and Epigenetics: Promising Therapeutic Approaches?" *Environmental Science and Pollution Research International* 28 (36): 49343.

Espinoza-Sánchez, Nancy Adriana, Eduardo Vadillo, Juan Carlos Balandrán, Alberto Monroy-García, Rosana Pelayo, and Ezequiel M. Fuentes-Pananá. 2017. "Evidence of Lateral Transmission of Aggressive Features Between Different Types of Breast Cancer Cells." *International Journal of Oncology* 51 (5): 1482.

Fang, D., H. Chen, J. Y. Zhu, W. Wang, Y. Teng, H-F Ding, Q. Jing, S.-B. Su, and S. Huang. 2016. "Epithelial–mesenchymal Transition of Ovarian Cancer Cells is Sustained by Rac1 Through Simultaneous Activation of MEK1/2 and Src Signaling Pathways." *Oncogene* 36 (11): 1546–58.

Fares, Jawad, Mohamad Y. Fares, Hussein H. Khachfe, Hamza A. Salhab, and Youssef Fares. 2020. "Molecular Principles of Metastasis: A Hallmark of Cancer Revisited." *Signal Transduction and Targeted Therapy* 5 (1): 1–17.

Feinberg, A. P., M. A. Koldobskiy, and A. Göndör. 2016. "Epigenetic Modulators, Modifiers and Mediators in Cancer Aetiology and Progression." *Nature Reviews. Genetics* 17 (5). https://doi.org/10.1038/nrg.2016.13.

Feng, Changjiang, Yi Zhao, Yunjing Li, Tong Zhang, Yongfu Ma, and Yang Liu. 2019. "LncRNA MALAT1 Promotes Lung Cancer Proliferation and Gefitinib Resistance by Acting as a miR-200a Sponge." *Archivos de Bronconeumologia* 55 (12): 627–33.

Feron, Olivier. 2019. "The Many Metabolic Sources of Acetyl-CoA to Support Histone Acetylation and Influence Cancer Progression." *Annals of Translational Medicine* 7 (Suppl 8). https://doi.org/10.21037/atm.2019.11.140.

Fischer, K. R., A. Durrans, S. Lee, J. Sheng, F. Li, S. T. Wong, H. Choi, et al. 2015. "Epithelial-to-Mesenchymal Transition Is Not Required for Lung Metastasis but Contributes to Chemoresistance." *Nature* 527 (7579). https://doi.org/10.1038/nature15748.

Flavahan, William A., Elizabeth Gaskell, and Bradley E. Bernstein. 2017. "Epigenetic Plasticity and the Hallmarks of Cancer." *Science*, July. https://doi.org/10.1126/science.aal2380.

Foss, A., L. Muñoz-Sagredo, J. Sleeman, and W. Thiele. 2020. "The Contribution of Platelets to Intravascular Arrest, Extravasation, and Outgrowth of Disseminated Tumor Cells." *Clinical & Experimental Metastasis* 37 (1). https://doi.org/10.1007/s10585-019-10009-y.

Fröhling, S., and H. Döhner. 2008. "Chromosomal Abnormalities in Cancer." *The New England Journal of Medicine* 359 (7). https://doi.org/10.1056/NEJMra0803109.

Fu, Rong, Xiaowan Jiang, Gang Li, Yi Zhu, and Huimin Zhang. 2022. "Junctional Complexes in Epithelial Cells: Sentinels for Extracellular Insults and Intracellular Homeostasis." *The FEBS Journal* 289 (23): 7314–33.

Fujie, Yujiro, Hirofumi Yamamoto, Chew Yee Ngan, Akimitsu Takagi, Taro Hayashi, Rei Suzuki, Koji Ezumi, et al. 2005. "Oxaliplatin, a Potent Inhibitor of Survivin, Enhances Paclitaxel-Induced Apoptosis and Mitotic Catastrophe in Colon Cancer Cells." *Japanese Journal of Clinical Oncology* 35 (8): 453–63.

Ganesan, A., P. B. Arimondo, M. G. Rots, C. Jeronimo, and M. Berdasco. 2019. "The Timeline of Epigenetic Drug Discovery: From Reality to Dreams." *Clinical Epigenetics* 11 (1). https://doi.org/10.1186/s13148-019-0776-0.

Gao, W., W. Li, T. Xiao, X. S. Liu, and W. G. Kaelin. 2017. "Inactivation of the PBRM1 Tumor Suppressor Gene Amplifies the HIF-Response in VHL-/- Clear Cell Renal Carcinoma." *Proceedings of the National Academy of Sciences of the United States of America* 114 (5). https://doi.org/10.1073/pnas.1619726114.

Garg, Minal. 2017. "Epithelial Plasticity and Cancer Stem Cells: Major Mechanisms of Cancer Pathogenesis and Therapy Resistance." *World Journal of Stem Cells* 9 (8): 118–26.

Gloushankova, Natalya A., Svetlana N. Rubtsova, and Irina Y. Zhitnyak. 2017. "Cadherin-Mediated Cell-Cell Interactions in Normal and Cancer Cells." *Tissue Barriers* 5 (3). https://doi.org/10.1080/21688370.2017.1356900.

Gomis, Roger R., and Sylwia Gawrzak. 2017. "Tumor Cell Dormancy." *Molecular Oncology* 11 (1): 62–78.

Grimm, Daniela, Johann Bauer, Petra Wise, Marcus Krüger, Ulf Simonsen, Markus Wehland, Manfred Infanger, and Thomas J. Corydon. 2020. "The Role of SOX Family Members in Solid Tumours and Metastasis." *Seminars in Cancer Biology* 67 (Pt 1): 122–53.

Guo, Dan, Yarui Li, Yifei Chen, Dan Zhang, Xin Wang, Guifang Lu, Mudan Ren, Xinlan Lu, and Shuixiang He. 2019. "DANCR Promotes HCC Progression and Regulates EMT by Sponging miR-27a-3p via ROCK1/LIMK1/COFILIN1 Pathway." *Cell Proliferation* 52 (4): e12628.

Guo, Lili, Xiuwen Zhang, Hongli Pan, Yang Li, Jing Wang, Lin Li, Yafang Dong, Xinxin Du, Jun Chen, and Fengjie Guo. 2021. "Prognostic and Immunological Significance of Metastasis Associated Lung Adenocarcinoma Transcript 1 Among Different Kinds of Cancers." *Bioengineered* 12 (1): 4247–58.

Guz, Małgorzata, Witold Jeleniewicz, Anna Malm, and Izabela Korona-Glowniak. 2021. "A Crosstalk Between Diet, Microbiome and microRNA in Epigenetic Regulation of Colorectal Cancer." *Nutrients* 13 (7): 2428.

Hakim, O., W. Resch, A. Yamane, I. Klein, K. R. Kieffer-Kwon, M. Jankovic, T. Oliveira, et al. 2012. "DNA Damage Defines Sites of Recurrent Chromosomal Translocations in B Lymphocytes." *Nature* 484 (7392). https://doi.org/10.1038/nature10909.

Hanahan, D. 2023. "The Biology of Cancer." *Medicine* 51 (1): 1–6.

Hanahan, D., and Robert A. Weinberg. 2011. "Hallmarks of Cancer: The Next Generation." *Cell* 144 (5): 646–74.

Harper, J. W., S. J. Elledge, K. Keyomarsi, B. Dynlacht, L. H. Tsai, P. Zhang, S. Dobrowolski, C. Bai, L. Connell-Crowley, and E. Swindell. 1995. "Inhibition of Cyclin-Dependent Kinases by p21." *Molecular Biology of the Cell* 6 (4): 387–400.

Hay, E. D. 2008. "An Overview of Epithelio-Mesenchymal Transformation." *Acta Anatomica* 154 (1): 8–20.

Hayashi, Makoto T., Anthony J. Cesare, James A. J. Fitzpatrick, Eros Lazzerini-Denchi, and Jan Karlseder. 2012. "A Telomere-Dependent DNA Damage Checkpoint Induced by Prolonged Mitotic Arrest." *Nature Structural & Molecular Biology* 19 (4): 387–94.

Heikenwalder, Mathias, and Anna Lorentzen. 2019. "The Role of Polarisation of Circulating Tumour Cells in Cancer Metastasis." *Cellular and Molecular Life Sciences: CMLS* 76 (19): 3765–81.

Hickey, Ryan, Michael Vouche, Daniel Y. Sze, Elias Hohlastos, Jeremy Collins, Todd Schirmang, Khairuddin Memon, et al. 2013. "Cancer Concepts and Principles: Primer for the Interventional Oncologist-Part II." *Journal of Vascular and Interventional Radiology: JVIR* 24 (8): 1167–88.

Ho, E., and R. H. Dashwood. 2010. "Dietary Manipulation of Histone Structure and Function." *World Review of Nutrition and Dietetics* 101. https://doi.org/10.1159/000314514.

Hobbs, G. Aaron, Channing J. Der, and Kent L. Rossman. 2016. "RAS Isoforms and Mutations in Cancer at a Glance." *Journal of Cell Science* 129 (7): 1287–92.

Hong, Sung Noh. 2018. "Genetic and Epigenetic Alterations of Colorectal Cancer." *Intestinal Research* 16 (3): 327–37.

Howard, A., and S. R. Pelc. 1953. "Synthesis of Deoxyribonucleic Acid in Normal and Irradiated Cells and its Relation to Chromosome Breakage." *Heredity* 6: 261–73.

Hussein, H. A. M., I. B. Okafor, L. R. Walker, U. M. Abdel-Raouf, and S. M. Akula. 2018. "Cellular and Viral Oncogenes: The Key to Unlocking Unknowns of Kaposi's Sarcoma-Associated Herpesvirus Pathogenesis." Archives of Virology 163 : 2633–643. https://doi.org/10.1007/s00705-018-3918-3.

Hydbring, Per, Marcos Malumbres, and Piotr Sicinski. 2016. "Non-Canonical Functions of Cell Cycle Cyclins and Cyclin-Dependent Kinases." *Nature Reviews. Molecular Cell Biology* 17 (5): 280–92.

Imodoye, Sikiru O., Kamoru A. Adedokun, Abdurrasheed Ola Muhammed, Ibrahim O. Bello, Musa A. Muhibi, Taofeeq Oduola, and Musiliu A. Oyenike. 2021. "Understanding the Complex Milieu of Epithelial-Mesenchymal Transition in Cancer Metastasis: New Insight Into the Roles of Transcription Factors." *Frontiers in Oncology* 11 (November): 762817.

Jayachandran, Aparna, Bijay Dhungel, and Jason C. Steel. 2016. "Epithelial-to-Mesenchymal Plasticity of Cancer Stem Cells: Therapeutic Targets in Hepatocellular Carcinoma." *Journal of Hematology & Oncology* 9 (1): 1–12.

Jerrell, Rachel J., Mitchell J. Leih, and Aron Parekh. 2020. "The ROCK Isoforms Differentially Regulate the Morphological Characteristics of Carcinoma Cells." *Small GTPases* 11 (2): 131–7.

Jiang, W. G., A. J. Sanders, M. Katoh, H. Ungefroren, F. Gieseler, M. Prince, S. K. Thompson, et al. 2015. "Tissue Invasion and Metastasis: Molecular, Biological and Clinical Perspectives." *Seminars in Cancer Biology* 35 Suppl (December). https://doi.org/10.1016/j.semcancer.2015.03.008.

Johnson, D. G., and C. L. Walker. 1999. "Cyclins and Cell Cycle Checkpoints." *Annual Review of Pharmacology and Toxicology* 39: 295–312.

Jones, Peter A., and Peter W. Laird. 1999. "Cancer-Epigenetics Comes of Age." *Nature Genetics* 21 (2): 163–7.

Kalluri, Raghu. 2009. "EMT: When Epithelial Cells Decide to Become Mesenchymal-Like Cells." *The Journal of Clinical Investigation* 119 (6): 1417–9.

Kalluri, Raghu, and Robert A. Weinberg. 2009. "The Basics of Epithelial-Mesenchymal Transition." *The Journal of Clinical Investigation* 119 (6): 1420–8.

Kang, Huijia, Di Wu, Tianyi Fan, and Yan Zhu. 2020. "Activities of Chromatin Remodeling Factors and Histone Chaperones and Their Effects in Root Apical Meristem Development." *International Journal of Molecular Sciences* 21 (3): 771.

Kastan, Michael B., and Jiri Bartek. 2004. "Cell-Cycle Checkpoints and Cancer." *Nature* 432 (7015): 316–23.

Khan, Kabir A., and Robert S. Kerbel. 2020. "A New Tie1 Targeted Antibody Blocks Tumor Cell Extravasation and Metastasis." *EMBO Molecular Medicine* 12 (6). https://doi.org/10.15252/emmm.202012355.

Kiefer, Julie C., Angela Nieto, and Jean Paul Thiery. 2008. "Primer and Interview: Epithelial to Mesenchymal Transition. [Interview by Julie Kiefer]." *Developmental Dynamics: An Official Publication of the American Association of Anatomists* 237 (10): 2769–74.

Kiesslich, Tobias, Martin Pichler, and Daniel Neureiter. 2013. "Epigenetic Control of Epithelial-Mesenchymal-Transition in Human Cancer (Review)." *Molecular and Clinical Oncology* 1 (1): 3–11.

Klemm, Florian, and Johanna A. Joyce. 2015. "Microenvironmental Regulation of Therapeutic Response in Cancer." *Trends in Cell Biology* 25 (4): 198–213.

Lagarde, Julien, Barbara Uszczynska-Ratajczak, Silvia Carbonell, Sílvia Pérez-Lluch, Amaya Abad, Carrie Davis, Thomas R. Gingeras, et al. 2017. "High-Throughput Annotation of Full-Length Long Noncoding RNAs With Capture Long-Read Sequencing." *Nature Genetics* 49 (12): 1731–40.

Lai, Xiaowei, Qian Li, Fang Wu, Jiechun Lin, Jiekai Chen, Hui Zheng, and Lin Guo. 2020. "Epithelial-Mesenchymal Transition and Metabolic Switching in Cancer: Lessons From Somatic Cell Reprogramming." *Frontiers in Cell and Developmental Biology* 8 (August): 760.

Lambert, A. W., Diwakar R. Pattabiraman, and Robert A. Weinberg. 2017. "Emerging Biological Principles of Metastasis." *Cell* 168 (4): 670–91.

Lambert, A. W., and R. A. Weinberg. 2021. "Linking EMT Programmes to Normal and Neoplastic Epithelial Stem Cells." *Nature Reviews. Cancer* 21 (5). https://doi.org/10.1038/s41568-021-00332-6.

Lamouille, Samy, Jian Xu, and Rik Derynck. 2014. "Molecular Mechanisms of Epithelial–Mesenchymal Transition." *Nature Reviews. Molecular Cell Biology* 15 (3): 178–96.

Lee, Ho-Sun. 2019. "The Interaction Between Gut Microbiome and Nutrients on Development of Human Disease Through Epigenetic Mechanisms." *Genomics & Informatics* 17 (3). https://doi.org/10.5808/GI.2019.17.3.e24.

Lee, Soyoung, and Clemens A. Schmitt. 2019. "The Dynamic Nature of Senescence in Cancer." *Nature Cell Biology* 21 (1): 94–101.

Li, G., Y. Tian, and W. G. Zhu. 2020. "The Roles of Histone Deacetylases and Their Inhibitors in Cancer Therapy." *Frontier in Cell and Developmental Biology* 29 (5): 76946. doi: 10.3389/fcell.2020.576946. PMID: 33117804; PMCID: PMC7552186.

Li, L., J. Xu, G. Qiu, J. Ying, Z. Du, T. Xiang, K. Y. Wong, et al. 2018. "Epigenomic Characterization of a p53-Regulated 3p22.2 Tumor Suppressor That Inhibits STAT3 Phosphorylation via Protein Docking and is Frequently Methylated in Esophageal and Other Carcinomas." *Theranostics* 8 (1). https://doi.org/10.7150/thno.20893.

Li, Rong-Hui, Min Chen, Jing Liu, Chang-Chun Shao, Cui-Ping Guo, Xiao-Long Wei, Yao-Chen Li, Wen-He Huang, and Guo-Jun Zhang. 2018. "Long Noncoding RNA ATB Promotes the Epithelial-Mesenchymal

Transition by Upregulating the miR-200c/Twist1 Axe and Predicts Poor Prognosis in Breast Cancer." *Cell Death & Disease* 9 (12): 1171.

Li, Yvonne Y., Glenn J. Hanna, Alvaro C. Laga, Robert I. Haddad, Jochen H. Lorch, and Peter S. Hammerman. 2015. "Genomic Analysis of Metastatic Cutaneous Squamous Cell Carcinoma." *Clinical Cancer Research: An Official Journal of the American Association for Cancer Research* 21 (6): 1447–56.

Liang, Haihai, Tong Yu, Yue Han, Hua Jiang, Chengyu Wang, Tianyi You, Xiaoguang Zhao, et al. 2018. "LncRNA PTAR Promotes EMT and Invasion-Metastasis in Serous Ovarian Cancer by Competitively Binding miR-101–3p to Regulate ZEB1 Expression." *Molecular Cancer* 17 (1): 119.

Lidzbarsky, Gabriel, Danielle Gutman, Huda Adwan Shekhidem, Lital Sharvit, and Gil Atzmon. 2018. "Genomic Instabilities, Cellular Senescence, and Aging: And Aging-Like Human Syndromes." *Frontiers of Medicine* 5 (April): 104.

Lin, Yueh-Te, and Kou-Juey Wu. 2020. "Epigenetic Regulation of Epithelial-Mesenchymal Transition: Focusing on Hypoxia and TGF-β Signaling." *Journal of Biomedical Science* 27 (1): 1–10.

Linder, B., A. V. Grozhik, A. O. Olarerin-George, C. Meydan, C. E. Mason, and S. R. Jaffrey. 2015. "Single-Nucleotide-Resolution Mapping of m6A and m6Am Throughout the Transcriptome." *Nature Methods* 12 (8). https://doi.org/10.1038/nmeth.3453.

Liu, Jinyang, Yaqin Zhu, and Chunlin Ge. 2020. "LncRNA ZFAS1 Promotes Pancreatic Adenocarcinoma Metastasis via the RHOA/ROCK2 Pathway by Sponging miR-3924." *Cancer Cell International* 20 (June): 249.

Liu, Yingjie, Peiyuan Zhang, Qiuyao Wu, Houqin Fang, Yuan Wang, Yansen Xiao, Min Cong, et al. 2021. "Author Correction: Long Non-Coding RNA NR2F1-AS1 Induces Breast Cancer Lung Metastatic Dormancy by Regulating NR2F1 and ΔNp63." *Nature Communications* 12 (1): 5973.

Lopez-Mejia, Isabel C., and Lluis Fajas. 2015. "Cell Cycle Regulation of Mitochondrial Function." *Current Opinion in Cell Biology* 33 (April): 19–25.

Lu, Yuanjun, Yau-Tuen Chan, Hor-Yue Tan, Sha Li, Ning Wang, and Yibin Feng. 2020. "Epigenetic Regulation in Human Cancer: The Potential Role of Epi-Drug in Cancer Therapy." *Molecular Cancer* 19 (1): 1–16.

Luchini, Claudio, Nicola Veronese, Shinichi Yachida, Liang Cheng, Alessia Nottegar, Brendon Stubbs, Marco Solmi, et al. 2016. "Different Prognostic Roles of Tumor Suppressor Gene BAP1 in Cancer: A Systematic Review With Meta-Analysis." *Genes, Chromosomes & Cancer* 55 (10): 741–9.

Lukas, Jiri, Claudia Lukas, and Jiri Bartek. 2004. "Mammalian Cell Cycle Checkpoints: Signalling Pathways and Their Organization in Space and Time." *DNA Repair* 3 (8–9): 997–1007.

Lund, Anders H., and Maarten van Lohuizen. 2004. "Epigenetics and Cancer." *Genes & Development* 18 (19): 2315–35.

Luo, N., S. Zhou, H. Miao, and J. A. Ferreira, eds. 2023. *Tumor Microenvironment in Cancer Hallmarks and Therapeutics*. Frontiers Media SA. doi: 10.3389/978-2-8325-2281-3.

Machesky, Laura M. 2008. "Lamellipodia and Filopodia in Metastasis and Invasion." *FEBS Letters* 582 (14): 2102–11.

Makohon-Moore, Alvin P., Ming Zhang, Johannes G. Reiter, Ivana Bozic, Benjamin Allen, Deepanjan Kundu, Krishnendu Chatterjee, et al. 2017. "Limited Heterogeneity of Known Driver Gene Mutations Among the Metastases of Individual Patients With Pancreatic Cancer." *Nature Genetics* 49 (3): 358–66.

Malladi, S., D. G. Macalinao, X. Jin, L. He, H. Basnet, Y. Zou, E. de Stanchina, and J. Massagué. 2016. "Metastatic Latency and Immune Evasion Through Autocrine Inhibition of WNT." *Cell* 165 (1). https://doi.org/10.1016/j.cell.2016.02.025.

Marjanovic, Nemanja D., Robert A. Weinberg, and Christine L. Chaffer. 2013. "Cell Plasticity and Heterogeneity in Cancer." *Clinical Chemistry* 59 (1): 168–79.

Maskey, Dipak, Shida Yousefi, Inès Schmid, Inti Zlobec, Aurel Perren, Robert Friis, and Hans-Uwe Simon. 2013. "ATG5 is Induced by DNA-Damaging Agents and Promotes Mitotic Catastrophe Independent of Autophagy." *Nature Communications* 4: 2130.

Massagué, Joan, and Anna C. Obenauf. 2016. "Metastatic Colonization by Circulating Tumour Cells." *Nature* 529 (7586): 298–306.

Matouk, Imad J., Eli Raveh, Rasha Abu-lail, Shaul Mezan, Michal Gilon, Eitan Gershtain, Tatiana Birman, et al. 2014. "Oncofetal H19 RNA Promotes Tumor Metastasis." *Biochimica et Biophysica Acta* 1843 (7): 1414–26.

Mattick, John S., Paulo P. Amaral, Piero Carninci, Susan Carpenter, Howard Y. Chang, Ling-Ling Chen, Runsheng Chen, et al. 2023. "Long Non-Coding RNAs: Definitions, Functions, Challenges and Recommendations." *Nature Reviews. Molecular Cell Biology* 24 (6): 430–47.

Mbeunkui, Flaubert, and Donald J. Johann Jr. 2009. "Cancer and the Tumor Microenvironment: A Review of an Essential Relationship." *Cancer Chemotherapy and Pharmacology* 63 (4): 571–82.

Meisenberg, G., and W. H. Simmons. 2012. "Cellular Growth Control and Cancer." *Principles of Medical Biochemistry*: 307–31. doi: 10.1016/B978-0-323-07155-0.00018-6.
Mendez, M. G., S. Kojima, and R. D. Goldman. 2010. "Vimentin Induces Changes in Cell Shape, Motility, and Adhesion During the Epithelial to Mesenchymal Transition." *FASEB Journal: Official Publication of the Federation of American Societies for Experimental Biology* 24 (6). https://doi.org/10.1096/fj.09-151639.
Miro-Blanch, Joan, and Oscar Yanes. 2019. "Epigenetic Regulation at the Interplay Between Gut Microbiota and Host Metabolism." *Frontiers in Genetics* 10 (July): 460718.
Moore, Patrick S., and Yuan Chang. 2010. "Why Do Viruses Cause Cancer? Highlights of the First Century of Human Tumour Virology." *Nature Reviews. Cancer* 10 (12): 878–89.
Morgan, David O. 1995. "Principles of CDK Regulation." *Nature* 374 (6518): 131–34.
Morgunova, Ekaterina, Yimeng Yin, Arttu Jolma, Kashyap Dave, Bernhard Schmierer, Alexander Popov, Nadejda Eremina, Lennart Nilsson, and Jussi Taipale. 2015. "Structural Insights into the DNA-Binding Specificity of E2F Family Transcription Factors." *Nature Communications* 6 (1): 1–8.
Moses, Colette, Benjamin Garcia-Bloj, Alan R. Harvey, and Pilar Blancafort. 2018. "Hallmarks of Cancer: The CRISPR Generation." *European Journal of Cancer* 93 (April): 10–8.
Musgrove, Elizabeth A., C. Elizabeth Caldon, Jane Barraclough, Andrew Stone, and Robert L. Sutherland. 2011. "Cyclin D as a Therapeutic Target in Cancer." *Nature Reviews. Cancer* 11 (8): 558–72.
Naab, Tammey J., Anita Gautam, Luisel Ricks-Santi, Ashwini K. Esnakula, Yasmine M. Kanaan, Robert L. DeWitty, Girmay Asgedom, Khepher H. Makambi, Massih Abawi, and Jan K. Blancato. 2018. "MYC Amplification in Subtypes of Breast Cancers in African American Women." *BMC Cancer* 18 (1): 1–7.
Nambiar, M., V. Kari, and S. C. Raghavan. 2008. "Chromosomal Translocations in Cancer." *Biochimica et Biophysica Acta* 1786 (2). https://doi.org/10.1016/j.bbcan.2008.07.005.
Narita, T., B. T. Weinert, and C. Choudhary. 2019. "Functions and Mechanisms of Non-Histone Protein Acetylation." *Nature Reviews. Molecular Cell Biology* 20 (3). https://doi.org/10.1038/s41580-018-0081-3.
Newman, Alice C., and Oliver D. K. Maddocks. 2017. "One-Carbon Metabolism in Cancer." *British Journal of Cancer* 116 (12): 1499–504.
Nieto, M. Angela. 2009. "Epithelial-Mesenchymal Transitions in Development and Disease: Old Views and New Perspectives." *The International Journal of Developmental Biology* 53 (8–10): 1541–47.
Nisticò, Paola, Mina J. Bissell, and Derek C. Radisky. 2012. "Epithelial-Mesenchymal Transition: General Principles and Pathological Relevance With Special Emphasis on the Role of Matrix Metalloproteinases." *Cold Spring Harbor Perspectives in Biology* 4 (2). https://doi.org/10.1101/cshperspect.a011908.
Oral, Didem, Pinar Erkekoglu, Belmar Kocer-Gumusel, and Ming-Wei Chao. 2016. "Epithelial-Mesenchymal Transition: A Special Focus on Phthalates and Bisphenol A." *Journal of Environmental Pathology, Toxicology and Oncology: Official Organ of the International Society for Environmental Toxicology and Cancer* 35 (1): 43–58.
Orth, James D., Alexander Loewer, Galit Lahav, and Timothy J. Mitchison. 2012. "Prolonged Mitotic Arrest Triggers Partial Activation of Apoptosis, Resulting in DNA Damage and p53 Induction." *Molecular Biology of the Cell* 23 (4): 567–76.
Oskarsson, T., E. Batlle, and J. Massagué. 2014. "Metastatic Stem Cells: Sources, Niches, and Vital Pathways." *Cell Stem Cell* 14 (3). https://doi.org/10.1016/j.stem.2014.02.002.
Otto, Tobias, and Piotr Sicinski. 2017. "Cell Cycle Proteins as Promising Targets in Cancer Therapy." *Nature Reviews. Cancer* 17 (2): 93–115.
Øvrebø, Jan Inge, Yiqin Ma, and Bruce A. Edgar. 2022. "Cell Growth and the Cell Cycle: New Insights About Persistent Questions." *BioEssays: News and Reviews in Molecular, Cellular and Developmental Biology* 44 (11): e2200150.
Pastushenko, I., and C. Blanpain. 2019. "EMT Transition States During Tumor Progression and Metastasis." *Trends in Cell Biology* 29 (3). https://doi.org/10.1016/j.tcb.2018.12.001.
Pattabiraman, Diwakar R., and Robert A. Weinberg. 2014. "Tackling the Cancer Stem Cells—What Challenges Do They Pose?"*Nature Reviews Drug Discovery* 13 (7): 497–512.
Pei, Hailong, Wentao Hu, Ziyang Guo, Huaiyuan Chen, Ji Ma, Weidong Mao, Bingyan Li, et al. 2018. "Long Noncoding RNA CRYBG3 Blocks Cytokinesis by Directly Binding G-Actin." *Cancer Research* 78 (16): 4563–72.
Perduca, V., H. Omichessan, L. Baglietto, and G. Severi. 2018. "Mutational and Epigenetic Signatures in Cancer Tissue Linked to Environmental Exposures and Lifestyle." *Current Opinion in Oncology* 30 (1). https://doi.org/10.1097/CCO.0000000000000418.
Plaks, Vicki, Niwen Kong, and Zena Werb. 2015. "The Cancer Stem Cell Niche: How Essential is the Niche in Regulating Stemness of Tumor Cells?"*Cell Stem Cell* 16 (3): 225–38.

Poli, Vittoria, Luca Fagnocchi, and Alessio Zippo. 2018. "Tumorigenic Cell Reprogramming and Cancer Plasticity: Interplay Between Signaling, Microenvironment, and Epigenetics." *Stem Cells International* 2018 (May). https://doi.org/10.1155/2018/4598195.

Prasanna, T., C. S. Karapetis, D. Roder, J. Tie, R. Padbury, T. Price, R. Wong, et al. 2018. "The Survival Outcome of Patients With Metastatic Colorectal Cancer Based on the Site of Metastases and the Impact of Molecular Markers and Site of Primary Cancer on Metastatic Pattern." *Acta Oncologica* 57 (11). https://doi.org/10.1080/0284186X.2018.1487581.

Pui, C. H., M. V. Relling, and J. R. Downing. 2004. "Acute Lymphoblastic Leukemia." *The New England Journal of Medicine* 350 (15). https://doi.org/10.1056/NEJMra023001.

Puneet, Hasan Raza Kazmi, Soni Kumari, Satendra Tiwari, A. Khanna, and Gopeshwar Narayan. 2018. "Epigenetic Mechanisms and Events in Gastric Cancer-Emerging Novel Biomarkers." *Pathology Oncology Research: POR* 24 (4): 757–70.

Quereda, V., E. Porlan, M. Cañamero, P. Dubus, and M. Malumbres. 2015. "An Essential Role for Ink4 and Cip/Kip Cell-Cycle Inhibitors in Preventing Replicative Stress." *Cell Death and Differentiation* 23 (3): 430–41.

Qureshi-Baig, Komal, Pit Ullmann, Serge Haan, and Elisabeth Letellier. 2017. "Tumor-Initiating Cells: A criTICal Review of Isolation Approaches and New Challenges in Targeting Strategies." *Molecular Cancer* 16 (1): 40.

Radisky, Derek C. 2005. "Epithelial-Mesenchymal Transition." *Journal of Cell Science* 118 (19): 4325–6.

Raghavan, S. C., and M. R. Lieber. 2006. "DNA Structures at Chromosomal Translocation Sites." *BioEssays: News and Reviews in Molecular, Cellular and Developmental Biology* 28 (5). https://doi.org/10.1002/bies.20353.

Ren, Bing, Hieu Cam, Yasuhiko Takahashi, Thomas Volkert, Jolyon Terragni, Richard A. Young, and Brian David Dynlacht. 2002. "E2F Integrates Cell Cycle Progression With DNA Repair, Replication, and G2/M Checkpoints." *Genes & Development* 16 (2): 245–56.

Revach, Or-Yam, and Benjamin Geiger. 2014. "The Interplay Between the Proteolytic, Invasive, and Adhesive Domains of Invadopodia and Their Roles in Cancer Invasion." *Cell Adhesion & Migration* 8 (3): 215–25.

Rhim, A. D., E. T. Mirek, N. M. Aiello, A. Maitra, J. M. Bailey, F. McAllister, M. Reichert, et al. 2012. "EMT and Dissemination Precede Pancreatic Tumor Formation." *Cell* 148 (1–2). https://doi.org/10.1016/j.cell.2011.11.025.

Ribatti, D., R. Tamma, and T. Annese. 2020. "Epithelial-Mesenchymal Transition in Cancer: A Historical Overview." *Translational Oncology* 13 (6). https://doi.org/10.1016/j.tranon.2020.100773.

Rigoutsos, Isidore, Sang Kil Lee, Su Youn Nam, Simone Anfossi, Barbara Pasculli, Martin Pichler, Yi Jing, et al. 2017. "N-BLR, a Primate-Specific Non-Coding Transcript Leads to Colorectal Cancer Invasion and Migration." *Genome Biology* 18 (1): 98.

Riihimäki, M., A. Hemminki, M. Fallah, H. Thomsen, K. Sundquist, J. Sundquist, and K. Hemminki. 2014. "Metastatic Sites and Survival in Lung Cancer." *Lung Cancer* 86 (1). https://doi.org/10.1016/j.lungcan.2014.07.020.

Roa, Iván, Gonzalo de Toro, Fernanda Fernández, Anakaren Game, Sergio Muñoz, Xabier de Aretxabala, and Milind Javle. 2015. "Inactivation of Tumor Suppressor Gene Pten in Early and Advanced Gallbladder Cancer." *Diagnostic Pathology* 10. https://doi.org/10.1186/s13000-015-0381-2.

Rosenzweig, Adam, John Blenis, and Ana P. Gomes. 2018. "Beyond the Warburg Effect: How Do Cancer Cells Regulate One-Carbon Metabolism?" *Frontiers in Cell and Developmental Biology* 6 (August): 402976.

Schulze, A., K. Zerfass, D. Spitkovsky, S. Middendorp, J. Bergès, K. Helin, P. Jansen-Dürr, and B. Henglein. 1995. "Cell Cycle Regulation of the Cyclin A Gene Promoter Is Mediated by a Variant E2F Site." *Proceedings of the National Academy of Sciences of the United States of America* 92 (24): 11264–8.

Schwartz, S., M. R. Mumbach, M. Jovanovic, T. Wang, K. Maciag, G. G. Bushkin, P. Mertins, et al. 2014. "Perturbation of m6A Writers Reveals Two Distinct Classes of mRNA Methylation at Internal and 5' Sites." *Cell Reports* 8 (1). https://doi.org/10.1016/j.celrep.2014.05.048.

Serrano-Gomez, Silvia Juliana, Mazvita Maziveyi, and Suresh K. Alahari. 2016. "Regulation of Epithelial-Mesenchymal Transition Through Epigenetic and Post-Translational Modifications." *Molecular Cancer* 15 (February): 18.

Shields, D. J., E. A. Murphy, J. S. Desgrosellier, A. Mielgo, S. K. M. Lau, L. A. Barnes, J. Lesperance, et al. 2011. "Oncogenic Ras/Src Cooperativity in Pancreatic Neoplasia." *Oncogene* 30 (18): 2123–34.

Singh Nanda, Jagpreet, Rahul Kumar, and Gajendra P. S. Raghava. 2016. "dbEM: A Database of Epigenetic Modifiers Curated From Cancerous and Normal Genomes." *Scientific Reports* 6 (1): 1–6.

Sökeland, G., and U. Schumacher. 2019. "The Functional Role of Integrins During Intra- and Extravasation Within the Metastatic Cascade." *Molecular Cancer* 18 (1). https://doi.org/10.1186/s12943-018-0937-3.

Son, Beomseok, Sungmin Lee, Hyesook Youn, Eungi Kim, Wanyeon Kim, and Buhyun Youn. 2016. "The Role of Tumor Microenvironment in Therapeutic Resistance." *Oncotarget* 8 (3): 3933–45.

Spiegel, A., M. W. Brooks, S. Houshyar, F. Reinhardt, M. Ardolino, E. Fessler, M. B. Chen, et al. 2016. "Neutrophils Suppress Intraluminal NK Cell-Mediated Tumor Cell Clearance and Enhance Extravasation of Disseminated Carcinoma Cells." *Cancer Discovery* 6 (6). https://doi.org/10.1158/2159-8290.CD-15-1157.

Strilic, B., and S. Offermanns. 2017. "Intravascular Survival and Extravasation of Tumor Cells." *Cancer Cell* 32 (3). https://doi.org/10.1016/j.ccell.2017.07.001.

Sun, Qian, Rui Xu, Hongbo Xu, Gengming Wang, Xueming Shen, and Hao Jiang. 2017. "Extracranial Metastases of High-Grade Glioma: The Clinical Characteristics and Mechanism." *World Journal of Surgical Oncology* 15 (1): 1–5.

Tanabe, Shihori, Sabina Quader, Horacio Cabral, and Ryuichi Ono. 2020. "Interplay of EMT and CSC in Cancer and the Potential Therapeutic Strategies." *Frontiers in Pharmacology* 11 (June): 495811.

Terashima, Minoru, Akihiko Ishimura, Sasithorn Wanna-Udom, and Takeshi Suzuki. 2018. "Long Noncoding RNA Contributes to Epigenetic Progression of the Epithelial-Mesenchymal Transition of Lung and Pancreatic Cancer Cells." *The Journal of Biological Chemistry* 293 (47): 18016–30.

Thiam, A., Z. Zhao, C. Quinn, and B. Barber. 2016. "Years of Life Lost due to Metastatic Melanoma in 12 Countries." *Journal of Medical Economics* 19 (3). https://doi.org/10.3111/13696998.2015.1115764.

Thompson, A. K., B. F. Kelley, L. J. Prokop, M. H. Murad, and C. L. Baum. 2016. "Risk Factors for Cutaneous Squamous Cell Carcinoma Recurrence, Metastasis, and Disease-Specific Death: A Systematic Review and Meta-Analysis." *JAMA Dermatology* 152 (4). https://doi.org/10.1001/jamadermatol.2015.4994.

Thwaites, Michael J., Matthew J. Cecchini, Daniel T. Passos, Ian Welch, and Frederick A. Dick. 2017. "Interchangeable Roles for E2F Transcriptional Repression by the Retinoblastoma Protein and p27KIP1–Cyclin-Dependent Kinase Regulation in Cell Cycle Control and Tumor Suppression." *Molecular and Cellular Biology*, January. https://doi.org/10.1128/MCB.00561-16.

Tominaga, Kaoru. 2015. "The Emerging Role of Senescent Cells in Tissue Homeostasis and Pathophysiology." *Pathobiology of Aging & Age Related Diseases* 5 (May): 27743.

Trybus, Wojciech, Ewa Trybus, and Teodora Król. 2022. "Emodin Sensitizes Cervical Cancer Cells to Vinblastine by Inducing Apoptosis and Mitotic Death." *International Journal of Molecular Sciences* 23 (15). https://doi.org/10.3390/ijms23158510.

Tsai, Jeff H., and Jing Yang. 2013. "Epithelial–mesenchymal Plasticity in Carcinoma Metastasis." *Genes & Development* 27 (20): 2192–206.

Tugues, Sonia, Laura Ducimetiere, Ekaterina Friebel, and Burkhard Becher. 2019. "Innate Lymphoid Cells as Regulators of the Tumor Microenvironment." *Seminars in Immunology* 41 (February): 101270.

Tulsyan, S., M. Aftab, S. Sisodiya, A. Khan, A. Chikara, P. Tanwar, and S. Hussain. 2022. "Molecular Basis of Epigenetic Regulation in Cancer Diagnosis and Treatment." *Frontiers in Genetics* 13 (August). https://doi.org/10.3389/fgene.2022.885635.

Uetake, Yumi, and Greenfield Sluder. 2010. "Prolonged Prometaphase Blocks Daughter Cell Proliferation Despite Normal Completion of Mitosis." *Current Biology: CB* 20 (18): 1666–71.

Undabeitia, J., M. Castle, M. Arrazola, C. Pendleton, I. Ruiz, and E. Úrculo. 2015. "Multiple Extraneural Metastasis of Glioblastoma Multiforme." *Anales Del Sistema Sanitario de Navarra* 38 (1): 157–61.

Vadillo, E., E. Dorantes-Acosta, R. Pelayo, and M. Schnoor. 2018. "T Cell Acute Lymphoblastic Leukemia (T-ALL): New Insights into the Cellular Origins and Infiltration Mechanisms Common and Unique Among Hematologic Malignancies." *Blood Reviews* 32 (1). https://doi.org/10.1016/j.blre.2017.08.006.

Vakifahmetoglu, H., M. Olsson, and B. Zhivotovsky. 2008. "Death Through a Tragedy: Mitotic Catastrophe." *Cell Death and Differentiation* 15 (7): 1153–62.

Vermeulen, Katrien, Dirk R. Van Bockstaele, and Zwi N. Berneman. 2003. "The Cell Cycle: A Review of Regulation, Deregulation and Therapeutic Targets in Cancer." *Cell Proliferation* 36 (3): 131–49.

Vitale, Ilio, Lorenzo Galluzzi, Maria Castedo, and Guido Kroemer. 2011. "Mitotic Catastrophe: A Mechanism for Avoiding Genomic Instability." *Nature Reviews Molecular Cell Biology* 12 (6): 385–92.

Waddington, C. H. 2012. "The Epigenotype 1942." *International Journal of Epidemiology* 41 (1): 10–13.

Wainwright, Elanor N., and Paola Scaffidi. 2017. "Epigenetics and Cancer Stem Cells: Unleashing, Hijacking, and Restricting Cellular Plasticity." *Trends in Cancer Research* 3 (5): 372.

Wang, Hui, Xisong Huo, Xin-Rong Yang, Jia He, Lijun Cheng, Na Wang, Xuan Deng, et al. 2017. "STAT3-Mediated Upregulation of lncRNA HOXD-AS1 as a ceRNA Facilitates Liver Cancer Metastasis by Regulating SOX4." *Molecular Cancer* 16 (1): 136.

Wang, Zhaoqing, Ming Fan, Demet Candas, Tie-Qiao Zhang, Lili Qin, Angela Eldridge, Sebastian Wachsmann-Hogiu, et al. 2014. "Cyclin B1/Cdk1 Coordinates Mitochondrial Respiration for Cell-Cycle G2/M Progression." *Developmental Cell* 29 (2): 217–32.

Wang, Zhiwei, Yiwei Li, Dejuan Kong, and Fazlul H. Sarkar. 2010. "The Role of Notch Signaling Pathway in Epithelial-Mesenchymal Transition (EMT) During Development and Tumor Aggressiveness." *Current Drug Targets* 11 (6): 745.

Weber, Anja, Helmut Klocker, Herbert Oberacher, Erich Gnaiger, Hannes Neuwirt, Natalie Sampson, and Iris E. Eder. 2018. "Succinate Accumulation Is Associated With a Shift of Mitochondrial Respiratory Control and HIF-1α Upregulation in PTEN Negative Prostate Cancer Cells." *International Journal of Molecular Sciences* 19 (7). https://doi.org/10.3390/ijms19072129.

Wichmann, C., I. Quagliano-Lo Coco, Ö. Yildiz, L. Chen-Wichmann, H. Weber, T. Syzonenko, C. Döring, et al. 2014. "Activating c-KIT Mutations Confer Oncogenic Cooperativity and Rescue RUNX1/ETO-Induced DNA Damage and Apoptosis in Human Primary CD34+ Hematopoietic Progenitors." *Leukemia* 29 (2): 279–89.

Woods, Catherine M., Jian Zhu, Patricia A. McQueney, Daniel Bollag, and Elias Lazarides. 1995. "Taxol-Induced Mitotic Block Triggers Rapid Onset of a p53-Independent Apoptotic Pathway." *Molecular Medicine* 1 (5): 506–26.

Wu, Wenjiao, Dequan Zhong, Zhan Zhao, Wentao Wang, Jun Li, and Wei Zhang. 2017. "Postoperative Extracranial Metastasis From Glioblastoma: A Case Report and Review of the Literature." *World Journal of Surgical Oncology* 15 (1): 1–5.

Yang, Juan, Wei-Gang Wang, and Ke-Qiang Zhang. 2020. "LINC00452 Promotes Ovarian Carcinogenesis Through Increasing ROCK1 by Sponging miR-501–3p and Suppressing Ubiquitin-Mediated Degradation." *Aging* 12 (21): 21129–46.

Yang, Juze, Qiongzi Qiu, Xinyi Qian, Jiani Yi, Yiling Jiao, Mengqian Yu, Xufan Li, et al. 2019. "Long Noncoding RNA LCAT1 Functions as a ceRNA to Regulate RAC1 Function by Sponging miR-4715–5p in Lung Cancer." *Molecular Cancer* 18 (1): 171.

Yeo-Teh, Nicole S. L., Yoshiaki Ito, and Sudhakar Jha. 2018. "High-Risk Human Papillomaviral Oncogenes E6 and E7 Target Key Cellular Pathways to Achieve Oncogenesis." *International Journal of Molecular Sciences* 19 (6): 1706.

Yoshida, Go J., and Hideyuki Saya. 2016. "Therapeutic Strategies Targeting Cancer Stem Cells." *Cancer Science* 107 (1): 5–11.

Youn, Young Hoon, Hyo Joo Byun, Jung-Ho Yoon, Chan Hyuk Park, and Sang Kil Lee. 2019. "Long Noncoding RNA N-BLR Upregulates the Migration and Invasion of Gastric Adenocarcinoma." *Gut and Liver* 13 (4): 421–9.

Yuan, Hang, Ewa Krawczyk, Jan Blancato, Christopher Albanese, Dan Zhou, Naidong Wang, Siddartha Paul, et al. 2017. "HPV Positive Neuroendocrine Cervical Cancer Cells are Dependent on Myc but Not E6/E7 Viral Oncogenes." *Scientific Reports* 7 (1): 1–11.

Zaccara, Sara, Ryan J. Ries, and Samie R. Jaffrey. 2019. "Reading, Writing and Erasing mRNA Methylation." *Nature Reviews Molecular Cell Biology* 20 (10): 608–24.

Zavyalova, M. V., E. V. Denisov, L. A. Tashireva, O. E. Savelieva, E. V. Kaigorodova, N. V. Krakhmal, and V. M. Perelmuter. 2019. "Intravasation as a Key Step in Cancer Metastasis." *Biochemistry. Biokhimiia* 84 (7). https://doi.org/10.1134/S0006297919070071.

Zeisberg, Michael, and Eric G. Neilson. 2009. "Biomarkers for Epithelial-Mesenchymal Transitions." *The Journal of Clinical Investigation* 119 (6): 1429–37.

Zhang, J., Hongmei Yao, Ge Song, Xia Liao, Yao Xian, and Weimin Li. 2015. "Regulation of Epithelial-Mesenchymal Transition by Tumor-Associated Macrophages in Cancer." *American Journal of Translational Research* 7 (10): 1699–711.

Zhang, J. J., T. T. Fan, Y. Z. Mao, J. L. Hou, M. Wang, M. Zhang, Y. Lin, et al. 2021. "Nuclear Dihydroxyacetone Phosphate Signals Nutrient Sufficiency and Cell Cycle Phase to Global Histone Acetylation." *Nature Metabolism* 3 (6). https://doi.org/10.1038/s42255-021-00405-8.

Zhao, Boyang, Michael T. Hemann, and Douglas A. Lauffenburger. 2016. "Modeling Tumor Clonal Evolution for Drug Combinations Design." *Trends in Cancer Research* 2 (3): 144–58.

Zhao, Guangfu, Fang He, Chenlu Wu, Pan Li, Nengzhang Li, Jinping Deng, Guoqiang Zhu, Wenkai Ren, and Yuanyi Peng. 2018. "Betaine in Inflammation: Mechanistic Aspects and Applications." *Frontiers in Immunology* 9 (May): 370622.

Zhao, Linjie, Gaili Ji, Xiaobing Le, Chenlu Wang, Lian Xu, Min Feng, Yaguang Zhang, et al. 2017. "Long Noncoding RNA LINC00092 Acts in Cancer-Associated Fibroblasts to Drive Glycolysis and Progression of Ovarian Cancer." *Cancer Research* 77 (6): 1369–82.

Zheng, Jie. 2013. "Oncogenic Chromosomal Translocations and Human Cancer (Review)." *Oncology Reports* 30 (5): 2011–9.

Zheng, X., J. L. Carstens, J. Kim, M. Scheible, J. Kaye, H. Sugimoto, C. C. Wu, V. S. LeBleu, and R. Kalluri. 2015. "Epithelial-to-Mesenchymal Transition is Dispensable for Metastasis but Induces Chemoresistance in Pancreatic Cancer." *Nature* 527 (7579). https://doi.org/10.1038/nature16064.

Zhou, B. B., H. Zhang, M. Damelin, K. G. Geles, J. C. Grindley, and P. B. Dirks. 2009. "Tumour-Initiating Cells: Challenges and Opportunities for Anticancer Drug Discovery." *Nature Reviews Drug Discovery* 8 (10). https://doi.org/10.1038/nrd2137.

Zhou, Yong, Ren-Gen Fan, Cheng-Lin Qin, Jing Jia, Xu-Dong Wu, and Wen-Zhang Zha. 2019. "LncRNA-H19 Activates CDC42/PAK1 Pathway to Promote Cell Proliferation, Migration and Invasion by Targeting miR-15b in Hepatocellular Carcinoma." *Genomics* 111 (6): 1862–72.

Zhu, Miaojun, Qin Chen, Xin Liu, Qian Sun, Xian Zhao, Rong Deng, Yanli Wang, et al. 2014. "lncRNA H19/miR-675 Axis Represses Prostate Cancer Metastasis by Targeting TGFBI." *The FEBS Journal* 281 (16): 3766–75.

Zhuang, Yan, Xiang Wang, Hong T. Nguyen, Ying Zhuo, Xinpeng Cui, Claire Fewell, Erik K. Flemington, and Bin Shan. 2013. "Induction of Long Intergenic Non-Coding RNA HOTAIR in Lung Cancer Cells by Type I Collagen." *Journal of Hematology &Oncology* 6 (May): 35.

2 Recent Patterns of Cancer Incidence and Mortality

Global and Indian Scenario

Dr. Sunita Saklani

ABBREVIATIONS

Acronym	Full Form
EPR	enhanced permeability and retention
WHO	World Health Organization
GDP	gross domestic product
CGDP	combined gross domestic product
HDI	human development index
HIV	human immunodeficiency virus
HBV	hepatitis B virus
HCV	hepatitis C virus
PSA	prostate-specific antigen
CRC	colon and rectum cancer

2.1 INTRODUCTION

Cancer is a prominent health issue faced by the world in recent times and a prime cause of death which acts as a significant hurdle in raising life expectancy in different regions of the world (Bray et al. 2021; Sung et al. 2021). It is accountable for approximately 10 million deaths in 2020 worldwide, and one out of every six deaths that occurred is due to cancer (Ferlay et al. 2020). Based on data released by the World Health Organization (WHO) in 2019, cancer is the leading cause of death for individuals under the age of 70 in 112 out of 183 countries. Cancer death ranks third or fourth in the remaining 23 countries, and fifth to eighth in 48. According to this data, cancer has surpassed heart disease and stroke as the leading cause of death, with the latter two conditions showing a minor decline in mortality (Sung et al. 2021). Lifestyle changes brought on by socioeconomic development, population growth, and the incidence and distribution of cancer risk factors are all being blamed for the rise in cancer-related mortality (Omran 1971; Gersten and Wilmoth 2002).

The lifestyle changes, along with the risk-contributing entities, enhance incidences of cancer, which is responsible for premature mortality worldwide and has required high economic and societal costs for its management (Bray et al. 2021). For example, premature deaths due to cancer increases productivity losses, the estimated costs of which were 0.62% of the GDP of Europe (Ortega-Ortega et al. 2018) and 0.33% of the CGDP (combined gross domestic product) countries of BRICS (Brazil, Russia, India, China, and South Africa) (Pearce et al. 2018).

As the number of cases of cancer is growing in all nations of the world, its prevention is a prime challenge for countries globally. It is estimated that approximately 40% of cancer cases can be avoided by controlling cancer-associated risk factors, including diet, nutrition, and physical activities (World Cancer Research Fund Organisation 2023). Premature death caused by cancer of a

DOI: 10.1201/9781003463191-3

specific nature can be prevented by proper and diligent public healthcare systems, but it does not take into account the heterogeneous nature of cancer associated with different histories, etiologies, and consequences (Martinez et al. 2020).

2.2 GLOBAL CANCER INCIDENCE AND PREVALENCE

Cancer incidence is increasing sharply at a significant rate worldwide. The data from Globocan revealed that there were 19.3 million cases in 2020, and it is expected that by 2040 the cases will rise to 28.4 million. Countries with a low human development index show a rapid increase in new cancer cases compared to countries with a high human development index. In addition, it is anticipated that in the 20 years between 2020 and 2040, the highest HDI countries will have the lowest rate of increase in cases, with 95% of cases likely to occur in low HDI, 64% in medium HDI, and 56% in high HDI (Figure 2.1). From this data, it is clear that cancer occurrence is expanding in all countries worldwide but sharply in middle- and low-income nations. The population aging and expansion in these countries are a major contributing reason to the increase in cancer incidence, with aging being the most significant contributor.

Based on data released by Globocan (2020) for 36 cancer types, there were 19.3 million newly diagnosed cases estimated (Table 2.3). Out of these, the top 10 cancers in which the newly diagnosed cases were high included female breast cancer and cancer related to the lung, prostate, skin (nonmelanoma), colon, stomach, liver, rectum, cervix uteri, and esophagus. Whereas the bottom 10 cancer types were of vagina, mesothelioma, sarcoma (Kaposi), penis, vulva, anus, salivary glands, testis, lymphoma (Hodgkin), and hypopharynx. Among the top 10 prevalent cancers, breast cancer has the highest number of diagnosed cases, that is, 11.7%, lung cancer having 11.4% and prostate cancers having 7.3%, followed by nonmelanoma of the skin, colon, stomach, liver, etc., whereas the diagnosed cases among the bottom 10 cancer comprise vaginal, having the least cancer incidence, that is, 0.1%, then mesothelioma, 0.2%; Kaposi's sarcoma, 0.2%; penis, 0.2%; vulva, 0.2%; anus, 0.3%; salivary gland, 0.3%; testis, 0.4%; lymphoma (Hodgkin), 0.4%; and hypopharynx, 0.4%.

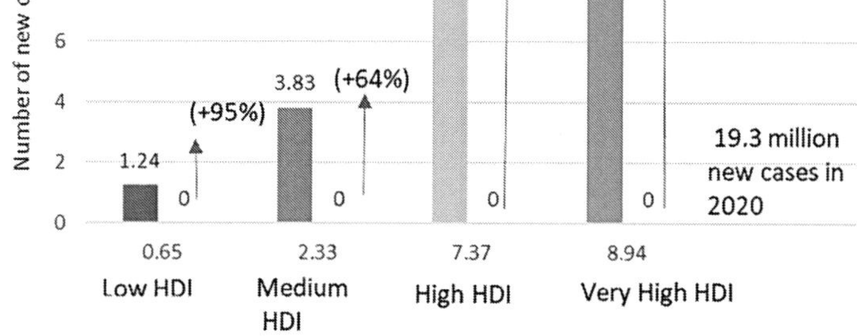

FIGURE 2.1 Estimated number of new cases for all cancer types in both sexes in 2040. The image shows the incidence of cancer prediction from 2020 to 2040. The maximum number of cancer incidences is expected in low- and middle-HDI countries.

Source: Globocan (2020).

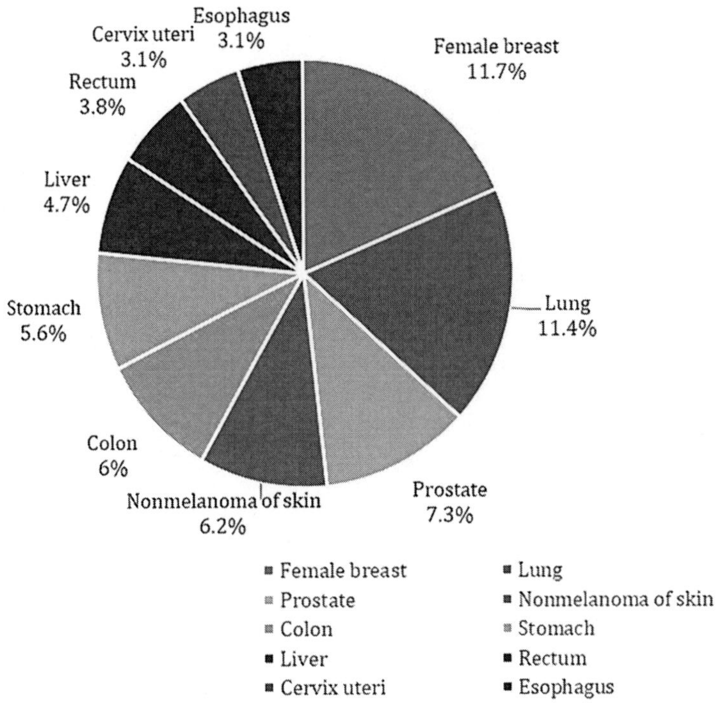

FIGURE 2.2 Top 10 cancers of high incidence and their percentage. The image shows the percentage of the top 10 cancer incidence. Female breast cancer has the highest rate of cancer incidence, followed by lung, prostate, skin (nonmelanoma), colon, etc.

Source: Globocan (2020).

Concerning the mortality among the top 10 highly prevalent cancers, the maximum mortality was caused by lung cancer, that is, at 18.0%, followed by liver at 8.3%, stomach at 7.7%, female breast cancer at 6.9%, colon at 5.8%, esophagus at 5.5%, prostate at 3.8%, rectum and cervix uteri at 3.4%, and nonmelanoma of skin responsible for 0.6% of the total deaths. In contrast, the least number of deaths was caused by penis, vagina, and testis, that is, 0.1% for all the 36 cancer types (Figure 2.2 and Figure 2.3). Collectively for both males and females, the first ten types of the most prevalent cancer cases accounted for more than 60% of incidences and 70% of the mortality caused.

2.3 PROMINENT CANCERS AMONG MALES WORLDWIDE IN 2020

The prevalent cancer types among the different regions of the world are shown in Table 2.1 and Table 2.2. Among cancer types in males, prostate cancer is widely distributed in the world, that is, 112 countries, including the countries of Northern and Southern America, Western Europe, Scandinavian countries, Central African Countries, South Africa, Australia, and New Zealand. It is responsible for high mortality. The high prevalence of prostate cancer is due to the age advancement of the population and the growth of the economy (Culp et al. 2020). In addition, there are ingrained risk factors related to Black ethnicity and family history. On the other hand, dietary patterns, vitamin E supplementation, obesity, diabetes, and changes in lifestyle may increase the risk of prostate cancer (Wang et al. 2022). In addition, the primary components of the human development index—life expectancy at birth, educational attainment, and gross national income—have an impact on the occurrence and fatality rate of this cancer (Center et al. 2012; Culp et al. 2020; UNDP 2020; Sung

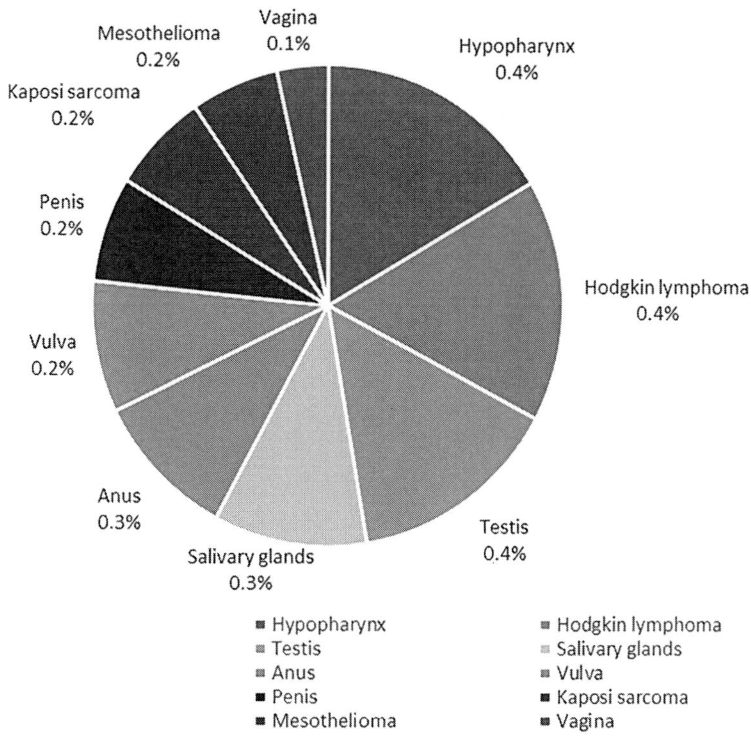

FIGURE 2.3 Bottom 10 cancers of low incidence. The image shows the bottom 10 cancers with low incidences. Vaginal cancer depicts the least number of diagnosed cases.

Source: Globocan (2020).

TABLE 2.1
Worldwide Distribution of Prominent Cancers of Males in 2020

Cancer Types of Males	Distribution in the World
Prostate cancer	Countries of North and South America, Western Europe, the Scandinavian region; some countries of Central Africa, South Africa, Australia, and New Zealand
Lung cancer	Russia, China, Central and Eastern European countries; some countries of Northern Africa; some Asian countries
Colon and rectum	Saudi Arabia, Yemen, Oman, UAE, Ethiopia
Liver	Mongolia, Laos, Vietnam, Cambodia, Thailand, Egypt, Niger, Sierra Leone, etc.
Stomach	Turkmenistan, Iran, Uzbekistan, Kyrgyzstan, Afghanistan, Tajikistan, Bhutan
Lip and oral cancer	Pakistan, India, Papua New Guinea
Kaposi's sarcoma	Mozambique, Malawi
Esophagus	Bangladesh

Source: Sung et al. (2021).

TABLE 2.2
Worldwide Distribution of Prominent Cancer in Females in 2020

Cancer Types in Females	Distribution in World
Breast cancer	North and South America (except Bolivia, Europe), Asian countries, Australia continent (except a few countries), most African countries
Cervix uteri	Bolivia, few Western African countries, Madagascar, South African countries (except Namibia and South Africa), Myanmar
Liver	Mongolia
Lung	North Korea
Thyroid	Some regions of North India, Western Sahara

Source: Sung et al. (2021).

et al. 2021). Several developed countries adopted prostate-specific antigen (PSA)–based screening, which somehow decreased the mortality trends in prostate cancer since 1990, and these countries are the USA, Canada, UK, and Japan (Wang et al. 2022). In the past few years, the incidence of prostate cancer increased, and the rate of mortality decreased (Wang et al. 2022). However, PSA is not extensively used, which means that incidence and death rates are not accurately calculated. This is because of overdiagnosis (false positive result) and issues arising from further biopsies.

Lung cancer is the second most prominent cancer in Russia, China, Central and Eastern European countries, some countries of North America, and a few Asian countries. Smoking is the major factor for lung cancer, along with environmental exposure–associated risks and genetic causes. The incidence of lung cancer greatly reflects smoking pattern trends which commonly vary with sex and economic development. Apart from this, occupational risk factors like biomass-related fuel, asbestos, arsenic, and radon can also cause cancer of the lung in some countries of the world (Leiter, Veluswamy, and Wisnivesky 2023). Colon and rectum cancer (CRC) is common in Saudi Arabia, Yemen, Oman, UAE, and Ethiopia. The reason for the high incidence of CRC are modifiable and nonmodifiable risk factors common in high-incidence countries (Wang et al. 2019). The modifiable risk factors are consumption of processed red meat, obesity, alcohol intake, smoking habits, and bowel diseases. Family or patient history and certain hereditary syndromes, ulcerative colitis, or Crohn's disease are nonmodifiable risk factors. In addition, the environment, food pattern modifications, and globalization all have an impact on the incidence rate (Almatroudi 2020). Liver cancer is prominent in Mongolia, Laos, Vietnam, Cambodia, Thailand, Egypt, Niger, Sierra Leone, etc. The risk factors accountable for liver cancer include alcohol drinking, smoking, chronic hepatitis virus, cirrhosis, type 2 diabetes, and carcinogenic substances exposure (Huang et al. 2021). Stomach cancer is prevalent in Turkmenistan, Iran, Uzbekistan, Kyrgyzstan, Afghanistan, Tajikistan, and Bhutan. Dietary patterns, tobacco, infection of *Helicobacter pylori*, obesity, and radiation are the main factors behind stomach cancer (Ilic and Ilic 2022). While Kaposi's sarcoma is more prevalent in Mozambique and Malawi, lip and mouth cancer is more common in Pakistan, India, and Papua New Guinea, and esophageal cancer is significantly more common in Bangladesh. Cigarette smoking, tobacco chewing, HPV (human papillomavirus) infection, chronic facial sun exposure, family history, inadequate nutrition, and genetic syndromes are the main risk factors for oral cancer. The risk factors for Kaposi's sarcoma include ethnicity, sex, HHV 8 (human herpesvirus 8) infection, immunological deficiencies, and sexual activity. Excessive nitrate uptake, exposure to natural as well as therapeutic radiation, iodine or selenium deficiency, and exposure to environmental pollution are the risk factors associated with thyroid cancer (Fiore et al. 2019).

2.4 PROMINENT CANCER TYPES AMONG FEMALES AROUND THE WORLD

Globally, female breast cancer affects nearly every region of the world, including most of Africa, Asia, Europe, Northern and Southern America (excluding Bolivia), the Australian continent (with a few exceptions), and Asia (Table 2.2). The two most common cancers affecting women include breast and cervical cancer, reported in 159 countries and 23 countries, respectively (Sung et al. 2021). Approximately 2.3 million cases of female breast cancer were reported in 2020, accounting for a share of 11.7% of total reported cases and standing on top, among 36 prominent cancer types, followed by cervix uteri, liver, lung, and thyroid. The incidence rate of breast cancer is higher in transitioned nations in comparison to non-transitioned nations, which is due to considerable changes in living standards and lifestyle-associated factors, such as increase in body weight, decrease in

TABLE 2.3
Number of Newly Reported Cases and New Fatalities for 36 Types of Cancers and Combined (For All Cancers) in 2020

Cancer Types	New Cases Reported (Shown in Blue) and New Deaths (Shown in Red)	Percentages
Female breast cancer	2,261,419	11.7%
	684,996	6.9%
Lung cancer	2,206,771	11.4%
	1,796,144	18.0%
Prostate	1,414,259s	7.3%
	375,304	3.8%
Nonmelanoma of skin	1,198,073	6.2%
	63,731	0.6%
Colon	1,148,515	6.0%
	576,858	5.8%
Stomach	1,089,103	5.6%
	768,793	7.7%
Liver	905,677	4.7%
	830,180	8.3%
Rectum	732,210	3.8%
	339,022	3.4%
Cervix uteri	604,127	3.1%
	341,831	3.4%
Esophagus	604,100	3.1%
	544,076	5.5%
Thyroid	586,202	3.0%
	43,646	0.4%
Bladder	573,278	3.0%
	212,536	2.1%
Non-Hodgkin's	544,352	2.8%
lymphoma	259,793	2.6%
Pancreas	495,773	2.6%
	466,003	4.7%
Leukemia	474,519	2.5%
	311,594	3.1%
Kidney	431,288	2.2%
	179,368	1.8%

(Continued)

TABLE 2.3 *(Continued)*
Number of Newly Reported Cases and New Fatalities for 36 Types of Cancers and Combined (For All Cancers) in 2020

Cancer Types	New Cases Reported (Shown in Blue) and New Deaths (Shown in Red)	Percentages
Corpus uteri	417,367	2.2%
	97,370	1.0%
Lip, oral cavity	377,713	2.0%
	177,757	1.8%
Melanoma of skin	324,635	1.7%
	57,043	0.6%
Ovary	313,959	1.6%
	207,252	2.1
Brain, nervous system	308,102	1.6%
	251,329	2.5%
Larynx	184,615	1.0%
	99,840	1.0%
Multiple myeloma	176,404	0.9%
	117,077	1.2%
Nasopharynx	133,354	0.7%
	80,008	0.8%
Gallbladder	115,949	0.6%
	84,695	0.9%
Oropharynx	98,412	0.5%
	48,143	0.5%
Hypopharynx	84,254	0.4%
	38,599	0.4%
Hodgkin's lymphoma	83,087	0.4%
	23,376	0.2%
Testis	74,458	0.4%
	9334	0.1%
Salivary glands	53,583	0.3%
	22,778	0.2%
Anus	50,865	0.3%
	19,293	0.2%
Vulva	45,240	0.2%
	17,427	0.2%
Penis	36,068	0.2%
	13,211	0.1%
Kaposi's sarcoma	34,270	0.2%
	15,086	0.2%
Mesothelioma	30,870	0.2%
	26,278	0.3%
Vagina	17,908	0.1%
	7995	0.1%
All sites, excluding	18,094,716	
nonmelanoma skin	9,894,402	
All sites	19,292,789	
	9,958,133	

Source: Globocan (2020).

physical activity, consumption of alcohol, delay in childbearing, a smaller number of childbirth, and decreasing trend in breastfeeding (Brinton, Gaudet, and Gierach 2018). Cervical cancer is the most reported cancer after breast cancer in women and is prevalent in Bolivia, a few Western African countries, Madagascar, South African countries, and Myanmar. It is caused by the human papillomavirus (HPV). The factors aggravating cervical cancer are infection with HIV and *Chlamydia trachomatis*, a larger number of childbirths, smoking, and prolonged use of contraceptives (Herrero and Murillo 2018). Its incidence rate also remains high in transitioning countries in comparison to non-transitioned countries (Sung et al. 2021). Cancer of the liver is common in women, as its diagnosed cases are threefold as compared to cervical cancer in Mongolia (Bridget Carter 2021). The risk factors responsible for this are HBV and HCV, along with alcohol consumption, type 2 diabetes, smoking, obesity, and food contaminated with aflatoxin (Thomas London et al. 2018). Cancer of the lung and thyroid is found in North Korea and in the region of North India, as well as in Western Sahara, respectively. The first one is considered the most prominent death-causing cancer for women in North Korea, where air pollution and smoking are the main contributors. Similarly, for cancer of the thyroid, the incidence rate is three times higher in women as compared to men. The risk factors associated with it include exposure to ionizing radiation in childhood, more body weight, greater height, environmental pollutants, etc. (Kitahara et al. 2018).

2.5 MORTALITY DUE TO CANCER

The comparison between incidence and mortality due to cancer in high–human development index countries and low/medium–human development index countries in both male and female (age-standardized rate) for 15 prominent cancers is shown in Table 2.4 and Table 2.5. When examining the cancer death rate among males in high-HDI nations, lung cancer comes in first place with 31.6 deaths per 100,000, followed by liver (15.1), colorectum (13.1), stomach (12.6), esophagus (8.9), and prostate (8.1), whereas in low- or medium-HDI countries, lung cancer stands on top with a 9.4 mortality rate per 100,000, followed by the liver (6.7), stomach (6.4), prostate (5.9), and lip and oral

TABLE 2.4
Occurrence and Death Rate of 15 Prominent Types of Cancer in Males Worldwide

	High HDI		Low, Medium HDI	
Type of Cancer	**Incidence**	**Mortality**	**Incidence**	**Mortality**
Lung	39.0	31.6	10.0	9.4
Prostate	37.5	8.1	11.3	5.9
Colorectum	29.0	13.1	7.4	4.7
Stomach	18.9	12.6	7.2	6.4
Liver	16.8	15.1	6.9	6.7
Esophagus	10.3	8.9	6.4	6.0
Bladder	11.7	3.7	3.1	1.8
Lip, oral cavity	3.8	1.4	10.2	5.7
Non-Hodgkin's lymphoma	7.9	3.4	4.0	2.5
Leukemia	7.6	4.4	3.8	3.0
Kidney	7.8	3.0	1.8	1.1
Pancreas	7.2	6.7	1.6	1.5
Larynx	3.4	1.7	3.9	2.5
Brain, nervous system	4.7	3.6	2.4	2.1
Melanoma of skin	5.2	0.9	0.4	0.2

Source: Sung et al. (2021).

TABLE 2.5
Occurrence and Death Rate of 15 Prominent Types of Cancer in Females Worldwide

	High HDI		Low, Medium HDI	
Type of Cancer	**Incidence**	**Mortality**	**Incidence**	**Mortality**
Breast	55.9	12.8	29.7	15.0
Cervix uteri	11.3	5.2	18.8	12.4
Colorectum	20.0	8.4	5.4	3.3
Lung	18.2	13.7	4.2	3.8
Thyroid	14.3	05	2.6	0.5
Corpus uteri	11.1	2.1	3.0	1.0
Ovary	7.1	4.1	5.8	4.2
Stomach	8.0	5.4	4.0	3.5
Liver	5.8	5.3	3.2	3.1
Leukemia	5.4	2.9	2.9	2.2
Non-Hodgkin's lymphoma	5.5	2.1	2.8	1.7
Esophagus	3.5	3.0	3.7	3.4
Pancreas	5.0	4.6	1.0	1.0
Brain, nervous system	3.8	2.8	1.7	1.4
Lip oral cavity	1.7	0.6	3.6	2.2

Source: Sung et al. (2021).

cavity (5.7), etc. Among women, the mortality rate of lung surpasses that of breast cancer, whose incidence rate is very high. Its mortality rate is 13.7; thereafter, breast cancer is at 12.8, colorectum at 8.4, stomach at 5.4, liver at 5.2, cervix uteri at 5.2, etc. in countries with the best human development index. Whereas in countries with low and medium human developed index the mortality rate for breast cancer stands on top, consequently, cervix uteri is at 12.4, ovary 4.2, lung 3.8, stomach 3.5, esophagus 3.4, etc. In totality, in all the 36 cancer types, the mortality rate for the males is 43% more than that of females, that is, 120.8 and 84.2 per 100,000, respectively (Sung et al. 2021).

2.6 INCIDENCE, PREVALENCE, AND MORTALITY IN INDIA

The country's lack of mass screening, growing population, longer life expectancies, and an increase in the number of old persons all contribute to the rising cancer incidence. Besides this, lifestyle alteration, Westernization, globalization, and control of communicable diseases accelerate its incidence. According to Dsouza et al. (2013), physical inactivity, a poor diet, and exposure to carcinogens and co-carcinogens found in tobacco are the main risk factors for cancer. The data released by Globocan 2020 (Table 2.6) indicates the number of new reported cases of cancer among men and women. The number of new cases in males and females was 646,030 and 678,383, respectively. The mortality rate is higher in males in comparison to females, that is, 438,297 in males and 413,381 in females. However, the incidence of cancer is higher in females. This may be attributed to more exposure of women to medical checkups, owing to pregnancy, childbirth, child-rearing, and common screening for breast and cervical cancer (Asiedu et al. 2014).

The five highly prominent types of cancer in males are the oral and lip, lung, stomach, colon and rectum, and esophagus, whereas in females, the breast, cervix uteri, ovary, oral cavity, and lip and colorectum are common (Globocan 2020). The incidence of breast cancer is high in females (age-standardized incidence rate), that is, 25.8 per 100,000, and lip oral cavity cancer is higher in

TABLE 2.6
Incidence and Death Rate in Males and Females in India in 2020

	Men	Women	Combined
Population	717,100,976	662,903,415	1,380,004,378
New cases found	646,030	678,383	1,324,413
Age-standardized rate around the globe	95.7	99.3	97.1
Percentage of getting cancer below 75-year age	10.4	10.5	10.4
Cancer deaths occurred	438,297	413,381	851,678
Age-standardized death rate around the globe	65.4	61.0	63.1
Percentage of death from cancer below 75-year age	7.4	6.7	7.1
Last 5-year cases reported	1,208,835	1,511,416	2,720,251

Source: Globocan (2020).

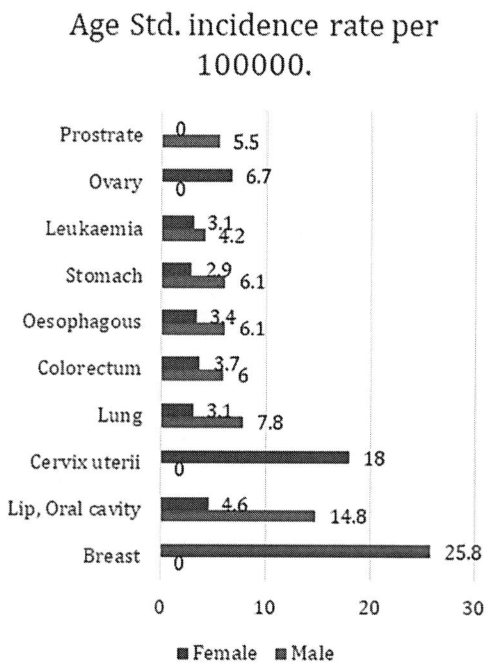

FIGURE 2.4 Age-standardized incidence rate (world) for males and females for the top 10 cancers in India. The image shows the occurrence rate of cancers for both sexes of the top 10 prevalent cancers in India. Prostate cancer has the highest incidence rate for males and breast cancer for females.

Source: Globocan (2020).

males, 14.8 per 100,000. The mortality rate for breast cancer is high in females, followed by cervix uteri. Risk factors associated with breast cancer among women in India comprise of increase in physical inactivity, overweight, obesity, aging, lack of breastfeeding, alcohol consumption or smoking, high consumption of nonvegetarian food, and a decrease in leafy vegetables diet (Pawar et al. 2023), whereas in males, it is high for the lip and oral cavity, followed by lung cancer (Figures 2.4 and 2.5). It is a result of the increasing consumption of tobacco, as chewing it is more prevalent among the illiterate population, who are ignorant of the risks for their health. Several

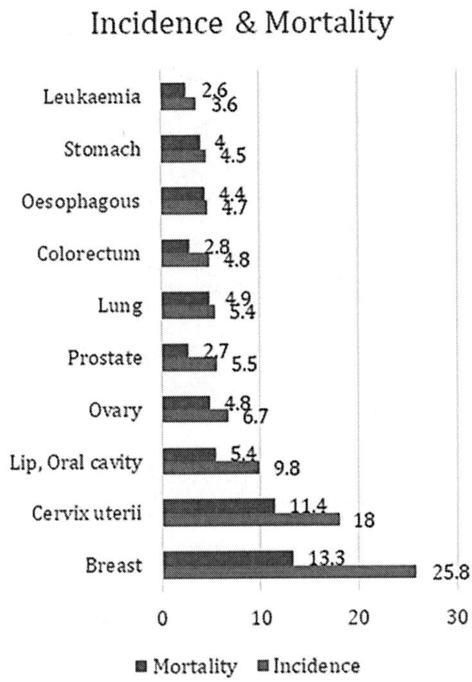

FIGURE 2.5 Incidence and mortality (world) for the top 10 prevalent cancers in India. The image shows the incidence and mortality rate of cancers for both sexes of the top 10 prevalent cancers in India. Breast cancer has the highest mortality rate, followed by cervix uteri.

Source: Globocan (2020).

studies showed the relationship between tobacco chewing and a high incidence of lip and oral cancer (Sharma et al. 2018).

For the year 2022, the number of cases of cancer and rough rate of incidence was 14,61,427 (100.4 per 100,000). Here also, the number of cases in females was again more than in males, 7,49,251 (105.4 per 100,000) and 7,12,176 (95.6 per 100,000), respectively.

In the age group between 0 and 14 years, the leading cancers for both genders are lymphoid leukemia, with boys at 29.3% and girls at 24.3% cases, followed by cancer of the brain and nervous system (NS), with boys at 12.4% and girls at 14.3% cases. For the age group 15–39 years, males have the principal cancer location of the mouth (12.0%), tongue (8.8%), and brain NS (7.0%) and myeloid leukemia (6.5%) and non-Hodgkin's lymphoma (NHL) (5.9%), whereas females of the same age group have cancer of the breast (27.3%), thyroid (12.2%), ovary (7.3%), cervix (7.1%), and myeloid leukemia (3.7%). In the 40–64 age group, the main sites of cancer comprise the lung (11.0%), mouth (10.9%), and tongue (7.3%) in males, and breast (33.0%), cervix (12.3%), and ovary (6.5%) in females. The high incidences of cancer cases found among this age group in men and females are 3,41,230 and 4,25,918, respectively. Lung (13.1%) and prostate (12.3%) cancer are on top, with one after the other in males, and breast (23.2%) and cervix (9.2%) in females of the "65 years old and above" age group. Cancer of the lung was ranked the major prominent cancer in males and breast cancer topped among women in the "40 and above" age group. The overall rate of incidence is expected to grow by 12.8% in 2025 compared to 2020 (Sathishkumar et al. 2022).

2.7 CONCLUSION

From the data of the world and India, it can be summarized that cancer incidence and mortality are linked with socioeconomic lifestyles, globalization, and industrialization. Based on trends observed from available data, the incidence and mortality rates sustain themselves on a steady state with time in developed countries, whereas unprecedented increase is seen in developing and low-income countries. Therefore, to conclude, it is quite clear that incidence and mortality rates are increasing and will be further expected to grow in the future. It is emphasized to innovate the new screening methods, techniques, and treatment methods for timely detection, treatment, and management. There is a need to tap into the latest fields of science and technology (like nanotechnology) to have a better solution to this growing menace.

REFERENCES

Almatroudi, Ahmad. 2020. "The Incidence Rate of Colorectal Cancer in Saudi Arabia: An Observational Descriptive Epidemiological Analysis." *International Journal of General Medicine* (13): 977–90. https://doi.org/10.2147/IJGM.S277272. PMID: 33149661; PMCID: PMC7605625.

Asiedu, Gladys B., Carmen Radecki Breitkopf, and Daniel M. Breitkopf. 2014. "Perceived Risk of Cervical Cancer Among Low-Income Women." *Journal of Lower Genital Tract Disease* 18(4): 304–8. https://doi.org/10.1097/LGT.0000000000000015.

Bray, Freddie, Mathieu Laversanne, Elisabete Weiderpass, and Isabelle Soerjomataram. 2021. "The Ever-Increasing Importance of Cancer as a Leading Cause of Premature Death Worldwide." *Cancer* 127(16): 3029–30. https://doi.org/10.1002/cncr.33587.

Bridget Carter. 2021. "Accurately Targeting Women's Cancers in Mongolia, With IAEA Support." *News, IAEA*. www.iaea.org/newscenter/news/accurately-targeting-womens-cancers-in-mongolia-with-iaea-support (accessed October 11, 2023).

Brinton, Louise A., Mia M. Gaudet, and Gretchen L. Gierach. 2018. "Breast Cancer." In *Cancer Epidemiology and Prevention*, eds. M. Thun, M. S. Linet, J. R. Cerhan, C. A. Haiman, and D. Schottenfeld, 861–88. Oxford University Press.

Center, Melissa M., Ahmedin Jemal, Joannie Lortet-Tieulent, Elizabeth Ward, Jacques Ferlay, Otis Brawley, and Freddie Bray. 2012. "International Variation in Prostate Cancer Incidence and Mortality Rates." *European Urology* 61(6): 1079–92. https://doi.org/10.1016/j.eururo.2012.02.054.

Culp, MaryBeth B., Isabelle Soerjomataram, Jason A. Efstathiou, Freddie Bray, and Ahmedin Jemal. 2020. "Recent Global Patterns in Prostate Cancer Incidence and Mortality Rates." *European Urology* 77(1): 38–52. https://doi.org/10.3389/fpubh.2022.811044. PMID: 35252092; PMCID: PMC8888523.

Dsouza, Neevan D. R., Nandagudi Srinivasa Murthy, and Radha Yeshwant Aras. 2013. "Projection of Cancer Incident Cases for India-Till 2026." *Asian Pacific Journal of Cancer Prevention* 14(7): 4379–86. PMID: 23992007.

Ferlay, J., M. Ervik, F. Lam, M. Colombet, L. Mery, M. Pineros, A. Znaor, I. Soerjomataram, and F. Bray. 2020. "Global Cancer Observatory: Cancer Today." *Lyon: International Agency for Research on Cancer* 2020. https://gco.iarc.fr/today (accessed February 2021).

Fiore, Maria, Gea Oliveri Conti, Rosario Caltabiano, Antonino Buffone, Pietro Zuccarello, Livia Cormaci, Matteo Angelo Cannizzaro, and Margherita Ferrante. 2019. "Role of Emerging Environmental Risk Factors in Thyroid Cancer: A Brief Review." *International Journal of Environmental Research and Public Health* 16(7): 1185. https://doi.org/10.3390/ijerph16071185. PMID: 30986998; PMCID: PMC6480006.

Gersten, O., and John R. Wilmoth. 2002. "The Cancer Transition in Japan Since 1951." *Demographic Research* 7: 271–306.

Globocan. 2020. "Global Cancer Observatory, Cancer Today." *International Agency for Research on Cancer, WHO*. https://gco.iarc.fr/today/en.12.2020 (accessed 22 October 2023).

Herrero, Ronaldo, and R. Murillo. 2018. "Cervical Cancer." In *Cancer Epidemiology and Prevention*, eds. M. Thun, M. S. Linet, J. R. Cerhan, C. A. Haiman, and D. Schottenfeld, 925–46. 4th ed. Oxford University Press.

Huang, Junjie, Veeleah Lok, Chun Ho Ngai, Cedric Chu, Harsh K. Patel, Viveksandeep Thoguluva Chandraseka, Lin Zhang, et al. 2021. "Disease Burden, Risk Factors, and Recent Trends of Liver Cancer: A Global Country-Level Analysis." *Liver Cancer* 10(4): 330–45. https://doi.org/10.1159/000515304. Epub 2021 Mar 30. PMID: 34414121; PMCID: PMC8339459.

Ilic, Milena, and Irena Ilic. 2022. "Epidemiology of Stomach Cancer." *World Journal of Gastroenterology* 28(12): 1187. https://doi.org/10.3748/wjg.v28.i12.1187. PMID: 35431510; PMCID: PMC8968487.

Kitahara, Cari M., Arthur B. Schneider, and A. V. Brenner. 2018. "Thyroid Cancer." In *Cancer Epidemiology and Prevention*. eds. M. Thun, M. S. Linet, J. R. Cerhan, C. A. Haiman, and D. Schottenfeld, 839–60. Oxford University Press.

Leiter, Amanda, Rajwanth R. Veluswamy, and Juan P. Wisnivesky. 2023. "The Global Burden of Lung Cancer: Current Status and Future Trends." *Nature Reviews Clinical Oncology* 20 (9): 624–39. https://doi.org/10.1038/s41571-023-00798-3.

Martinez, Ramon, Peter Lloyd-Sherlock, Patricia Soliz, Shah Ebrahim, Enrique Vega, Pedro Ordunez, and Martin McKee. 2020. "Trends in Premature Avertable Mortality From Non-Communicable Diseases for 195 Countries and Territories, 1990–2017: A Population-Based Study." *The Lancet Global Health* 8 (4): e511–23. www.thelancet.com/action/showPdf?pii=S2214-109X%2820%2930035-8.

Omran, A. R. 1971. "The Epidemiologic Transition: A Theory of the Epidemiology of Population Change." *The Milbank Memorial Fund Quarterly* 49: 509–38.

Ortega-Ortega, Marta, Paul Hanly, Alison Pearce, Isabelle Soerjomataram, and Linda Sharp. 2018. "Paid and Unpaid Productivity Losses Due to Premature Mortality From Cancer in Europe in 2018." *International Journal of Cancer* 150 (4): 580–93.

Pawar Prashant A., Neha K. Pandit, Pratik B. Suryawanshi, Presenjit G. Sarvade, Mayuri S. Khaparde, Snehal A. Gojare, and Swateja S. Bhosale. 2023. "Awareness and Assessment of Risk Factors Associated With Breast Cancer Among Indian Women: A Questionnaire Survey." *Bulletin of Environment Pharmacology Life Science* 12 (5): 66–73.

Pearce, Alison, Linda Sharp, Paul Hanly, Anton Barchuk, Freddie Bray, Marianna de Camargo Cancela, Prakash Gupta, et al. 2018. "Productivity Losses Due to Premature Mortality From Cancer in Brazil, Russia, India, China, and South Africa (BRICS): A Population-Based Comparison." *Cancer Epidemiology* 53: 27–34.

Sathishkumar, Krishnan, Meesha Chaturvedi, Priyanka Das, S. Stephen, and Prashant Mathur. 2023. "Cancer Incidence Estimates for 2022 & Projection for 2025: Result From National Cancer Registry Programme, India." *Indian Journal of Medical Research* 156 (4&5): 598–607. https://doi.org/10.4103/ijmr.ijmr_1821_22.

Sharma, Swati, L. Satyanarayana, Smitha Asthana, K. K. Shivalingesh, Bala Subramanya Goutham, and Sujatha Ramachandra. 2018. "Oral Cancer Statistics in India on the Basis of First Report of 29 Population-Based Cancer Registries." *Journal of Oral and Maxillofacial Pathology* 22 (1): 18–26. https://doi.org/10.4103/jomfp.JOMFP_113_17. PMID: 29731552; PMCID: PMC5917535.

Sung, Hyuna, Jacques Ferlay, Rebecca L. Siegel, Mathieu Laversanne, Isabelle Soerjomataram, Ahmedin Jemal, and Freddie Bray. 2021. "Global Cancer Statistics 2020: GLOBOCAN Estimates of Incidence and Mortality Worldwide for 36 Cancers in 185 Countries." *CA: A Cancer Journal for Clinicians* 71 (3): 209–49. https://doi.org/10.3322/caac.21660.

Thomas London, W., Jessica L. Petrick, and Katherine A. McGlynn. 2018. "Liver Cancer." In *Cancer Epidemiology and Prevention*, eds. M. Thun, M. S. Linet, J. R. Cerhan, C. A. Haiman, and D. Schottenfeld, 635–60. Oxford University Press.

UNDP (United Nations Development Programme). 2020. "Human Development Report 2020." *The Next Frontier: Human Development and the Anthropocene*. http://hdr.undp.org/sites/default/files/hdr2020.pdf (accessed August 15, 2021).

Wang, Le, Bin Lu, Mengjie He, Youqing Wang, Zongping Wang, and Lingbin Du. 2022. "Prostate Cancer Incidence And Mortality: Global Status and Temporal Trends in 89 Countries From 2000 to 2019." *Frontiers in Public Health* 10: 176.

Wang, Xiaoliang, Kelli O'Connell, Jihyoun Jeon, Mingyang Song, David Hunter, Michael Hoffmeister, Yi Lin, et al. 2019. "Combined Effect of Modifiable and Non-Modifiable Risk Factors for Colorectal Cancer Risk in a Pooled Analysis of 11 Population-Based Studies." *BMJ Open Gastroenterology* 6 (1): e000339.

3 Nano–Bio Dynamics
Mechanisms and Challenges in Shaping Nanomaterials for Biomedical Use

Gagandeep Singh, L. Preethi, and Neelam Thakur

ABBREVIATIONS

Acronym	**Full Form**
ROS	reactive oxygen species
NPs	nanoparticles
DNA	deoxyribonucleic acid
mRNA	messenger ribonucleic acid
AML	acute myeloid leukemia
2DG	2-deoxy-D-glucose
BPTES	bis-2-(5-phenylacetamido-1,3,4-thiadiazol-2-yl)ethyl sulfide

3.1 INTRODUCTION

The complex interaction between nanomaterials and biological systems, known as nano–bio interactions, is of critical importance in biomedical applications. These interactions serve as the fundamental link that bridges the promising potential of nanomaterials to revolutionize medicine with the actual clinical translation of these innovations (Bettencourt and Gonçalves 2022). Nanoparticles, as innovative systems in medicine, are subject to rigorous evaluation from their very inception. It is imperative to understand that inherent physicochemical properties, such as shape, size, and surface charge, possess the potential to significantly influence cellular uptake, intracellular trafficking, exocytosis, as well as cyto- or geno-compatibility (Bettencourt and Gonçalves 2022). However, the evaluation of these nanoparticles is a formidable challenge, often yielding controversial results. Hence, a comprehensive understanding of nano–bio interactions becomes essential in order to develop nanomaterials that are both safe and effective for biomedical purposes (Tian, Chong, and Ge 2020). To deepen our comprehension of these intricate interactions and their potential applications, a highly controllable model for nano–bio interaction studies has been conceived through the programmable assembly of nucleic acids into framework nucleic acids. This model allows for the meticulous examination of "nanostructure–activity relationships," shedding light on how nanomaterials can be harnessed for selective biomedical purposes (Wang et al. 2022). Furthermore, nano–bio interactions offer multifunctional platforms with diverse applications in biomedicine (Tian, Chong, and Ge 2020). For instance, rare earth doped nanoparticles, distinguished by their unique spectral properties, have emerged as superior in vivo optical probes compared to conventional quantum dots and organic dyes (Chouryal et al. 2020). The multifunctionality of these platforms extends the scope of nanomedicine, promising innovative solutions in areas like diagnostics and targeted therapies. To advance nanomedicine, we need a systematic way to foresee how nanoparticles and cells interact.

DOI: 10.1201/9781003463191-4

Nanoparticles have remarkable potential for applications in biomedicine and environment, which demands a quantitative and accurate description and characterization of the surface chemistry of nanomaterials. Yet this task is far from trivial, owing to the complex interplay of nanoparticle mechanisms with the intricate biological environments they encounter (Allen et al. 2017).

In this review, we will delve into the essential components that make up the intricate terrain of nano–bio interactions. We will explore the factors influencing these interactions, dissect the underlying mechanisms, and examine the biological responses they elicit. Moreover, we will confront the challenges hindering our full understanding and clinical translation of these interactions. By the review's conclusion, we aim to envision the future of this captivating field within the ever-progressing landscape of nanomedicine.

3.2 FACTORS INFLUENCING NANO–BIO INTERACTIONS

Comprehending the nuanced interactions between nanomaterials and biological systems is imperative in shaping the future of biomedical applications. Nano–bio interactions encompass an intricate web of influences which, when comprehended, have the potential to optimize the safety, efficacy, and clinical viability of nanomaterials. This section delves into the multifaceted factors governing nano–bio interactions, exploring surface modification, particle size, nanoparticle shape, composition, nanoparticle concentration, and synthesis methods, each playing a distinctive role in shaping the landscape of nanomaterials for biomedical applications (Figure 3.1).

3.2.1 Surface Modification

Surface modification of nanoparticles plays a pivotal role in shaping their interactions with biological systems, constituting a critical dimension in the field of nano–bio interactions (Greskovich et al. 2023). One of the key aspects influenced by surface modification is colloidal stability, where alterations in nanoparticles' surface properties can impact their aggregation and dispersion in biological environments, influencing their overall behavior and functionality (Greskovich et al. 2023). Surface coatings also exert significant control over the composition of acquired protein corona in the biological settings, a dynamic layer that forms on the nanoparticle surface upon interaction with biological fluids. This corona composition directly affects the interactions of nanoparticles with the local biological environment, adding a layer of complexity to the nano–bio interface (Greskovich et al. 2023). Furthermore, surface modifications expand the potential functionalities of the ligand layer on nanoparticles, enabling the targeting of specific intracellular organelles, an essential feature for applications in drug delivery and intracellular therapies (Greskovich et al. 2023). The implications of surface modification extend to nanoparticle toxicity, an area of paramount importance in safety assessment. While surface modification can enhance the activity of nanoparticles, it may also lead to increased toxicity, both in terms of human health and environmental impacts (Yadav and Chaudhary 2021). Evaluating this toxicity is a highly complex undertaking and has yielded some controversial results, highlighting the intricate balance between surface modification and safety in the context of nano–bio interactions (Bettencourt and Gonçalves 2022).

3.2.2 Particle Size

The size of nanoparticles is a fundamental parameter that exerts a significant impact on their interaction with biological systems. It significantly impacts aspects such as cellular uptake, intracellular distribution, toxicity, and stability, each with distinct implications for biomedical applications (Pelka et al. 2009; Lichtenstein et al. 2015). The cellular uptake of nanoparticles is intricately linked to their size. Smaller nanoparticles are more readily taken up by cells compared to their larger counterparts. For example, platinum nanoparticles with a size distribution of <20 nm were found to be taken up into human colon carcinoma cells in their particulate form (Pelka et al. 2009). This

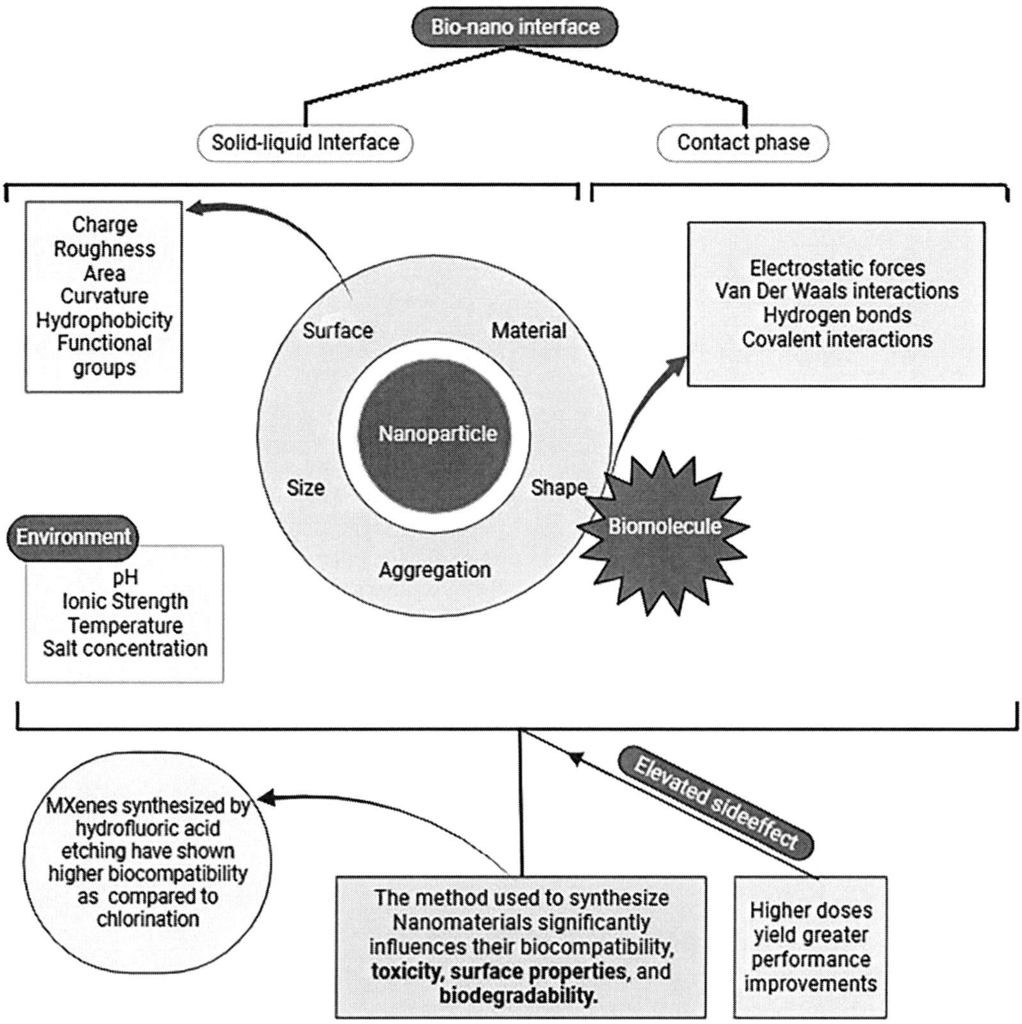

FIGURE 3.1 Factors influencing nano–bio interactions. A schematic representation intricately depicts the dynamics of bio-interface interactions in a biological setting, where elements such as material, surface, and nanoparticle size play pivotal roles, shaping the mechanism of interaction. Surface modification parameters, encompassing charge, roughness, area, curvature, hydrophobicity, and functional groups, are illustrated as influential factors. Environmental considerations, including pH, ionic strength, temperature, and salt concentration, are highlighted for their impact on the bio-interface. The contact interface is influenced by electrostatic forces, van der Waals interactions, hydrogen bonds, and covalent interactions, presenting a comprehensive overview of the complex interplay within the biological milieu. Additionally, precise control over nanoparticle dose proves crucial in balancing therapeutic benefits and potential side effects in various biomedical applications. Furthermore, the method used to synthesize nanomaterials significantly influences their biocompatibility, toxicity, surface properties, and biodegradability, emphasizing the need for careful consideration in optimizing nanomaterials for safety and efficacy in biomedicine.

size-dependent cellular uptake is of immense importance in the realm of drug delivery, as it directly influences the target cell drug delivery efficiency. Additionally, nanoparticle size plays a pivotal role in determining their intracellular distribution. Smaller particles may localize differently within cells, which has significant consequences for the release of drugs from nanoparticles and their overall efficacy, for example, hyaluronan-grafted liposomes possessing a mean nanoparticle size ranging from 120 to 180 nm were found to localize primarily to endosomes and lysosomes once inside cells (Qhattal and Liu 2011). Smaller nanoparticles may undergo different processing in biological systems, potentially leading to variations in cellular effects and biopersistence. For example, ceria nanoparticles were found to undergo in vivo processing in the liver, resulting in the formation of ultrafines with increased free radical scavenging potential. This variation directly affects the safety of nanomaterials and their potential effects on cells and tissues (Graham et al. 2014). Stability in biological environments is yet another dimension where nanoparticle size comes into play. Silver nanoparticles with radii from 3.6 to 16.0 nm were found to be stable and comparably taken up by Caco-2 cells, whereas the uptake of particles with larger sizes was decreased by 60% (Lichtenstein et al. 2015), which lead us to conclude that smaller particles may exhibit enhanced stability and cellular uptake compared to their larger counterparts, thus playing a pivotal role in designing nanomaterials for biomedical applications, where stability directly affects performance and efficacy.

3.2.3 Nanoparticle Shape

The shape of nanoparticles is a key determinant of their interactions with biological entities, significantly impacting cellular uptake, protein adsorption, toxicity, targeting, and surface area. Each aspect has unique implications for their applications in biomedicine. The shape of nanoparticles has a direct bearing on their cellular uptake. Distinct shapes may be taken up more readily by cells. For example, rod-shaped nanoparticles are found to exhibit higher cellular uptake rates compared to spherical counterparts (Reichenfelser et al. 2020). This facet is pivotal in the context of drug delivery, where efficient uptake directly influences the efficacy of drug delivery to target cells. Protein adsorption onto nanoparticle surfaces is also influenced by their shape. Certain shapes demonstrate more efficient protein adsorption than others. For instance, compared to gold nanospheres, protein adsorption onto gold nanorods was found to be more effective (Bilardo et al. 2022). This factor has a big impact on how biocompatible nanomaterials are, since protein adsorption can alter how well the body removes nanomaterials from the body and cause immunological reactions. Some shapes may exhibit higher toxicity compared to others, with notable variations in cellular effects and biopersistence, as it was found that silver nanowires were more toxic than silver nanospheres (Mudunkotuwa and Grassian 2015). This variation directly impacts the safety of nanomaterials and their potential cellular effects. Moreover, nanoparticle shape can be strategically harnessed to enhance targeting of specific cells or tissues. For instance, rod-shaped nanoparticles demonstrate superior penetration of tumor tissue compared to spherical counterparts. This finding holds significant implications for designing nanomaterials for targeted drug delivery, enhancing specificity and efficacy (Reichenfelser et al. 2020). Distinct shapes may result in varying surface areas, a factor that has direct consequences for designing nanomaterials in biomedicine. Surface area influences their overall performance and efficacy, becoming crucial in applications across various biomedical domains (Bilardo et al. 2022).

3.2.4 Composition

The composition of nanomaterials plays a critical role in determining their compatibility with biological systems, influencing biocompatibility, toxicity, surface properties, and biodegradability. Each aspect is integral to their applications in biomedicine. Biocompatibility is a foundational aspect influenced by the composition of nanomaterials. Certain compositions like hydroxyapatite/titanium dioxide exhibit good biocompatibility and antimicrobial properties, directly affecting the safety and efficacy of these materials in biomedical applications (Mirković et al. 2022). Toxicity varies based on the composition of nanomaterials, with distinct materials demonstrating varying levels of cytotoxicity. This diversity ranges from relatively non-toxic to those inducing oxidative DNA damage, significantly impacting the safety and potential effects of nanomaterials on cells and tissues (Jedrzejczak-Silicka and Mijowska 2018). Surface properties such as charge, coating, and aspect ratio are directly affected by the composition of nanomaterials. For example, specific compositions like DNA-stabilized silver nanoclusters have shown exceptional potential for biosensing and genetic mutation detection due to their small size, tunable spectra, and biocompatibility (Bonis-O'Donnell and Travis 2016). Biodegradability, an essential aspect in determining the compatibility of nanomaterials with biological systems, is significantly influenced by their composition. Some compositions, like Ti3C2TxMXene composite 3D hydrogel, promote biodegradability, addressing environmental concerns while enhancing safety in regenerative medicine as well as tissue engineering applications (Zhang et al. 2022).

3.2.5 Dose-Dependent Effects of Nanoparticle Concentration

The dose-dependent effects of nanoparticle concentration hold significant importance in various biomedical contexts, wherein precise control over the administered dose is essential to balance therapeutic efficacy with potential adverse outcomes. A multitude of studies across diverse domains shed light on the nuanced relationship between dose and its consequences. For instance, investigations into creatine nitrate supplementation in exercise performance have revealed that higher doses yield greater performance improvements, albeit with an elevated risk of side effects (Galvan et al. 2016). Similarly, studies focusing on the efficacy of gold clusters for rheumatoid arthritis treatment emphasize the heightened effectiveness of higher doses in symptom alleviation, juxtaposed with greater toxicity and side effects (Yuan et al. 2019). The context extends to menopausal symptom management, where *Cimicifuga racemosa* extract showcases superior results with higher doses, despite the accompanying increase in side effects (Schellenberg et al. 2012). Furthermore, research exploring the use of strontium ranelate in bone marrow cells and endothelial cells underscores the greater potential of higher doses in promoting osteogenesis and angiogenesis, although it comes at the cost of increased toxicity (Guo et al. 2016). Dose-dependent effects have implications for hormonal therapy as well. For instance, studies on testosterone administration show that higher doses can effectively suppress sperm production, but they also increase the risk of side effects (Matsumoto 1990). Similarly, exenatide, a drug for diabetes management, has dose-dependent effects on glycemic control. Higher doses of exenatide lower hemoglobin A1c levels more, but they also raise the chances of side effects, such as hypoglycemia, nausea, and diarrhea (Kadowaki et al. 2009). These findings underscore the importance of finding a balance between therapeutic efficacy and safety. Dose-dependent effects can help fine-tune treatment regimens in various biomedical applications.

3.2.6 Synthesis Method

The method used to synthesize nanomaterials influences biocompatibility, toxicity, surface properties, and biodegradability, each with direct implications for the performance of nanomaterials in biomedicine. Biocompatibility is significantly affected by the synthesis method. For example, MXenes synthesized by hydrofluoric acid etching have shown higher biocompatibility than those synthesized by chlorination (Vasyukova et al. 2022). Therefore, the choice of synthesis method can have significant implications for the safety and efficacy of nanomaterials. Certain methods may yield less-toxic nanomaterials, directly affecting their biopersistence and cellular effects. For example, silver nanoparticles synthesized using a green synthesis method have demonstrated lower toxicity than those synthesized using a chemical reduction method (Danish et al. 2022). The synthesis method significantly affects surface properties, such as charge, coating, and aspect ratio, directly impacting the interactional interplay of nanomaterials with biological entities. For example, the choice of synthesis method can influence surface area and photocatalytic activity, directly affecting the performance and efficacy of nanomaterials in various biomedical and environmental applications (Pragatisheel and Prakash 2020). Biodegradability is another vital consideration influenced by the synthesis method. The choice of method can directly impact the biodegradability of nanomaterials, making them more suitable for regenerative medicine and tissue engineering. For example, hydroxyapatite nanoparticles synthesized using a wet chemical method have shown enhanced biodegradability, promoting biocompatibility and safety (Bhandari et al. 2021).

3.3 MECHANISMS GOVERNING NANO–BIO INTERACTIONS

Nano–bio interactions at the cellular level are governed by intricate processes and dynamic relationships between nanoparticles (NPs) and biological environments. At the heart of these interactions lies the concept of the protein corona, a layer of biomolecules, predominantly proteins, enveloping NPs when exposed to biological contexts (Kokkinopoulou et al. 2017; Mahmoudi et al. 2023). This corona's formation is a complex endeavor, influenced significantly by NP attributes such as size, surface chemistry, and charge (Park 2020; Kopac 2021). The composition of the protein corona, in turn, plays a pivotal role in determining the cellular fate of NPs, affecting their uptake, internalization, and pathway activation (Yan et al. 2013; Fleischer and Payne 2014). Consequently, the protein corona wields the power to bestow NPs with new identities, altering their bioactivity, stability, and ultimate destination (Kokkinopoulou et al. 2017; Bashiri et al. 2023). Thus, the protein corona formation and composition stand as key determinants in shaping cellular interactions of NPs, a critical facet of understanding nano–bio interactions.

Internalization of NPs by cells encompasses a variety of mechanisms, notably endocytosis, phagocytosis, and macropinocytosis (Bannunah et al. 2014; Kuhn et al. 2014; Mazumdar, Chitkara, and Mittal 2021). The method of internalization is heavily contingent on NP characteristics, encompassing shape, size, and surface charge (Bannunah et al. 2014). Among these, endocytosis prevails as the most prevalent mechanism, further subcategorized into caveolae-mediated, clathrin-mediated, and lipid raft–mediated endocytosis (Bannunah et al. 2014; Kuhn et al. 2014). The manner in which NPs are internalized can profoundly influence drug delivery, influencing intracellular trafficking and drug cargo release. For instance, the endocytic pathway chosen by NPs can impact the efficiency of delivering drugs to the cytosol or nucleus (Rennick, Johnston, and Parton 2021). Furthermore, the chosen internalization mechanism can significantly affect the cellular uptake efficiency of NPs, directly impacting the therapeutic effectiveness of the drug (Feng et al. 2022). Hence, comprehension of NP internalization mechanisms stands as a pivotal linchpin in the development of effective drug delivery systems.

Nanoparticles' interactions extend beyond cellular uptake, encompassing various intracellular organelles, including the plasma membrane, endosomes, mitochondria, lysosomes, and nucleus (Augustine et al. 2020; Villanueva-Flores et al. 2020; Migliaccio et al. 2023). These interactions bear the potential to influence intracellular trafficking, distribution, and biological function (Augustine et al. 2020; Villanueva-Flores et al. 2020). To illustrate, interactions with the plasma membrane can directly impact cellular uptake efficiency and internalization mechanisms (Yameen et al. 2014). Concurrently, interactions with endosomes and lysosomes can influence drug cargo degradation and release. Furthermore, interactions with mitochondria can alter cellular metabolism and oxidative stress (Migliaccio et al. 2023), while interactions with the nucleus can impact gene expression and DNA integrity (Villanueva-Flores et al. 2020). These interactions carry substantial implications, capable of molding the therapeutic efficacy and safety of nanoparticle-based drug delivery systems. Therefore, comprehending the nuances of interactions between NPs and intracellular organelles is instrumental in the rational design of medical nanodevices. Redox reactions ignited by NPs result from their interactions with the cellular milieu, sparking the generation of reactive oxygen species (ROS) as well as oxidative stress, wielding a profound impact on cellular responses and cytotoxicity (Manke, Wang, and Rojanasakul 2013; Sims et al. 2017; Mortezaee et al. 2019). The redox properties of NPs can lean toward pro-oxidative, fostering the generation of ROS, instigating cellular damage and DNA impairment (Mortezaee et al. 2019). Essential factors driving NP-induced ROS include pro-oxidant functional groups on NP surfaces and active redox cycling at NP interfaces (Manke, Wang, and Rojanasakul 2013). Redox imbalances can cascade into cellular damage and dysfunction, playing a pivotal role in the onset and progression of numerous diseases (Shi et al. 2023). Consequently, the significance of NP-induced redox reactions lies in their potential to influence the therapeutic efficacy and safety of nanoparticle-based drug delivery systems. The influence of redox reactions on cellular responses and cytotoxicity can be encapsulated through the following points: firstly, redox reactions can culminate in oxidative stress, precipitating cellular damage and DNA injury (Mortezaee et al. 2019). Secondly, the generation of ROS can impact cellular signaling pathways, perturbing cellular responses (Sims et al. 2017). Thirdly, redox reactions can influence the intracellular trafficking and distribution of NPs, directly shaping their therapeutic effectiveness (Sims et al. 2017). Finally, the redox properties of NPs can be harnessed for therapeutic purposes, exemplified in the development of redox nanomaterials for disease therapy (Holmila et al. 2021; Shi et al. 2023). This comprehensive understanding of the mechanisms governing nano–bio interactions is vital for realizing the full potential of nanomaterials in medical applications and disease therapy.

3.4 BIOLOGICAL RESPONSES TO NANOMATERIALS

Understanding the biological responses to nanomaterials is paramount in harnessing their potential for various applications and managing their associated risks. The reactions observed are shaped by a blend of factors, encompassing the physicochemical characteristics of the nanomaterials, the method and route of administration, and the biological obstacles they confront (Figure 3.2) (Zhu, Perrett, and Nie 2013; Liu, Workalemahu, and Jiang 2017).

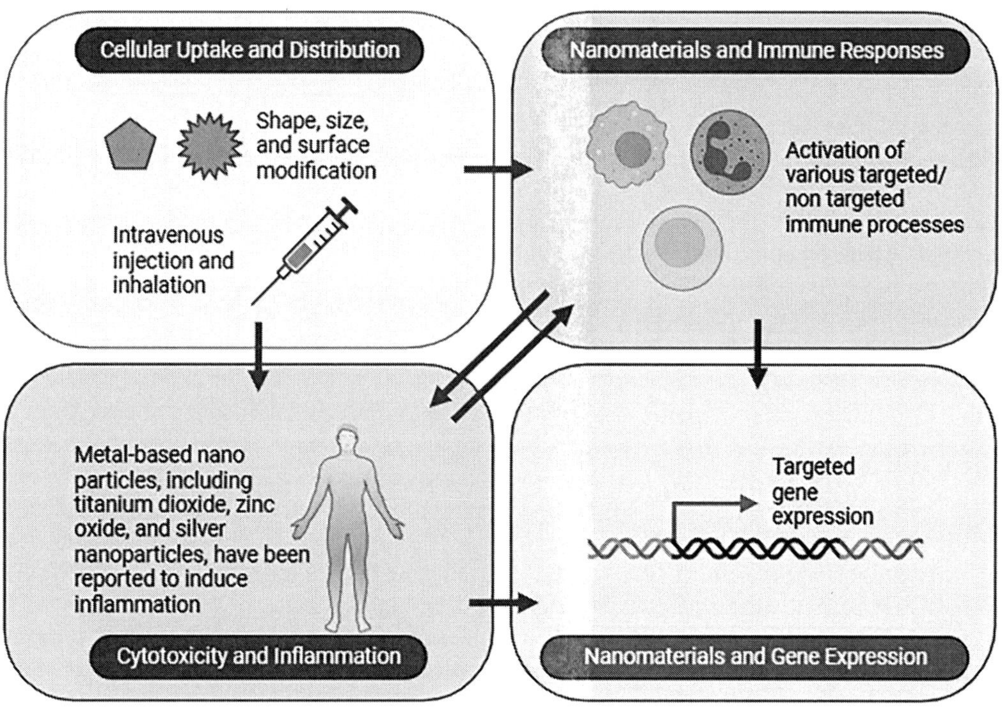

FIGURE 3.2 Biological responses to nanomaterials: interconnected pathways. This diagram illustrates the intricate relationships in the biological responses to nanomaterials. Divided into four sections—"cellular uptake and distribution," "cytotoxicity and inflammation," "nanomaterials and immune responses," and "nanomaterials and gene expression"—the arrows depict the dynamic interplay between these domains. Arrows from "cellular uptake and distribution" to "cytotoxicity and inflammation" and "nanomaterials and immune responses" emphasize the influence of nanomaterial characteristics on cellular health. Conversely, arrows from "cytotoxicity and inflammation" delineate pathways to both "nanomaterials and immune responses" and "nanomaterials and gene expression," illustrating the interconnected nature of cytotoxic effects, immune reactions, and genetic modulation induced by nanomaterials.

3.4.1 Cellular Uptake and Distribution of Nanomaterials in Vivo

As already discussed, the size, shape, rigidity, and surface modification of nanomaterials play a pivotal role in determining their cellular uptake and in vivo distribution (Liu, Workalemahu, and Jiang 2017). Smaller nanoparticles are generally more readily internalized by cells than their larger counterparts, and those with a positively charged surface may exhibit a stronger interaction with negatively charged cell membranes (Zhu, Perrett, and Nie 2013). Such nuances in physicochemical properties underscore the importance of careful design and engineering when developing nanomaterials for biomedical or environmental applications. The method by which nanomaterials are introduced into the body significantly influences their uptake and distribution. For example, intravenous injection often results in rapid liver and spleen uptake, while inhalation may lead to nanomaterial deposition in the lungs (Zhu, Perrett, and Nie 2013). This knowledge underscores the necessity of tailoring administration routes based on the intended target and desired outcomes. Nanomaterials must navigate biological barriers as they traverse the body, including the formidable blood–brain barrier and the intricate gastrointestinal tract (Lefebvre et al. 2015; Lin et al. 2022). These barriers act as gatekeepers, regulating nanomaterial distribution to specific tissues or organs. Understanding these physiological boundaries is critical for efficient drug delivery and the safe deployment of nanomaterials. The use of carrier systems, such as liposomes or nanoparticles, further influences cellular uptake and distribution (Zhu, Perrett, and Nie 2013). Liposomes, for example, can be engineered to specifically target cells or tissues, enhancing drug delivery efficiency and reducing the risk of cytotoxicity (Liang et al. 2014).

3.4.2 Cytotoxicity and Inflammation

Nanomaterials can induce cytotoxicity and inflammation through diverse mechanisms, emphasizing the need for caution in their applications (Zimmer et al. 2014; Danielsen et al. 2015; Chen et al. 2017; Xie et al. 2022; Salama et al. 2023). Mesoporous carbon nanomaterials have been shown to inhibit pulmonary surfactants, which can lead to cytotoxicity, inflammation, and lung fibrosis (Chen et al. 2017). Metal-based nanomaterials, including titanium dioxide, zinc oxide, and silver nanoparticles, have been reported to induce oxidative stress and inflammation in various cell types, potentially causing cell damage, inflammation, and apoptosis (Figure 3.2) (Danielsen et al. 2015; Salama et al. 2023). Innovative approaches, such as single-cell mechanics, reveal the potential of certain nanoparticles to alter cellular mechanics, indicating cytotoxicity (Zimmer et al. 2014). Moreover, exposure to nanomaterials can cause genotoxicity, leading to DNA damage and mutations (Xie et al. 2022). To mitigate these adverse effects of nanomaterials, several strategies have been developed (Anwe 2014; Dharsana et al. 2015; Gheata et al. 2022; Jasrotia et al. 2022). Surface modification, involving the application of biocompatible polymers or proteins, can reduce interactions with cells and tissues, subsequently decreasing cytotoxicity (Anwe 2014). Targeted delivery to specific cells or tissues minimizes exposure to non-target areas, reducing overall toxicity (Gheata et al. 2022). Chemical transformations have been successful in reducing nanomaterial toxicity, for example, sulfidation of copper nanoparticles has been shown to reduce their toxicity in zebrafish by reducing oxidative stress and micronucleus formation (Dharsana et al. 2015). Combining nanomaterials with conventional therapies offers a promising approach, decreasing systemic toxicity while enhancing therapeutic efficacy (Jasrotia et al. 2022). A study found that supplementation of vitamin E alone is effective in reducing inflammation, oxidative stress, cytotoxicity, and genotoxicity in cells and animals exposed to nanomaterials, making it a cost-effective option for preventing nanomaterial-induced injuries (Xie et al. 2022).

3.4.3 Nanomaterials and Immune Responses

Nanoparticles can trigger diverse immune responses based on their physicochemical properties and applications. This versatility can be harnessed for both healthcare and environmental applications. Nanoparticles can serve as effective delivery platforms for vaccines, eliciting humoral and cellular immune responses against specific antigens (Kim et al. 2023; Hussein et al. 2023). For instance, mRNA vaccines delivered via polymeric nanoparticles have demonstrated the ability to induce cellular and humoral immunity in mice (Kim et al. 2023). In aquaculture, nanoparticle-based vaccines have emerged as a superior alternative for combating fish pathogens, inciting robust cellular and humoral immune responses (Harshitha et al. 2023). While some nanoparticles induce inflammation and oxidative stress, potentially leading to cell damage and apoptosis (Kim et al. 2016), their design can also mitigate these effects. Coating nanoparticles with biocompatible polymers or proteins can reduce inflammation and oxidative stress (Hussein et al. 2023), enhancing their safety and applications. Nanoparticles are also pivotal in diagnostic applications, such as the detection of sepsis-derived hyperdegranulation in neutrophilic granulocytes (Santopolo et al. 2021). Innovative plasmonic nanosensors enable the colorimetric detection of septic cell degranulation, offering a promising method for diagnosing sepsis in decentralized healthcare systems (Santopolo et al. 2021).

3.4.4 Nanomaterials and Gene Expression

Research suggests that nanomaterials can significantly impact gene expression and cellular metabolism, holding therapeutic promise. Oxidative stress can alter gene expression and cellular metabolism, contributing to various diseases (Grune 2005). Antioxidant treatments can mitigate the adverse effects of oxidative stress, improving cellular function. Nanomaterials have demonstrated the ability to regulate gene expression in diverse cell types. For example, gold nanoparticles upregulate genes related to cell proliferation and differentiation, while silver nanoparticles downregulate genes associated with oxidative stress as well as inflammation (Chun, Yuk, and Um 2018). Nanomaterials can be harnessed to silence gene expression, offering therapeutic potential. DNAzymes delivered via nanoparticles have proven efficient in degrading messenger RNA transcripts, facilitating persistent gene silencing in mammalian cells (Wang et al. 2021). Metabolic inhibitors targeting various pathways can modulate gene expression and cellular metabolism, presenting a promising therapeutic approach for diseases like acute myeloid leukemia. Substances like metformin, 2DG, BPTES, 6AN, and ST1326 have demonstrated strong antiproliferative as well as proapoptotic effects on AML cells that were derived from patients (Grønningsæter et al. 2020).

3.5 CHALLENGES IN UNDERSTANDING NANO–BIO INTERACTIONS

In our quest to understand nano–bio interactions, a multitude of formidable challenges looms large, each presenting its unique hurdle. Foremost among these hurdles is the intrinsic complexity of biological systems, where the intricate dance of nanoparticles remains unpredictable. An array of factors, encompassing nanoparticle size, shape, surface charge, and surface chemistry, wields influence over these interactions, rendering the task of anticipation a formidable undertaking (Ouyang et al. 2022). The lack of standardized methods for investigating these interactions emerges as another substantial impediment, casting a shadow over comparative analysis across diverse studies (Ouyang et al. 2022). Furthermore, the dearth of knowledge concerning nanoparticle toxicity contributes an added dimension of complexity, particularly in the realm of drug development, where the assurance of drug safety is paramount (Qamar et al. 2019).

The permeability of the BBB (blood–brain barrier), notably low in Alzheimer's disease drug development, further obstructs the delivery of therapeutics to their intended target within the brain (Ouyang et al. 2022). Scarce resources allocated to the development of treatment strategies for conditions like hand, foot, and mouth disease have contributed to the sluggish progress of promising drug as well as vaccine candidates in the clinical pipeline (Lim et al. 2020). Moreover, the inherent heterogeneity within the patient population, coupled with diversity in Alzheimer's disease drugs, treatment protocols, and analytical techniques, presents a formidable challenge, particularly in the design and execution of platform trials aimed at advancing the quest for effective Alzheimer's disease treatments (Aisen et al. 2021). These multifaceted challenges underscore the need for meticulous research, innovative methodologies, and substantial resources to navigate the intricate realm of nano–bio interactions and the development of novel therapies in the field of biotechnology.

3.6 FUTURE DIRECTIONS

The burgeoning use of nanomaterials is accompanied by an array of scientific challenges, compelling researchers to delve into uncharted territories. Safety remains a paramount concern, as these minute entities can infiltrate the human body through inhalation, ingestion, or skin contact, and their unique properties may induce unforeseen interactions with biological systems (Martinez et al. 2013). Thus, rigorous evaluations of nanomaterial safety are essential to safeguard human health. Moreover, the environmental impact of nanomaterials cannot be overlooked, as their entry into the ecosystem via various routes, such as wastewater, has the potential to perturb soil microorganisms and plants (Schlich et al. 2018). The consequences of long-term exposure could be detrimental, necessitating investigations to prevent environmental damage. Regulatory agencies underscore the importance of safety assessments for nanomaterials prior to their integration into commercial products, which necessitates comprehensive, long-term studies to meet regulatory requirements (Martinez et al. 2013). Beyond safety, the relation between nanomaterials and biological systems remains a field of fervent exploration. Understanding long-term interactions offers a gateway to unravel the intricacies of their impact on cellular and tissue responses, potentially unlocking the secrets to developing safer and more effective nanomaterials across diverse applications (Martinez et al. 2013).

Recent technological advancements have paved the way for innovative methodologies and tools to navigate this intricate terrain. Biofabrication, encompassing 3D printing and related techniques, serves as a burgeoning field for creating biological structures and models that facilitate the study of nanomaterial–biological system interactions (Sun and Forgacs 2011). Simulation techniques enable the examination of nanomaterial behavior within biological systems, offering invaluable insights into long-term effects (Foffi and Kahl 2010). Proteomics, dedicated to unraveling the structure and function of proteins, lends its expertise to scrutinizing nanomaterial–protein interactions, providing insights into their biological implications (Brusniak et al. 2009; Zellner 2015). The demand for improved techniques for nanoparticle characterization has led to the development of novel methodologies for detecting and localizing nanoparticles in biological systems, enhancing our understanding of nanomaterial dynamics (Zellner 2015). Integrated bio-micro and bio-nano fabrication leverages micro- and nanofabrication techniques to engineer biological models that facilitate the study of nanomaterial interactions with biological systems (Sun and Forgacs 2011).

Translating research findings on nano–bio interactions into clinical practice presents a transformative opportunity to enhance healthcare outcomes through more effective and targeted therapies. The design of effective nanoparticle delivery systems, capable of surmounting biological roadblocks, promises to improve therapeutic cargo delivery to specific cells or tissues, amplifying the efficacy of therapies (Simpson et al. 2019). The development of reliable and validated numerical tools, utilizing multiscale imaging techniques, offers the potential for predicting age-related bone fractures, enabling early diagnosis and intervention (Buccino, Colombo, and Vergani 2021). The control of the nanomaterial interface in fundamental interactions with the biological environment paves the way for beneficial biomedical applications, underpinning advancements in nanomedicine (Gagner et al. 2012). Standardizing analytical characterization methodology not only bolsters the reliability of the nanomedicine literature but also enhances the accuracy and reproducibility of research findings, culminating in more effective therapies (Sharifi et al. 2022).

3.7 CONCLUSION

In conclusion, this review has illuminated the complex realm of nano–bio interactions, highlighting key factors influencing these interactions and their profound impact on biomedicine and environmental science. From surface modification to particle size, shape, composition, and synthesis methods, we have elucidated the multifaceted elements that shape nanomaterial behavior within biological systems. We have also delved into the mechanisms guiding nano–bio interactions at the cellular level, revealing how nanoparticles traverse cellular pathways, influence gene expression, and initiate redox reactions, all of which significantly impact the therapeutic potential of these materials. The responses of biological systems to nanomaterials, including cellular uptake, distribution, cytotoxicity, and inflammation, have been examined in detail, emphasizing the importance of precise design and engineering to achieve therapeutic efficacy while mitigating potential risks. Additionally, we have explored how nanomaterials trigger immune responses and impact gene expression, offering innovative opportunities in healthcare and environmental applications. Nonetheless, challenges persist in understanding these interactions, stemming from the complexity of biological systems, the lack of standardized investigation methods, and the elusive nature of nanoparticle toxicity.

Looking forward, safety assessments and environmental considerations must remain paramount, ensuring that the integration of nanomaterials into commercial products is both safe and eco-friendly. Innovative methodologies, such as biofabrication, simulations, proteomics, and advanced nanoparticle characterization techniques, provide valuable tools for unraveling the intricacies of nano–bio interactions. Translating research findings into clinical practice offers transformative potential for more effective and targeted therapies. Standardizing analytical characterization methodologies will enhance the reliability and reproducibility of research findings.

REFERENCES

Aisen, P. S., R. J. Bateman, M. Carrillo, R. Doody, K. Johnson, J. R. Sims, R. Sperling, B. Vellas, and EU/US CTAD Task Force. 2021. "Platform Trials to Expedite Drug Development in Alzheimer's Disease: A Report From the EU/US CTAD Task Force." *The Journal of Prevention of Alzheimer's Disease* 8 (3): 306.

Allen, Caley, Tian A. Qiu, Sunipa Pramanik, Joseph T. Buchman, Miriam O. P. Krause, and C. Murphy. 2017. "Research Highlights: Investigating the Role of Nanoparticle Surface Charge in Nano–Bio Interactions." *Environmental Science: Nano*. https://doi.org/10.1039/C7EN90014G.

Anwe, Chen. 2014. "Advance in Research on Toxicity of Metal Nanomaterials." *Huan Jing Hua Xue = Environmental Chemistry*. www.semanticscholar.org/paper/5b2b5757f5c99bc40d78cd686d098eed26084082.

Augustine, Robin, Anwarul Hasan, Rosita Primavera, Rudilyn Joyce Wilson, Avnesh S. Thakor, and Bhavesh D. Kevadiya. 2020. "Cellular Uptake and Retention of Nanoparticles: Insights on Particle Properties and Interaction With Cellular Components." *Materials Today Communications* 25 (December): 101692.

Bannunah, A. M., D. Vllasaliu, J. Lord, and S. Stolnik. 2014. "Mechanisms of Nanoparticle Internalization and Transport Across an Intestinal Epithelial Cell Model: Effect of Size and Surface Charge." *Molecular Pharmaceutics* 11 (12). https://doi.org/10.1021/mp500439c.

Bashiri, Ghazal, Marshall S. Padilla, Kelsey L. Swingle, Sarah J. Shepherd, Michael J. Mitchell, and Karin Wang. 2023. "Nanoparticle Protein Corona: From Structure and Function to Therapeutic Targeting." *Lab on a Chip* 23 (6): 1432–66.

Bettencourt, A., and L. M. Gonçalves. 2022. "Trends in the Design and Evaluation of Polymeric Nanocarriers: The In Vitro Nano-Bio Interactions." *Advances in Experimental Medicine and Biology* 1357. https://doi.org/10.1007/978-3-030-88071-2_2.

Bhandari, N. L., Sunita Bista, T. Gautam, K. Bist, G. Bhandari, Sumita Subedi, and K. Dhakal. 2021. "An Overview of Synthesis Based Biomedical Applications of Hydroxyapatite Nanomaterials." *Journal of Nepal Chemical Society*. https://doi.org/10.3126/JNCS.V42I1.35333.

Bilardo, Roberta, Federico Traldi, Alena Vdovchenko, and Marina Resmini. 2022. “Influence of Surface Chemistry and Morphology of Nanoparticles on Protein Corona Formation.” *Wiley Interdisciplinary Reviews: Nanomedicine and Nanobiotechnology* 14 (4). https://doi.org/10.1002/wnan.1788.

Bonis-O’Donnell, Del, and J. Travis. 2016. “DNA-Stabilized Fluorescent Silver Nanoclusters: A Versatile Nanomaterial for the Specific Detection of DNA.” www.semanticscholar.org/paper/a4104264df49d3b60a631b2982c9ff6c0ba923d2.

Brusniak, M., D. Campbell, J. Chen, M. Christiansen, E. Deutsch, C. Kwok, S. Letarte, et al. 2009. “Epitope Tagging of Endogenous Proteins in Human Cells for Discovery of Novel Protein/Protein Interactions Quantitative Analysis of the Phosphoproteome of Resting and Activated Human Primary T Cells.” www.semanticscholar.org/paper/a5bc0ceaaa01b21e0de9cdd9fd0db01ad2a03082.

Buccino, Federica, Chiara Colombo, and Laura Maria Vergani. 2021. “A Review on Multiscale Bone Damage: From the Clinical to the Research Perspective.” *Materials* 14 (5). https://doi.org/10.3390/ma14051240.

Chen, Y., Y. Yang, B. Xu, S. Wang, B. Li, J. Ma, J. Gao, Y. Y. Zuo, and S. Liu. 2017. “Mesoporous Carbon Nanomaterials Induced Pulmonary Surfactant Inhibition, Cytotoxicity, Inflammation and Lung Fibrosis.” *Journal of Environmental Sciences* 62 (December). https://doi.org/10.1016/j.jes.2017.08.018.

Chouryal, Y. N., S. Nema, R. K. Sharma, H. L. Kewat, A. Pandey, P. Ghosh, and Y. Bhargava. 2020. “The Nano-Bio Interactions of Rare-Earth Doped BaF2 Nanophosphors Shape the Developmental Processes of Zebrafish.” *Biomaterials Science* 8 (23). https://doi.org/10.1039/d0bm01282c.

Chun, Sang Hun, Ji Soo Yuk, and Soong Ho Um. 2018. “Regulation of Cellular Gene Expression by Nanomaterials.” *Nano Convergence* 5 (December). https://doi.org/10.1186/s40580-018-0166-x.

Danielsen, P. H., Y. Cao, M. Roursgaard, P. Møller, and S. Loft. 2015. “Endothelial Cell Activation, Oxidative Stress and Inflammation Induced by a Panel of Metal-Based Nanomaterials.” *Nanotoxicology* 9 (7). https://doi.org/10.3109/17435390.2014.980449.

Danish, M., Liezel L. Estrella-Pajulas, Ivy Michelle A. Alemaida, M. Grilli, A. Mikhaylov, and T. Senjyu. 2022. “Green Synthesis of Silver Oxide Nanoparticles for Photocatalytic Environmental Remediation and Biomedical Applications.” *Metals*. https://doi.org/10.3390/met12050769.

Dharsana, U. S., M. S. Varsha, Ayaz Ahmed Khan Behlol, Anbazhagan Veerappan, and R. Thiagarajan. 2015. “Sulfidation Modulates the Toxicity of Biogenic Copper Nanoparticles.” *RSC Advances*. https://doi.org/10.1039/C4RA17322H.

Feng, Yun Hao, Bo Zhi Chen, Wen Min Fei, Yong Cui, Can Yang Zhang, and Xin Dong Guo. 2022. “Mechanism Studies on the Cellular Internalization of Nanoparticles Using Computer Simulations: A Review.” *AIChE Journal* 68 (2): e17507.

Fleischer, Candace C., and Christine K. Payne. 2014. “Nanoparticle–Cell Interactions: Molecular Structure of the Protein Corona and Cellular Outcomes.” July. https://doi.org/10.1021/ar500190q.

Foffi, G., and G. Kahl. 2010. “New Trends in Simulating Colloids and Self-Assembling Systems.” *Journal of Physics: Condensed Matter: An Institute of Physics Journal* 22 (10). https://doi.org/10.1088/0953-8984/22/10/100301.

Gagner, J. E., S. Shrivastava, X. Qian, J. S. Dordick, and R. W. Siegel. 2012. “Engineering Nanomaterials for Biomedical Applications Requires Understanding the Nano-Bio Interface: A Perspective.” *The Journal of Physical Chemistry Letters* 3 (21). https://doi.org/10.1021/jz301253s.

Galvan, Elfego, Dillon K. Walker, Sunday Y. Simbo, Ryan Dalton, Kyle Levers, Abigail O’Connor, Chelsea Goodenough, et al. 2016. “Acute and Chronic Safety and Efficacy of Dose Dependent Creatine Nitrate Supplementation and Exercise Performance.” *Journal of the International Society of Sports Nutrition* 13. https://doi.org/10.1186/s12970-016-0124-0.

Gheata, Adrian, Geoffrey Gaulier, Gabriel Campargue, Jérémy Vuilleumier, Simon Kaiser, Ivan Gautschi, Florian Riporto, et al. 2022. “Photoresponsive Nanocarriers Based on Lithium Niobate Nanoparticles for Harmonic Imaging and On-Demand Release of Anticancer Chemotherapeutics.” *ACS Nanoscience Au* 2 (4): 355.

Graham, U. M., M. T. Tseng, J. B. Jasinski, R. A. Yokel, J. M. Unrine, B. H. Davis, A. K. Dozier, et al. 2014. “In Vivo Processing of Ceria Nanoparticles Inside Liver: Impact on Free-Radical Scavenging Activity and Oxidative Stress.” *ChemPlusChem* 79 (8). https://doi.org/10.1002/cplu.201402080.

Greskovich, K. M., K. M. Powderly, M. M. Kincanon, N. B. Forney, C. A. Jalomo, A. Wo, and C. J. Murphy. 2023. “The Landscape of Gold Nanocrystal Surface Chemistry.” *Accounts of Chemical Research* 56 (12). https://doi.org/10.1021/acs.accounts.3c00109.

Grønningsæter, Ida Sofie, Håkon Reikvam, Elise Aasebø, Sushma Bartaula-Brevik, Tor Henrik Tvedt, Øystein Bruserud, and Kimberley Joanne Hatfield. 2020. “Targeting Cellular Metabolism in Acute Myeloid Leukemia and the Role of Patient Heterogeneity.” *Cells* 9 (5). https://doi.org/10.3390/cells9051155.

Grune, Tilman. 2005. *Free Radicals and Diseases: Gene Expression, Cellular Metabolism and Pathophysiology*. IOS Press.

Guo, Xiaojing, Silong Wei, Mengmeng Lu, Zhengwei Shao, Jiayu Lu, Lunguo Xia, Kaili Lin, and Derong Zou. 2016. "Dose-Dependent Effects of Strontium Ranelate on Ovariectomy Rat Bone Marrow Mesenchymal Stem Cells and Human Umbilical Vein Endothelial Cells." *International Journal of Biological Sciences* 12 (12): 1511.

Harshitha, Mave, Ashwath Nayak, Somanath Disha, Uchangi Satyaprasad Akshath, Saurabh Dubey, H. Munang'andu, Anirban Chakraborty, I. Karunasagar, and B. Maiti. 2023. "Nanovaccines to Combat Aeromonas Hydrophila Infections in Warm-Water Aquaculture: Opportunities and Challenges." *Vaccines*. https://doi.org/10.3390/vaccines11101555.

Holmila, Reetta, Hanzhi Wu, Jingyun Lee, Allen W. Tsang, Ravi Singh, and Cristina M. Furdui. 2021. "Integrated Redox Proteomic Analysis Highlights New Mechanisms of Sensitivity to Silver Nanoparticles." *Molecular & Cellular Proteomics: MCP* 20 (January). https://doi.org/10.1016/j.mcpro.2021.100073.

Hussein, M., M. Mumtaz, Iqra Nasir, and Anisa Abdullahi. 2023. "Nanotechnology-Based Vaccines." *Biology, Medicine, & Natural Product Chemistry*. https://pdfs.semanticscholar.org/1179/1a9b92c5c69a19cdeb0a305956b8f2eb524b.pdf.

Jasrotia, P., M. Nagpal, C. Mishra, Ajay Sharma, Satish Kumar, Umesh Kamble, A. Bhardwaj, P. L. Kashyap, Sudheer Kumar, and G. Singh. 2022. "Nanomaterials for Postharvest Management of Insect Pests: Current State and Future Perspectives." https://doi.org/10.3389/fnano.2021.811056.

Jedrzejczak-Silicka, Magdalena, and Ewa Mijowska. 2018. "General Cytotoxicity and Its Application in Nanomaterial Analysis." *Cytotoxicity*. https://pdfs.semanticscholar.org/1cb9/9f9e75c21dfc7c4245c74ccc163c12aaed29.pdf.

Kadowaki, T., M. Namba, A. Yamamura, H. Sowa, A. M. Wolka, and R. G. Brodows. 2009. "Exenatide Exhibits Dose-Dependent Effects on Glycemic Control Over 12 Weeks in Japanese Patients With Suboptimally Controlled Type 2 Diabetes." *Endocrine Journal* 56 (3). https://doi.org/10.1507/endocrj.k08e-296.

Kim, H., A. R. Kirtane, N. Y. Kim, N. U. Rajesh, C. Tang, K. Ishida, A. M. Hayward, R. Langer, and G. Traverso. 2023. "Gastrointestinal Delivery of an mRNA Vaccine Using Immunostimulatory Polymeric Nanoparticles." *The AAPS Journal* 25 (5). https://doi.org/10.1208/s12248-023-00844-z.

Kim, H., Lin Niu, Peter G. Larson, K. Murphy, T. Kucaba, D. Ferguson, T. Griffith, and J. Panyam. 2016. "Abstract 2348: Nanovaccine: A Novel Immunotherapeutic Strategy to Treat Bladder Cancer." *Cancer Research*. https://doi.org/10.1158/1538-7445.AM2016-2348.

Kokkinopoulou, Maria, Johanna Simon, Katharina Landfester, Volker Mailänder, and Ingo Lieberwirth. 2017. "Visualization of the Protein Corona: Towards a Biomolecular Understanding of Nanoparticle-Cell-Interactions." *Nanoscale* 9 (25): 8858–70.

Kopac, T. 2021. "Protein Corona, Understanding the Nanoparticle-Protein Interactions and Future Perspectives: A Critical Review." *International Journal of Biological Macromolecules* 169 (February). https://doi.org/10.1016/j.ijbiomac.2020.12.108.

Kuhn, Dagmar A., Dimitri Vanhecke, Benjamin Michen, Fabian Blank, Peter Gehr, Alke Petri-Fink, and Barbara Rothen-Rutishauser. 2014. "Different Endocytotic Uptake Mechanisms for Nanoparticles in Epithelial Cells and Macrophages." *Beilstein Journal of Nanotechnology* 5 (1): 1625–36.

Lefebvre, D. E., K. Venema, L. Gombau, L. G. Valerio, J. Raju, G. S. Bondy, H. Bouwmeester, et al. 2015. "Utility of Models of the Gastrointestinal Tract for Assessment of the Digestion and Absorption of Engineered Nanomaterials Released From Food Matrices." *Nanotoxicology* 9 (4). https://doi.org/10.3109/17435390.2014.948091.

Liang, Hao, Xiao-Bing Zhang, Yifan Lv, Liang Gong, Ruowen Wang, Xiaoyan Zhu, Ronghua Yang, and Weihong Tan. 2014. "Functional DNA-Containing Nanomaterials: Cellular Applications in Biosensing, Imaging, and Targeted Therapy." *Accounts of Chemical Research* 47 (6): 1891.

Lichtenstein, D., J. Ebmeyer, P. Knappe, S. Juling, L. Böhmert, S. Selve, B. Niemann, A. Braeuning, A. F. Thünemann, and A. Lampen. 2015. "Impact of Food Components During In Vitro Digestion of Silver Nanoparticles on Cellular Uptake and Cytotoxicity in Intestinal Cells." *Biological Chemistry* 396 (11). https://doi.org/10.1515/hsz-2015-0145.

Lim, Z. Q., Q. Y. Ng, J. W. Q. Ng, V. Mahendran, and S. Alonso. 2020. "Recent Progress and Challenges in Drug Development to Fight Hand, Foot and Mouth Disease." *Expert Opinion on Drug Discovery* 15 (3). https://doi.org/10.1080/17460441.2019.1659241.

Lin, Zhoumeng, Santosh Aryal, Yi-Hsien Cheng, and Andre J. Gesquiere. 2022. "Integration of In Vitro and In Vivo Models to Predict Cellular and Tissue Dosimetry of Nanomaterials Using Physiologically Based Pharmacokinetic Modeling." *ACS Nano* 16 (12): 19722.

Liu, Y., B. Workalemahu, and X. Jiang. 2017. "The Effects of Physicochemical Properties of Nanomaterials on Their Cellular Uptake In Vitro and In Vivo." *Small* 13 (43). https://doi.org/10.1002/smll.2017 01815.

Mahmoudi, Morteza, Markita P. Landry, Anna Moore, and Roxana Coreas. 2023. "The Protein Corona From Nanomedicine to Environmental Science." *Nature Reviews Materials* 8 (7): 422–38.

Manke, Amruta, Liying Wang, and Yon Rojanasakul. 2013. "Mechanisms of Nanoparticle-Induced Oxidative Stress and Toxicity." *BioMed Research International* 2013. https://doi.org/10.1155/2013/942916.

Martinez, J. O., C. Boada, I. K. Yazdi, M. Evangelopoulos, B. S. Brown, X. Liu, M. Ferrari, and E. Tasciotti. 2013. "Short and Long Term, in Vitro and in Vivo Correlations of Cellular and Tissue Responses to Mesoporous Silicon Nanovectors." *Small* 9 (9–10). https://doi.org/10.1002/smll.201201939.

Matsumoto, A. M. 1990. "Effects of Chronic Testosterone Administration in Normal Men: Safety and Efficacy of High Dosage Testosterone and Parallel Dose-Dependent Suppression of Luteinizing Hormone, Follicle-Stimulating Hormone, and Sperm Production." *The Journal of Clinical Endocrinology and Metabolism* 70 (1). https://doi.org/10.1210/jcem-70-1-282.

Mazumdar, Samrat, Deepak Chitkara, and Anupama Mittal. 2021. "Exploration and Insights into the Cellular Internalization and Intracellular Fate of Amphiphilic Polymeric Nanocarriers." *Acta Pharmaceutica Sinica* 11 (4): 903–24.

Migliaccio, Vincenzo, NaymBlal, Micaela De Girolamo, Valentina Mastronardi, Federico Catalano, Ilaria Di Gregorio, Lillà Lionetti, Pier Paolo Pompa, and Daniela Guarnieri. 2023. "Inter-Organelle Contact Sites Mediate the Intracellular Antioxidant Activity of Platinum Nanozymes: A New Perspective on Cell–Nanoparticle Interaction and Signaling." *ACS Applied Materials & Interfaces* 15 (3): 3882.

Mirković, Miljana, Suzana Filipović, Ana Kalijadis, Pavle Mašković, Jelena Mašković, Branislav Vlahović, and Vladimir Pavlović. 2022. "Hydroxyapatite/TiO2 Nanomaterial With Defined Microstructural and Good Antimicrobial Properties." *Antibiotics* 11 (5). https://doi.org/10.3390/antibiotics11050592.

Mortezaee, K., M. Najafi, H. Samadian, H. Barabadi, A. Azarnezhad, and A. Ahmadi. 2019. "Redox Interactions and Genotoxicity of Metal-Based Nanoparticles: A Comprehensive Review." *Chemico-Biological Interactions* 312 (October): 108814.

Mudunkotuwa, Imali A., and V. Grassian. 2015. "Biological and Environmental Media Control Oxide Nanoparticle Surface Composition: The Roles of Biological Components (proteins and Amino Acids), Inorganic Oxyanions and Humic Acid." *Environmental Science: Nano*. https://doi.org/10.1039/C4EN00215F.

Ouyang, Q., Y. Meng, W. Zhou, J. Tong, Z. Cheng, and Q. Zhu. 2022. "New Advances in Brain-Targeting Nano-Drug Delivery Systems for Alzheimer's Disease." *Journal of Drug Targeting* 30 (1). https://doi.org/10.1080/1061186X.2021.1927055.

Park, Sung Jean. 2020. "Protein–Nanoparticle Interaction: Corona Formation and Conformational Changes in Proteins on Nanoparticles." *International Journal of Nanomedicine* 15: 5783.

Pelka, J., H. Gehrke, M. Esselen, M. Türk, M. Crone, S. Bräse, T. Muller, et al. 2009. "Cellular Uptake of Platinum Nanoparticles in Human Colon Carcinoma Cells and Their Impact on Cellular Redox Systems and DNA Integrity." *Chemical Research in Toxicology* 22 (4). https://doi.org/10.1021/tx800354g.

Pragatisheel, and J. Prakash. 2020. "Silver Nanostructures, Chemical Synthesis Methods, and Biomedical Applications." https://doi.org/10.1007/978-3-030-44176-0_11.

Qamar, Zufika, Farheen Fatima Qizilbash, Mohammad Kashif Iqubal, Asgar Ali, Jasjeet Kaur Narang, Javed Ali, and Sanjula Baboota. 2019. "Nano-Based Drug Delivery System: Recent Strategies for the Treatment of Ocular Disease and Future Perspective." *Recent Patents on Drug Delivery & Formulation* 13 (4): 246.

Qhattal, H. S., and X. Liu. 2011. "Characterization of CD44-Mediated Cancer Cell Uptake and Intracellular Distribution of Hyaluronan-Grafted Liposomes." *Molecular Pharmaceutics* 8 (4). https://doi.org/10.1021/mp2000428.

Reichenfelser, R., E. Punz, I. Joubert, M. Geppert, and M. Himly. 2020. "Nano-Bio Interactions." https://doi.org/10.12681/osj.22599.

Rennick, Joshua J., Angus P. R. Johnston, and Robert G. Parton. 2021. "Key Principles and Methods for Studying the Endocytosis of Biological and Nanoparticle Therapeutics." *Nature Nanotechnology* 16 (3): 266–76.

Salama, B., K. J. Alzahrani, K. S. Alghamdi, O. Al-Amer, K. E. Hassan, M. A. Elhefny, A. J. A. Albarakati, et al. 2023. "Silver Nanoparticles Enhance Oxidative Stress, Inflammation, and Apoptosis in Liver and Kidney Tissues: Potential Protective Role of Thymoquinone." *Biological Trace Element Research* 201 (6). https://doi.org/10.1007/s12011-022-03399-w.

Santopolo, G., A. Clemente, M. Aranda, A. Socias, A. Del Castillo, A. Chica, M. Borges, and R. de la Rica. 2021. "Colorimetric Detection of Sepsis-Derived Hyperdegranulation With Plasmonic Nanosensors." *ACS Sensors* 6 (12). https://doi.org/10.1021/acssensors.1c01884.

Schellenberg, Ruediger, Reinhard Saller, Lorenzo Hess, Jörg Melzer, Christian Zimmermann, Juergen Drewe, and Catherine Zahner. 2012. "Dose-Dependent Effects of the Cimicifuga Racemosa Extract Ze 450 in the Treatment of Climacteric Complaints: A Randomized, Placebo-Controlled Study." *Evidence-Based Complementary and Alternative Medicine: eCAM* 2012. https://doi.org/10.1155/2012/260301.

Schlich, K., M. Hoppe, M. Kraas, J. Schubert, M. Chanana, and K. Hund-Rinke. 2018. "Long-Term Effects of Three Different Silver Sulfide Nanomaterials, Silver Nitrate and Bulk Silver Sulfide on Soil Microorganisms and Plants." *Environmental Pollution* 242 (Pt B). https://doi.org/10.1016/j.envpol.2018.07.082.

Sharifi, Shahriar, Nouf N. Mahmoud, Elizabeth Voke, Markita P. Landry, and Morteza Mahmoudi. 2022. "Importance of Standardizing Analytical Characterization Methodology for Improved Reliability of the Nanomedicine Literature." *Nano-Micro Letters* 14 (December). https://doi.org/10.1007/s40820-022-00922-5.

Shi, Xiaolu, Ye Tian, Shaobo Zhai, Yang Liu, Shunli Chu, and Zhengrong Xiong. 2023. "The Progress of Research on the Application of Redox Nanomaterials in Disease Therapy." *Frontiers in Chemistry* 11 (February): 1115440.

Simpson, Joshua D., Samuel A. Smith, Kristofer J. Thurecht, and Georgina Such. 2019. "Engineered Polymeric Materials for Biological Applications: Overcoming Challenges of the Bio–Nano Interface." *Polymers* 11 (9). https://doi.org/10.3390/polym11091441.

Sims, Christopher M., Shannon K. Hanna, Daniel A. Heller, Christopher P. Horoszko, Monique E. Johnson, Antonio R. Montoro Bustos, Vytas Reipa, Kathryn R. Riley, and Bryant C. Nelson. 2017. "Redox-Active Nanomaterials for Nanomedicine Applications." *Nanoscale* 9 (40): 15226.

Sun, W., and G. Forgacs. 2011. "The 2010 International Conference on Biofabrication (BF2010) Special Issue." *Biofabrication* 3 (3). https://doi.org/10.1088/1758-5082/3/3/030201.

Tian, Xin, Yu Chong, and Cuicui Ge. 2020. "Understanding the Nano-Bio Interactions and the Corresponding Biological Responses." *Frontiers in Chemistry* 8 (June): 446.

Vasyukova, Inna A., Olga V. Zakharova, Denis V. Kuznetsov, and Alexander A. Gusev. 2022. "Synthesis, Toxicity Assessment, Environmental and Biomedical Applications of MXenes: A Review." *Nanomaterials* 12 (11). https://doi.org/10.3390/nano12111797.

Villanueva-Flores, Francisca, Andrés Castro-Lugo, Octavio T. Ramírez, and Laura A. Palomares. 2020. "Understanding Cellular Interactions With Nanomaterials: Towards a Rational Design of Medical Nanodevices." *Nanotechnology* 31 (13). https://doi.org/10.1088/1361-6528/ab5bc8.

Wang, H., Q. Liu, X. Lan, and D. Jiang. 2022. "Framework Nucleic Acids in Nuclear Medicine Imaging: Shedding Light on Nano-Bio Interactions." *Angewandte Chemie* 61 (8). https://doi.org/10.1002/anie.202111980.

Wang, Y., K. Nguyen, R. C. Spitale, and J. C. Chaput. 2021. "A Biologically Stable DNAzyme That Efficiently Silences Gene Expression in Cells." *Nature Chemistry* 13 (4). https://doi.org/10.1038/s41557-021-00645-x.

Xie, Dongli, Jianchen Hu, Zhenhua Yang, Tong Wu, Wei Xu, Qingyang Meng, Kangli Cao, and Xiaogang Luo. 2022. "Vitamin Supplementation Protects Against Nanomaterial-Induced Oxidative Stress and Inflammation Damages: A Meta-Analysis of In Vitro and In Vivo Studies." *Nutrients* 14 (11). https://doi.org/10.3390/nu14112214.

Yadav, Ram Dhan, and Abha Chaudhary. 2021. "Nano–bio Surface Interactions, Cellular Internalisation in Cancer Cells and E-data Portals of Nanomaterials: A Review." *IET Nanobiotechnology/IET* 15 (6): 519.

Yameen, Basit, Won Il Choi, Cristian Vilos, Archana Swami, Jinjun Shi, and Omid C. Farokhzad. 2014. "Insight into Nanoparticle Cellular Uptake and Intracellular Targeting." *Journal of Controlled Release: Official Journal of the Controlled Release Society* 190 (September): 485.

Yan, Yan, Katelyn T. Gause, Marloes M. J. Kamphuis, Ching-Seng Ang, Neil M. O'Brien-Simpson, Jason C. Lenzo, Eric C. Reynolds, Edouard C. Nice, and Frank Caruso. 2013. "Differential Roles of the Protein Corona in the Cellular Uptake of Nanoporous Polymer Particles by Monocyte and Macrophage Cell Lines." November. https://doi.org/10.1021/nn404481f.

Yuan, Qing, Yao Zhao, Pengju Cai, Zhesheng He, Fuping Gao, Jinsong Zhang, and Xueyun Gao. 2019. "Dose-Dependent Efficacy of Gold Clusters on Rheumatoid Arthritis Therapy." *ACS Omega* 4 (9): 14092.

Zellner, Reinhard. 2015. "Biological Responses to Nanoscale Particles." *Beilstein Journal of Nanotechnology* 6: 380.

Zhang, Zhong, Shan Gao, Yang-nan Hu, Xin Chen, Cheng Cheng, Xiao-long Fu, Sha-sha Zhang, et al. 2022. "Ti3C2TxMXene Composite 3D Hydrogel Potentiates mTOR Signaling to Promote the Generation of Functional Hair Cells in Cochlea Organoids." *Advanced Science Letters* 9 (32). https://doi.org/10.1002/advs.202203557.

Zhu, M., S. Perrett, and G. Nie. 2013. "Understanding the Particokinetics of Engineered Nanomaterials for Safe and Effective Therapeutic Applications." *Small* 9 (9–10). https://doi.org/10.1002/smll.201201630.

Zimmer, Christopher C., Ying X. Liu, Joshua T. Morgan, Guohua Yang, Kang-Hsin Wang, Ian M. Kennedy, Abdul I. Barakat, and Gang-Yu Liu. 2014. "New Approach to Investigate the Cytotoxicity of Nanomaterials Using Single Cell Mechanics." *The Journal of Physical Chemistry. B* 118 (5): 1246.

Part II

Nanoparticles in Cancer Diagnosis

4 Conventional Methods of Cancer Diagnosis

Dr. Sunita Saklani

ABBREVIATIONS

Acronym	Full Form
EPR	enhanced permeability and retention
CT	computed tomography
MRI	magnetic resonance imaging
PET	positron emission tomography
GEPNENs	gastroenteropancreatic neuroendocrine neoplasms
CtDNA	circulating DNA
BMA	bone marrow aspiration
BMB	bone marrow biopsies
EcPKA	extracellular protein kinase A
NNMT	nicotinamide A-methyltransferase
IHC	immunohistochemistry
HER 2	human epidermal growth factor 2 receptor
CBC	complete blood count
AFP	alpha-fetoprotein
CA125	cancer antigen for ovarian cancer
CEA	carcinoembryonic antigen for colorectal cancer
CTC	circulating tumor cells
CRC	colorectal cancer
HPV	human papillomavirus
TAAbs	tumor-associated antigens

4.1 INTRODUCTION

Cancer is the unrestricted cell growth developed in any body organ that spreads to nearby tissue and causes impairment (Borse, Konwar, and Buragohain 2020). In other words, the growth of cells in these tissues and organs is stopped, and the cells become uncontrollable for its division. These cells sustain their division at a fast pace till either their deportation through operation, drug delivery, hormonal or radiation therapy, or their natural vanishing. Natural recovery or vanishing occurs in cancers like cancer of the kidney and skin (Tufail et al. 2021). There are more than 150 cancer types that are prevalent worldwide (Tufail et al. 2021). Among the most widely occurring cancers are of the breast, oral lip, thyroid, and cervical, whereas the most infrequent cancer comprises Ewing's sarcoma, osteosarcoma, male breast cancer, chondrosarcoma, mesothelioma, gastrointestinal stromal tumors, adrenocortical carcinoma, cholangiocarcinoma, pheochromocytoma kidney chromophobe carcinoma, and paraganglioma and sarcoma that account for >20% of cancer type (Roy and Saikia 2016; Torre et al. 2016; Baust et al. 2018; Abbas-Aghababazadeh et al. 2020; Tufail et al. 2021).

DOI: 10.1201/9781003463191-6

Being a genetically associated disease, cancer results from alterations in the vital affairs of the cell cycle, such as mitosis, replication, and formation of reactive oxygen species, which subsequently lead to cancer progression (Aggarwal et al. 2019). This progression continues in the origin of cancerous cells up to their death. Simultaneously, cancer cells acquire mass with the help of mesenchymal stromal support cells, endothelial cells, and cells of the immune system (Tufail et al. 2021). All these cells gathered to develop into cancerous masses, owing to the presence of cancerous-related stress ligands and antigens. Metabolic changes (which result from mitochondrial dysfunctioning that plays an essential role in energetic pathways), nucleotides' displaced acid, and proteotoxicity are other cancer-based stress components. All these stresses and changes are controlled by the genes that represent the systematic arrangement of nucleotides (Hammoudi et al. 2011; Balajee and Hande 2018; Lichtenstein 2018; Seelige et al. 2018).

The fast growth and new clone formation of cancerous cells are ignited by sugar, which is an essential component of their meal, ensuring expansions and mass formation. Some prevalent bacteria that are related to cancers include *Chlamydia trachomatis*, *Helicobacter pylori*, *Serovar typhi*, *Salmonella enterica*, enterotoxigenic *Bacteroides fragilis*, *Fusobacterium nucleatum*, *Koribacteraceae*, etc. (Dasgupta et al. 2016; Marx 2019; Parida, Sheetal, and Sharma 2021).

Being a main cause of serious human health hazards, cancer causes maximum mortality worldwide. According to the data revealed by WHO, it stands in the first or second rank for death caused in the pre-70 age group in 112 out of 183 countries and, in the other 23, in the third or fourth position (Sung et al. 2021). The control of cancer depends on early and precise diagnostic techniques, and effective cognitive efficiency is needed for its management. A lower cancer survival rate is brought on by cognitive deficiencies that delay early treatment due to a lack of timely and effective diagnostic methods.

4.2 TECHNIQUES OF CANCER DIAGNOSIS

Cancer has persisted from long ago in humans. Up to the early twentieth century, its diagnosis relied on the examination of visible and physical symptoms that involve certain outgrowth or lumps. But in the middle of the twentieth century, with the availability of X-ray techniques, physicians were able to diagnose inner abnormalities, outgrowth, or tumors, and this technique was quite helpful in developing a new technique of screening breast cancers, known as mammography, in the 1960s (Nicosia et al. 2023). Similarly, a method was introduced for identifying abnormalities in cervical cells, known as Pap smear tests, which transform the examining method of cervical cancer in earlier stages. With time, numerous other advancements in the detection of cancer have taken place. The proper diagnostic technique plays an important role in clinical diagnosis, in monitoring of effective toxicity, and subsequently, for accurate and effective treatment of cancers (Wu and Qu 2015). The methods of cancer diagnosis depend on symptoms experienced by the patients, medical history, suspect type, and location type where it exists. These are also varied with the type and location of cancer. Based on available information about cancer diagnostics, tumors can be classified typically into two large groups. The first group is usually non-life-threatening, as it exists as noncancerous tumors, known as benign tumors, and such tumors do not move from one part to another in the body. The other type, known as malignant tumors, can spread from one part to another nearby tissue or organ and become cancerous. Cancer diagnosis and treatment mainly revolve around malignant tumors. In present times, different methods are used for cancer diagnosis, that is, imaging techniques, laboratory tests, biopsy techniques, cytology and histology, and genetic and molecular techniques (Figure 4.1).

4.2.1 Imaging Techniques

For characterizing and managing treatment plan for in-time cancer diagnosis, imagining techniques come out as a better option that gives precise information about tumor size and location. For this,

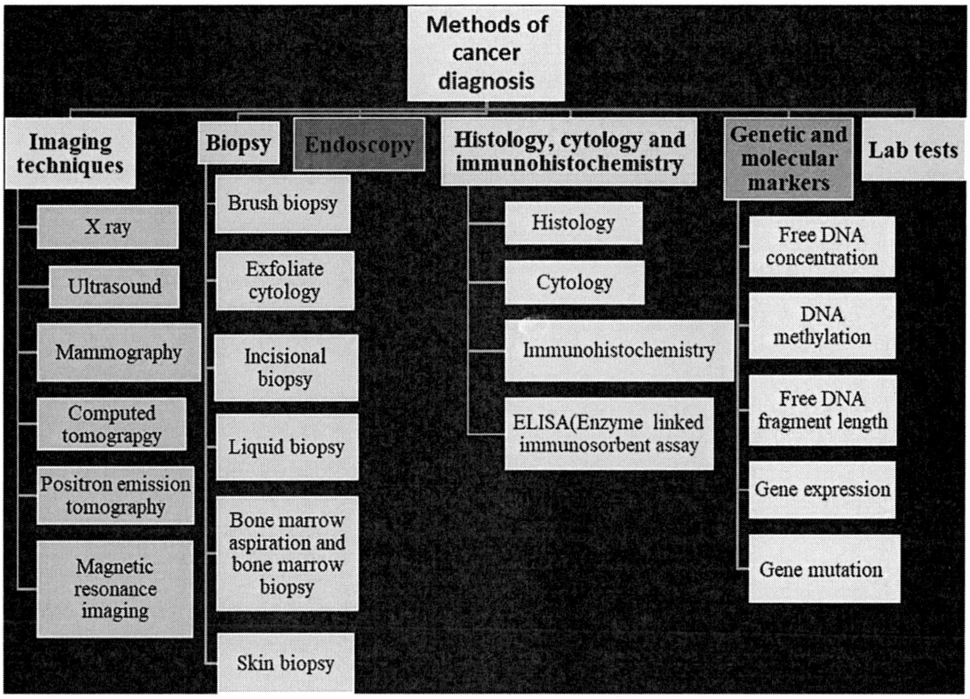

FIGURE 4.1 Conventional methods used for cancer diagnosis and their different categories. This image depicts the different diagnostic techniques for cancer detection, like imaging techniques, biopsy, endoscopy, histology cytology immunohistochemistry, etc., which are further subdivided into available techniques

a number of imaging techniques are used. The most common techniques are X-ray imaging, CT (computed tomography) scan, MRI (magnetic resonance imaging), PET (positron emission tomography) scan, ultrasound, mammography, and endoscopy.

4.2.1.1 X-rays

These are electromagnetic radiation used on areas such as bones, breasts, or chest to create a shadow image on a film, called a radiograph. As the density of various tissues varies, so do their X-ray images (Astrakhantsev et al. 2004). Thus, we obtain denser images of cancerous outgrowth around healthy tissue. These images help identify the localized characteristics and size of the tumors and for comparison before and after treatment (Malik et al. 2016). Bone metastasis and lung and breast cancers are usually detected with the help of this technique. It is a faster and painless technique. However, ionizing radiation exposure may involve cancer risk in children, and it is not suitable for soft tissue cancer detection (Malik et al. 2016).

4.2.1.2 Mammography

It is a special X-ray technique where low-intensity X-rays are used for earlier detection of breast cancer in females. It is of two types: film mammography and digital mammography. Although they both provide early detection of breast cancer, the digital method is better as it provides higher diagnosis (Khalkhali, Mena, and Diggles 1994; Heywang-Köbrunner et al. 2011; Ramani, Suthanthira, and Vanitha 2014). Despite these, it also involves exposure to ionizing radiation.

4.2.1.3 Ultrasound

This technique involves the use of high-frequency sound waves on the areas of interest after applying a thin layer of gel through the transducer. Depending on the strength and time of reflected sound waves, images of concerned organs are prepared for diagnosis (Malik et al. 2016). Here, the images of internal organs are seen using a device that can be seen on a computer monitor. It is also of two types: 3D ultrasound and Doppler ultrasound (Gregg et al. 1997). This technique is also helpful in biopsy by indicating the place of the tumor (Bailey et al. 2003). As there is no use of ionizing radiation in this technique, the soft tissue's images can be obtained without harming it. But it can't identify certain kinds of cancer unless there are adequately trained specialists to operate it, and that's not always the case.

4.2.1.4 Computed Tomography

It is also an X-ray-based technique where a cross-sectional 2D sliced image of an internal organ can be prepared, and all these images could be used to prepare 3D images, which are studied by an experienced radiologist to identify the approximate size and location of tumor outgrowth (Malik et al. 2016). It also helps us compare before and after treatment situations. The latest technique provides very efficient detection and location as compared to earlier CT scan techniques. As this technique involves a higher dose of radiation exposure, it can therefore cause damage to designated areas (Hashemi, Pilevar, and Rafeh 2013; Xing and Wang 2011).

4.2.1.5 Magnetic Resonance Imaging

It is used to get the image of soft tissues, internal body organs, bone ligaments, and cartilage, where the properties of hydrogen, radio waves, and the powerful magnetic field are used to generate images of higher information, where dark gray and black areas indicate areas of low signal and light gray and white areas indicate high signal. Brain tumors and abdominal tumors can be detected through this technique; moreover, experts can also identify the malignant or non-malignant tumors (Jhamb et al. 2015). Although it is a painless procedure, it is noisy, takes more time, and sometimes patients feel uncomfortable due to claustrophobia (Malik et al. 2016).

4.2.1.6 Positron Emission Tomography

This technique helps determine the cancerous nature of a tumor by introducing a radioactive substance through an injection in the body lying in a still condition. The given radioactive component accumulates in higher concentration in tumor cells in comparison to normal cells. The images are captured by the PET scanner and interpreted by the radiologist to analyze the abnormal growth, because cancerous cells have more radioactive components. The result obtained through PET is exact for large tumors and also helpful in confirming whether the given treatment is working or not. The early-stage detection of cancer is quite effective through this imaging technique; however, the use of radioactive substances limits the frequency of PET scans for the patient (Cabeza and Nyberg 2000; Glaser, Luthra, and Brady 2003).

4.2.2 Endoscopy

In this imaging technique, a flexible tube known as an endoscope fitted with a tiny camera is used to examine the digestive tract of a patient for abnormal growth on the monitor. It can easily move through the mouth, esophagus, stomach, and upper part of the small intestine. Likewise, for examining the large intestine, it can pass through the colon and rectum. GEP-NENs, also known as gastroenteropancreatic neuroendocrine neoplasms, are effectively and accurately detected by endoscopic ultrasonography and standard axial endoscopy (Rossi et al. 2022). For observing the gastric, esophageal, and duodenal NENs, gastrointestinal endoscopy is perfect, whereas ileocolonoscopy is for the colon, rectum, and far-placed lesions of the ileum. For the detection of small bowel NENs, video capsule endoscopy, and double balloon endoscopy have proved quite useful (Rossi et al. 2022).

4.2.3 Lab Test for Cancer Diagnosis

Blood and urine are two important constituents of lab tests that give the initial conviction about the cancer signs and progression. Acute cancerous cells are seen under the microscope in the blood, and it may also find some cancerous cell proteins, such as PSA (protein-specific antigens for prostate cancer), AFP (alpha-fetoprotein for liver and ovarian cancer), CA125 (cancer antigen for ovarian cancer, CEA (carcinoembryonic antigen for colorectal cancer), etc. and other cancer-related substances present in the blood (Landegren and Hammond 2021). Some blood tests, if not used for cancer detection, give the ideas that help the expert make the other diagnosis, which helps in identifying cancer and also indicates the working of organs. Blood tests used to detect cancer comprise (1) blood cell counting test, (2) blood proteins test, (3) blood chemicals (formed by cancerous cells test), (4) presence of cancerous cells test, (5) cancerous cells genetic material test, etc.

4.2.3.1 Blood Cell Counting Test

It is the most common test performed to evaluate the total number of cells, such as RBC and WBC, and the counting of platelets to give the overall health of individuals. The risk of cancer can be predicted using CBC (complete blood count). CBC gives an approximation of acute or chronic infection, that is, an increase in WBC in the case of leukemia (Seo and Lee 2022).

4.2.3.2 Blood Protein Test

Blood protein tests are used to detect the proteins made by the immune system of the body to fight germs. Their level increases in the blood during cancer progression. This test is used to detect multiple myeloma by making use of M-proteins formed by the plasma cells in the blood (Barnidge et al. 2014).

4.2.3.3 Blood Chemicals Tests

It is used to detect the chemicals made by cancerous cells and is also known as tumor markers test. Some important tumor markers used include PSA (protein-specific antigens for prostate cancer), AFP (alpha-fetoprotein for liver and ovarian cancer), CA125 (cancer antigen for ovarian cancer), CEA (carcinoembryonic antigen for colorectal cancer), etc. (Landegren and Hammond 2021).

4.2.3.4 Cancerous Cell Test

CTC (circulating tumor cell) is considered important in cancer diagnosis and disease management. CTC spreads from tumors into the bloodstream and conveys important information regarding tumor initiation, progression, and metastasis (Habli et al. 2020). The potential of CTC cell test is used to diagnose breast, prostate, CRC, lung, and pancreatic ductal adenocarcinoma (Lawrence et al. 2023).

4.2.3.5 Cancerous Cells Genetic Material Tests

This test utilizes the genetic material of cancer cells in diagnosing the cancer type. Cancer-related genetic alteration, known as genetic tumor markers, such as cell-free DNA and RNA, can be detected in the blood by using digital PCR, real-time quantitative PCR, fluorescent dye method, and other molecular biological techniques (Quraish et al. 2023).

Similarly, urine tests can also be used for the diagnosis of cancer. Cancerous cells release some molecules that go to the kidneys through blood. Out of these, only small cancerous proteins are allowed to pass through the kidney's filtering system, which acts as a barrier for large molecules. These small cancerous cell proteins are therefore used in cancer detection. The HPV-based (human papillomavirus, which causes cervical cancer) urine screening test is performed to detect the virus present in cervical cancer patients (Poljak et al. 2023).

4.2.4 Biopsy Technique

The biopsy includes the surgical removal of cells, tissue, or fluid from any part of the body, then observed through a microscope for detection of cancer. Oral or oropharyngeal cancer is only detected through this technique (Borse, Konwar, and Buragohain 2020). The proper handling of the concerned tissue is an essential requirement for the biopsy, failure of which can lead to repetition of the whole procedure due to defective biopsy. Exfoliate cytological biopsy and incisional biopsy may be performed based on requirements (Borse, Konwar, and Buragohain 2020).

4.2.4.1 Brush Biopsy

In this method, transepithelial cells from surface mucosa are taken for examination by scrapping. It is a pain-free, cheap, and sensitive method for the detection of oral cancer and is quite helpful in detecting small red and white suspicious lesions. It is a telemedicine-based screening technique due to its coupling with tablet-based portable microscopes for digital detection. Therefore, results are interpreted by clinicians at far or remote places, and it has vast scope for application in India (Mehrotra et al. 2011; Skandarajahet al. 2017).

4.2.4.2 Exfoliate Cytology

It is based on characteristics related to morphology and staining of individual cells and therefore needs a cytopathological expert. Though it is non-invasive and easy, it is not highly sensitive. Therefore, it is mainly appropriate for the preliminary diagnosis of premalignant lesions. It is suitable for screening of large-scale populations (Jaitley, Agarwal, and Upadhyay 2015; Shaila, Shetty, and Pai 2016).

4.2.4.3 Incisional Biopsy

It is carried out after oral exfoliative cytology and is focused on small representative tissue taken from large lesions. It is accurate in comparison to other biopsies because of its dependence on small areas. Various cancer types are detected by experts that are based on structural modification. Different types of specific staining agents are used for the sample in differentiating and categorizing the cancer types of cells (Sylvie Louise Avon and Kleib 2012).

4.2.4.4 Liquid Biopsies

Liquid biopsies are used for the diagnosis of lung, breast, prostate, and colorectal cancer. This method relies on tumor cells and their products, like circulating DNA (ctDNA) released in the main location and present in the blood or fluid of the body. It gives information regarding the evolution of tumor cells, the target of therapy, and the resistance mechanism of therapy. It is easy to isolate ctDNA using these methods. However, diagnosing brain lesions with this technology is not easy (Heidrich et al. 2020).

4.2.4.5 Bone Marrow Aspiration (BMA) and Bone Marrow Biopsies (BMB)

BMA and BMB are the techniques to detect cancer related to blood, such as leukemia and lymphoma (Trejo-Ayala et al. 2015). For collection, processing, and sample interpretation in BMA and BMB, good technical skills are an essential requirement. It is used to detect the bone marrow's health for making blood cells normally. The liquid (needle used) and solid sample collection are needed in BMA and BMB to analyze the tissue. It is a painful process, and specimen size is the main problem for interpretation, as the large volume of collected sample has the possibility of hemodilution (Trejo-Ayala et al. 2015).

4.2.4.6 Skin Biopsy

Skin biopsy is used to detect skin cancer and melanoma. This technique is an easy, safe outpatient process for diagnosis. The methods of skin biopsies depend upon the lesion's size, site, and clinical suspicion. Though it is a safe method, sometimes problems of infections, bleeding, and scarring may occur with a lack of suitable infrastructure. It ensures substantial evidence for diagnosis and starting of treatment (Nischal, Nischal, and Khopkar 2008).

4.2.5 Histopathology, Cytopathology, and Immunohistochemistry

Histopathology and cytopathology have been essential tools for the diagnosis of cancer from the days of hematoxylin and eosin (H&E) staining and, more recently, immunohistochemistry. Immunohistochemistry (IHC) is used for the diagnosis of cancer based on markers of cancer cells that are detected by using antibodies, a protein type that binds to the markers or antigens (Magaki et al. 2019). In IHC detection, specific antibodies are utilized to identify the markers. The binding of antibodies to antigen/markers produces the colored dye that reveals the specific cell type that enables the expert to make conclusions about the exact cancer type. IHC is not included in standard diagnosis methods; however, the choice of IHC is made by an expert after examining the biopsy sample under the microscope and if it is not possible to conclude the cancer type. IHC is usually performed to diagnose invasive, metastatic, and recurrent breast cancer, gastrointestinal cancer, prostate cancer, lung cancer, and lymphoma (Birkman et al. 2018; Carneiro et al. 2018; Inamura 2018; Cho 2022; Ding et al. 2022). In patients having breast cancer, an IHC test is used to diagnose/determine the presence or absence of human epidermal growth factor 2 receptor (HER 2) that reveals the fueling nature of cancer and shows the possibility of treating it with target therapy that inhibits the HER 2 proteins effect (Iqbal and Iqbal 2014). It is also used routinely to detect Lynch syndrome, which may lead to cancer or increases the chances of causing cancer. It is generally associated with colorectal cancer and causes cancer of the stomach, liver, brain, kidney, and uterus. Experts advise the use of IHC to identify the markers of Lynch syndrome in women less than 70 years old (Sarode and Robinson 2019). Similarly, some specific cytokeratins, such as CK7 and CK27, are epithelial cell markers used for the characterization of different epithelial tumors, like carcinoma of transitional cells, urothelial cells, pancreas, colon and rectum, prostate, renal, hepatocellular, Merkel cell, etc. Vimetin is an intermediate filament of sarcoma, and melanoma is variable in lymphomas and co-expressed along with vimentin in renal, endometrial, thyroid, and ovarian carcinoma, and CD45 is a good marker for hemopoietic neoplasm. However, IHC staining results may vary in anaplastic and preliminary neoplasm; therefore, a broad screening panel requires to differentiate the cell type, that is, CD3 (Tcell), CD79a (Bcell), and/or PAX-5 (Bcell) stains are used to identify lymphoid cell type, and CD4 and CD8 markers are used to distinguish neoplastic T cells subsets (Painter, Clayton, and Herbert 2010).

4.2.5.1 Enzyme-Linked Immunosorbent Assay (ELISA)

ELISA, also known as enzyme-linked immunosorbent assay, utilizes the enzyme's catalytic properties to identify and quantify the proteins. In this technique, a solid phase like a microtiter well, magnetic particle, or plastic bead is used to bind or adsorb one of the reaction components covalently. This binding accelerates the bound and free labelled reactants separation on microtiter. Commonly, samples containing antigen (Ag) that need to be quantified are added and conceded to bind with antibodies to the solid phase. After that, unbound antigens are removed through washing, and antibodies labeled to enzymes are added to form a solid-phase Ab-Ag-Ab enzyme sandwich complex. Enzyme substrate is added after washing unbound antibodies, and the generated product is proportional to the antigen quantity present in the sample. The specific antibodies can also be quantified by binding antigen to microtiter or solid phase in place of antibodies. The other reagent used is antibodies (enzyme-labeled) specific to analyte antibodies. Additionally, ELISA has been widely used to identify antibodies specific to autoantigens or viruses in whole blood or serum. Moreover, ELISA-type assays have been developed by coupling substrate-producing visible products to the enzyme conjugate, and the result can be visually analyzed. Such assays are beneficial in screening and home testing applications (Engvall 2010; Aydin 2015; Shah and Maghsoudlou 2016; Konstantinou 2017).

TABLE 4.1
Biomarkers Used in the Detection of Different Cancer Types

S. No.	Cancer Type	Biomarker	Reference
1	Breast cancer	Rab31 and mucin-1 (CA15–3)	Kotzsch et al. (2017)
2	Prostate cancer	Integrin alpha V	Zemskov et al. (2021)
3	Liver cancer	Alpha-fetoprotein (AFP)	Li et al. (2021)
4	Renal carcinoma	Vim3, Mxi-2	von Brandenstein et al. (2021)
5	Hepatocellular carcinoma	Midkine	Guo et al. (2021)
6	Lung cancer	Tumor-associated antigens (TAAbs)	Jiang et al. (2021)
7	Cervical cancer	HPV E6 and E7 oncoproteins	Falcucci et al. (2021)
8	Pancreatic cancer	LRG1, TTR, CA 19–9	Choi et al. (2021)
9	Thyroid cancer	Marker 8 (ANTXR1) SAS1B	Yang et al. (2021)
10	Ovarian cancer	Annexin A2, DKK3	Lokman et al. (2021); Nie et al. (2021)

The use of ELISA in the detection of cancer by identifying the protein biomarkers of cancer in physiological samples is a benchmark in the diagnosis of cancer. It can be used in early diagnosis of colorectal cancer by identifying and quantifying the biomarker present in the serum, that is, extracellular protein kinase A (ecPKA) and nicotinamide A-methyltransferase (NNMT), by spotting the auto-antibodies specific to these biomarkers in the serum of humans (Štefatić et al. 2008). Similarly, other important biomarkers of different cancer types have been detected by using ELISA (Table 4.1)

4.2.6 Genetic and Molecular Markers Technique

Loss of genetic stability in the cell is a key factor associated with the origin of tumor or cancer. Therefore, instability in the genetic material of the cells gives rise to heterogeneity in the genetic material of tumors and, consequently, diversity in the cancer type. The alteration in genetic material known, as mutation, is identified by different detection methods available in molecular biology and acts as authentic genetic molecular markers for in-time diagnosis of anomalous changes in the body cells that lead to cancer. This is a fast cancer diagnostic method in comparison to other available techniques, and thus, in-time therapeutic substitution or alteration of these mutations can be feasible and efficient, and specific cancer treatment against target cells or tissue is feasible, devoid of any negative impact related to chemotherapeutic treatment. The genetic test available for cancer detection comprises free DNA concentration, DNA methylation, gene expression, gene mutation, and free DNA fragment length (Figure 4.2) (Quraish et al. 2023).

4.2.6.1 Free DNA Concentration

In the free DNA concentration detection technique, free DNA, termed circulating free DNA (also known as circulating tumor DNA), is detected. Usually, cancer patients have large amounts of cfDNA, that is, 3–10 times more in plasma as compared to normal persons (Minciacchi et al. 2017; Vidal, Taus, and Mantergut 2020; Papatheodoridi et al. 2021). In cancerous patients, the concentration of free DNA is 80 ng/mL on average, whereas in healthy persons, it is 30 ng/mL. By making use of this concentration, the free DNA is measured and quantified with the help of PCR techniques like real-time quantitative and digital, fluorescent dye method, and other techniques related to molecular biology (Agassi et al. 2015; Condappa et al. 2020; Hsu et al. 2022).

4.2.6.2 DNA Methylation

It is an epigenetic change that comprises methylation of cytosine at the fifth position of the CpG island of promoter and therefore plays an important role in epigenetic regulations comprising proliferation

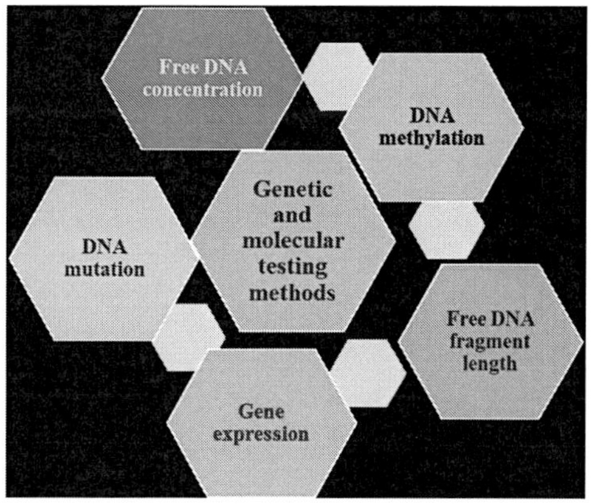

FIGURE 4.2 Diagnosis of cancer by making use of alterations in genetic level that act as genetic molecular markers. This image shows the different genetic and molecular testing methods for cancer diagnosis, which include free DNA concentration, DNA fragment length, gene expression, DNA methylation, etc.

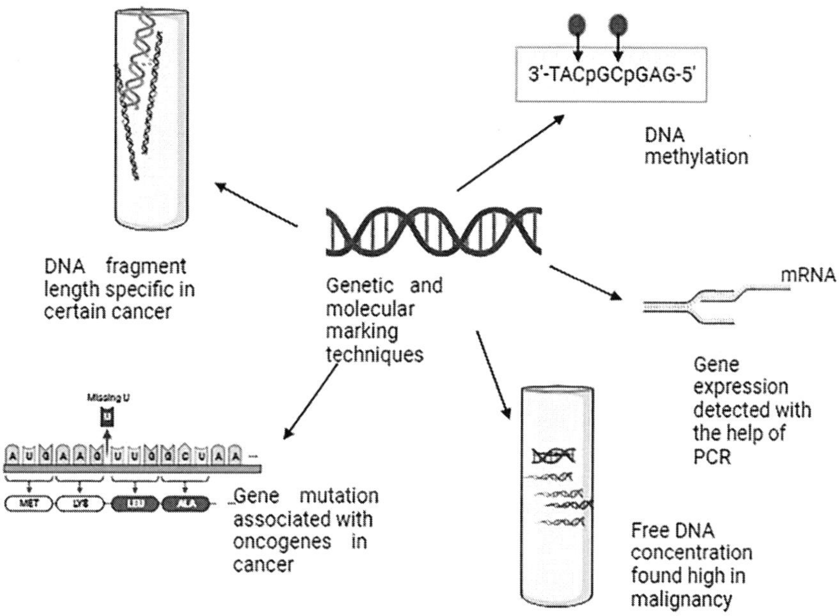

FIGURE 4.3 Different genetic markers that act as bases for the diagnosis of cancer. This image depicts the different genetic and molecular alterations that act as molecular markers, such as DNA methylation, gene expression, free DNA concentration, DNA fragment length, gene mutation, and DNA methylation, that are detected by using molecular biological techniques like PCR.

of cells, gene expression, inactivation of X chromosome, embryonic development, genomic imprinting, and carcinogenesis (Fienberg 2018; Skvortsova, Stirzaker, and Taberlay 2019). The changes or disruptions in epigenetic regulation can give rise to the initiation, progression, and maintenance of cancer. Therefore, there are changes in the expression of genes and the development of neoplastic transformation. The control by DNA methylation is crucial for regulating the transcription of genes sustaining the genome integrity and attuning the immune response (Figure 4.4) (Skvortsova, Stirzaker, and Taberlay 2019). DNA methylation can act as a biomarker for in-time cancer detection,

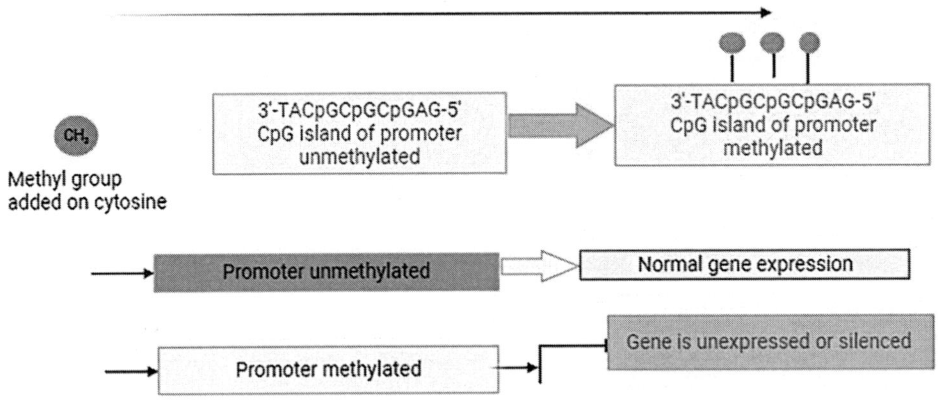

FIGURE 4.4 Methylation of promoter and silencing of gene. This image shows the hypermethylation of the promoter that prevents the expression of the gene and silences it. When the promoter is unmethylated, gene is expressed normally. Methylation of promoter, sometimes called hypermethylation, is an important factor in carcinogenesis when preventing proper expression of tumor suppressor gene.

as distorted DNA hypermethylation may lead to tumor formation and progression when occurring in the promoter's place of particular transcriptional factors (Luo et al. 2020).

4.2.6.3 Gene Expression

Change in the expression of genes can be a useful marker for the early detection of cancer, as it is seen in most cancer types, as hyperexpression of genes is very frequent in cancerous cells or tissue. Specific cancer types having a change in the level of gene expression of a particular gene, that is, increased or decreased gene expression, can be identified with the help of PCR techniques, such as real-time and digital PCR, or by using microarray techniques or northern blot (Jin and Da 2013; Rao et al. 2013; Koul and Manvi 2021). The increase or decrease in expression of genes is known as differential gene expression in cancer types. Research has also been carried out to find out the hub genes, by using the genetic database to analyze the expression of genes related to various tissue tumors. By identifying different hub genes associated with different cancers, potential therapeutic targets can be obtained. There are ten hub genes (Table 4.2) that have common characteristics of gene expression associated with multiple cancers, like lung cancer, liver cancer, kidney cancer, cervical cancer, and breast cancer. Their expression is upregulated in these cancers. The expression level of CDK1 and ASPM was found substantially high in tumor tissue in comparison to normal tissue (Xue et al. 2020).

4.2.6.4 Gene Mutation

Mutations are consequences of defective DNA replication, mutation exposure to DNA, and viral infection (Sfeir and Symington 2015). The mutation is an essential genetic marker, and change in DNA sequence during mutation can show the carcinogenic progress. DNA sequencing in molecular genetics can enable the identification of variation in the gene at the level of nucleotides. The mutation associated with the oncogene is present in all types of cancer, and it is an important tumor marker that can be used for the early detection of cancer and pre- and post-cancer progress before and after cancer treatment (Quraish et al. 2023).

4.2.6.5 Free DNA Fragment Length

DNA of different fragment lengths is released by normal as well as cancerous cells. DNA fragments of cancer cells are not uniform in size because of faulty and irregular digestion of genomic DNA by nuclease. In normal and healthy people generally, DNA fragments of 185–200 bp are released mainly during apoptosis; in cancer patients, however, long and variable-length DNA fragments

TABLE 4.2
The Higher Expression Level of Ten Hub Genes and Cancer Types

Hub Genes	Cancer Type
TOP2, ECT2, RRM2, NEK2, BUB12, CDK1, DTL, PRC1, ANLN, ASPM	Sarcoma, esophageal cancer, gastric cancer, colon cancer, pancreatic cancer, bladder cancer, thyroid cancer, oral cancer, glioma, ovarian cancer, and lymphoma

are released due to necrosis. This variable DNA fragment length is used for early detection and cancer prognosis in oncology. In some specific cancer types, like hepatocellular carcinomas, small DNA fragments along with longer DNA fragments of base pairs in thousands have been reported (Krishnamurthy et al. 2017; Abe et al. 2020; Shi et al. 2020; Rapado-González et al. 2022).

4.3 LIMITATIONS OF CONVENTIONAL METHODS AND HOW NANOTECHNOLOGY CAN HELP IN OVERCOMING THESE

Conventional methods of cancer diagnosis have been used by humans for a long time and help in managing cancer; however, each method has its advantages or disadvantages. The conventional methods of cancer diagnosis, like imaging techniques, endoscopy, biopsy, lab test, IHC, and genetic and molecular techniques, prove quite useful for well-timed and efficient disease management. However, their efficiency is limited by certain associated impediments that need to be addressed, like the use of ionizing radiation in most of the imaging techniques, claustrophobia, associated noise, precise tissue handling, associated pain (BMA and BMB), suitable infrastructure, tediousness, precise tissue requirement for screening, need of expert trainer, and high sensitivity involved in genetic and molecular techniques. The screening efficiency of all these techniques are highly dependent on precise precursor lesion identification for preventing cancer invasives and prognosis improvement. In addition, the optimal target definition of deep-rooted tumors, artifact requirements, high cost, and high signal-to-background ratio also seems critical for the efficiency of conventional methods (Pulumati et al. 2023).

In recent times, nanotechnology has been gaining popularity in its use in different cancer diagnosis imaging techniques, owing to its physical properties, small size, and efficient diagnostic probe loading. Quantum dots possessing high-tissue-penetration capacity, combined with biological probes associated with tumors (antibodies, peptides, and other smaller molecules), have been used for visual improvement, and silver-rich Ag2Te quantum dots for improvement of spatial resolution (Parungo et al. 2004; Zhang et al. 2020). Likewise, gold nanoparticles having better biocompatibility and nanoshells have also been a good option for tumor imaging for in-time malignancy detectors (Jin et al. 2020). Therefore, nanotechnology is proving useful in the nanomedicine landscape with inventions of contemporary nanostructures that can help in cancer diagnosis in a better way. It is the physiochemical properties of nanoparticles that help them bind, absorb, and transport DNA, proteins, and RNAs and probe small drug molecules to their target tissue. These are proving quite appealing in the wide field of oncology due to their magnificent durability, their great carrier potential, their integrating ability with both hydrophobic and hydrophilic compounds, and their various transport routes compatibilities (Mosleh-Shirazi et al. 2022).

4.4 CONCLUSION AND FUTURE PROSPECTS

In-time cancer diagnosis and screening are critical for cancer management and comprehension of prognosis. Effective screening is itself dependent on resource requirements, cost, and impact that vary with different diagnostic techniques. It is the type and tumor location that determine the appropriate diagnostic techniques. However, the efficiency of each technique has limitations, determined by resources, infrastructure, substances used, and experts involved. Some techniques are quite useful to detect certain specific cancer types, whereas others only give approximations or detection up to a certain extent. Among conventional methods, IHC and ELISA are proven benchmarks for cancer types, whereas genetic and molecular markers techniques give fast diagnosis for the origin. In today's technologically advanced world, there is wide scope for an update of these conventional techniques for better and efficacious diagnosis and for emerging techniques, like nanotechnology, to become powerful tools for in-time and precise cancer detection.

REFERENCES

Abbas-Aghababazadeh, Farnoosh, Qianxing Mo, and Brooke L. Fridley. 2020. "Statistical Genomics in Rare Cancer." *Seminars in Cancer Biology* 61: 1–10. Academic Press.

Abe, Tomonori, Chiho Nakashima, Akemi Sato, Yohei Harada, Eisaburo Sueoka, Shinya Kimura, Atsushi Kawaguchi, and Naoko Sueoka-Aragane. 2020. "Origin of Circulating Free DNA in Patients With Lung Cancer." *PLoS One* 15(7): e0235611.

Agassi, Ravit, David Czeiger, Gad Shaked, Avital Avriel, Jony Sheynin, Konstantin Lavrenkov, Samuel Ariad, and Amos Douvdevani. 2015. "Measurement of Circulating Cell-Free DNA Levels by a Simple Fluorescent Test in Patients With Breast Cancer." *American Journal of Clinical Pathology* 143 (1): 18–24.

Aggarwal, Vaishali, Hardeep Singh Tuli, Ayşegül Varol, Falak Thakral, Mukerrem Betul Yerer, Katrin Sak, Mehmet Varol, Aklank Jain, Md Asaduzzaman Khan, and Gautam Sethi. 2019. "Role of Reactive Oxygen Species in Cancer Progression: Molecular Mechanisms and Recent Advancements." *Biomolecules* 9(11): 735. https://doi.org/10.3390/biom9110735.

Astrakhantsev, F. A., A. V. Ivanov, and N. V. Erdneeva. 2004. "X-Ray Diagnosis of Lung Cancer and Its Morphological Variants." *VestnikRentgenologiiiRadiologii* 3: 26–31.

Aydin, Suleyman. 2015. "A Short History, Principles, and Types of ELISA, and Our Laboratory Experience With Peptide/Protein Analyses Using ELISA." *Peptides* 72: 4–15.

Bailey, M. R., V. A. Khokhlova, O. A. Sapozhnikov, S. G. Kargl, and L. A. Crum. 2003. "Physical Mechanisms of the Therapeutic Effect of Ultrasound (A Review)." *Acoustical Physics* 49 (4): 369–88.

Balajee, Adayabalam S., and M. Prakash Hande. 2018. "History and Evolution of Cytogenetic Techniques: Current and Future Applications in Basic and Clinical Research." *Mutation Research/Genetic Toxicology and Environmental Mutagenesis* 836: 3–12.

Barnidge, David R., Renee C. Tschumper, Jason D. Theis, Melissa R. Snyder, Diane F. Jelinek, Jerry A. Katzmann, Angela Dispenzieri, and David L. Murray. 2014. "Monitoring M-Proteins in Patients With Multiple Myeloma Using Heavy-Chain Variable Region Clonotypic Peptides and LC–MS/MS." *Journal of Proteome Research* 13(4): 1905–10.

Baust, John M., Yoed Rabin, Thomas J. Polascik, Kimberly L. Santucci, Kristi K. Snyder, Robert G. Van Buskirk, and John G. Baust. 2018. "Defeating Cancers' Adaptive Defensive Strategies Using Thermal Therapies: Examining Cancer's Therapeutic Resistance, Ablative, and Computational Modeling Strategies as a Means for Improving Therapeutic Outcome." *Technology in Cancer Research & Treatment* 17 (2018). https://doi.org/10.1177/1533033818762207.

Birkman, Eva-Maria, Naziha Mansuri, Samu Kurki, Annika Ålgars, Minnamaija Lintunen, Raija Ristamäki, Jari Sundström, and Olli Carpén. 2018. "Gastric Cancer: Immunohistochemical Classification of Molecular Subtypes and Their Association With Clinicopathological Characteristics." *VirchowsArchiv* 472: 369–82.

Borse, Vivek, Aditya Narayan Konwar, and Pronamika Buragohain. 2020. "Oral Cancer Diagnosis and Perspectives in India." *Sensors International* 1: 2666–3511. https://doi.org/10.1016/j.sintl.2020.100046.

Cabeza, Roberto, and Lars Nyberg. 2000 "Imaging Cognition II: An Empirical Review of 275 PET and fMRI Studies." *Journal of Cognitive Neuroscience* 12 (1): 1–47.

Carneiro, Arie, Álan Roger Gomes Barbosa, Lucas Seiti Takemura, Paulo Priante Kayano, Natasha Kouvaleski Saviano Moran, Carolina Ko Chen, Marcelo Langer Wroclawski, et al. 2018. "The Role of Immunohistochemical Analysis as a Tool for the Diagnosis, Prognostic Evaluation and Treatment of Prostate Cancer: A Systematic Review of the Literature." *Frontiers in Oncology* 8: 377.

Cho, Junhun. 2022. "Basic Immunohistochemistry for Lymphoma Diagnosis. *Blood Research* 57 (S1): 55–61.

Choi, Yoo Jin, Woongchang Yoon, Areum Lee, Youngmin Han, Yoonhyeong Byun, Jae Seung Kang, Hongbeom Kim, et al. 2021. "Diagnostic Model for Pancreatic Cancer Using a Multi-Biomarker Panel." *Annals of Surgical Treatment and Research* 100 (3): 144–53.

Condappa, Andrew, Donovan McGrowder, William Aiken, Wayne McLaughlin, and Maxine Gossell-Williams. 2020. "Evaluation of Plasma Circulating Cell-Free DNA Concentration and Integrity in Patients With Prostate Cancer in Jamaica: A Preliminary Study." *Diseases* 8 (3): 34.

Dasgupta, Atreyi, Motonari Nomura, Ryan Shuck, and Jason Yustein. "Cancer's Achilles' Heel: Apoptosis and Necroptosis to the Rescue. 2016. "*International Journal of Molecular Sciences* 18 (1): 23.

Ding, Qingqing, Lei Huo, Yan Peng, Esther C. Yoon, Zaibo Li, and Aysegul A. Sahin. 2022." Immunohistochemical Markers for Distinguishing Metastatic Breast Carcinoma From Other Common Malignancies: Update and Revisit." *Seminars in Diagnostic Pathology* 39 (5): 313–21.

Engvall, E. 2010. "The ELISA, Enzyme-Linked Immunosorbent Assay." *Clinical Chemistry* 56 (2): 319–20.

Falcucci, Susanna, Francesca Paolini, Anna Maria Mileo, Rosella Franconi, Silvia Massa, Antonio Rinaldi, and Aldo Venuti. 2021. "ePCL Electrospun Microfibrous Layers for Immune Assays: Sensitive ELISA for the Detection of Serum Antibodies Against HPV16 E7 Oncoprotein." *ACS Omega* 6 (13): 8778–83.

Feinberg, Andrew P. 2018. "The Key Role of Epigenetics in Human Disease Prevention and Mitigation." *New England Journal of Medicine* 378 (14): 1323–34.

Glaser, Matthias, Sajinder K. Luthra, and Frank Brady. 2003. "Applications of Positron-Emitting Halogens in PET Oncology." *International Journal of Oncology* 22 (2): 253–67.

Gregg, Edward W., Andrea M. Kriska, Loran M. Salamone, Matthew M. Roberts, S. J. Aderson, Robert E. Ferrell, Lewis H. Kuller, and Jane A. Cauley. 1997. "The Epidemiology of Quantitative Ultrasound: A Review of the Relationships With Bone Mass, Osteoporosis and Fracture Risk." *Osteoporosis International* 7 (2): 89–99.

Guo, Xinyue, Zhang Zhang, Maosheng Yang, Pibin Bing, Xin Yan, Qili Yang, Dequan Wei, Longhai Liu, Lanju Liang, and Jianquan Yao. 2021. "Time-Frequency Double Domain Resolving by Electromagnetically Induced Transparency Metasensors for Rapid and Label-Free Detection of Cancer Biomarker Midkine." *Optics and Lasers in Engineering* 142: 106566.

Habli, Zeina, Walid AlChamaa, Raya Saab, Humam Kadara, and Massoud L. Khraiche. 2020. "Circulating Tumor Cell Detection Technologies and Clinical Utility: Challenges and Opportunities." *Cancers* 12 (7): 1930.

Hammoudi, Naima, Kausar Begam Riaz Ahmed, Celia Garcia-Prieto, and Peng Huang. 2011. "Metabolic Alterations in Cancer Cells and Therapeutic Implications." *Chinese Journal of Cancer* 30 (8): 508.

Hashemi, Atiyeh, Abdol Hamid Pilevar, and Reza Rafeh. 2013. "Mass Detection in Lung CT Images Using Region Growing Segmentation and Decision Making Based on Fuzzy Inference System and Artificial Neural Network." *International Journal of Image, Graphics and Signal Processing* 5 (6): 16–24. https://doi.org/10.5815/ijigsp.2013.06.03.

Heidrich, Isabel, Lucija Ačkar, Parinaz Mossahebi Mohammadi, and Klaus Pantel. 2020. "Liquid Biopsies: Potential and Challenges." *International Journal of Cancer* 148 (3): 528–45.

Heywang-Köbrunner, Sylvia H., Astrid Hacker, and Stefan Sedlacek. 2011. "Advantages and Disadvantages of Mammography Screening." *Breast Care* 6 (3): 199–207.

Hsu, Phillip J., Khushboo Singh, Ankit Dhiman, Hunter D. D. Witmer, Chuan He, Oliver S. Eng, Daniel V. T. Catenacci, Mitchell C. Posner, and Kiran K. Turaga. 2022. "Utility of Perioperative Measurement of Cell-Free DNA and Circulating Tumor DNA in Informing the Prognosis of GI Cancers: A Systematic Review." *JCO Precision Oncology* 6: e2100337.

Inamura, Kentaro. 2018 "Update on Immunohistochemistry for the Diagnosis of Lung Cancer." *Cancers* 10 (30): 72.

Iqbal, Nida, and Naveed Iqbal. 2014. "Human Epidermal Growth Factor Receptor 2 (HER2) in Cancers: Overexpression and Therapeutic Implications." *Molecular Biology International* 2014: 852748. https://doi.org/10.1155/2014/852748.

Jaitley, Shweta, Pankaj Agarwal, and Ramballabh Upadhyay. 2015. "Role of Oral Exfoliative Cytology in Predicting Premalignant Potential of Oral Submucous Fibrosis: A Short Study." *Journal of Cancer Research and Therapeutics* 11 (2): 471–4. https://doi.org/10.4103/0973-1482.151421.

Jhamb, Tanuj Kumar, Vinith Rejathalal, and V. K. Govindan. 2015. "A Review on Image Reconstruction Through MRI k-Space Data." *International Journal of Image, Graphics and Signal Processing* 7 (7): 42. https://doi.org/10.5815/ijigsp.2015.07.06.

Jiang, Di, Xue Zhang, Man Liu, Yulin Wang, Tingting Wang, Lu Pei, Peng Wang, et al. 2021. "Discovering Panel of Autoantibodies for Early Detection of Lung Cancer Based on Focused Protein Array." *Frontiers in Immunology* 12: 658922.

Jin, Cancan, Kankai Wang, Anthony Oppong-Gyebi, and Jiangnan Hu. 2020. "Application of Nanotechnology in Cancer Diagnosis and Therapy-A Mini-Review." *International Journal of Medical Sciences* 17 (18): 2964–73.

Jin, Yong, and Wei Da. 2013. "RETRACTED ARTICLE: Screening of Key Genes in Gastric Cancer With DNA Microarray Analysis." *European Journal of Medical Research* 18: 1–7.

Khalkhali Iraj, Ismael Mena, and Linda Diggles. 1994. "Review of Imaging Techniques for the Diagnosis of Breast Cancer: A New Role of Prone Scintimammography Using Technetium-99m Sestamibi." *European Journal of Nuclear Medicine* 21 (4): 357–62.

Konstantinou, George N. 2017. "Enzyme-Linked Immunosorbent Assay (ELISA)." *Food Allergens: Methods and Protocols* 79–94.

Kotzsch, Matthias, Thomas Kirchner, Susanne Soelch, Sonja Schäfer, Katrin Friedrich, Gustavo Baretton, Viktor Magdolen, and Thomas Luther. 2017. "Inverse Association of rab31 and Mucin-1 (CA15-3) Antigen Levels in Estrogen Receptor-Positive (ER+) Breast Cancer Tissues With Clinicopathological Parameters and Patients' Prognosis." *American Journal of Cancer Research* 7 (9): 1959.

Koul, Nimrita, and Sunilkumar S. Manvi. 2021. "Framework for Classification of Cancer Gene Expression Data Using Bayesian Hyper-Parameter Optimization." *Medical & Biological Engineering & Computing* 59: 2353–71.

Krishnamurthy, Nithya, Emily Spencer, Ali Torkamani, and Laura Nicholson. 2017. "Liquid Biopsies for Cancer: Coming to a Patient Near You." *Journal of Clinical Medicine* 6 (1): 3.

Landegren, U., and M. Hammond. 2021. "Cancer Diagnostics Based on Plasma Protein Biomarkers: Hard Times But Great expectations." *Molecular Oncology* 15 (6): 1715–26. doi: 10.1002/1878-0261.12809.

Lawrence, Rachel, Melissa Watters, Caitlin R. Davies, Klaus Pantel, and Yong-Jie Lu. 2023. "Circulating Tumour Cells for Early Detection of Clinically Relevant Cancer." *Nature Reviews Clinical Oncology* 1–14.

Li, Shan-Shan, Yuan-Yuan Tan, Yan Zhang, Mingjun Liu, and Aihua Liu. 2021. "A Simple Electrochemical Immunosensor Based on Worm-Like Platinum for Highly Sensitive Determination of Alpha-Fetoprotein." *Bioelectrochemistry* 140: 107804.

Lichtenstein, Anatoly V. 2018. "Genetic Mosaicism and Cancer: Cause and Effect." *Cancer Research* 78 (6): 1375–8.

Lokman, Noor A, Carmela Ricciardelli, Andrew N. Stephens, Thomas W. Jobling, Peter Hoffmann, and Martin K. Oehler. 2021. "Diagnostic Value of Plasma Annexin a2 in Early-Stage High-Grade Serous Ovarian Cancer." *Diagnostics* 11 (1): 69.

Luo, Huiyan, Qi Zhao, Wei Wei, Lianghong Zheng, Shaohua Yi, Gen Li, Wenqiu Wang, et al. 2020. "Circulating Tumor DNA Methylation Profiles Enable Early Diagnosis, Prognosis Prediction, and Screening for Colorectal Cancer." *Science Translational Medicine* 12 (524): eaax7533.

Magaki, Shino, Seyed A. Hojat, Bowen Wei, Alexandra So, and William H. Yong. 2019. "An Introduction to the Performance of Immunohistochemistry." *Biobanking: Methods and Protocols* 1897: 289–98. https://doi.org/10.1007/978-1-4939-8935-5_25.

Malik, Showkat Hassan, Tariq Ahmad Lone, and S. M. K. Quadri. 2016. "Imaging Techniques for Cancer Diagnosis and Scope for Enhancement." *International Journal of Image, Graphics and Signal Processing* 8 (5): 83–91. https://doi.org/10.5815/ijigsp.2016.05.08.

Marx, V. 2019. "How to Follow Metabolic Clues to Find Cancer's Achilles Heel." *Nature Methods* 16 (3): 221–4.

Mehrotra, Ravi, Sanjay Mishra, Mamta Singh, and Mangal Singh. 2011. "The Efficacy of Oral Brush Biopsy With Computer-Assisted Analysis in Identifying Precancerous and Cancerous Lesions." *Head & Neck Oncology* 3 (1): 1–8.

Minciacchi, V. R., A. Zijlstra, Mark Andrew Rubin, and D. Di Vizio. 2017. "Extracellular Vesicles for Liquid Biopsy in Prostate Cancer: Where are We and Where are We Headed?." *Prostate Cancer and Prostatic Diseases* 20 (3): 251–8.

Mosleh-Shirazi, Sareh, Milad Abbasi, Mohammad reza Moaddeli, Ahmad Vaez, Mostafa Shafiee, Seyed Reza Kasaee, Ali Mohammad Amani, and Saeid Hatam. 2022. "Nanotechnology Advances in the Detection and Treatment of Cancer: An Overview." *Nanotheranostics* 6 (4): 400.

Nicosia, Luca, Giulia Gnocchi, Ilaria Gorini, Massimo Venturini, Federico Fontana, Filippo Pesapane, Ida Abiuso, et al. 2023. "History of Mammography: Analysis of Breast Imaging Diagnostic Achievements Over the Last Century." *Healthcare* 11 (11): 1596. https://doi.org/10.3390/healthcare11111596.

Nie, Xiao-Cui, Fang He, Chong Lan, Ju-Min Niu, and Pu Xia. 2021. "Combined Serum DKK3 and Circulating CD133 Cells as Prognostic Biomarkers for Ovarian Cancer Patients." *OncoTargets and Therapy* 427–34.

Nischal, U., K. C. Nischal, and U. Khopkar. 2008. "Techniques of Skin Biopsy and Practical Considerations." *Journal of Cutaneous Aesthetic Surgery* 1 (2): 107–11. doi: 10.4103/0974-2077.44174.

Painter, J, T., N. P. Clayton, and R. A. Herbert. 2010. "Useful Immunohistochemical Markers of Tumor Differentiation." *Toxicologic Pathology* 38 (1): 131–41.

Papatheodoridi, Alkistis, Nikolaos Karakousis, Panagiotis Lembessis, Antonios Chatzigeorgiou, and George V. Papatheodoridis. 2021. "The Significance of Circulating Cell-Free DNA Markers in Chronic Hepatitis B Patients With Hepatocellular Carcinoma." *Pathogens* 10 (11): 1524.

Parida, Sheetal, and Dipali Sharma. 2021. "The Microbiome and Cancer: Creating Friendly Neighborhoods and Removing the Foes Within." *Cancer Research* 81 (4): 790–800.

Parungo, Cherie P., Shunsuke Ohnishi, Alec M. De Grand, Rita G. Laurence, Edward G. Soltesz, Yolonda L. Colson, Peter M. Kang, Tomislav Mihaljevic, Lawrence H. Cohn, and John V. Frangioni. 2004. "In Vivo Optical Imaging of Pleural Space Drainage to Lymph Nodes of Prognostic Significance." *Annals of Surgical Oncology* 11: 1085–92. https://doi.org/10.1245/ASO.2004.03.054.

Poljak, Mario, Kate Cuschieri, Laia Alemany, and Alex Vorsters. 2023. "Testing for Human Papillomaviruses in Urine, Blood, and Oral Specimens: An Update for the Laboratory." *Journal of Clinical Microbiology* 61 (8): e01403–22.

Pulumati, Akhil, Anika Pulumati, Bilikere S. Dwarakanath, Amit Verma, and Rao V. L. Papineni. 2023. "Technological Advancements in Cancer Diagnostics: Improvements and Limitations." *Cancer Reports* 6(2): e1764.

Quraish, Reeshanul, Tetsuyuki Hirahata, Afraz ul Quraish, and Shahan ul Quraish. 2023. "An Overview: Genetic Tumor Markers for Early Detection and Current Gene Therapy Strategies." *Cancer Informatics* 22 (2023). https://doi.org/10.1177/11769351221150772.

Ramani, R., N. Suthanthira, and Vanitha. 2014. "Computer Aided Detection of Tumours in Mammograms." *International Journal of Image Graphics and Signal Processing* 6 (4): 54–9. https://doi.org/10.5815/ijigsp.2014.04.07.

Rao, Priya, Guy Lahat, Christina Arnold, Alde Carlo Gavino, Sharon Lahat, Jason L. Hornick, Dina Lev, and Alexander J. Lazar. 2013. "Angiosarcoma: A Tissue Microarray Study With Diagnostic Implications." *The American Journal of Dermatopathology* 35 (4): 432–7.

Rapado-González, Óscar, José Luis López-Cedrún, Ramón Manuel Lago-Lestón, Alicia Abalo, Guillermo Rubin-Roger, Ángel Salgado-Barreira, Rafael López-López, Laura Muinelo-Romay, and María Mercedes Suárez-Cunqueiro. 2022. "Integrity and Quantity of Salivary Cell-Free DNA as a Potential Molecular Biomarker in Oral Cancer: A Preliminary Study." *Journal of Oral Pathology & Medicine* 51 (5): 429–35.

Rossi, Roberta Elisa, Alessandra Elvevi, Camilla Gallo, Andrea Palermo, Pietro Invernizzi, and Sara Massironi. 2022. "Endoscopic Techniques for Diagnosis and Treatment of Gastro-Entero-Pancreatic Neuroendocrine Neoplasms: Where We are." *World Journal of Gastroenterology* 28 (26): 3258. https://doi.org/10.3748/wjg.v28.i26.3258. PMID: 36051341; PMCID: PMC9331536.

Roy, P. S., and B. J. Saikia. 2016. "Cancer and Cure: A Critical Analysis." *Indian Journal of Cancer* 53 (3): 441–2.

Sarode, Venetia R., and Linda Robinson. 2019. "Screening for Lynch Syndrome by Immunohistochemistry of Mismatch Repair Proteins: Significance of Indeterminate Result and Correlation With Mutational Studies." *Archives of Pathology & Laboratory Medicine* 143 (10): 1225–33.

Seelige, Ruth, Stephen Searles, and Jack D. Bui. 2018. "Innate Sensing of Cancer's Non-Immunologic Hallmarks." *Current Opinion in Immunology* 50: 1–8.

Seo, In-Ho, and Yong-Jae Lee. 2022. "Usefulness of Complete Blood Count (CBC) to Assess Cardiovascular and Metabolic Diseases in Clinical Settings: A Comprehensive Literature Review." *Biomedicines* 10 (11): 2697.

Sfeir, Agnel, and Lorraine S. Symington. 2015. "Microhomology-Mediated End Joining: A Back-Up Survival Mechanism or Dedicated Pathway?." *Trends in Biochemical Sciences* 40 (11): 701–14.

Shah, Karishma, and Panagiotis Maghsoudlou. 2016. "Enzyme-Linked Immunosorbent Assay (ELISA): The Basics." *British Journal of Hospital Medicine* 77 (7): C98–101.

Shaila, M., P. Shetty, and P. Pai. "2016. A New Approach to Exfoliative Cytology: A Comparative Cytomorphometric Study." *Indian Journal of Cancer* 53 (1): 193–8.

Shi, Jiping, Runling Zhang, Jinming Li, and Rui Zhang. 2020. "Size Profile of Cell-Free DNA: A Beacon Guiding the Practice and Innovation of Clinical Testing." *Theranostics* 10 (11): 4737–48.

Skandarajah, Arunan, Sumsum P. Sunny, Praveen Gurpur, Clay D. Reber, Michael V. D'Ambrosio, Nisheena Raghavan, Bonney Lee James, et al. 2017. "Mobile Microscopy as a Screening Tool for Oral Cancer in India: A Pilot Study." *PLoS One* 12 (11): e0188440. https://doi.org/10.1371/journal.pone.0188440.

Skvortsova, K., C. Stirzaker, and P. Taberlay. 2019. The DNA Methylation Landscape in Cancer. *Essays Biochem* 63: 797–811. [PMC free article] [PubMed] [Google Scholar].

Štefatić, Daria, Monika Riederer, Marija Balić, Nadia Dandachi, Stefanie Stanzer, Birgit Janesch, Margit Resel, Darko Ler, Hellmut Samonigg, and Thomas Bauernhofer. 2008. "Optimization of Diagnostic ELISA-Based

Tests for the Detection of Auto-Antibodies Against Tumor Antigens in Human Serum." *Bosnian Journal of Basic Medical Sciences* 8 (3): 245. https://doi.org/10.17305/bjbms.2008.2926.

Sung, H., J. Ferlay, R. L. Siegel, M. Laversanne, I. Soerjomataram, A. Jemal, and F. Bray. 2021. "Global Cancer Statistics 2020: GLOBOCAN Estimates of Incidence and Mortality Worldwide for 36 Cancers in 185 Countries." *CA Cancer Journal for Clinicians* 71 (3): 209–49. doi: 10.3322/caac.21660.

Sylvie-Louise Avon, D., and H. B. Klieb. 2012. "Oral Soft-Tissue Biopsy: An Overview." *Journal of the Canadian Dental Association* 78: c75.

Torre, Lindsey A., Rebecca L. Siegel, Elizabeth M. Ward, and Ahmedin Jemal. 2016. "Global Cancer Incidence and Mortality Rates and Trends—an Update." *Cancer Epidemiology, Biomarkers & Prevention* 25 (1): 16–27.

Trejo-Ayala, R. A., M. Luna-Pérez, M. Gutiérrez-Romero, J. Collazo-Jaloma, M. C. Cedillo-Pérez, and C. O. Ramos-Peñafiel. 2015. "Bone Marrow Aspiration and Biopsy. Technique and Considerations." *RevistaMédica Del Hospital General De México* 78 (4): 196–201. https://doi.org/10.1016/j.hgmx.2015.06.006.

Tufail, Ahsan Bin, Yong-Kui Ma, Mohammed K. A. Kaabar, Francisco Martínez, A. R. Junejo, Inam Ullah, and Rahim Khan. 2021. "Deep Learning in Cancer Diagnosis and Prognosis Prediction: A Minireview on Challenges, Recent Trends, and Future Directions." *Computational and Mathematical Methods in Medicine* 2021 (2021). https://doi.org/10.1155/2021/9025470.

Vidal, Joana, Alvaro Taus, and Clara Montagut. 2020. "Dynamic Treatment Stratification Using ctDNA." *Tumor Liquid Biopsies* 263–73.

Von Brandenstein, Melanie, Jan Herden, Barbara Köditz, Manuel Huerta, Tim Nestler, Axel Heidenreich, and Jochen W. U. Fries. 2021. "Non-Invasive Urine Markers for the Differentiation Between RCCs and Oncocytoma." *Journal of Clinical Laboratory Analysis* 35 (5): e23762.

Wu, Li, and Xiaogang Qu. 2015. "Cancer Biomarker Detection: Recent Achievements and Challenges." *Chemical Society Reviews* 44 (10): 2963–97.

Xing, Li, and Ruiping Wang. 2011. "A New Efficient 2D Combined With 3D CAD System for Solitary Pulmonary Nodule Detection in CT Images." *International Journal of Image, Graphics and Signal Processing* 3 (4): 18–24.

Xue, Jin-min, Yi Liu, Ling-hong Wan, and Yu-xi Zhu. 2020. "Comprehensive Analysis of Differential Gene Expression to Identify Common Gene Signatures in Multiple Cancers." *Medical Science Monitor: International Medical Journal of Experimental and Clinical Research* 26: e919953–1.

Yang, H.-X., Y. Yang, X.-D. Li, X.-M. Miao, C. Yang, D.-F. Zhi, H. Su, et al. 2021. "The Detection of SAS1B in Serum Provides Clues for Early Diagnosis of Thyroid Cancer." *European Review for Medical & Pharmacological Sciences* 25 (3) (2021).

Zemskov, M. Y., M. V. Marinets, A. V. Sivkov, J. V. Pavlova, A. N. Shibaev, and K. S. Sorokin. 2021. "Integrin Alpha V in Urine: A Novel Noninvasive Marker for Prostate Cancer Detection." *Frontier in Oncology* 10 (10): 610647. doi: 10.3389/fonc.2020.610647.

Zhang, Yejun, Hongchao Yang, Xinyi An, Zan Wang, Xiaohu Yang, Mengxuan Yu, Rong Zhang, Ziqiang Sun, and Qiangbin Wang. 2020. "Controlled Synthesis of Ag2Te@ Ag2S Core–Shell Quantum Dots With Enhanced and Tunable Fluorescence in the Second Near-Infrared Window." *Small* 16 (14): 2001003.

5 Uncovering the Impact of Nanoparticles in Cancer Diagnosis

Priyanka Chambial, Asvin Suresh Babu, and Neelam Thakur

ABBREVIATIONS

Acronym	Full Form
GNPs	gold nanoparticles
CTCs	circulating tumor cells
LPs	liposomes
SPION	superparamagnetic iron oxide NPs
EPR	enhanced permeability and retention effect
PNPs	polymeric nanoparticles
QDs	quantum dots
Co and Ni	cobalt and nickel
GO	graphene
MNPs	magnetic nanoparticles
AuNPs	gold nanoparticles
LTLD	magnetic resonance imaging
CT	computed tomography
NPs	nanoparticles
CNTs	carbon nanotubes
NPs	nanoparticles

5.1 INTRODUCTION

Tumor incidence and mortality rates are still very high all around the world. Cancer is the primary cause of mortality on a global scale, resulting in around 8 million deaths per year (Liu et al. 2019). Conventional methods of treating malignancies have faced criticism due to their inefficiency, high likelihood of undesirable side effects, and mediocre rates of effectiveness. In the current circumstances, it is of utmost importance to ascertain a carrier that is both safer and more efficient (Herma et al. 2019). The utilization of nanoparticles (NPs) as carriers in innovative tumor treatment strategies has gained significant popularity due to their diminutive dimensions, biosafety considerations, drug-loading capabilities, and physical features that might facilitate physical therapy. Nanoparticle-based pharmaceuticals possess the capacity to concurrently address many medical problems, exhibit reduced incidence of undesirable effects, and demonstrate enhanced overall efficacy (Woodman et al. 2021). Many medical imaging systems rely on nanoparticles to enhance clarity and precision, which aids in accurate tumor diagnosis (Israel et al. 2020). As nanotechnology and medical technology have progressed, a wide variety of materials, including gold, silver, liposomes, etc., has been utilized in the development of NPs.

DOI: 10.1201/9781003463191-7

The field of cancer diagnostics and treatments places significant emphasis on the timely identification and suppression of malignant cell proliferation and metastasis. Nanotechnology's contributions to the development of cutting-edge diagnostic tools have opened the door to a new era of innovation in medicine. However, it is important to consider that early diagnosis is key to better prognosis and better quality of life for patients (Kim et al. 2010). Despite the emergence of various imaging modalities such as computed tomography, ultrasound, and magnetic resonance imaging (MRI) as potential early diagnostic tools for cancer, their effectiveness is limited due to a lack of comprehensive clinical data across different stages of cancer (Wang et al. 2010).

In addition, there are limitations with conventional imaging techniques that make it difficult to distinguish between benign and malignant tumors, necessitating confirmation of cancer through histology or cytology. Nanotechnology has enabled the development of cutting-edge molecular contrast media and materials that have greatly improved the speed and accuracy of both the initial diagnosis and ongoing assessment of cancer treatment. Particularly in spotting the initial stage of cancer, nanoparticle imaging of tumor tissue has been used (Bicak et al. 2021). Using MRI, cancer metastases can be located with the use of immune superparamagnetic iron oxide NPs (SPIONs) that target cancer cell lines. Recent studies have shown that SPIONs are an ideal building block for aerosols in MRI imaging of lung cancer due to their high specificity and minimum side effects (Pramanik 2019). These developments have great promise for giving in-depth diagnoses of diseases and facilitating the administration of targeted treatments (Wan et al. 2016). When used for cancer diagnosis, nanotechnology's incorporation into existing diagnostic methods holds great promise for more accurate early detection and better overall patient care. The application of nanotechnology has significant promise in enhancing cancer therapy and enhancing patients' quality of life (Sherry and Woods 2008).

Chemotherapy, surgery, radiation therapy, and their many combinations are currently the gold standard for treating cancer. Nonspecificity and toxicity are just two of the many difficulties with these methods. The goal of contemporary medicine is to optimize drug pharmacological action while minimizing unwanted side effects. To reduce side effects, the drug must be administered at a higher dosage directly to the tumor and at a lower concentration to surrounding healthy tissue (Figure 5.1) (Gmeiner and Ghosh 2016). The utilization of nanotechnology in cancer treatment is already beyond the limitations of what was previously achievable. Using nanotechnology, we can decrease the overall dose of drugs needed for treatment while raising the drug concentration directly at the site of the tumor without affecting healthy tissue. This novel approach holds promise of significantly augmenting the effectiveness of cancer therapies and improving patient prognoses (Singh 2005).

This review will look into the different ways in which nanotechnology is changing the face of oncology and explore the enormous promise it has for cancer treatment. Exploring this cutting-edge area will help improve cancer diagnosis (Mazahir et al. 2023). Imaging procedures, laboratory tests, and morphological inspection of tissues and cells are today able to diagnose the vast majority of malignancies in a patient. Immunohistochemistry analysis, histological changes, mutation analysis, and molecular genetics research are all examples of pathological features that can be used to identify cancer (Zhang et al. 2020).

Magnetic, polymeric, quantum dots, graphene, liposome, carbon nanotube, and dendrimer are a few examples of NPs utilized in cancer detection (Figure 5.2). These NPs also serve important functions in several imaging techniques. Nanoparticles stay for a long time in the bloodstream before they can access the target cells and pass past the many barriers they encounter along the way (Bhardwaj and Rasool 2023). In the same way as the composition of nanoparticles can vary, the composition of their beginning ingredients, such as biological lipids, dextran, chitosan, or chemicals like silica, etc., can also vary. Because of their profound influence on nanodrug transport efficiency and, by extension, on the regulation of therapeutic efficacy, the sizes, surface features, and shapes of the nanoparticles used in medical therapy

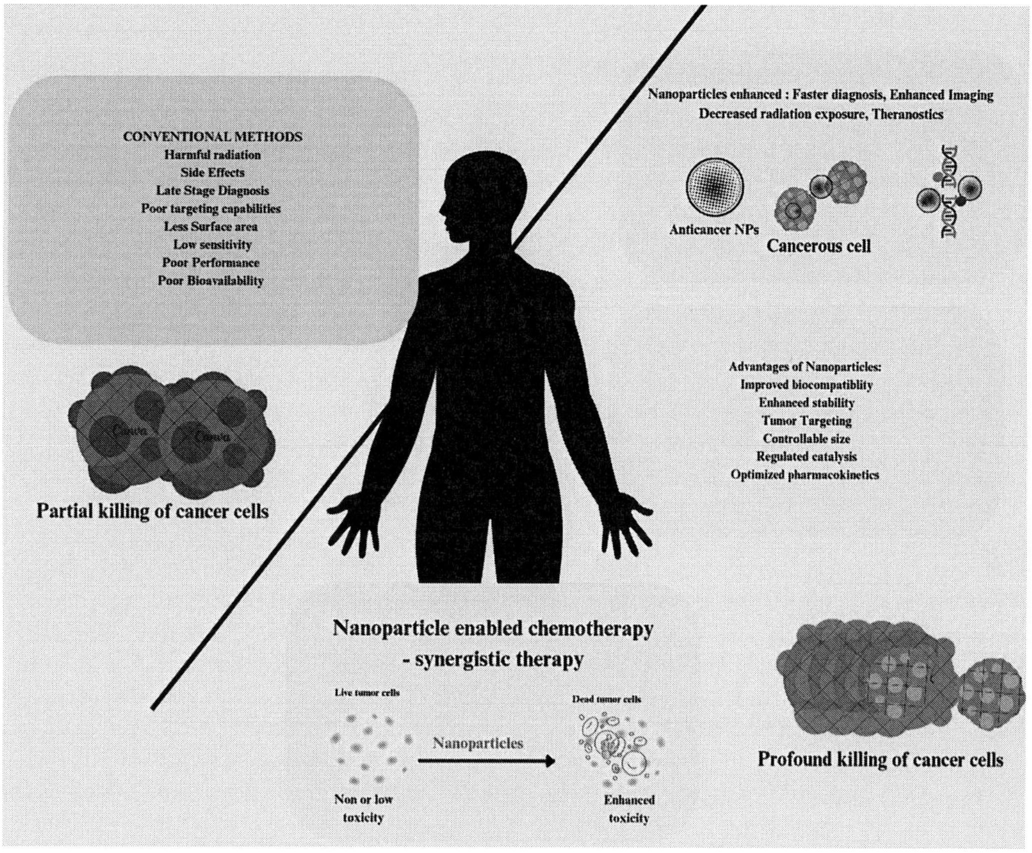

FIGURE 5.1 Benefits of using NPs to boost cancer diagnosis compared to traditional methods of cancer diagnosis. Nanoparticles offer increased biocompatibility, enhanced stability, optimized pharmacokinetics, and regulated catalysis.

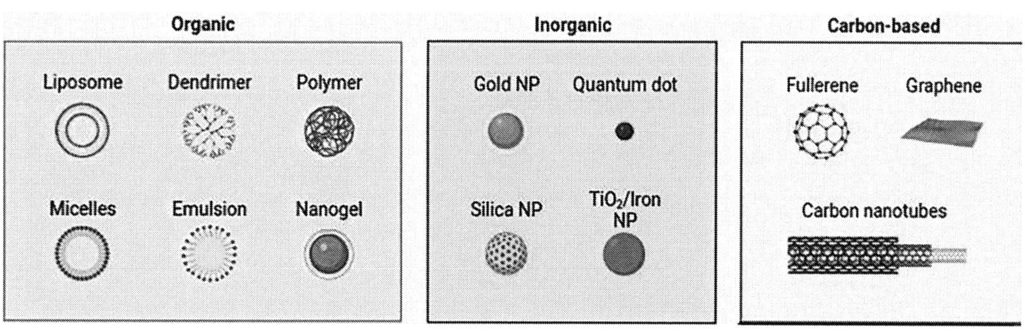

FIGURE 5.2 The following are various categories of nanoparticles employed in the diagnosis of cancer. There are three main categories into which the entities fall: organic, inorganic, and carbon-based.

are of enormous relevance (Beriso 2017). Cancer therapy typically employs NPs with a diameter between 10 and 100 nm due to their capacity to efficiently transport drugs and produce an enhanced permeability and retention (EPR) effect. However, particles with less than 10 nm diameter are not effectively filtered by the kidneys and can rapidly infiltrate the normal vasculature, where they may damage healthy cells (Marques et al. 2020).

5.2 COMMONLY USED NANOPARTICLES IN CANCER DIAGNOSIS

5.2.1 Polymeric Nanoparticles (PNPs)

Active compounds can be surface-adsorbed onto the polymeric core of 1 to 1,000 nm polymeric nanoparticles or loaded inside of them (Ahmed et al. 2020). Despite their physical differences, nanospheres and nanocapsules are both commonly referred to as "nanoparticles" (Soppimath et al. 2001). The utilization of polymeric nanoparticles has exhibited encouraging outcomes in the context of targeted medication delivery for the therapeutic intervention of numerous ailments Owens and Peppas 2006). The surface properties of PNPs can be altered through the attachment of certain polymers or the utilization of diverse polymer endgroups. PNPs have demonstrated efficacy in mitigating cytotoxic adverse effects. A diverse range of polymers, which are biocompatible and biodegradable, have been granted approval by the FDA for their application in the field of human medicine (Dang and Guan 2020). Nanoparticles based on polymers might be either organic or synthetic. They have many benefits over other nanocarriers (Duncan 2003), including liposomes, micelles, and inorganic nanosystems. Several chemotherapeutics have been encased in polymeric delivery systems to boost antitumor efficacy, prevent metastases, reduce the effective dose, and lessen unwanted effects (Miyata et al. 2011). Polymers can either encapsulate an active material in their structure or adsorb it to their surfaces. In cancer nanomedicine, PNPs have attracted a lot of interest because of their potential to overcome the difficulty of drug delivery while causing few undesirable side effects or leading to drug resistance (Marques et al. 2020). These PNPs have demonstrated promising results in the creation of nanotechnology-based cancer medicines. For instance, adriamycin-conjugated nanomaterials have shown significant therapeutic effects when used to treat several forms of cancer (Feng and Zhao 2016). Furthermore, there has been research conducted on the utilization of near-infrared fluorescent polymeric nanoparticles that are loaded with the anticancer drug doxorubicin, to employ them in the fields of cancer imaging and therapy. The research team has also developed a study on the biodistribution of nanoparticle in non–small cell lung cancer (Huang 2022).

5.2.2 Liposomes (LPs)

Liposomes are the most widely employed nanocarriers for a variety of hydrophobic and hydrophilic substances with potential biological activity because of their remarkable biocompatibility and minimal immunogenicity (Figure 5.3) (Olusanya et al. 2018). There is a wide range of diversity in liposome attributes, including lipid composition, size, and surface charge. The potential of liposomes as nanocarriers is growing as a means to improve patient outcomes through earlier diagnosis and more effective, highly focused, and safe treatment. Liposomes, tiny spherical structures made up of lipid bilayers, have garnered considerable interest in the field of cancer diagnostics (Shah et al. 2017). Targeted medication administration and imaging in cancer diagnostics are facilitated by various advantages they provide. Liposomes have the capability to include contrast agents, such as fluorescent dyes or nanoparticles, in order to improve imaging techniques like fluorescence imaging or MRI (Raza et al. 2023). In addition, liposomes can be modified with precise targeting ligands, such as antibodies, to specifically concentrate in tumor tissues. This facilitates enhanced visualization of tumors and permits accurate identification of cancer cells. Liposomes offer a regulated discharge of enclosed imaging chemicals, enabling extended imaging and enhanced sensitivity (Saraf et al. 2020). In summary, liposomes have significant potential in the field of cancer diagnostics since they enhance imaging capabilities and facilitate the precise administration of contrast chemicals to tumor tissues.

5.2.3 Dendrimers

Dendrimers are special nanoscale molecules with a specified, monodisperse, and radially symmetric structure. They have a symmetrical core, an outer shell, and an inner shell. They are versatile and

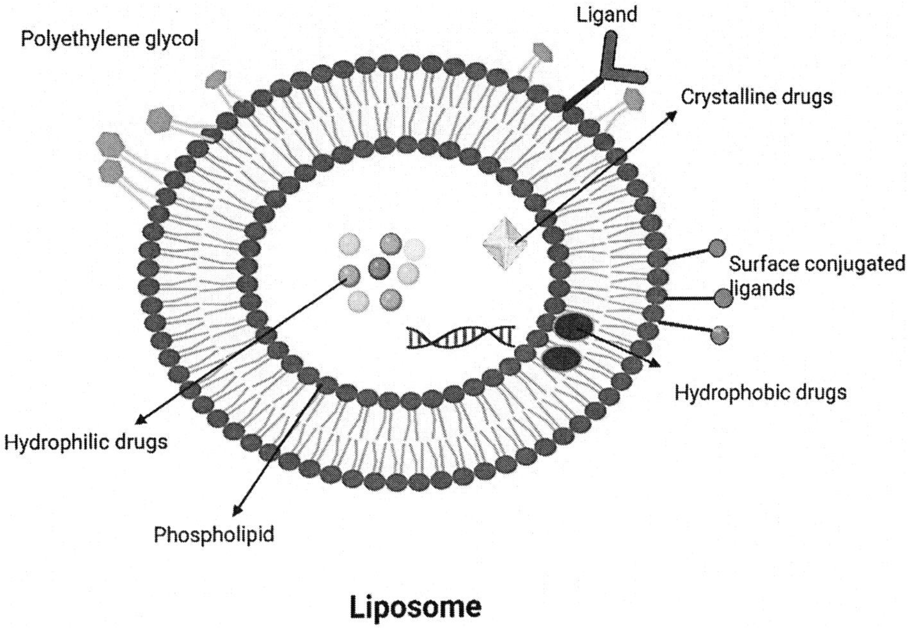

FIGURE 5.3 A quick overview of the liposome structure. The ability of liposomes to encapsulate drug molecules in their aqueous interior or in their lipophilic membrane, together with their hydrophobic and hydrophilic characteristics, makes them an attractive candidate for drug delivery vehicles.

useful in many contexts (Abbasi et al. 2014). When possessing a hydrophobic core and a hydrophilic outer layer, these entities are capable of operating as micelles, which are single-molecule structures with a variety of uses. Dendrimers have been used successfully to enclose and dissolve hydrophobic drugs inside their intramolecular cavity using this feature. Cationic dendrimers have also shown promise as a non-viral means of transporting genes. Dendrimers modified with metal chelates are extremely useful in MRI contrast agents (Han et al. 2017). Drug–dendrimer conjugates are another common application of dendrimers. The selective accumulation of these conjugates in solid tumors, together with their high solubility and minimal systemic toxicity, renders them potential candidates for the administration of drugs. Multiple approaches have been suggested to include colors, genetic material, targeting agents, and pharmaceutical compounds within the dendrimer structure. These methods include encapsulation, complexation, and conjugation (Agarwal et al. 2009).

Because of its affinity for CD44 receptors, hyaluronic acid–coupled PAMAM dendrimer has shown improved tumor-penetrating characteristics. As mannose can only bind to mannose receptors expressed on the macrophages, a liver-X-receptor-coupled PAMAM dendrimer has been designed for the selective delivery of ligands to macrophages (Ghai et al. 2018). Potential applications of dendrimers span numerous fields, from medical imaging to gene therapy. They are extremely applicable for many applications in nanomedicine due to their well-defined shapes and distinctive characteristics (Kolhe et al. 2006). The potential applications of dendrimers in cancer diagnosis are shown in Table 5.1.

5.2.4 Quantum Dots (QDs)

QDs are artificially synthesized nanoscale crystals that possess unique optical properties, including the capacity to transport electrons and the potential to emit diverse hues of light upon exposure to ultraviolet rays (Fang et al. 2017). Synthetic semiconductor nanoparticles possess a wide range of potential applications, including fluorescent biological tagging, displays, illumination, and medical

TABLE 5.1
Cancer Diagnosis Using Dendrimers

Complex	Treatment	Uses	Outcomes	Reference
PAMAM G4.5 dendrimer	Breast cancer	Diagnosis	Uptake studies (both in vivo and in vitro)	Teow et al. (2011)
Cisplatin and human antigen	Encapsulation of chemotherapeutic drugs	Drug delivery	In vitro development of multifunctional dendrimer-based nanoparticles	Bulbake et al. (2019)
5-aminolevulinic acid–based dendrimers	Bladder cancer	Diagnosis	A novel in vivo strategy for the diagnosis of fluorescence diagnosis	Singla et al. (2019)
PG4 and cationic dendrimer generation	Breast cancer	Analysis of cell cycle	Dendrimers as carrier delivery in in vitro breast cancer	Harish et al. (2022)

imaging. The effective application of QDs in many demonstrations can be attributed to their notable photostability, high extinction coefficient, and brightness, as well as their significant stroke shift (Peng and Li 2010). Organic dyes are unsuitable for many imaging and biosensing applications because of their inability to exhibit all these characteristics. They have a high surface area and can be tracked visually in vitro. When developing multimodal/multifunctional probes, QDs may offer an advantage over much bigger silica and polymer-based nanoparticles (Wang and Chen 2011). In a variety of cancers, overexpressed receptors are critical for target identification and bioimaging. By attaching QDs to antibodies or ligands specific to cancer, it is possible to detect cancer cells (Tholouli et al. 2008). These cancers include prostate, breast, and pancreatic cancer metastatic tumors, glioblastoma, bone marrow, and tongue cancers. QDs need to be monodisperse, be small enough to preserve the intrinsic properties of the molecules they are tagging, and have a low level of nonspecific adsorption if they are to consistently label their targets (True and Gao 2007).

5.2.5 Graphene (GO)

Graphene, a two-dimensional carbon crystal, has recently attracted interest as a tool for monitoring and modulating neuronal activity in the laboratory and living organisms. GO, a versatile carbon nanomaterial, may be exploited to develop platform technologies for cancer diagnosis (Wang et al. 2011). GO, the oxidized form of graphene, is the most investigated form of graphene in drug carrier applications because it is simple to produce and disperse in aqueous solutions. Graphene nanocarriers are being developed to release their cargo inside tumors based on the tumor's pH or other chemical conditions (Eskiizmir et al. 2018). The surface of the material can undergo covalent functionalization with anticancer medications and functional groups that possess a special affinity for cancer cells and tissues. This modification enhances the effectiveness of treatment. Its physicochemical properties are also useful for stimulus-responsive medicine and drug delivery (Karki et al. 2020). Magnetic GO nanoparticles were coated with polylactic acid/glycolic acid to facilitate the delivery of 5-iodo-2-deoxyuridine and enhance radiosensitizing effects in glioblastoma patients. Nanocomposites based on functionalized GO have been produced to deliver anticancer drugs (Shirvalilou et al. 2020). The use of folic acid–functionalized reduced GO nanosheets was employed to fabricate a nanocarrier possessing exceptional biocompatibility properties. This nanocarrier was designed to deliver the anticancer medication chlorambucil (Sun et al. 2008).

5.2.6 Fullerene

The extraordinary properties of fullerene and its derivatives have recently attracted a lot of attention, making them very attractive nanomaterials with many potential medical uses.

Malignant tumors were transplanted into mice of different strains and monitored for their progress (Chen et al. 2012). Water-soluble C60 fullerenes can be found. C60 fullerenes have been found to effectively inhibit the progression of transplanted cancerous tumors. They can transport therapeutic drugs to the tumor cells (Martin et al. 2017). Functionalized fullerenes have anticancer capabilities beyond tumor inhibition, including the ability to combat systemic toxicity and drug resistance, both of which are common in conventional chemotherapeutic approaches. The effective photosensitizer pure C60 fullerene (C60) was studied in sonodynamic therapy for cancer (Serpe et al. 2012). C60 fullerene has also found application in the creation of biosensors. Gd@C82(OH)22 endohedral metallofullerenols show low doses and toxicity but high antineoplastic efficacy when they are not loaded with drugs. They also have strong antiproliferative effects on various cell lines of breast cancer, carcinoma, MCF-7, lung, and liver. Gadolinium metallofullerene is an appropriate MRI contrast agent due to its extraordinarily high relaxivity (Ye et al. 2021).

5.2.7 Magnetic Nanoparticles

Magnetic nanoparticles (MNPs) have great potential for targeted drug administration and hyperthermia therapy in cancer treatment due to their advantageous properties, such as strong magnetic moments and high surface-to-volume ratios (Table 5.2). Furthermore, aside from their application as contrast agents in MRI, they possess the capability to enhance the sensitivity of biosensors and diagnostic devices (Rahman 2023). MNPs are a significant subset of nanoparticles, commonly synthesized using pure metals, such as Fe, Co, and Ni (Bossmann et al. 2017). The contrast of images of certain tissues can be improved by using MNPs in magnetic resonance imaging. Targeting MNPs to the site of tissue interest can enhance proton relaxation and visibility. Imaging nanocrystalline particles that can be further functionalized with biocompatible coatings and ligands are viewed as next-generation MRI material (Sun et al. 2008). Nanoparticles can be made by a variety of techniques. Spray pyrolysis, laser ablation, and the chemical sol-gel method are all viable options for their production. What qualities the nanoparticles should have will determine which method is used to create them. Alterations can be implemented to the dimensions, morphology, and chemical makeup of the nanoparticles (Angelakeris 2017). This provides an opportunity for the development of particles possessing distinct characteristics, such as enhanced efficacy in delivering drugs or heightened magnetic potency.

5.2.8 Gold Nanoparticles (GNPs)

GNPs have surface plasmon resonance, which is an interesting physicochemical property. For the reasons that they can bind certain chemicals, are biocompatible, have a high atomic number, and are relatively small (Patra et al. 2010), GNPs possess the capability to serve as contrast agents. The utilization of iodine and other contrast materials has been observed to augment the demarcation of

TABLE 5.2
MNPs in Cancer Screening and Detection

Nanoparticle	Cancer Cell	Uses	References
Magnetic nanoparticles	Liver	In vitro detection of liver cancer cells	Kim et al. (2009)
	Brain	MNs as contrasting agents in cancer diagnosis	
Surface-modified magnetic nanoparticles	Colon	In vitro detection	Kim et al. (2009); Gao et al. (2009)
Magnetic gold nanoparticles	Breast	HER2 breast cancer detection and ELISA	Gao et al. (2009)
Super magnetic iron oxide nanoparticles	Pancreas	Diagnosis using MRI	Arami et al. (2015)

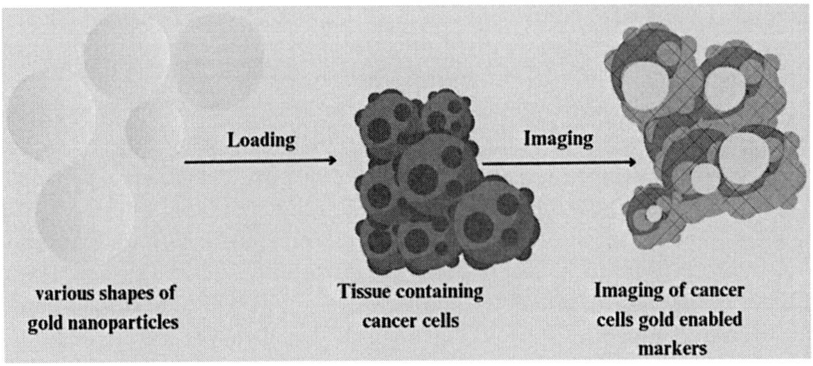

FIGURE 5.4 Gold nanoparticles application in cancer diagnosis and imaging. More accurate cancer diagnoses may be possible with the use of gold nanoparticles because of their ability to enhance tumor targeting and prolong circulation times in the bloodstream

TABLE 5.3
Widely Explored Utilization of GNPs in Cancer Imaging and Their Demonstrated Significant Potential

Nanoparticles	Type	Application	Reference
Gold nanoparticle	Spheres	X-ray imaging	Zhang et al. (2017)
	Spheres, stars	Surface-enhanced Raman spectroscopy imaging	Qiu et al. (2018)
	Primarily spheres	Optical imaging	
	Rods	Fluorescence imaging	Qiu et al. (2018)
	Shells		
	Clusters	Photoacoustic imaging	He et al. (2022)

Source: Qiu et al. (2018).

tumors that exhibit a high degree of vascularity, hence resulting in more accurate cancer diagnoses (Figure 5.4) (Fan et al. 2020). The use of 5 nm GNPs as a delivery system in the context of pancreatic cancer is a prime example of the potential of multifunctional GNPs in medication administration. These GNPs are chemically linked to cetuximab, an active targeting agent, and gemcitabine, a therapeutic payload (Wei et al. 2013). Research findings indicate that the growth of stomach cancer cells can be notably suppressed through the use of gold nanorods that have been engineered with a polypeptide capable of attaching to low-density lipoprotein binding domain (He et al. 2022).

Furthermore, researchers have demonstrated much greater antitumor activity when utilizing these compounds for tumor treatment, as well as enhanced in vivo biosafety, in comparison to the unbound drug doxorubicin (Essig et al. 2000). Pancreatic cancer was avoided with a cocktail of rubescensine A, gold nanocages, anti-GPC-1 antibody, and hyaluronic acid HA. The multimodal imaging capabilities of gold nanocages, encompassing near-infrared fluorescence and MRI, contribute to the timely identification of pancreatic cancer (Zhang et al. 2017). Radiotherapy, photoacoustic imaging, and medication delivery are just a few of the many uses for gold nanoparticles. As a result of their excellent biocompatibility and little cytotoxicity, AuNPs are promising therapeutic possibilities (Table 5.3).

5.2.9 Carbon Nanotubes (CNTs)

CNTs are widely used in cancer diagnostics because of their distinctive physicochemical features. These nanomaterials are highly regarded for their potential to both identify malignant cells and transport medications or therapeutic compounds to these cells. Nanotubes exhibit exceptional electrical and thermal conductivity, rendering them highly suitable for a wide range of electronic nanodevices (Shiba 2003). Additionally, they have remarkable resilience and a low weight, rendering them appropriate for use in composite materials and hydrogen storage. The performance of single-wall nanotubes, which are far longer and have a diameter of only 1 nm, is much better than that of multi-wall nanotubes. Nanotubes have diverse uses in several industries, such as rechargeable lithium batteries, biosensors, touch displays, and even as cardiac electrodes (Hasanzade and Raissi 2019). Moreover, they may be employed in combination with gold nanoparticles for diverse applications, such as detecting acetylcholinesterase enzymes and fabricating sensor electrodes. To optimize their performance, they can be coated with Nafion. When applied atop carboxylic single-walled nanotubes, they exhibit exceptional efficacy as sensing electrodes (Amreddy et al. 2019).

5.3 NANOPARTICLES IN MEDICAL IMAGING METHODS

To enhance image contrast and reveal previously unseen details, contrast agents are increasingly utilized in medical imaging (Nayak et al. 2021). Various types of NPs are being developed, such as gold nanoparticles for enhancing X-ray contrast, magnetic nanoparticles for enhancing MRI contrast, and even hybrid nanoparticles comprising iron oxide and gold in a polymer covering. These nanoparticles are useful as MRI and CT contrast agents (Thirugnanasambandan 2021). Using NPs in immunoimaging applications may have far-reaching implications for tailoring therapies to individual patients and keeping tabs on their responses in real time. It is possible to create contrast agents in a wide variety of shapes (spheres, cubes, stars, rods, etc.), encapsulate them in materials like porous silica nanoparticles, or embed them in lipid or protein nanovesicles like dendrimers or liposomes or micelles. With or without a targeting moiety, NP-based imaging agents have the potential to be employed for the monitoring of T cells and dendritic cells and as well as the detection of immune checkpoint receptors. Preclinical investigations have utilized iron oxide NPs and perfluorocarbon nanoemulsions to evaluate the capacity of MRI in monitoring immune cells (Ahrens and Bulte 2013). Optical imaging comprises a diverse range of methodologies, including fluorescence, bioluminescence, and photoacoustics-based approaches. Protein nanoparticles can facilitate the transportation of fluorescent dyes, hence enabling their utilization in fluorescence imaging conducted within living organisms (Rosenthal et al. 2002). By using biomarker chemicals that are exclusively produced by cancer cells, molecular imaging holds the promise of improving the accuracy of cancer diagnosis. This approach involves employing probes that are directed by ligands capable of recognizing and interacting with target molecules, hence facilitating the imaging process. Recently, optical, radioactive, and magnetic probes that can specifically target tumors have been developed, and their efficacy has been evaluated in animal cancer models and a small number of clinical studies (Wilson et al. 2016). Cancer imaging applications can make use of imaging agents based on NP and nanomaterials, which can have tunable properties. To get around the drawbacks of conventional imaging contrast agents, NPs can be mixed with imaging agents used in a variety of imaging modalities and resolutions (Figure 5.5) (Ma et al. 2017).

5.3.1 Magnetic Resonance Imaging (MRI)

The initial study on nanoparticles for imaging applications documented the use of iron oxide NPs. By MRI targeting asialoglycoprotein receptors, the researchers developed iron oxide NPs with the express purpose of detecting liver cancer (Orel 2003). Next, a rat model was used to assess the effects of these nanoparticles. Oral administration of iron oxide NPs as an imaging agent for abdominal imaging was the primary focus of the earliest clinical investigation using these particles in 1991. The first FDA approval for the use of iron oxide NPs was in 1993, following this experiment. Various types of iron oxide NPs that were authorized by the FDA or in Europe from 1993 to 2001 were subsequently recalled due to concerns about their toxicity (Haris et al. 2015). For the treatment of iron deficiency anemia, ferumoxytol is the only iron

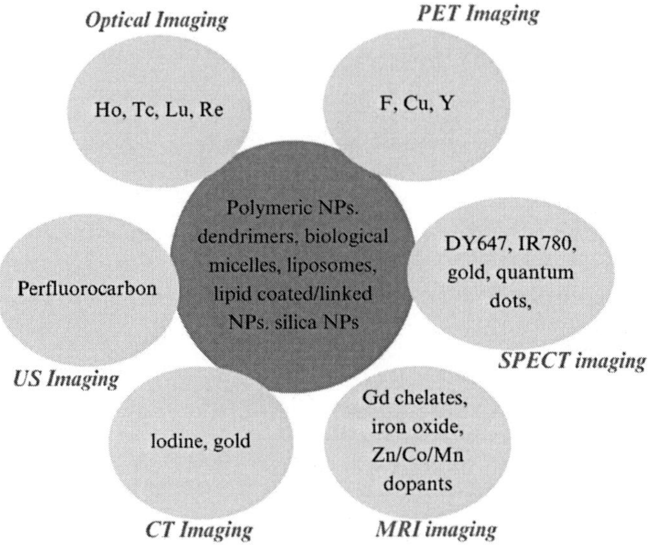

FIGURE 5.5 Optical imaging, PET, SPECT, CT, MRI, US, and other imaging modalities can use NPs with a variety of labels. *Ho* represents the isotope holmium-166, *Lu* represents the isotope lutetium-177, *Re* represents the isotope rhenium-188, *F* represents the isotope fluorine-18, *Cu* represents the isotope copper-64, and *Y* represents the isotope yttrium-86. *Co* is the chemical symbol for cobalt. *Zn* represents zinc, and *Mn* represents manganese. DY647 is a fluorescent compound, and IR780 is a fluorescent probe (Ma et al. 2017).

oxide nanoparticle that has been approved by the FDA at this time. In various stages of clinical trials, ferumoxytol is used as an MRI contrast agent despite not having been licensed for this purpose (Luo et al. 2020).

The utilization of MRI has significantly increased in non-invasive clinical diagnosis due to its notable attributes, including spatial resolution and depth of penetration. T1 and T2 relaxation durations of protons in water in vivo are linked to the strength of the MRI signal (Mehta et al. 2016). To improve image clarity, "contrast agents" consisting of different inorganic nanoparticles and complexes are provided before scanning. Increasing the relaxation rates, 1/T1 and 1/T2, causes more intense and less intense signals to be generated in a shorter amount of time, respectively, when T1 and T2 are shortened. Although MRI has great potential as a cancer diagnostic tool, its low specificity has prevented it from being used to its fullest extent. Small amounts of superparamagnetic NPs can be used to compensate for MRI's lack of specificity when tagged with cell-specific markers. Placing SPIONs in a magnetic field disrupts the field, accelerating the relaxation of water's proton and making MRI detection possible (Blasiak et al. 2013). SPIONs have been the subject of substantial research as prospective MRI contrast agents, owing to their favorable amalgamation of superparamagnetic characteristics, biodegradability, and surface qualities that can be readily altered to enhance in vivo kinetics and multifunctionality (Farncombe 2017). Some cancers, including those of the stomach, kidneys, and brain, may be detectable with the use of iron oxide NPs. The modification of nanoparticles with specific antibodies against epidermal growth factor receptor and short peptides can facilitate the achievement of this purpose. They have been modified for use in a variety of settings apart from cancer detection, including the early identification of thrombosis and the detection of brain inflammation (Avasthi et al. 2020). To detect immune checkpoint receptors, mark and monitor T cells, dendritic cells, etc. NP-based imaging agents can be used with or without a targeting moiety. Iron oxide NPs and perfluorocarbon nanoemulsions have been used in preclinical studies to track immune cell activity with MRI (Hoeks et al. 2011).

5.3.2 Computed Tomography (CT)

To attain the requisite circulation durations, biodistribution, solubility in biological fluids, and biocompatibility, nanoparticle contrast agents designed for CT commonly feature a central core that is laden with atoms capable of producing contrast, which is subsequently enveloped by polymers, proteins, or other similar substances. Incorporation of other attributes, such as the ability to selectively target specific entities through the use of antibodies, the potential therapeutic benefits achieved through the use of pharmaceuticals or nucleic acids, or the capability to enable multimodal imaging by employing different contrast-generating substances, can frequently be achieved through straightforward alterations to the coating layers (Kambali and Suryanto 2020). Long blood pool residence durations, the ability to follow cells, and specialized imaging applications are just a few of how nanoparticles outperform small molecule CT contrast agents. Notable examples of NPs that have been modified for use as CT contrast agents include lipoproteins and micelles. Contrast agents based on iodine are frequently utilized for this purpose. Some people are iodine-intolerant due to disorders of the thyroid gland, and it has been discovered that iodine-based contrast agents are harmful to the environment. Researchers from a variety of disciplines work to create new contrast agents that can replace those that use iodine. Due to their high density, metallic nanoparticles could be employed as a CT contrast agent. Nanoscale metal particles are thought to be poisonous to living things. Nanoparticles' biocompatibility and safety can be improved by having organic molecules coat them (Aslan et al. 2020). Researchers also hypothesized that, like other inflammatory disorders, inflammatory bowel disease would promote accumulation in inflammation sites if cerium oxide nanoparticles were coated with dextran. Because of their unique biological and physical properties, metal nanoparticles show great promise as CT contrast agents. There is a direct relationship between the cube of the atomic number (Z^3) and the computed tomography contrast, which is improved as the atomic number of the contrast agent increases. Iodine possesses an atomic number of 53, whereas the metals tantalum (73) and bismuth (83) that have been recently proposed exhibit far greater atomic numbers. Hence, the aforementioned metals have the potential to induce a more substantial level of X-ray attenuation (Shilo et al. 2012).

For CT contrast agents, tantalum's great radioactivity and biocompatibility make it a great candidate. Stents and implants made of tantalum are often used in hospitals and clinics. Tantalum oxide nanoparticles may be synthesized using a sol-gel process using tantalum ethoxide and then easily modified with different silane agents. Due to the similarity in the synthetic techniques of tantalum oxide nanoparticles and silica nanoparticles, it is possible to manufacture a wide range of multifunctional nanomaterials (Seo et al. 2019).

5.3.3 Optical Imaging

The use of optical imaging to detect tissues in image-guided therapeutic operations has recently shown great promise. Monitoring the progress of a condition or treatment can be achieved simply. At first, regular fluorophores were utilized. These included fluorescent dyes and fluorescent proteins. While their predecessors were not suitable for imaging-guided therapy, recent advances in the creation of fluorescent NPs have made them promising options (Jiang et al. 2009). Unless they are innately luminous nanoparticles, nanomaterials add imaging functionality by covalently attaching standard fluorescent dyes. Recently, several different kinds of nanomaterials with intrinsic fluorescence have been described, and not just quantum dots. Nanoparticles made of carbon have great fluorescence, cheap cost, and minimal toxicity, and they are physically and photochemically stable. Since AuNPs have distinct plasmonic capabilities, they have been the subject of extensive studies for improving optical imaging. Darkfield (DF) microscopy is a viable approach for detecting AuNPs in biological systems due to the substantial difference in scattering signals between AuNPs and the scattering background originating from tissues. Adding AuNPs to a molecule's surface can significantly boost its Raman signal. Ultrasensitive single-molecule detection (down to 10–15 M) is made possible by surface-enhanced Raman scattering, which achieves more than ten orders of signal augmentation (Wu et al. 2019).

One sort of fluorescent semiconductor nanoparticle with unique electrical and optical characteristics is the QD. Because of the phenomena of quantum confinement, their characteristics differ from their bulk states. By adjusting their size, their emission wavelength may be easily controlled (Fang et al. 2016). They have remarkable optical characteristics that enable long-term fluorescence imaging without photobleaching, including a high quantum yield, absorption coefficient, and photostability. Moreover, the QDs possess a significant multi-photon absorption coefficient, which enables the achievement of high-resolution fluorescence imaging by minimizing excitation that occurs outside the intended focal point. Nevertheless, due to the presence of hazardous metals like cadmium in the originally created QDs, there have been significant apprehensions over their safety (Ramezani et al. 2023).

5.4 UTILIZATION OF NANOTECHNOLOGY TOOLS IN CANCER DIAGNOSIS

In continuing research, nanotechnology has the potential to validate cancer imaging on a molecular, cellular, and tissue level (Jin et al. 2020). Researchers found that this was achieved by exploring the tumor's environment using nanotechnology applications. One such approach is to detect tumor-associated fibroblasts activated protein-a on their cell membrane using pH-responsive fluorescent nanoprobes. In this section, we will explore nanotechnology-based methods that enable precise tracking of living cells and monitoring of dynamic biological processes within tumors (Garrigue et al. 2018).

5.4.1 NIR Quantum Dots

Visible spectrum imaging has limited applicability due to its inability to penetrate objects. To solve this problem, quantum dots have been made to emit light in the 700–1,000 nm range, which is part of the near-infrared (NIR) spectrum (Dubertret et al. 2002). This modification enhances their applicability for seeing colorectal cancer, pancreatic cancer, and lymphoma. Another NIR range, known as NIR-ii (900–1,700 nm), has been created to enhance cancer imaging by offering more tissue penetration depth, as well as improved spatial resolution. Furthermore, a study has documented the creation of QDs composed of silver-rich compound, which incorporate a sulfur source. This innovation enables the production of high-resolution pictures with improved spatial accuracy across a broad spectrum of infrared wavelengths (Zhang et al. 2020).

5.4.2 Nanoshells

Nanoshells are often employed in many nanotechnology applications. Nanoshells are tiny dielectric cores with dimensions ranging from 10 to 300 nm. Typically, they consist of silicon and are encased in a thin metal shell, commonly made of gold (Hirsch et al. 2003). These nanoshells operate by converting electrical energy, facilitated by plasma, into light energy. Their optical characteristics may be modified by utilizing arrays that emit or absorb light ranging from ultraviolet (UV) to infrared (IR). Nanoshells are attractive due to their imaging capabilities that are free from heavy metal toxicity but are restricted by their significant dimensions (Nunes et al. 2019).

5.5 NANOPARTICLES FOR CANCER CELL DETECTION

5.5.1 Detecting Tumor Cells in the Blood

The term "circulating tumor cells" (CTCs) refers to cancer cells that have detached from the primary tumor and exist as either individual or grouped masses circulating inside the bloodstream.

Metastasis is widely believed to be the primary cause of around 90% of fatalities resulting from solid tumors. Metastasis is a biological phenomenon characterized by the infiltration of cancerous cells originating from the main tumor into adjacent tissues, followed by their further dissemination through the microvessels of the lymphatic systems (Hu et al. 2016). When the cells reach their destination in the microvessels of distant tissue, they can survive outside of the bloodstream (extravasate) and continue their existence. The potential of CTCs in liquid biopsies has been extensively studied. The detection of CTCs provides a non-invasive method of learning about the molecular architecture of cancers. CTCs detach from primary tumors and circulate in the bloodstream, reflecting metastasis (Yao 2016). Several studies have shown the therapeutic and prognostic usefulness of CTCs. CTC detection benefits from nanoparticles' capacity to adsorb targeted ligands. CTC separations improve detection sensitivity because of their high specificity and recoverability. Therefore, one therapeutic strategy could be to interfere with the spread of cancer cells (Andree et al. 2015). Various nanomaterials, including MNPs, AuNPs, QDs, nanowires, dendrimers, carbon nanotubes, polymers, etc., have been reported by researchers for the purpose of detecting CTCs (Table 5.4).

5.5.2 Detection by Identifying Cell Surface Proteins

Specific surface proteins are the principal targets of CTCs. CTCs that undergo EMT are unable to be positively sorted based on EpCAM expression. Hence, it is beneficial to look for other EpCAM indicators (Powell et al. 2012). Several cell surface markers have been investigated for their potential use in the detection of CTCs, including major vault protein, glycans, vimentin, and fibroblast activation protein (Table 5.5).

TABLE 5.4
Utilizing Nanotechnology for the Identification of Cancer Cells

Nanoparticles	Ligand	Affinity	Cancer	References
Gold nanoparticles	Her2	Aptamer Antibody	Breast Leukemia	Zhu et al. 2013
Nanorod arrays	EpCAM	DNA aptamer	Breast	Wen et al. 2013
Magnetic nanoparticles	EpCAM	Antibody	Colon	Burinaru et al. 2019
Nanofibers	EpCAM	Antibody	Breast	Sun et al. 2016
Quantum dots	PTK7	Aptamer	Leukemia	Pang et al. 2018
Carbon nanotubes	EpCAM	Antibody	Liver	Zhang et al. 2018
Nanoparticle-coated silicon bead	EpCAM	Antibody	Colorectal	Chen et al. 2019

TABLE 5.5
Indicators of Cell Surface Proteins for CTC Detection

Marker	Cell Type	Cancer	Detection Strategy	Reference
EpCAM	CTC	Breast and colorectal cancer	Cell search	Powell et al. (2012)
Bmi1	CTC	Lung and breast cancer	Polymerase chain reaction (RT-PCR)	
Vimentin	CTC	Gastrointestinal	Confocal microscopy	Zhang et al. (2019)
Glycan	CTC	Breast	Flow cytometry	Zhang et al. (2019)
EpCam and FR	CTC	Lung cancer	Cell search	Guan and Zhang 2020

Source: Zhang et al. (2019).

Comparison of DNA, mRNA, protein, or antibody reactivity in tumor and non-tumor tissues, cell lines, or other biological components is often necessary for target identification. Next, during target validation, antibodies are used to determine the antigen's expression profile in normal and cancerous tissue and to verify that the antigen is found exclusively on the surface of tumor cells. While certain physical attributes of cells, such as size and density, may occasionally be utilized, the primary method of cell trapping typically relies on the capacity of cell surface chemicals to bind to CTCs and be identified by molecules such as antibodies (Akbarzadeh et al. 2012).

5.5.3 mRNA-Based Detection

Gold nanoparticles are a distinct category of probes that have been modified with oligonucleotides and subjected to hybridization for amplification. These modified probes are further labeled with a fluorophore, enabling them to function as transfection agents. The aforementioned probes, referred to as "nanoflares," have exhibited the capability to identify mRNA within viable cells. Nanoflares exhibit notable attributes, such as efficiency, sensitivity, and a substantial signal-to-noise ratio, enabling them to overcome diverse obstacles and demonstrate sensitivity toward alterations in cellular RNA transcripts. They have the unique advantage of high directivity and cell entry without the need for cytotoxic transfection chemicals, making them valuable for intracellular mRNA detection (Katsarou et al. 2022). In recent studies, researchers have developed multiplexed nanoflares capable of simultaneously detecting multiple mRNA transcripts within cells. This was achieved by hybridizing short complementary reporter strands to AuNPs functionalized with 2–3 DNA recombination strands. The use of mRNA-based immunotherapies has shown good results in clinical studies, particularly in the fields of therapeutic vaccines, cytokine therapy, checkpoint inhibition, and chimeric antigen receptor (CAR) cell therapy (Chehelgerdi and Chehelgerdi 2023). Given their potential applications and success in various immunotherapeutic approaches, nanoflares hold significant promise as powerful tools for detecting and studying intracellular mRNA. Further research and development in this field can potentially lead to advancements in precision medicine and targeted therapies (Kuhlmann et al. 2014).

A further strategy to improve screening is to augment the sensitivity of mass spectrometry by using nanocarriers. The unique optical and thermal properties of carbon nanotubes enhance the efficiency of energy transfer in the analyte, so accelerating its absorption and ionization, while also minimizing the interference produced by naturally occurring matrix ions. An alternative approach is utilizing nanotechnology to manufacture lab-on-a-chip microfluidics devices, which may be used for immuno-screening or the analysis of tumor cell properties (Zhai et al. 2022). A noteworthy device showcasing considerable promise is the lab-on-a-chip for advanced and efficient detection of numerous proteins simultaneously. This system employs quantum dots consisting of a core made of cadmium selenide (CdSe) and a shell made of zinc sulfide (ZnS). The quantum dots are then linked to antibodies that are specific to carcinoembryonic antigen, cancer antigen, and Her-2/Neu. Another example is the discovery that cells grown on nanometer-sized surfaces may discriminate between tumor cells. It is important to highlight that screening biomarkers using nanotechnology still produces both false-positive and false-negative findings. Therefore, it is necessary to enhance the sensitivity of the screening process without sacrificing specificity (Seferos et al. 2007).

5.6 CONTRAST AGENTS USED IN CANCER DIAGNOSIS

5.6.1 Iron Oxide Contrast Agents

Superparamagnetic iron oxide (SPIO) and ultrasmall superparamagnetic iron oxide (USPIO) are two distinct categories of iron oxide contrast agents. SPIO and USPIO are composed of colloids containing iron oxide nanoparticles that attenuate the T2 signals in tissues when used in imaging procedures (Na et al. 2009). SPIO, the initial nanoparticulate MRI contrast agent, was initially launched for liver imaging and continues to be employed in clinical practice. Approved SPIO and USPIO agents include Resovist, Sinerem, and Clariscan. Presently, with the exception of the oral iron oxide contrast agent Lumirem/GastroMARK, these agents are not currently accessible. These contrast agents have exhibited encouraging outcomes in the detection of liver cancers (Nakamura et al. 2000). The small size and distinctive particle morphologies of iron oxide contrast agents have clear benefits in terms of how they are distributed in the body and their potential uses, as compared to other contrast agents. Presently, nanoparticulate iron oxide is widely favored in clinical practice. Nevertheless, progress in molecular and cellular imaging has sparked a greater fascination with alternative nanoparticles that might serve as MRI contrast agents. The nanoparticles possess the capability to render disease-specific biomarkers detectable at both microscopic and molecular scales. Recent progress in nanotechnology has led to the creation of innovative MRI contrast agents at the nanoscale, which exhibit enhanced contrast capabilities and offer supplementary functionality. These advancements create opportunities for improved imaging and diagnostics in the medical imaging industry (Xiao et al. 2016).

5.6.2 Gadolinium-Based Contrast Agents

Due to their exceptional imaging capabilities, gadolinium-based contrast agents are extensively utilized in clinical MRI. Considerable endeavors have been undertaken to create and produce innovative Gd(III) contrast agents that possess a high relaxivity, little toxicity, and a particular affinity for tumor binding (Gries 2002). Chemical changes can increase the relaxivity of Gd(III) contrast agents. In order to decrease toxicity, the stability of Gd(III) contrast agents is enhanced both thermodynamically and kinetically, while also optimizing their pharmacokinetic characteristics (S. Al-Showiman 2021). Clinical MRI contrast agents that include Gd(III) provide significant augmentation of positive contrast and are efficiently cleared from the body following MRI procedures. The agents may be divided into two groups: linear Gd(III) chelates and macrocyclic chelates. Generally, macrocyclic chelates have better stability. Presently, MRI contrast agents that are based on Gd(III) are widely utilized in clinical practice (Yigitaslan and Erol 2021).

5.6.3 Gold Nanoparticles-Based Contrast Agents

AuNPs have several advantageous properties that render them very suitable for CT imaging applications. Firstly, they possess the capacity to transport substantial amounts of contrast-generating material, which results in improved imaging sensitivity. In addition, AuNPs possess a high ability to absorb X-rays, allowing them to greatly increase contrast in CT imaging. Furthermore, AuNPs exhibit exceptional biocompatibility, guaranteeing few negative consequences when employed in vivo. AuNPs may be modified to optimize their surface chemistry for precise targeting and improved stability in physiological environments (Luo et al. 2021). Furthermore, the dimensions and configurations of AuNPs may be accurately regulated, allowing for customization to meet specific imaging needs. The combination of these features makes AuNPs particularly desirable for enhancing CT imaging (Vankayala and Hwang 2018).

AuNPs have attracted interest for enhancing CT imaging due to their 2.7 times greater X-ray mass attenuation compared to iodine-based contrast agents. This is advantageous because iodine-based treatments have rapid renal clearance and may cause renal toxicity (Daniel and Astruc 2004). Multiple scientific studies have examined the use of AuNPs as contrast agents in cancer detection with CT. These studies have utilized the nanoparticles' passive targeting abilities, which exploit the EPR effect (Dou et al. 2016). The primary objective of these investigations has been to comprehend the correlation between the dimensions of AuNPs and their ability to enhance CT imaging, while also examining their behavior within living organisms. AuNPs show potential as prospective CT contrast agents for enhanced cancer imaging (Oraevsky 2017).

5.7 CHALLENGES IN NANOPARTICLE-BASED CANCER DIAGNOSIS

Nanotechnology-based cancer diagnostics raise concerns about accuracy and efficiency. For nanotechnology-based systems to be deployed in hospitals, they must produce accurate findings (Parra-Cabrera, Samitier, and Homs-Corbera 2016). Nanoparticle-based detection signals can be reliable and reproducible, but they face obstacles such as nanoparticle aggregation, nonspecific probe binding, and erroneous detection. Large pools of clinical samples are required for careful evaluation of these obstacles in clinical trial applications. Another difficulty is the mass manufacture of nanoprobes that can be stored for an extended period and are highly sensitive, reproducible, and inexpensive. The shape, charge, size, and surface-coating nanoprobes all play very important roles in cancer detection and diagnosis (Conde 2020). To reduce variability across batches, it is necessary to optimize the synthesis methods and streamline the functionalization of nanoprobe. In addition, nanoprobes tend to group when they are stored. The last difficulty to jump is the production of NP-based goods that are sensitive, user-friendly, and cheap (Dessale et al. 2022). While several NP-based evaluations have been developed in research settings, not all of them have undergone validation for clinical use. The effective advancement of point-of-care systems utilizing NPs will greatly streamline the implementation of nanotechnology in cancer diagnosis (Syedmoradi et al. 2017). When employing cutting-edge NP probes for in vivo imaging, it is imperative to consider the potential occurrence of NP toxicity resulting from their systemic injection. Before employing these NP probes, it is imperative to assess any potential toxicity (Sharaf et al. 2023). As a result, the application of nanotechnology in cancer diagnosis relies heavily on solving the problems of reliability and reproducibility, mass production, efficient detection, and toxicity assessment.

5.8 CONCLUSION

Nanotechnology in the fight against cancer aims to develop safer and more efficient methods of diagnosis. Conventional cancer treatment and diagnosis have many drawbacks, including a low rate of success

TABLE 5.6
Utilizations of Nanoparticles in Cancer Detection

Nanoparticles	Applications	Properties	Example in Diagnosis
Polymeric NPs	Detection Drug delivery	Enclosed in a polymer shell	Targeted delivery of dye molecules and RGD peptide–conjugated block copolymer–coated nanoparticles for tumor localization.
Metallic NPs	Imaging Detection	Identification and safeguarding against metastatic breast cancer	AuNPs for Raman imaging.
Carbon-based NPs	Detection Diagnosis	Physiochemical features of this substance exceptional, characterized by its ability to easily penetrate the cell membrane, and drug loading capacity	Both in vivo and in vitro investigations demonstrate that nanodroplets serve as a very efficient contrast agent for both photoacoustic and ultrasonic imaging.
Lipid-based NPs	Diagnosis Drug carrier	Low toxicity Better incompatibility	The process of attaching anti-HER2 antibodies to phospholipid-coated QDs demonstrated the capability to specifically target tumors that express HER2.
Dendrimers	Drug delivery	Low toxicity Chemical stability	Precise delivery. Efficiency of diagnosis is doubled.

Source: Alrushaid et al. (2023).

in curing the disease, insufficient ability to target specific tumors, a wide range of unpleasant side effects, and the possibility of serious biological risk. As a result of its superior selectivity and sensitivity, NP-based assays have emerged as a game-changing development in cancer diagnosis (Table 5.6). These assays not only improve the precision and consistency of cancer detection but also usher in previously impossible capabilities. These developments may greatly increase the survival rate of cancer patients by allowing for earlier diagnosis. Because of developments in molecular cell biology and contemporary nanotechnology, NPs are gaining prominence in the realm of cancer treatment. Nanotechnology has the potential to dramatically improve healthcare and should get continued funding.

REFERENCES

Abbasi, Elham, Sedigheh Fekri Aval, Abolfazl Akbarzadeh, Morteza Milani, Hamid Tayefi Nasrabadi, Sang Woo Joo, Younes Hanifehpour, Kazem Nejati-Koshki, and Roghiyeh Pashaei-Asl. 2014. "Dendrimers: Synthesis, Applications, and Properties." *Nanoscale Research Letters* 9 (1). https://doi.org/10.1186/1556-276x-9-247.

Agarwal, Abhinav, Umesh Gupta, Abhay Asthana, and Narendra K. Jain. 2009. "Dextran Conjugated Dendritic Nanoconstructs as Potential Vectors for Anti-Cancer Agent." *Biomaterials* 30 (21): 3588–96. https://doi.org/10.1016/j.biomaterials.2009.03.016.

Ahmed, Arsalan, Shumaila Sarwar, Yong Hu, Muhammad Usman Munir, Muhammad Farrukh Nisar, Fakhera Ikram, Anila Asif, Saeed Ur Rahman, Aqif Anwar Chaudhry, and Ihtasham Ur Rehman. 2020. "Surface-Modified Polymeric Nanoparticles for Drug Delivery to Cancer Cells." *Expert Opinion on Drug Delivery* 18 (1): 1–24. https://doi.org/10.1080/17425247.2020.1822321.

Ahrens, Eric T., and Jeff W. Bulte. 2013. "Tracking Immune Cells in Vivo Using Magnetic Resonance Imaging." *Nature Reviews Immunology* 13 (10): 755–63. https://doi.org/10.1038/nri3531.

Akbarzadeh, Abolfazl, Mohammad Samiei, and Soodabeh Davaran. 2012. "Magnetic Nanoparticles: Preparation, Physical Properties, and Applications in Biomedicine." *Nanoscale Research Letters* 7 (1). https://doi.org/10.1186/1556-276x-7-144.

Alrushaid, Noor, Firdos Alam Khan, Ebtesam Abdullah Al-Suhaimi, and Abdelhamid Elaissari. 2023. "Nanotechnology in Cancer Diagnosis and Treatment." *Pharmaceutics* 15 (3): 1025. https://doi.org/10.3390/pharmaceutics15031025.

Al-Showiman, Sami S. 2021. *Contrast Agents (Gadolinium).* https://doi.org/10.14293/s2199-1006.1.sor-.pp3c6gs.v1.

Amreddy, Narsireddy, Rebaz A. Ahmed, Anupama Munshi, and Rajagopal Ramesh. 2019. "Tumor-Targeted Dendrimer Nanoparticles for Combinatorial Delivery of Sirna and Chemotherapy for Cancer Treatment." *Drug Delivery Systems* 167–89. https://doi.org/10.1007/978-1-4939-9798-5_8.

Andree, Kiki C., Guus van Dalum, and Leon W. M. M. Terstappen. 2015. "Challenges in Circulating Tumor Cell Detection by the Cell Search System." *Molecular Oncology* 10 (3): 395–407. https://doi.org/10.1016/j.molonc.2015.12.002.

Angelakeris, M. 2017. "Magnetic Nanoparticles: A Multifunctional Vehicle for Modern Theranostics." *Biochimica et Biophysica Acta (BBA)—General Subjects* 1861 (6): 1642–51. https://doi.org/10.1016/j.bbagen.2017.02.022.

Arami, Hamed, Amit P. Khandhar, Asahi Tomitaka, Elaine Yu, Patrick W. Goodwill, Steven M. Conolly, and Kannan M. Krishnan. 2015. "In Vivo Multimodal Magnetic Particle Imaging (MPI) With Tailored Magneto/Optical Contrast Agents." *Biomaterials* 52: 251–61. https://doi.org/10.1016/j.biomaterials.2015.02.040.

Aslan, Naim, Burhan Ceylan, Mümin Mehmet Koç, and Fehim Findik. 2020. "Metallic Nanoparticles as X-Ray Computed Tomography (CT) Contrast Agents: A Review." *Journal of Molecular Structure* 1219: 128599. https://doi.org/10.1016/j.molstruc.2020.128599.

Avasthi, Ashish, Carlos Caro, Esther Pozo-Torres, Manuel Pernia Leal, and María Luisa García-Martín. 2020. "Magnetic Nanoparticles as MRI Contrast Agents." *Topics in Current Chemistry* 378 (3). https://doi.org/10.1007/s41061-020-00302-w.

Beriso, Adem. 2017. "Early Cancer Detection and Treatment With Nanotechnology." *Journal of Nanomaterials & Molecular Nanotechnology* 6 (5). https://doi.org/10.4172/2324-8777.1000233.

Bhardwaj, Mansavi, and Shafaq Rasool. 2023. "Nanotechnology for the Treatment of Cancer: Progress and Challenges." *Nanotechnology and Human Health* 285–307. https://doi.org/10.1016/b978-0-323-90750-7.00010-7.

Bicak, Bilge, Serda Kecel Gunduz, and Aysen E. Ozel. 2021. "Advancements in Cancer Therapeutics." *Handbook of Research on Advancements in Cancer Therapeutics* 382–412. https://doi.org/10.4018/978-1-7998-6530-8.ch013.

Blasiak, Barbara, Frank C. van Veggel, and Boguslaw Tomanek. 2013. "Applications of Nanoparticles for MRI Cancer Diagnosis and Therapy." *Journal of Nanomaterials* 2013: 1–12. https://doi.org/10.1155/2013/148578.

Bossmann, Stefan, Viktor Chikan, and Raj Kumar Dani. 2017. "Biosensing and Cancer Treatment With Magnetic Nanoparticles." *Biosensors Based on Nanomaterials and Nanodevices* 397–430. https://doi.org/10.1201/b16234-19.

Bulbake, Upendra, Nagavendra Kommineni, Maksim Ionov, Maria Bryszewska, and Wahid Khan. 2019. "Comparison of Cationic Liposome and Pamam Dendrimer for Delivery of Anti-Plk1 Sirna in Breast Cancer Treatment." *Pharmaceutical Development and Technology* 25 (1): 9–19. https://doi.org/10.1080/10837450.2019.1567763.

Burinaru, T., M. Volmer, M. Avram, Vasilica Schiopu-Tucureanu, A. Avram, B. Tincu, C. Mărculescu, M. Alina, R. Marinescu, and Manuella Militaru. 2019. "Antibody Functionalized Magnetic Nanoparticles for Circulating Tumor Cells Detection and Capture using Magnetophoresis." *IOP Conference Series: Materials Science and Engineering* 485: 012005. 10.1088/1757-899X/485/1/012005.

Chehelgerdi, M., and M. Chehelgerdi. 2023. "The Use of RNA-Based Treatments in the Field of Cancer Immunotherapy." *Molecular Cancer* 22 (1): 106. doi: 10.1186/s12943-023-01807-w.

Chen, Kun, Ting Fu, Weidi Sun, Qin Huang, Pengge Zhang, Zilong Zhao, Xiaobing Zhang, and Weihong Tan. 2019. "DNA-Supramolecule Conjugates in Theranostics." *Theranostics* 9 (11): 3262–79. https://doi.org/10.7150/thno.31885.

Chen, Zhiyun, Ruoqing Mao, and Ying Liu. 2012. "Fullerenes for Cancer Diagnosis and Therapy: Preparation, Biological and Clinical Perspectives." *Current Drug Metabolism* 13 (8): 1035–45. https://doi.org/10.2174/138920012802850128.

Conde, João. 2020. "Above and Beyond Cancer Therapy: Translating Biomaterials into the Clinic." *Trends in Cancer* 6 (9): 730–2. https://doi.org/10.1016/j.trecan.2020.04.008.

Dang, Yu, and Jianjun Guan. 2020. "Nanoparticle-Based Drug Delivery Systems for Cancer Therapy." *Smart Materials in Medicine* 1: 10–9. https://doi.org/10.1016/j.smaim.2020.04.001.

Daniel, Marie-Christine, and Didier Astruc. 2004. "Gold Nanoparticles: Assembly, Supramolecular Chemistry, Quantum-Size-Related Properties, and Applications Toward Biology, Catalysis, and Nanotechnology." *ChemInform* 35 (16). https://doi.org/10.1002/chin.200416213.

Dessale, Mesfin, Getachew Mengistu, and Hylemariam Mihiretie Mengist. 2022. "Nanotechnology: A Promising Approach for Cancer Diagnosis, Therapeutics and Theragnosis." *International Journal of Nanomedicine* 17: 3735–49. https://doi.org/10.2147/ijn.s378074.

Dou, Yan, Yanyan Guo, Xiaodong Li, Xue Li, Sheng Wang, Lin Wang, Guoxian Lv et al. 2016. "Size-Tuning Ionization to Optimize Gold Nanoparticles for Simultaneous Enhanced CT Imaging and Radiotherapy." *ACS Nano* 10 (2): 2536–48. https://doi.org/10.1021/acsnano.5b07473.

Dubertret, Benoit, Paris Skourides, David J. Norris, Vincent Noireaux, Ali H. Brivanlou, and Albert Libchaber. 2002. "In Vivo Imaging of Quantum Dots Encapsulated in Phospholipid Micelles." *Science* 298 (5599): 1759–62. https://doi.org/10.1126/science.1077194.

Duncan, Ruth. 2003. "The Dawning Era of Polymer Therapeutics." *Nature Reviews Drug Discovery* 2 (5): 347–60. https://doi.org/10.1038/nrd1088.

Eskiizmir, Görkem, Yasemin Baskın, and Kerim Yapıcı. 2018. "Graphene-Based Nanomaterials in Cancer Treatment and Diagnosis." *Fullerens, Graphenes and Nanotubes* 331–74. https://doi.org/10.1016/b978-0-12-813691-1.00009-9.

Essig, Marco, Jürgen Debus, Heinz-Peter Schlemmer, Hans Hawighorst, Michael Wannenmacher, and Gerhard van Kaick. 2000. "Verbesserter Tumorkontrast Und -Abgrenzung in Der Stereotaktischen Strahlentherapieplanung Zerebraler Gliome Und Metastasen Mit Kontrastmittelunterstützter Flair-Bildgebung." *Strahlentherapie Und Onkologie* 176 (2): 84–94. https://doi.org/10.1007/pl00002333.

Fan, M., Yu Han, Shutao Gao, Hongyu Yan, Lingzhi Cao, Zhenhua Li, Xing-Jie Liang, and Jinchao Zhang. 2020. "Ultrasmall Gold Nanoparticles in Cancer Diagnosis and Therapy." *Theranostics* 10 (11): 4944–57. https://doi.org/10.7150/thno.42471.

Fang, Min, Ming Chen, Lulu Liu, and Yan Li. 2017. "Applications of Quantum Dots in Cancer Detection and Diagnosis: A Review." *Journal of Biomedical Nanotechnology* 13 (1): 1–16. https://doi.org/10.1166/jbn.2017.2334.

Fang, Min, Dai-Wen Pang, and Yan Li. 2016. "Quantum Dots for Cancer Diagnosis." *Biomedical Nanomaterials* 207–26. https://doi.org/10.1002/9783527694396.ch8.

Farncombe, Troy H. 2017. "Multimodality Imaging With Mr/PET and Mr/SPECT." *Medical Imaging* 359–402. https://doi.org/10.1201/b15511-14.

Feng, Tao, and Yanli Zhao. 2016. "Nanomaterial-Based Drug Delivery Carriers for Cancer Therapy." *Nanomaterial-Based Drug Delivery Carriers for Cancer Therapy* 15–54. https://doi.org/10.1007/978-981-10-3299-8_3.

Gao, Jinhao, Hongwei Gu, and Bing Xu. 2009. "Multifunctional Magnetic Nanoparticles: Design, Synthesis, and Biomedical Applications." *Accounts of Chemical Research* 42 (8): 1097–1107. https://doi.org/10.1021/ar9000026.

Garrigue, Philippe, Jingjie Tang, Ling Ding, Ahlem Bouhlel, Aura Tintaru, Erik Laurini, Yuanyu Huang, et al. 2018. "Self-Assembling Supramolecular Dendrimer Nanosystem for PET Imaging of Tumors." *Proceedings of the National Academy of Sciences* 115 (45): 11454–9. https://doi.org/10.1073/pnas.1812938115.

Ghai, Anchal, Natasha Singh, Shalini Chopra, and Baljinder Singh. 2018. "Radiolabeled Dendrimers as Potential PET Agents for Molecular Imaging of Tumor Angiogenesis." *Dendrimers—Fundamentals and Applications*. https://doi.org/10.5772/intechopen.71189.

Gmeiner, William H., and Supratim Ghosh. 2016. "Nanotechnology for Cancer Treatment." *Nano Online*. https://doi.org/10.1515/nano.0034.00077.

Gries, H. 2002. "Extracellular MRI Contrast Agents Based on Gadolinium." *Topics in Current Chemistry* 1–24. https://doi.org/10.1007/3-540-45733-x_1.

Guan, B., and Xingwang Zhang. 2020. "Aptamers as Versatile Ligands for Biomedical and Pharmaceutical Applications." *International Journal of Nanomedicine* 15: 1059–71. https://doi.org/10.2147/ijn.s237544.

Han, Min, Ming-Yi Huang-Fu, Wang-Wei Guo, Ning-Ning Guo, JieJian Chen, Hui-Na Liu, Zhi-Qi Xie, Meng-Ting Lin, Qi-Chun Wei, and Jian-Qing Gao. 2017. "MMP-2-Sensitive Ha End-Conjugated Poly(Amidoamine) Dendrimers via Click Reaction to Enhance Drug Penetration into Solid Tumor." *ACS Applied Materials & Interfaces* 9 (49): 42459–70. https://doi.org/10.1021/acsami.7b10098.

Haris, Mohammad, Santosh K. Yadav, Arshi Rizwan, Anup Singh, Ena Wang, Hari Hariharan, Ravinder Reddy, and Francesco M. Marincola. 2015. "Molecular Magnetic Resonance Imaging in Cancer." *Journal of Translational Medicine* 13 (1). https://doi.org/10.1186/s12967-015-0659-x.

Harish, Vancha, Md Mustafiz Ansari, Devesh Tewari, Manish Gaur, Awadh Bihari Yadav, María-Luisa García-Betancourt, Fatehy M. Abdel-Haleem, Mikhael Bechelany, and Ahmed Barhoum. 2022. "Nanoparticle and Nanostructure Synthesis and Controlled Growth Methods." *Nanomaterials* 12 (18): 3226. https://doi.org/10.3390/nano12183226.

Hasanzade, Zohre, and Heidar Raissi. 2019. "Carbon and Boron Nanotubes as a Template Material for Adsorption of 6-Thioguanine Chemotherapeutic: A Molecular Dynamics and Density Functional Approach." *Journal of Biomolecular Structure and Dynamics* 38 (3): 697–707. https://doi.org/10.1080/07391102.2019.1585951.

He, Wei, Guanyu Ma, Quanli Shen, and Zhenghua Tang. 2022. "Engineering Gold Nanostructures for Cancer Treatment: Spherical Nanoparticles, Nanorods, and Atomically Precise Nanoclusters." *Nanomaterials* 12 (10): 1738. https://doi.org/10.3390/nano12101738.

Herma, Regina, Dominika Wrobel, Michaela Liegertová, Monika Müllerová, Tomáš Strašák, Marek Maly, Alena Semerádtová, Marcel Štofik, Dietmar Appelhans, and Jan Maly. 2019. "Carbosilane Dendrimers With Phosphonium Terminal Groups are Low Toxic Non-Viral Transfection Vectors for Sirna Cell Delivery." *International Journal of Pharmaceutics* 562: 51–65. https://doi.org/10.1016/j.ijpharm.2019.03.018.

Hirsch, L. R., R. J. Stafford, J. A. Bankson, S. R. Sershen, B. Rivera, R. E. Price, J. D. Hazle, N. J. Halas, and J. L. West. 2003. "Nanoshell-Mediated Near-Infrared Thermal Therapy of Tumors Under Magnetic Resonance Guidance." *Proceedings of the National Academy of Sciences* 100 (23): 13549–54. https://doi.org/10.1073/pnas.2232479100.

Hoeks, Caroline M., Jelle O. Barentsz, Thomas Hambrock, Derya Yakar, Diederik M. Somford, Stijn W. Heijmink, Tom W. Scheenen, et al. 2011. "Prostate Cancer: Multiparametric MR Imaging for Detection, Localization, and Staging." *Radiology* 261 (1): 46–66. https://doi.org/10.1148/radiol.11091822.

Hu, Yanjie, Jin'e Zheng, and Shiang Huang. 2016. "Detection of Circulating Tumor Cells and Circulating Tumor Stem Cells in Breast Cancer by Using Flow Cytometry." *Tumor Metastasis*. https://doi.org/10.5772/63423.

Huang, Yingbo. 2022. "Review for an Overview of Polymeric Nanoparticles-Based Drug Delivery System in Cancer Treatment." https://doi.org/10.1177/15330338231152083/v2/review2.

Israel, Liron L., Anna Galstyan, Eggehard Holler, and Julia Y. Ljubimova. 2020. "Magnetic Iron Oxide Nanoparticles for Imaging, Targeting and Treatment of Primary and Metastatic Tumors of the Brain." *Journal of Controlled Release* 320: 45–62. https://doi.org/10.1016/j.jconrel.2020.01.009.

Jiang, Shan, Muthu Kumara Gnanasammandhan, and Yong Zhang. 2009. "Optical Imaging-Guided Cancer Therapy With Fluorescent Nanoparticles." *Journal of The Royal Society Interface* 7 (42): 3–18. https://doi.org/10.1098/rsif.2009.0243.

Jin, Cancan, Kankai Wang, Anthony Oppong-Gyebi, and Jiangnan Hu. 2020. "Application of Nanotechnology in Cancer Diagnosis and Therapy—A Mini-Review." *International Journal of Medical Sciences* 17 (18): 2964–73. https://doi.org/10.7150/ijms.49801.

Kambali, Imam, and Hari Suryanto. 2020. "Cancer Imaging Using Positron Emission Tomography/Computed Tomography." *2020 International Seminar on Intelligent Technology and Its Applications (ISITIA)*. https://doi.org/10.1109/isitia49792.2020.9163740.

Karki, Neha, Anita Rana, Himani Tiwari, Pushpa Negi, and Nanda Gopal Sahoo. 2020. "Theranostics Application of Graphene-Based Materials in Cancer Imaging, Targeting and Treatment." *Tumor Progression and Metastasis*. https://doi.org/10.5772/intechopen.91331.

Katsarou, Spyridoula D., Ippokratis Messaritakis, Anastasia Voumvouraki, Stavros Kakavogiannis, Athanasios Kotsakis, Saad Alkahtani, Christos Stournaras, Stuart S. Martin, Vassilis Georgoulias, and Galatea Kallergi. 2022. "Detyrosinated α-Tubulin, Vimentin and PD-L1 in Circulating Tumor Cells (Ctcs) Isolated From Non-Small Cell Lung Cancer (NSCLC) Patients." *Journal of Personalized Medicine* 12 (2): 154. https://doi.org/10.3390/jpm12020154.

Kim, Dongkyu, Yong Yeon Jeong, and Sangyong Jon. 2010. "A Drug-Loaded Aptamer–Gold Nanoparticle Bioconjugate for Combined CT Imaging and Therapy of Prostate Cancer." *ACS Nano* 4 (7): 3689–96. https://doi.org/10.1021/nn901877h.

Kim, Jaeyun, Yuanzhe Piao, and Taeghwan Hyeon. 2009. "Multifunctional Nanostructured Materials for Multimodal Imaging, and Simultaneous Imaging and Therapy." *Chemical Society Reviews* 38 (2): 372–90. https://doi.org/10.1039/b709883a.

Kolhe, Parag, Jayant Khandare, Omathanu Pillai, Sujatha Kannan, Mary Lieh-Lai, and Rangaramanujam M. Kannan. 2006. "Preparation, Cellular Transport, and Activity of Polyamidoamine-Based Dendritic Nanodevices With a High Drug Payload." *Biomaterials* 27 (4): 660–9. https://doi.org/10.1016/j.biomaterials.2005.06.007.

Kuhlmann, Jan Dominik, Pauline Wimberger, Agnes Bankfalvi, Thomas Keller, Sarah Schöler, Bahriye Aktas, Paul Buderath, Siegfried Hauch, Friedrich Otterbach, Rainer Kimmig, Sabine Kasimir-Bauer. 2014. "ERCC1-Positive Circulating Tumor Cells in the Blood of Ovarian Cancer Patients as a Predictive Biomarker for Platinum Resistance." *Clinical Chemistry* 60 (10): 1282–89. https://doi.org/10.1373/clinchem.2014.224808.

Liu, Yijing, Pravin Bhattarai, Zhifei Dai, and Xiaoyuan Chen. 2019. "Photothermal Therapy and Photoacoustic Imaging *via* Nanotheranostics in Fighting Cancer." *Chemical Society Reviews* 48 (7): 2053–108. https://doi.org/10.1039/c8cs00618k.

Luo, Dong, Andrew Johnson, Xinning Wang, Hao Li, Bernadette O. Erokwu, Sarah Springer, Jason Lou et al. 2020. "Targeted Radiosensitizers for MR-Guided Radiation Therapy of Prostate Cancer." *Nano Letters* 20 (10): 7159–67. https://doi.org/10.1021/acs.nanolett.0c02487.

Luo, Dong, Xinning Wang, Clemens Burda, and James P. Basilion. 2021. "Recent Development of Gold Nanoparticles as Contrast Agents for Cancer Diagnosis." *Cancers* 13 (8): 1825. https://doi.org/10.3390/cancers13081825.

Ma, Ying-Yu, Ke-Tao Jin, Shi-Bing Wang, Hui-Ju Wang, Xiang-Min Tong, Dong-Sheng Huang, and Xiao-Zhou Mou. 2017. "Molecular Imaging of Cancer With Nanoparticle-Based Theranostic Probes." *Contrast Media & Molecular Imaging* 2017: 1–11. https://doi.org/10.1155/2017/1026270.

Marques, A. C., P. J. Costa, S. Velho, and M. H. Amaral. 2020. "Functionalizing Nanoparticles With Cancer-Targeting Antibodies: A Comparison of Strategies." *Journal of Controlled Release* 320: 180–200. https://doi.org/10.1016/j.jconrel.2020.01.035.

Martin, Jacob W., Grant J. McIntosh, Rakesh Arul, Reece N. Oosterbeek, Markus Kraft, and Tilo Söhnel. 2017. "Giant Fullerene Formation Through Thermal Treatment of Fullerene Soot." *Carbon* 125: 132–8. https://doi.org/10.1016/j.carbon.2017.09.045.

Mazahir, Farhan, Anchal Pathak, Ujala Gupta, and Awesh K. Yadav. 2023. "Nanotechnology for Cancer Treatment: An Introduction." *Therapeutic Nanocarriers in Cancer Treatment: Challenges and Future Perspective* 31–63. https://doi.org/10.2174/9789815080506123010005.

Mehta, Arnav, Ketan Ghaghada, and Srinivasan Mukundan. 2016. "Molecular Imaging of Brain Tumors Using Liposomal Contrast Agents and Nanoparticles." *Magnetic Resonance Imaging Clinics of North America* 24 (4): 751–63. https://doi.org/10.1016/j.mric.2016.06.004.

Miyata, Kanjiro, R. James Christie, and Kazunori Kataoka. 2011. "Polymeric Micelles for Nano-Scale Drug Delivery." *Reactive and Functional Polymers* 71 (3): 227–34. https://doi.org/10.1016/j.reactfunctpolym.2010.10.009.

Na, Hyon Bin, In Chan Song, and Taeghwan Hyeon. 2009. "Inorganic Nanoparticles for MRI Contrast Agents." *Advanced Materials* 21 (21): 2133–48. https://doi.org/10.1002/adma.200802366.

Nakamura, Hiroshi, Naoki Ito, Fumio Kotake, Yuji Mizokami, and Takeshi Matsuoka. 2000. "Tumor-Detecting Capacity and Clinical Usefulness of Spio-MRI in Patients With Hepatocellular Carcinoma." *Journal of Gastroenterology* 35 (11): 849–55. https://doi.org/10.1007/s005350070022.

Nayak, Pratyusha, Reetuparna Nanda, and Monalisa Mishra. 2021. "Role of Nanoparticles in Medical Imaging." *Medical Imaging Methods* 107–44. https://doi.org/10.1201/9781003112068-5.

Nunes, Toni, Thomas Pons, Xue Hou, Khanh Van Do, Benoît Caron, Marthe Rigal, Mélanie Di Benedetto, et al. 2019. "Pulsed-Laser Irradiation of Multifunctional Gold Nanoshells to Overcome Trastuzumab Resistance in HER2-Overexpressing Breast Cancer." *Journal of Experimental & Clinical Cancer Research* 38 (1). https://doi.org/10.1186/s13046-019-1305-x.

Olusanya, Temidayo, Rita Haj Ahmad, Daniel Ibegbu, James Smith, and Amal Elkordy. 2018. "Liposomal Drug Delivery Systems and Anticancer Drugs." *Molecules* 23 (4): 907. https://doi.org/10.3390/molecules 23040907.

Oraevsky, Alexander A. 2017. "Gold and Silver Nanoparticles as Contrast Agents for Optoacoustic Tomography." *Photoacoustic Imaging and Spectroscopy* 373–86. https://doi.org/10.1201/9781420059922-40.

Orel, Susan Greenstein. 2003. "Magnetic Resonance Imaging (MRI) and MRI-Guided Intervention in the Detection and Diagnosis of Breast Cancer." *Image-Guided Diagnosis and Treatment of Cancer* 75–100. https://doi.org/10.1007/978-1-59259-422-1_4.

Owens III, D., and N. Peppas. 2006. "Opsonization, Biodistribution, and Pharmacokinetics of Polymeric Nanoparticles." *International Journal of Pharmaceutics* 307 (1): 93–102. https://doi.org/10.1016/j.ijpharm.2005.10.010.

Pang, Xuehui, Cheng Cui, Minhui Su, Yaoguang Wang, Qin Wei, and Weihong Tan. 2018. "Construction of Self-Powered Cytosensing Device Based on Zno Nanodisks@g-C3N4 Quantum Dots and Application in the Detection of CCRF-Cem Cells." *Nano Energy* 46: 101–9. https://doi.org/10.1016/j.nanoen.2018.01.018.

Parra-Cabrera, C., J. Samitier, and A. Homs-Corbera. 2016. "Multiple Biomarkers Biosensor With Just-in-time Functionalization: Application to Prostate Cancer Detection." *Bioelectronics/Biosensors & Bioelectronics* (Online) 77 (March): 1192–200. https://doi.org/10.1016/j.bios.2015.10.064.

Patra, Chitta Ranjan, Resham Bhattacharya, Debabrata Mukhopadhyay, and Priyabrata Mukherjee. 2010. "Fabrication of Gold Nanoparticles for Targeted Therapy in Pancreatic Cancer." *Advanced Drug Delivery Reviews* 62 (3): 346–61. https://doi.org/10.1016/j.addr.2009.11.007.

Peng, Chun-Wei, and Yan Li. 2010. "Application of Quantum Dots-Based Biotechnology in Cancer Diagnosis: Current Status and Future Perspectives." *Journal of Nanomaterials* 2010: 1–11. https://doi.org/10.1155/2010/676839.

Powell, Ashley A., AmirAli H. Talasaz, Haiyu Zhang, Marc A. Coram, Anupama Reddy, Glenn Deng, Melinda L. Telli, et al. 2012. "Single Cell Profiling of Circulating Tumor Cells: Transcriptional Heterogeneity and Diversity From Breast Cancer Cell Lines." *PLoS One* 7 (5). https://doi.org/10.1371/journal.pone.0033788.

Pramanik, Arindam. 2019. "Recent Advancements on Nano-Based Drug Delivery System for Targeted Cancer Therapy." *Nanotechnology in Biology and Medicine* 133–41. https://doi.org/10.1201/9780429259333-10.

Qiu, Wenli, Rong Chen, Xiao Chen, Huifeng Zhang, Lina Song, Wenjing Cui, Jingjing Zhang, Dandan Ye, Yifen Zhang, and Zhongqiu Wang. 2018. "Oridonin-Loaded and GPC1-Targeted Gold Nanoparticles for Multimodal Imaging and Therapy in Pancreatic Cancer." *International Journal of Nanomedicine* 13: 6809–27. https://doi.org/10.2147/ijn.s177993.

Rahman, M. 2023. "Magnetic Resonance Imaging and Iron-Oxide Nanoparticles in the Era of Personalized Medicine." *Nanotheranostics* 7 (4): 424–49. https://doi.org/10.7150/ntno.86467.

Ramezani, Zahra, Michael Thompson, and Elaheh Mohammadi. 2023. "Quantum Dots in Imaging, Diagnosis, and Targeted Drug Delivery to Cancer Cells." *Quantum Dots in Bioanalytical Chemistry and Medicine* 107–41. https://doi.org/10.1039/9781839169564-00107.

Raza, Faisal, Lauren Evans, Mahzad Motallebi, Hajra Zafar, Miguel Pereira-Silva, Kalsoom Saleem, Diana Peixoto et al. 2023. "Liposome-Based Diagnostic and Therapeutic Applications for Pancreatic Cancer." *Acta Biomaterialia* 157: 1–23. https://doi.org/10.1016/j.actbio.2022.12.013.

Rosenthal, David I., Sue S. Yom, Li Liu, Mitchell Machtay, Kenneth Algazy, Randal S. Weber, Gregory S. Weinstein, et al. 2002. "A Phase I Study of SPI-077 (Stealth® Liposomal Cisplatin) Concurrent With Radiation Therapy for Locally Advanced Head and Neck Cancer." *Investigational New Drugs* 20 (3): 343–9. https://doi.org/10.1023/a:1016201732368.

Saraf, Shivani, Ankit Jain, Ankita Tiwari, Amit Verma, Pritish Kumar Panda, and Sanjay K. Jain. 2020. "Advances in Liposomal Drug Delivery to Cancer: An Overview." *Journal of Drug Delivery Science and Technology* 56: 101549. https://doi.org/10.1016/j.jddst.2020.101549.

Seferos, Dwight S., David A. Giljohann, Haley D. Hill, Andrew E. Prigodich, and Chad A. Mirkin. 2007. "Nano-Flares: Probes for Transfection and Mrna Detection in Living Cells." *Journal of the American Chemical Society* 129 (50): 15477–9. https://doi.org/10.1021/ja0776529.

Seo, Nieun, Joon Seok Lim, and Arthur Cho. 2019. "Radiologic Diagnosis (CT, MRI, & Pet-CT)." *Surgery for Gastric Cancer* 67–86. https://doi.org/10.1007/978-3-662-45583-8_4.

Serpe, Loredana, Federica Foglietta, and Roberto Canaparo. 2012. "Nanosonotechnology: The Next Challenge in Cancer Sonodynamic Therapy." *Nanotechnology Reviews* 1 (2): 173–82. https://doi.org/10.1515/ntrev-2011-0009.

Shah, Muhammad Raza, Muhammad Imran, and Shafi Ullah. 2017. "Liposomes." *Lipid-Based Nanocarriers for Drug Delivery and Diagnosis* 63–110. https://doi.org/10.1016/b978-0-323-52729-3.00003-2.

Sharaf, M., Ali A. Alhamad, Olfa O. Ltaief, and Ilham B. Amor. 2023. "Challenges of Nanomaterials-Based Cancer Therapy: A Future Destination." *International Journal of Surgery* 109 (6): 1819–20. https://doi.org/10.1097/js9.0000000000000412.

Sherry, A. Dean, and Mark Woods. 2008. "Chemical Exchange Saturation Transfer Contrast Agents for Magnetic Resonance Imaging." *Annual Review of Biomedical Engineering* 10 (1): 391–411. https://doi.org/10.1146/annurev.bioeng.9.060906.151929.

Shiba, Kiyotaka. 2003. "Nanotubes, Nanowires, Nanocantilevers and Nanorods in Cancer Treatment and Diagnosis." *Nanotechnologies for the Life Sciences*. https://doi.org/10.1002/9783527610419.ntls0078.

Shilo, Malka, Tobi Reuveni, Menachem Motiei, and Rachela Popovtzer. 2012. "Nanoparticles as Computed Tomography Contrast Agents: Current Status and Future Perspectives." *Nanomedicine* 7 (2): 257–69. https://doi.org/10.2217/nnm.11.190.

Shirvalilou, Sakine, SamidehKhoei, Sepideh Khoee, Seied Rabi Mahdavi, Nida Jamali Raoufi, Manijeh Motevalian, and Mohammad Yahya Karimi. 2020. "Enhancement Radiation-Induced Apoptosis in C6 Glioma Tumor-Bearing Rats via PH-Responsive Magnetic Graphene Oxide Nanocarrier." *Journal of Photochemistry and Photobiology B: Biology* 205: 111827. https://doi.org/10.1016/j.jphotobiol.2020.111827.

Singh, Keshav K. 2005. "Nanotechnology in Cancer Detection and Treatment." *Technology in Cancer Research & Treatment* 4 (6): 583. https://doi.org/10.1177/153303460500400601.

Singla, Rubbel, Chandni Sharma, Ashish K. Shukla, and Amitabha Acharya. 2019. "Toxicity Concerns of Therapeutic Nanomaterials." *Journal of Nanoscience and Nanotechnology* 19 (4): 1889–907. https://doi.org/10.1166/jnn.2019.16502.

Soppimath, Kumaresh S., Tejraj M. Aminabhavi, Anandrao R. Kulkarni, and Walter E. Rudzinski. 2001. "Biodegradable Polymeric Nanoparticles as Drug Delivery Devices." *Journal of Controlled Release* 70 (1–2): 1–20. https://doi.org/10.1016/s0168-3659(00)00339-4.

Sun, Conroy, Jerry S. H. Lee, and Miqin Zhang. 2008. "Magnetic Nanoparticles in MR Imaging and Drug Delivery." *Advanced Drug Delivery Reviews* 60 (11): 1252–65. https://doi.org/10.1016/j.addr.2008.03.018.

Sun, Na, Xinpan Li, Zhili Wang, Ruihua Zhang, Jine Wang, Kewei Wang, and Renjun Pei. 2016. "A Multiscale Tio2 Nanorod Array for Ultrasensitive Capture of Circulating Tumor Cells." *ACS Applied Materials & Interfaces* 8 (20): 12638–43. https://doi.org/10.1021/acsami.6b02178.

Syedmoradi, Leila, Maryam Daneshpour, Mehrdad Alvandipour, Frank A. Gomez, Hassan Hajghassem, and Kobra Omidfar. 2017. "Point of Care Testing: The Impact of Nanotechnology." *Biosensors and Bioelectronics* 87: 373–87. https://doi.org/10.1016/j.bios.2016.08.084.

Teow, Yiwei, P. V. Asharani, M. Prakash Hande, and Suresh Valiyaveettil. 2011. "Health Impact and Safety of Engineered Nanomaterials." *Chemical Communications* 47 (25): 7025. https://doi.org/10.1039/c0cc05271j.

Thirugnanasambandan, Theivasanthi. 2021. "Nanoparticles for Biomedical Imaging Advancements." *Nanoparticles in Analytical and Medical Devices* 127–54. https://doi.org/10.1016/b978-0-12-821163-2.00008-x.

Tholouli, E., E. Sweeney, E. Barrow, V. Clay, J. A. Hoyland, and R. J. Byers. 2008. "Quantum Dots Light Up Pathology." *The Journal of Pathology* 216 (3): 275–85. https://doi.org/10.1002/path.2421.

True, Lawrence D., and Xiaohu Gao. 2007. "Quantum Dots for Molecular Pathology." *The Journal of Molecular Diagnostics* 9 (1): 7–11. https://doi.org/10.2353/jmoldx.2007.060186.

Vankayala, Raviraj, and Kuo Chu Hwang. 2018. "Near-Infrared-Light-Activatable Nanomaterial-Mediated Phototheranostic Nanomedicines: An Emerging Paradigm for Cancer Treatment." *Advanced Materials* 30 (23). https://doi.org/10.1002/adma.201706320.

Wan, Xinyuan, Yuanqing Song, Nijia Song, Jiehua Li, Lie Yang, Yuan Li, and Hong Tan. 2016. "The Preliminary Study of Immune Superparamagnetic Iron Oxide Nanoparticles for the Detection of Lung Cancer in Magnetic Resonance Imaging." *Carbohydrate Research* 419: 33–40. https://doi.org/10.1016/j.carres.2015.11.003.

Wang, Jianqiu, Meihua Sui, and Weimin Fan. 2010. "Nanoparticles for Tumor Targeted Therapies and Their Pharmacokinetics." *Current Drug Metabolism* 11 (2): 129–41. https://doi.org/10.2174/138920010791110827.

Wang, Ying, Zhaohui Li, Jun Wang, Jinghong Li, and Yuehe Lin. 2011. "Graphene and Graphene Oxide: Biofunctionalization and Applications in Biotechnology." *Trends in Biotechnology* 29 (5): 205–12. https://doi.org/10.1016/j.tibtech.2011.01.008.

Wang, Yunqing, and Lingxin Chen. 2011. "Quantum Dots, Lighting up the Research and Development of Nanomedicine." *Nanomedicine: Nanotechnology, Biology and Medicine* 7 (4): 385–402. https://doi.org/10.1016/j.nano.2010.12.006.

Wei, A., M. Thomas, J. Mehtala, and J. Wang. 2013. "Gold Nanoparticles (Gnps) as Multifunctional Materials for Cancer Treatment." *Biomaterials for Cancer Therapeutics*. https://doi.org/10.1533/9780857096760.3.349.

Wen, Cong-Ying, Ling-Ling Wu, Zhi-Ling Zhang, Yu-Lin Liu, Shao-Zhong Wei, Jiao Hu, Man Tang, et al. 2013. "Quick-Response Magnetic Nanospheres for Rapid, Efficient Capture and Sensitive Detection of Circulating Tumor Cells." *ACS Nano* 8 (1): 941–9. https://doi.org/10.1021/nn405744f.

Wilson, Katheryne E., Keerthi S. Valluru, and Jürgen K. Willmann. 2016. "Nanoparticles for Photoacoustic Imaging of Cancer." *Design and Applications of Nanoparticles in Biomedical Imaging* 315–35. https://doi.org/10.1007/978-3-319-42169-8_15.

Woodman, Christopher, Gugulethu Vundu, Alex George, and Cornelia M. Wilson. 2021. "Applications and Strategies in Nanodiagnosis and Nanotherapy in Lung Cancer." *Seminars in Cancer Biology* 69: 349–64. https://doi.org/10.1016/j.semcancer.2020.02.009.

Wu, Yue, Moustafa R. K. Ali, Kuangcai Chen, Ning Fang, and Mostafa A. El-Sayed. 2019. "Gold Nanoparticles in Biological Optical Imaging." *Nano Today* 24: 120–40. https://doi.org/10.1016/j.nantod.2018.12.006.

Xiao, Yu-Dong, Ramchandra Paudel, Jun Liu, Cong Ma, Zi-Shu Zhang, and Shun-Ke Zhou. 2016. "MRI Contrast Agents: Classification and Application (Review)." *International Journal of Molecular Medicine* 38 (5): 1319–26. https://doi.org/10.3892/ijmm.2016.2744.

Yao, Ying. 2016. *Detection of Ovarian Cancer Circulatng Tumor Cells to Monitor the Metastasis of Ovarian Cancer*. https://doi.org/10.26226/morressier.5770e29cd462b80290b4bf19.

Ye, Lianjie, Larwubah Kollie, Xing Liu, Wei Guo, Xiangxian Ying, Jun Zhu, Shengjie Yang, and Meilan Yu. 2021. "Antitumor Activity and Potential Mechanism of Novel Fullerene Derivative Nanoparticles." *Molecules* 26 (11): 3252. https://doi.org/10.3390/molecules26113252.

Yigitaslan, Semra, and Kevser Erol. 2021. "Chemistry, Physicochemical Properties and Pharmacokinetics of Gadolinium-Based Contrast Agents." *Medical Imaging Contrast Agents: A Clinical Manual* 63–9. https://doi.org/10.1007/978-3-030-79256-5_7.

Zhai, Guijin, Liping Yang, Qun Luo, Kui Wu, Yao Zhao, and Fuyi Wang. 2022. "Serum Phosphopeptide Profiling for Colorectal Cancer Diagnosis Using Liquid Chromatography–Mass Spectrometry." *Rapid Communications in Mass Spectrometry* 36 (15). https://doi.org/10.1002/rcm.9316.

Zhang, Dan, Xin-Lei Ma, Yan Gu, He Huang, and Guang-Wei Zhang. 2020. "Green Synthesis of Metallic Nanoparticles and Their Potential Applications to Treat Cancer." *Frontiers in Chemistry* 8 (October). https://doi.org/10.3389/fchem.2020.00799.

Zhang, Nan, Dongxue Zhu, Feng Li, Haiying Hua, Xin Tian, and Yongxing Zhao. 2017. "Low Density Lipoprotein Peptide-Conjugated Gold Nanorods for Combating Gastric Cancer." *Journal of Biomedical Nanotechnology* 13 (2): 134–43. https://doi.org/10.1166/jbn.2017.2330.

Zhang, P., W. Yi, J. Hou, S. Yoo, W. Jin, and Q. Yang. 2018. "A Carbon Nanotube-Gemcitabine-Lentinan Three-Component Composite for Chemo-photothermal Synergistic Therapy of Cancer." *International Journal of Nanomedicine* 25 (13): 3069–80. doi: 10.2147/IJN.S165232.

Zhu, Y., P. Chandra, and Y. B. Shim. 2013. "Ultrasensitive and Selective Electrochemical Diagnosis of Breast Cancer Based on a Hydrazine-Au Nanoparticle-Aptamer Bioconjugate." *Analytical Chemistry* 85 (2): 1058–64. doi: 10.1021/ac302923k [PubMed].

6 Nano Contrast Agents
Illuminating Cancer Pathways for Precise Diagnosis

Gagandeep Singh, Arshiya Sood, and Neelam Thakur

ABBREVIATIONS

Acronym	Full Form
MRI	magnetic resonance imaging
SPIONs	superparamagnetic iron oxide nanoparticles
CT	computed tomography
PET	positron emission tomography
SERS	surface-enhanced Raman spectroscopy
FI/OI	fluorescence/optical imaging
PAI	photoacoustic imaging
PTT	photothermal therapy
ROS	reactive oxygen species
BBB	blood–brain barrier
GBCAs	gadolinium-based contrast agents
FDA	Food and Drug Administration
FTIR	Fourier transform infrared spectroscopy
T1	longitudinal relaxation time
T2	transverse relaxation time
GON	gadolinium oxide nanocrystals
AN	albumin nanoparticles
FA	folic acid
TPL	two-photon photoluminescence

6.1 INTRODUCTION

Cancer, a relentless and potentially fatal disease, presents an imposing challenge to modern medicine. To enhance patient outcomes and elevate survival rates, the early diagnosis and effective treatment of this insidious adversary are imperative. This review embarks on a journey through the ever-evolving landscape of contrast agents for cancer diagnosis. It focuses on nanoparticles and their potential to revolutionize the field. In doing so, we aim to underscore the significance of early detection, precision, and tailored therapy, drawing from recent studies and research papers. In the domain of cancer, gastric cancer, while relatively rare in young patients, often emerges at an advanced stage, resulting in a bleak prognosis. Evaluating *Helicobacter pylori* infection and employing eradication therapy can play a pivotal role in its prevention and early detection (Kono et al. 2020). Meanwhile, bladder cancer, another formidable foe, could significantly benefit from the development of exosomal biomarkers found in urine, offering essential tools for its management, diagnosis, and surveillance (Georgantzoglou et al. 2021). Cervical cancer, on the other hand, is linked to aberrant DNA

DOI: 10.1201/9781003463191-8

methylation and hydroxymethylation in specific genes. Profiling these genetic patterns emerges as a vital strategy for early prevention, diagnosis, prognosis, and treatment (Zhu et al. 2020). Shifting the focus to breast cancer, a primary contributor to cancer-related deaths in women, a novel hybrid deep learning model holds potential for classifying histopathological images of breast cancer. This innovation could potentially result in earlier and more precise diagnoses (Burçak and Uguz 2022). Early detection is equally critical for lung cancer, and a multiple-instance learning algorithm with deep attention, incorporating radiomics as input features, has shown significant promise, providing optimism for both patients and clinicians (Chen et al. 2021).

This review delves into the transformative potential of nanoparticles as contrast agents in cancer diagnosis, transitioning from conventional diagnostic methods to the forefront of nanotechnology. These nanostructures hold immense promise, as our comprehensive review illustrates. Each type of nanoparticle—magnetic, iron oxide, polymer, nanocomposites, peptide-coated, and gold—has a special function in the arsenal for addressing and diagnosing cancer (Table 6.1). A new age of precision medicine has been ushered in by the functional modification of magnetic nanoparticles to behave as carriers and targeting motifs for therapeutic medicines (Gallo, Long, and Aboagye 2013). Ultrasmall iron oxide nanoparticles, often employed as MRI contrast agents, offer exceptional diagnostic potential, potentially surpassing the limitations of conventional gadolinium-based agents (Amraee et al. 2022). Polymer nanoparticles have emerged as contrast-enhancing agents for cervical tumor imaging and photothermal therapy, showcasing their versatility and utility (Qiu et al. 2021). Additionally, nanocomposites have opened up new avenues for cancer diagnostics and therapeutics with multifaceted applications in sensing, imaging, and drug delivery (Subramanian, Jaganathan, and Supriyanto 2015). Peptide-coated nanoparticles are poised to revolutionize targeted anticancer therapy, showing a particular affinity for mitochondrial accumulation, enhancing their effectiveness (Poursharifi et al. 2020). Gold nanoparticles, renowned for their versatility, have played a substantial role in advancing laboratory-based clinical diagnosis and in vivo characterization methodologies, leading to early detection and therapeutic interventions (Vijayakumar and Paulsi 2013).

We shall go into more detail about these contrast agents based on nanoparticles in the upcoming sections of this review. We will specifically examine magnetic nanoparticles, gold nanoparticles, superparamagnetic iron oxide nanoparticles, and gadolinium oxide nanocrystal–based autofluorescent composite nanoparticles. Our exploration will encompass their descriptions, applications, and recent advancements. These nanoparticles offer immense promise in enhancing the precision and efficacy of cancer diagnosis, further strengthening our arsenal in the ongoing battle against this formidable adversary.

6.2 MAGNETIC NANOPARTICLES

Magnetic nanoparticles, distinguished by their potent magnetization but absence of permanent magnetism, have emerged as indispensable tools in the realm of medical diagnostics, particularly in the enhancement of magnetic resonance imaging (MRI) contrast (Issa and Obaidat 2019). These nanoparticles, most notably iron oxide nanoparticles, have been employed as contrast agents in MRI due to their superparamagnetic properties. These nanoparticles are often coated with polymers and functional particles, rendering them versatile for a range of biomedical applications (Issa and Obaidat 2019) (Figure 6.1). The intrinsic properties of magnetic nanoparticles, including size, shape, and surface coating, significantly influence their efficacy as MRI relaxation enhancers, with a particular emphasis on T2 relaxation (Issa and Obaidat 2019). Their tunable relaxivity enables the creation of high-contrast MRI images, facilitating the delineation of pathological tissues (Vuong et al. 2012). Furthermore, the biocompatibility of functionalized magnetic nanoparticles, as assessed through their interaction with lipid bilayers mimicking plasma cellular membranes, ensures their safe use in clinical applications (Luchini 2016).

TABLE 6.1
Comparison of Contrast Agents for Cancer Diagnosis and Therapy

Contrast Agent	Magnetic Properties	Biocompatibility	Specificity	Cytotoxicity	Imaging Modalities Supported	Clinical Applications	References
Magnetic nanoparticles	Superparamagnetic	Yes	High	Low	MRI	Cancer therapy, drug delivery, imaging enhancement	Luchini (2016); Issa and Obaidat (2019); Kaliamurthi et al. (2019); Cortés-Llanos et al. (2021); Etli and Akar (2022); Onishi et al. (2022)
Gold nanoparticles	Gold nanoparticles	Yes	High	Low	CT, MRI, PET, PAI, TPL, SERS	Early-phase clinical trials, radiation therapy, drug carriers	Jain, Hirst, and O'Sullivan (2012); Butterworth et al. (2013); Dorsey et al. (2013); Cabral and Baptista (2014); Liu et al. (2015); Ning, Zhu, and Gao (2017)
Superparamagnetic iron oxide	Superparamagnetic	Yes	High	Low	MRI	MRI contrast enhancement, hyperthermia, drug delivery	Crimi et al. (2013); Fattahi, Eghbali, and Oskoei (2015); Luchini (2016)
Gadolinium-based contrast agents	Paramagnetic ions	Yes	High	Low	MRI	MRI diagnostics, neurological disorders	Fattahi, Eghbali, and Oskoei (2015); Pinter, Klein, and Mechtler (2016); Asadollahzade et al. (2022)
Gadolinium oxide nanocrystal–based autofluorescent composite nanoparticles	–	Yes	High	Low	MRI, autofluorescence	Early tumor detection, MRI sensitivity enhancement	Shen, Ma, and Wu (2015)

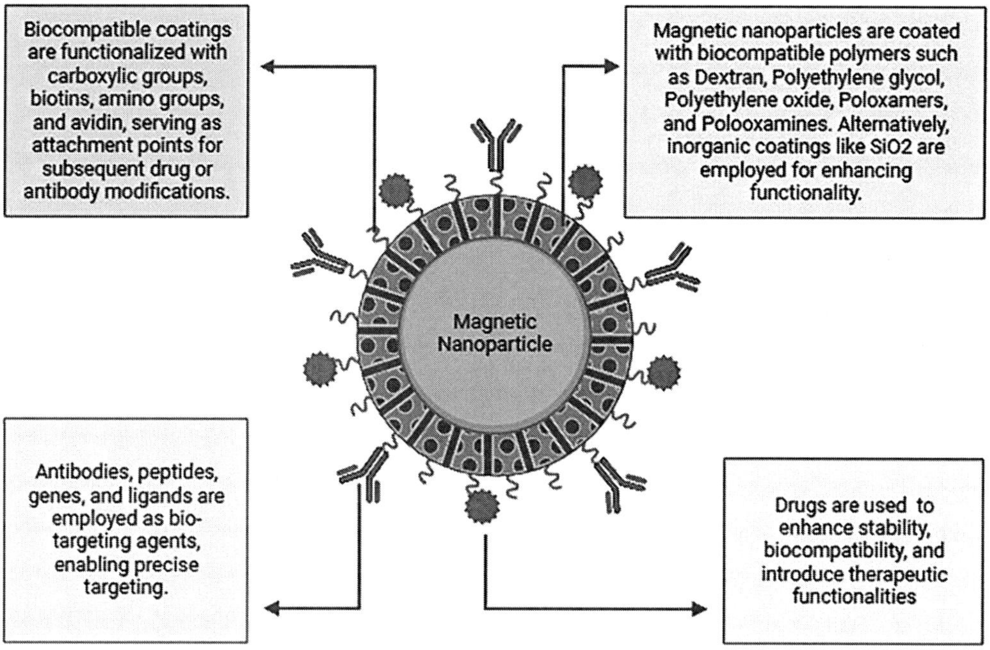

FIGURE 6.1 Multifunctional surface-stabilized magnetic nanoparticles for theranostic applications. This image illustrates the innovative surface stabilization of magnetic nanoparticles (MNPs) through the strategic application of peptides, antibodies, ligands, genes, and drugs. The purpose is to fabricate multifunctional MNPs, showcasing their potential in theranostic applications—integrating both therapeutic and diagnostic functionalities for advanced biomedical uses.

6.2.1 Clinical Applications of Magnetic Nanoparticles

Expanding the scope of their utility, magnetic nanoparticles have garnered considerable attention for their potential in cancer diagnosis and treatment. Notably, they offer an accelerated and safer approach to oncological investigations, enabling the detection of cancer biomarkers and immunostaining over a wide spectrum of applications (Onishi et al. 2022). In clinical settings, superparamagnetic iron oxide nanoparticles (SPIONs) have demonstrated their utility in the detection of sentinel lymph nodes, a critical component of breast cancer diagnosis, and have shown promise for gallbladder cancer in animal models. The rapidity of these diagnostic capabilities positions them as valuable tools for use during surgery, enhancing precision and minimizing invasiveness (Onishi et al. 2022). Moreover, magnetic nanoparticles hold the promise of earlier cancer detection compared to conventional imaging methods, presenting an opportunity for improved prognosis and therapeutic interventions (Gobbo et al. 2015). Their multifunctional nature allows for their application as non-invasive, ligand-conjugated nano-imaging vehicles for targeted drug delivery, presenting a groundbreaking approach to cancer diagnosis and therapy (Kaliamurthi et al. 2019). The concepts of active and passive targeting drug delivery, encompassing magnetic drug targeting and targeting ligand-conjugated magnetic nanoparticles, open new avenues for precision medicine in oncology (Kaliamurthi et al. 2019; Onishi et al. 2022). In MRI, magnetic nanoparticles are not confined to their role as positive contrast agents. They can also serve as negative contrast agents, and their relaxivity can be finely tuned to enhance the contrast in MRI images, further extending their utility in diagnostic imaging (Cortés-Llanos et al. 2021; Onishi et al. 2022). Optimal results have been achieved by employing magnetic nanoparticles with a core size ranging between 12 and 14 nm and coated with DMSA (dimercaptosuccinic acid), yielding enhanced contrast (Cortés-Llanos et al. 2021).

Beyond diagnostics, magnetic nanoparticles have penetrated the field of cancer therapy, offering versatile applications. Hyperthermia treatments, drug release systems, and imaging are among the promising avenues that have been explored, highlighting their multifaceted potential in the battle against cancer (Etli and Akar 2022).

6.2.2 Advancements in Functionalization and Therapeutic Drug Inclusion

Advancements in the functionalization and inclusion of therapeutic drugs in magnetic nanoparticles have ushered in promising developments in targeted drug delivery for various medical applications, particularly cancer treatment and brain cancer therapy. Recent research has unveiled several notable breakthroughs in this domain, further emphasizing the transformative potential of magnetic nanoparticles in the field of medical oncology. An innovative therapeutic platform designed for glioblastoma (GBM) therapy represents a notable advancement. This platform synergizes the magnetic targeting properties and drug delivery capabilities of magnetic nanoparticles with engineered exosomes. These exosomes enable the encapsulation of siRNA and the efficient penetration of the blood–brain barrier (BBB). Achieving enrichment within the brain via localized magnetic targeting, the platform utilizes angiopep-2 peptide-modified engineered exosomes for transcytosis. This allows the particles to traverse the blood–brain barrier, targeting glioblastoma cells by recognizing the LRP-1 receptor (B. Li et al. 2022). In the context of breast cancer, chitosan-coated magnetic nanoparticles have demonstrated effectiveness as drug delivery vehicles, presenting a potential avenue for targeted treatment of this malignancy (Taherian, Esfandiari, and Rouhani 2021). Additionally, in the context of colorectal cancer therapy, the utilization of magnetic functionalized nanoparticles has been instrumental in achieving responsive and targeted drug delivery. This approach leverages the interplay between inorganic nanoparticles and conjugated targeting ligands, promising efficient delivery and enhanced therapeutic outcomes (Darroudi et al. 2021). Brain cancer, a formidable adversary, has also witnessed significant strides in the form of polymeric magnetic nanoparticles. A multi-therapeutic strategy for drug delivery and imaging is to use polymeric nanoparticles that carry magnetic iron oxide nanoparticles. This can deliver drugs for chemotherapy, imaging, and magnetic targeting and induce hyperthermia (Joshi and Joshi 2022). In the context of bone marrow–related disorders, such as bone metastases, inorganic nanoparticles functionalized with glutamate ligands have demonstrated high affinity toward NMDA receptors on bone cells. These nanoparticles, for example, Fe_2O_3, have the potential to generate photo-induced reactive oxygen species, presenting a novel therapeutic opportunity for these challenging conditions (Ghosh et al. 2022).

6.3 GOLD NANOPARTICLES

Gold nanoparticles have become compelling contenders in cancer diagnosis and therapy, owing to their distinctive physicochemical and optical characteristics. Their versatile applications encompass roles as diagnostic reagents, drug carriers, contrast agents, photothermal agents, and radiosensitizers (Ning, Zhu, and Gao 2017). Positioned at the forefront of advanced platforms for combined diagnostic and therapeutic approaches, gold nanoparticles showcase an array of capabilities driven by their exquisite properties (Cabral and Baptista 2014). In the realm of cancer therapy, gold nanoparticles have garnered substantial attention and are currently under investigation in early-phase clinical trials (Jain, Hirst, and O'Sullivan 2012). A notable feature lies in their rich surface functionalization chemistry and high surface-area-to-volume ratio, enabling precise targeting while minimizing adverse effects on normal tissues associated with traditional treatments (Ning, Zhu, and Gao 2017). Designated as multifunctional tools for controlled drug release, gene therapy, photothermal therapy, and contrast imaging, they facilitate continuous monitoring in real time of both the progression of diseases and the effectiveness of therapeutic interventions, marking a significant stride in personalized medicine (Cabral and Baptista 2014). Furthermore, gold nanoparticles are uniquely suited to enhance the efficacy of radiation therapy due to their high atomic number (Z), resulting in significantly improved contrast compared to soft tissue (Butterworth et al. 2013; Dorsey et al. 2013). Their role as radiation sensitizers holds the potential to revolutionize cancer treatment strategies. The versatility of gold nanoparticles extends to their function as multimodal contrast agents. Gold nanostars (AuNS) showcase a noteworthy cross-platform adaptability, functioning as contrast agents across diverse imaging modalities, including macroscopic X-ray computer tomography (CT), PET, and MRI. Furthermore, they serve as nanoprobes in applications such as two-photon photoluminescence (TPL), photoacoustic tomography (PAT), and surface-enhanced Raman spectroscopy (SERS) (Liu et al. 2015).

6.3.1 Unique Advantages in Biomedical Applications

Gold nanoparticles offer an array of unique advantages in biomedical applications, further underscoring their significance in the field. Their high biocompatibility and low toxicity render them suitable for various medical applications, aligning with the stringent safety requirements of modern medicine (Wani 2017; Milan, Niemczyk, and Kus-Liśkiewicz 2022). The ease of synthesis and functionalization of gold nanoparticles allows for tailored customization, optimizing their utility for specific applications and diagnostic requirements (Wani 2017; Milan, Niemczyk, and Kus-Liśkiewicz 2022). Their high surface-area-to-volume ratio, a critical parameter, enhances their interaction with biological molecules and cells, facilitating their role as targeted agents in cancer diagnosis and therapy (Wani 2017; Milan, Niemczyk, and Kus-Liśkiewicz 2022). Gold nanoparticles showcase unique optical properties, including strong absorption as well as scattering of light, making them valuable as contrast agents in imaging techniques such as computed tomography (CT) and optical imaging (Wani 2017; Milan, Niemczyk, and Kus-Liśkiewicz 2022). Additionally, their ability to encapsulate and release drugs in a controlled manner positions them as versatile drug delivery systems (Wani 2017; Milan, Niemczyk, and Kus-Liśkiewicz 2022; Abdellatif et al. 2023). Photothermal therapy, a promising avenue for destroying cancer cells through light-induced heating, has seen significant advancements with the application of gold nanoparticles (Grigore et al. 2019; Milan, Niemczyk, and Kus-Liśkiewicz 2022). Furthermore, gold nanoparticles serve as photosensitizers in photodynamic therapy, generating reactive oxygen species to selectively target and eliminate cancer cells (Grigore et al. 2019). Their synergy with other materials, such as cyclodextrins, enhances their drug delivery capabilities, presenting a multifaceted approach to cancer management (Abdellatif et al. 2023).

6.3.2 Recent Applications in Imaging Diagnosis

The remarkable attributes of gold nanoparticles have spurred their recent utilization in diverse cancer imaging modalities. These nanoparticles have evolved into theranostic nanoplatforms, contributing to computed tomography (CT), surface-enhanced Raman spectroscopy imaging (SERS), fluorescence/optical imaging (FI/OI), photoacoustic imaging (PAI), and photothermal therapy (PTT). These applications underscore their potential for comprehensive cancer diagnosis and treatment (X. Liet al. 2022). In the realm of cancer diagnosis, gold nanoparticles have played a significant role as contrast agents across various imaging modalities. Their impact extends to MRI, CT, nuclear imaging, photoacoustic imaging, fluorescence imaging, and X-ray fluorescence imaging, showcasing their versatility and effectiveness in diverse diagnostic platforms (Luo et al. 2021). Notably, their application as contrast agents in CT imaging stands out, leveraging their high X-ray attenuation coefficient as well as biocompatibility to ensure effective enhancement of contrast in medical imaging (Luo et al. 2021). In MRI, gold nanoparticles leverage their unique magnetic properties to enhance image contrast, facilitating the identification of pathological tissues (Luo et al. 2021). As contrast agents in fluorescence imaging, their strong fluorescence and specific cell-targeting capabilities prove pivotal in advancing precision medicine (Luo et al. 2021). For photoacoustic imaging, their robust light absorption properties enable the generation of acoustic waves, aiding in visualizing tissue abnormalities (Luo et al. 2021). Gold nanoparticles deployed as contrast agents in X-ray fluorescence imaging further expand the toolkit for cancer diagnosis and research, emitting characteristic X-rays when excited by X-rays (Luo et al. 2021).

6.4 SUPERPARAMAGNETIC IRON OXIDE NANOPARTICLES (SPIONS)

SPIONs have emerged as potent contrast agents in MRI, finding extensive applications across various medical fields. Typically synthesized through the thermal decomposition method, these nanoparticles necessitate surface modification to ensure stability in aqueous media and biocompatibility (Luchini 2016). Application of functionalization strategies to SPIONs results in the production of monodispersed, biocompatible nanoparticles that effectively serve as MRI contrast agents (Luchini 2016). SPIONs showcase remarkable magnetic characteristics, responding precisely to both low-frequency (magneto-mechanical therapy) and high-frequency (magnetic hyperthermia) alternating magnetic fields (Figure 6.2). Additionally, their capacity to intrinsically produce ROS or respond to various stimuli positions them as highly favorable candidates for cancer therapy (Vangijzegem et al. 2023). Efforts to enhance the utility of SPIONs have led to the development of SPION-loaded iodinated nanoemulsions (NEs) as dual-modal injectable contrast agents for both X-ray and MRI imaging. This innovation not only provides dual-modal contrast but also simplifies nanoparticulate assembly, rendering it highly promising for imaging applications. In vivo investigations have

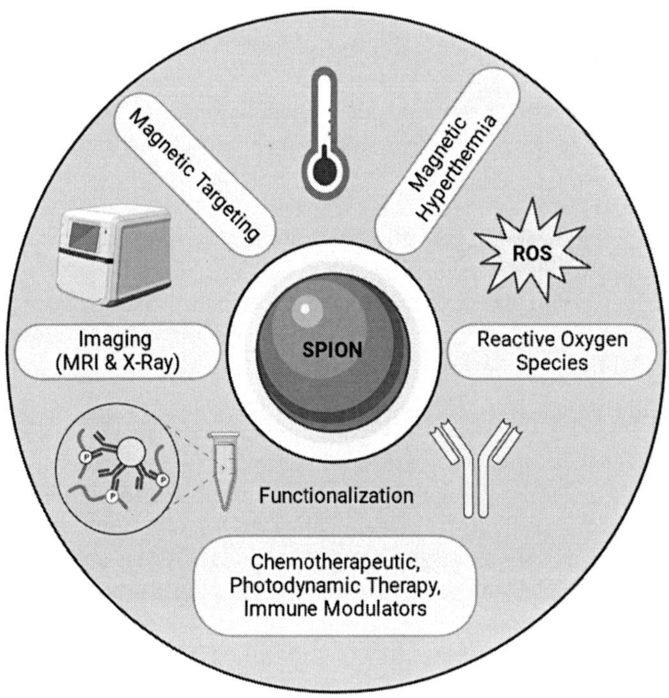

FIGURE 6.2 SPIONs as versatile nanoparticle platform. This image highlights the significance of superparamagnetic iron oxide nanoparticles (SPIONs) as a versatile nanoparticle platform for multimodal tumor therapy. SPIONs are capable of being functionalized with diverse cargos, including cytotoxic agents for chemotherapy, photosensitizers for photodynamic therapy, and immune modulators for immunotherapy. The image illustrates the enhancement of treatment efficacy through magnetic hyperthermia induced in alternating magnetic fields. Additionally, radiation triggers the release of reactive oxygen species (ROS) on the particle surface. The controlled therapy is visualized through magnetic resonance imaging (MRI), allowing for imaging-guided interventions.

demonstrated excellent contrast enhancement with the selected NEs in both MRI and X-ray imaging (Wallyn et al. 2019).

6.4.1 Contrast Mechanisms and Classification in MRI

Magnetic resonance imaging (MRI) serves as a fundamental clinical tool for diagnosing various medical conditions, including cancer. Contrast agents play a pivotal role in numerous MRI experiments, enhancing the precision of lesion detection by modifying the magnetic properties of surrounding tissue, thus improving the contrast between different tissues (Fattahi, Eghbali, and Oskoei 2015). Two broad categories of MRI contrast agents exist: positive and negative. Positive contrast agents, containing paramagnetic ions like gadolinium, aim to increase the signal intensity of the surrounding tissue, thereby improving visibility in MRI images. Conversely, negative contrast agents consist of SPIONs, causing a decrease in the signal intensity of the surrounding tissue, enhancing the contrast with healthy tissue. SPIONs, notably significant in cancer diagnosis (Fattahi, Eghbali, and Oskoei 2015), possess unique magnetic properties enabling specific responses to magnetic fields. They can generate ROS either autonomously or when triggered by various stimuli, making them notably suitable for applications in cancer therapy (Crimi et al. 2013; Fattahi, Eghbali, and Oskoei 2015). The stability and biocompatibility of SPIONs depend on appropriate surface modifications (Fattahi, Eghbali, and Oskoei 2015).

6.4.2 Gadolinium-Based Contrast Agents and Safety Concerns

Gadolinium-based contrast agents (GBCAs) have played a vital role in MRI diagnostics, enhancing the early and accurate detection of neurological disorders since 1988 (Asadollahzade et al. 2022). While GBCAs have benefited millions of patients, minor side effects have been noted, including injection site, discomfort, itching, nausea, headaches, rash, and dizziness. Patients with significant renal issues are at risk of experiencing more severe, albeit rare, side effects, like gadolinium poisoning and nephrogenic systemic fibrosis (Asadollahzade et al. 2022). Recent years have expressed concerns regarding the safety of GBCAs in MRI due to the discovery of gadolinium deposits in the brain following repeated administration (Pinter, Klein, and Mechtler 2016; Asadollahzade et al. 2022). These deposits correlate with the number of GBCAs administered, prompting a substantial debate in the radiology community about the safety of these agents (Asadollahzade et al. 2022). In response to these concerns, the FDA (Food and Drug Administration) has mandated a new class warning as well as additional safety precautions for all GBCAs used in MRI. The agency points out that gadolinium stays in patients' bodies for months to years, even in their brains, following the administration of the medication. This is of particular importance for patients with renal insufficiency, as they lack the ability to effectively filter gadolinium from their bodies, necessitating careful monitoring of GBCA usage (Chehabeddine et al. 2019; Asadollahzade et al. 2022).

6.4.3 Synthesis, Surface Modification, and Characterization of SPIONs

Superparamagnetic iron oxide nanoparticles (SPIONs) have attracted considerable attention for their versatile applications in various biomedical domains, including cell sorting, magnetic resonance imaging, drug delivery, hyperthermia, and more. The distinctive properties of SPIONs are significantly influenced by the synthesis method and surface modifications applied. Among synthetic techniques, the hydrothermal method stands out for its simplicity and uniformity, producing iron oxide nanoparticles with exceptional magnetic properties (Ahmad and Phul 2015). To maintain stability and prevent undesirable clumping, employing diverse capping agents for surface modification of SPIONs is crucial. Precise control over the shape, size, and surface properties of SPIONs is attainable through these surface coatings (Ahmad and Phul 2015). Oleic acid (OA), along with other stabilizers, plays a crucial role in preventing agglomeration, and the hydrodynamic size of

SPIONs can be customized by adjusting OA concentrations and stirring conditions (Wulandari, Sutriyo, and Rahmasari 2022). For instance, introducing 1.5%v/v oleic acid and stirring at a rate of 750 rpm yield SPIONs with the smallest hydrodynamic size, along with a low polydispersity index, underscoring the paramount importance of these parameters in nanoparticle design (Wulandari, Sutriyo, and Rahmasari 2022). The potential of SPIONs as contrast agents is promising due to their biocompatibility, non-toxic nature, and expansive surface area. It is noteworthy that the biocompatibility of SPIONs is significantly enhanced through surface coatings and modifications (Ahmad and Phul 2015). These nanoparticles exhibit a magnetic cubic crystal structure, with the size of Fe_3O_4 crystallite varying based on synthesis parameters (Suter et al. 2023). Fourier transform infrared spectroscopy (FTIR) reveals a high-intensity peak at 546.28 cm^{-1}, due to the Fe–O stretching bond, further characterizing the SPIONs (Suter et al. 2023).

6.5 GADOLINIUM OXIDE NANOCRYSTAL-BASED AUTOFLUORESCENT COMPOSITE NANOPARTICLES

In our quest for early cancer diagnosis, gadolinium oxide nanocrystal–based autofluorescent composite nanoparticles have emerged as a compelling type of contrast agent, facilitating the detection of early tumors through magnetic resonance imaging (MRI) techniques. These nanoparticles are meticulously designed to amplify MRI sensitivity for the early identification of malignancies while maintaining exceptional biocompatibility. The core of these nanoparticles is formed by gadolinium oxide nanocrystals (GON), which are encapsulated within albumin nanoparticles (AN) and cross-linked with glutaraldehyde (Shen, Ma, and Wu 2015). A remarkable feature of these nanoparticles is their inherent bright and stable autofluorescence, requiring no additional conjugation with fluorescent agents. The surface of these nanoparticles is further modified with folic acid (FA), enhancing their targeting capability to construct GON-AN-FA composite nanoparticles. Importantly, these nanoparticles exhibit high biocompatibility and stability in serum, demonstrating their suitability for clinical applications. These nanoparticles are almost non-cytotoxic (Shen, Ma, and Wu 2015).

6.5.1 Limitations of Traditional Positive MRI Contrast Agents

Traditional positive MRI contrast agents, though valuable, exhibit several limitations that can hinder their efficacy in enhancing MRI sensitivity for early tumor detection. These limitations include their inherent low sensitivity to signal changes in conventional T1 or T2 MRI, which restricts their ability to detect early tumors effectively (Zhou et al. 2019). Moreover, these agents often maintain a constant signal, resulting in reduced sensitivity and specificity, potentially leading to false-positive signals and suspicious artifacts in MRI images, which can compromise the accuracy of diagnoses (Fu, Cai, and Ai 2021). Additionally, concerns regarding cytotoxicity have arisen, particularly with certain agents like Magnevist, casting doubt on their clinical suitability (Zhou et al. 2019). Furthermore, traditional contrast agents may have limited capabilities in enhancing image contrast, thereby impacting their ability to improve MRI sensitivity for early tumor detection (Alzola-Aldamizetxebarria et al. 2022). Finally, precise dosing of these agents can be challenging, with the potential for over- or under-dosage, which can lead to adverse outcomes, such as syncope, worsened renal function, or early hospital readmission, consequently affecting diagnostic accuracy and treatment effectiveness for specific medical conditions (Beckmann 2022).

6.5.2 Design of Gadolinium Oxide Nanocrystal-Based MRI Contrast Agents for Early Cancer Diagnosis

The development and crafting of MRI contrast agents utilizing gadolinium oxide nanocrystals (GON) for targeted imaging and early cancer diagnosis encompass a systematic sequence of procedures, as illustrated by Ma et al. (2013) and Shen, Ma, and Wu (2015). Initially, GON is precisely synthesized using the polyol method, ensuring both their integrity and compatibility with subsequent phases. Subsequently, the encapsulation of GON within albumin nanoparticles (AN) takes place, and these AN particles are cross-linked using glutaraldehyde to ensure both structural stability and biocompatibility. A notable attribute of AN is their capacity to display bright and stable autofluorescence, even without the incorporation of any external fluorescent agents, augmenting the nanoparticles' suitability for improved MRI imaging. To enhance targeting capabilities further, a specific molecule, such as folic acid (FA), is conjugated to the GON-loaded AN surface, forming GON-AN-FA composite nanoparticles. The resultant composite nanoparticles exhibit remarkable biocompatibility and stability when exposed to serum, emphasizing their suitability for clinical applications. Significantly, these composite nanoparticles demonstrate markedly higher longitudinal relaxivity (rl) compared to conventional positive MRI contrast agents, such as Magnevist, thereby substantially contributing to their efficacy in heightening MRI sensitivity. Moreover, GON-AN and GON-AN-FA composite nanoparticles demonstrate noteworthy non-cytotoxicity, minimizing the potential adverse effects on biological systems (Ma et al. 2013; Shen, Ma, and Wu 2015).

6.6 CONCLUSION

This book review underscores the transformative potential of contrast agents, specifically nanoparticles, in the context of cancer diagnosis and therapy. Cancer, a relentless adversary, demands early detection and precise treatment, and the diverse array of nanoparticles discussed herein offers promising solutions to these critical challenges. Magnetic nanoparticles, with their superparamagnetic properties, are instrumental in enhancing magnetic resonance imaging (MRI) contrast, enabling the identification of pathological tissues and fostering precision medicine. Their multifunctionality, including targeted drug delivery, positions them as valuable tools in the ongoing battle against cancer. Gold nanoparticles, distinguished by their unique physicochemical properties, open new horizons in cancer diagnosis and therapy. They serve as versatile drug carriers, contrast agents, and radiation sensitizers, offering real-time monitoring of disease progression and therapeutic efficacy. Their high atomic number enhances the efficacy of radiation therapy, potentially revolutionizing cancer treatment strategies. The advent of gadolinium oxide nanocrystal–based autofluorescent composite nanoparticles introduces a novel contrast agent for early tumor detection through MRI. These nanoparticles exhibit remarkable biocompatibility, providing a promising avenue for clinical applications. In light of the limitations of traditional positive MRI contrast agents, the innovative design and synthesis of these novel contrast agents offer significant advantages. Their non-cytotoxic nature and superior effectiveness in enhancing MRI sensitivity mark a substantial advancement in early cancer diagnosis and personalized therapy. In essence, this review illuminates the path toward enhanced precision and efficacy in the ongoing battle against cancer, with nanoparticles serving as formidable allies in the quest for early detection and tailored treatment.

REFERENCES

Abdellatif, Ahmed A. H., Fatma Ahmed, Ahmed M. Mohammed, Mansour Alsharidah, Amal Al-Subaiyel, Waad A. Samman, Aisha A. Alhaddad, et al. 2023. "Recent Advances in the Pharmaceutical and Biomedical Applications of Cyclodextrin-Capped Gold Nanoparticles." *International Journal of Nanomedicine* 18: 3247.

Ahmad, Tokeer, and Ruby Phul. 2015. "Magnetic Iron Oxide Nanoparticles as Contrast Agents: Hydrothermal Synthesis, Characterization and Properties." *Diffusion and Defect Data-Solid State Data, Pt. B: Solid State Phenomena*. https://doi.org/10.4028/www.scientific.net/SSP.232.111.

Alzola-Aldamizetxebarria, Saioa, Laura Fernández-Méndez, Daniel Padro, Jesús Ruíz-Cabello, and Pedro Ramos-Cabrer. 2022. "A Comprehensive Introduction to Magnetic Resonance Imaging Relaxometry and Contrast Agents." *ACS Omega* 7 (42): 36905.

Amraee, A., S. Khoei, M. Bahreyni-Toossi, H. Azimian, F. Ansari, F. Fallahi, N. Robatmili, S. Teshnizi, and L. Darvish. 2022. "Evaluation of Ultra-Small Iron Oxide Nanoparticles as T1-Weighted MRI Contrast in Cancerous Tissues: A Meta-Analysis." *Clinical and Translational Imaging*. https://doi.org/10.1007/s40336-022-00491-y.

Asadollahzade, E., F. Ghadiri, Z. Ebadi, and A. N. Moghadasi. 2022. "The Benefits and Side Effects of Gadolinium-Based Contrast Agents in Multiple Sclerosis Patients." *Revista Da AssociaçãoMédica Brasileira* 68 (8): 979.

Beckmann, N. 2022. "Editorial for 'Evaluation of Dynamic Contrast-Enhanced MRI Measures of Lung Congestion and Endothelial Permeability in Heart Failure: A Prospective Method Validation Study.' " *Journal of Magnetic Resonance Imaging: JMRI* 56 (2). https://doi.org/10.1002/jmri.27906.

Burçak, Kadir Can, and Harun Uguz. 2022. "A New Hybrid Breast Cancer Diagnosis Model Using Deep Learning Model and ReliefF." *Traitement Du Signal*. https://doi.org/10.18280/ts.390214.

Butterworth, K., S. McMahon, Laura Taggart, and K. Prise. 2013. "Radiosensitization by Gold Nanoparticles: Effective at Megavoltage Energies and Potential Role of Oxidative Stress." *Translational Cancer Research*. https://doi.org/10.3978/J.ISSN.2218-676X.2013.08.03.

Cabral, R. M., and P. V. Baptista. 2014. "Anti-Cancer Precision Theranostics: A Focus on Multifunctional Gold Nanoparticles." *Expert Review of Molecular Diagnostics* 14 (8). https://doi.org/10.1586/14737159.2014.965683.

Chehabeddine, L., T. Al Saleh, M. Baalbaki, E. Saleh, S. J. Khoury, and S. Hannoun. 2019. "Cumulative Administrations of Gadolinium-Based Contrast Agents: Risks of Accumulation and Toxicity of Linear vs Macrocyclic Agents." *Critical Reviews in Toxicology* 49 (3). https://doi.org/10.1080/10408444.2019.1592109.

Chen, Junhua, Haiyan Zeng, Chong Zhang, Zhenwei Shi, Andre Dekker, Leonard Wee, and Inigo Bermejo. 2021. "Lung Cancer Diagnosis Using Deep Attention Based on Multiple Instance Learning and Radiomics." April. https://doi.org/10.1002/mp.15539.

Cortés-Llanos, Belén, Sandra M. Ocampo, Leonor de la Cueva, Gabriel F. Calvo, Juan Belmonte-Beitia, Lucas Pérez, Gorka Salas, and Ángel Ayuso-Sacido. 2021. "Influence of Coating and Size of Magnetic Nanoparticles on Cellular Uptake for In Vitro MRI." *Nanomaterials* 11 (11). https://doi.org/10.3390/nano11112888.

Crimi, A., O. Commowick, J. Ferré, A. Maarouf, G. Edan, and C. Barillot. 2013. "Semi-Automatic Classification of Lesion Patterns in Patients With Clinically Isolated Syndrome." *2013 IEEE 10th International Symposium on Biomedical Imaging*. http://ieeexplore.ieee.org/stamp/stamp.jsp?tp=&arnumber=6556671.

Darroudi, Mahdieh, Mehrdad Gholami, Majid Rezayi, and Majid Khazaei. 2021. "An Overview and Bibliometric Analysis on the Colorectal Cancer Therapy by Magnetic Functionalized Nanoparticles for the Responsive and Targeted Drug Delivery." *Journal of Nanobiotechnology* 19. https://doi.org/10.1186/s12951-021-01150-6.

Dorsey, J. F., L. Sun, D. Y. Joh, A. Witztum, G. D. Kao, M. Alonso-Basanta, S. Avery, S. M. Hahn, A. Al Zaki, and A. Tsourkas. 2013. "Gold Nanoparticles in Radiation Research: Potential Applications for Imaging and Radiosensitization." *Translational Cancer Research* 2 (4). https://doi.org/10.3978/j.issn.2218-676X.2013.08.09.

Etli, Elif, and A. Akar. 2022. "Magnetic Nanoparticles for Diagnosis and Treatment." *McGill Journal of Medicine: MJM: An International Forum for the Advancement of Medical Sciences by Students*. https://pdfs.semanticscholar.org/c745/857ca982b77f6c1e64524eb58925fdb3e56a.pdf.

Fattahi, H., P. Eghbali, and Yones Mosaei Oskoei. 2015. "MRI Contrast Agents Based on Superparamagnetic Iron Oxide Nanoparticles for Cancer Diagnosis." www.semanticscholar.org/paper/6bcf6a4faa456d92104f4cc4cc1b353c978ed9c2.

Fu, S., Z. Cai, and H. Ai. 2021. "Stimulus-Responsive Nanoparticle Magnetic Resonance Imaging Contrast Agents: Design Considerations and Applications." *Advanced Healthcare Materials* 10 (5). https://doi.org/10.1002/adhm.202001091.

Gallo, J., N. J. Long, and E. O. Aboagye. 2013. "Magnetic Nanoparticles as Contrast Agents in the Diagnosis and Treatment of Cancer." *Chemical Society Reviews* 42 (19). https://doi.org/10.1039/c3cs60149h.

Georgantzoglou, Natalia, Alexandros Pergaris, Christos Masaoutis, and Stamatios Theocharis. 2021. "Extracellular Vesicles as Biomarkers Carriers in Bladder Cancer: Diagnosis, Surveillance, and Treatment." *International Journal of Molecular Sciences* 22 (5). https://doi.org/10.3390/ijms22052744.

Ghosh, R., S. Mondal, D. Mukherjee, A. Adhikari, M. Bhattacharyya, and S. K. Pal. 2022. "Inorganic-Organic Synergy in Nano-Hybrids Makes a New Class of Drug With Targeted Delivery: Glutamate

Functionalization of Iron Nanoparticles for Potential Bone Marrow Delivery and X-Ray Dynamic Therapy." *Current Drug Delivery* 19 (10). https://doi.org/10.2174/1567201819666220328142620.
Gobbo, Oliviero L., Kristine Sjaastad, Marek W. Radomski, Yuri Volkov, and Adriele Prina-Mello. 2015. "Magnetic Nanoparticles in Cancer Theranostics." *Theranostics* 5 (11): 1249.
Grigore, M., R. Ion, L. Iancu, and R. Grigorescu. 2019. "Tailored Porphyrin–Gold Nanoparticles for Biomedical Applications." *Porphyrin Science by Women*. https://doi.org/10.1142/S108842461930012X.
Issa, B., and I. Obaidat. 2019. "Magnetic Nanoparticles as MRI Contrast Agents." *Magnetic Resonance Imaging*. https://pdfs.semanticscholar.org/b1f7/494986159056cb72e6aa50f3ca31c141aec6.pdf.
Jain, S., D. G. Hirst, and J. M. O'Sullivan. 2012. "Gold Nanoparticles as Novel Agents for Cancer Therapy." *The British Journal of Radiology* 85 (1010). https://doi.org/10.1259/bjr/59448833.
Joshi, B., and A. Joshi. 2022. "Polymeric Magnetic Nanoparticles: A Multitargeting Approach for Brain Tumour Therapy and Imaging." *Drug Delivery and Translational Research* 12 (7). https://doi.org/10.1007/s13346-021-01063-9.
Kaliamurthi, S., A. Demir-Korkmaz, G. Selvaraj, E. Gokce-Polat, Y. K. Wei, M. A. Almessiere, A. Baykal, K. Gu, and D. Q. Wei. 2019. "Viewing the Emphasis on State-of-the-Art Magnetic Nanoparticles: Synthesis, Physical Properties, and Applications in Cancer Theranostics." *Current Pharmaceutical Design* 25 (13). https://doi.org/10.2174/1381612825666190523105004.
Kono, Y., H. Kanzaki, M. Iwamuro, S. Kawano, Y. Kawahara, and H. Okada. 2020. "Reality of Gastric Cancer in Young Patients: The Importance and Difficulty of the Early Diagnosis, Prevention and Treatment." *Acta Medica Okayama* 74 (6). https://doi.org/10.18926/AMO/61204.
Li, Boyan, Xin Chen, Wei Qiu, Rongrong Zhao, Jiazhi Duan, Shouji Zhang, Ziwen Pan, et al. 2022. "Synchronous Disintegration of Ferroptosis Defense Axis via Engineered Exosome-Conjugated Magnetic Nanoparticles for Glioblastoma Therapy." *Advanced Science Letters* 9 (17). https://doi.org/10.1002/advs.202105451.
Li, Xinxin, Yiwei Zhang, Guangkuo Liu, Ziyi Luo, Lu Zhou, Yanan Xue, and Min Liu. 2022. "Recent Progress in the Applications of Gold-Based Nanoparticles Towards Tumor-Targeted Imaging and Therapy." *RSC Advances* 12 (13): 7635.
Liu, Yang, Hsiangkuo Yuan, Andrew M. Fales, Janna K. Register, and Tuan Vo-Dinh. 2015. "Multifunctional Gold Nanostars for Molecular Imaging and Cancer Therapy." *Frontiers in Chemistry* 3. https://doi.org/10.3389/fchem.2015.00051.
Luchini, A. 2016. "Iron Oxide Nanoparticles as MRI Contrast Agents: A Physico-Chemical Insight." www.semanticscholar.org/paper/30ee8d11f39c3e1fce983c6cdd9f811c1f4e13bb.
Luo, Dong, Xinning Wang, Clemens Burda, and James P. Basilion. 2021. "Recent Development of Gold Nanoparticles as Contrast Agents for Cancer Diagnosis." *Cancers* 13 (8). https://doi.org/10.3390/cancers13081825.
Ma, X. H., A. Gong, L. C. Xiang, T. X. Chen, Y. X. Gao, X. J. Liang, Z. Y. Shen, and A. G. Wu. 2013. "Biocompatible Composite Nanoparticles With Large Longitudinal Relaxivity for Targeted Imaging and Early Diagnosis of Cancer." *Journal of Materials Chemistry. B, Materials for Biology and Medicine* 1 (27). https://doi.org/10.1039/c3tb20648c.
Milan, Justyna, Klaudia Niemczyk, and Małgorzata Kus-Liśkiewicz. 2022. "Treasure on the Earth—Gold Nanoparticles and Their Biomedical Applications." *Materials* 15 (9). https://doi.org/10.3390/ma15093355.
Ning, L., B. Zhu, and T. Gao. 2017. "Gold Nanoparticles: Promising Agent to Improve the Diagnosis and Therapy of Cancer." *Current Drug Metabolism* 18 (11). https://doi.org/10.2174/1389200218666170925122513.
Onishi, Tatsuya, Kisyo Mihara, Sachiko Matsuda, Satoshi Sakamoto, Akihiro Kuwahata, Masaki Sekino, Moriaki Kusakabe, Hiroshi Handa, and Yuko Kitagawa. 2022. "Application of Magnetic Nanoparticles for Rapid Detection and In Situ Diagnosis in Clinical Oncology." *Cancers* 14 (2). https://doi.org/10.3390/cancers14020364.
Pinter, N. K., J. P. Klein, and L. L. Mechtler. 2016. "Potential Safety Issues Related to the Use of Gadolinium-Based Contrast Agents." *Continuum: Neuroimaging* 22 (5). https://doi.org/10.1212/CON.0000000000000378.
Poursharifi, Mina, Sylwia A. Dragulska, Ying Chen, J. Martignetti, and A. Mieszawska. 2020. "The Development of Peptide-coated Nanoparticles for Targeting and Drug Delivery to Cancer Cells." *The FASEB Journal*. https://doi.org/10.1096/fasebj.2020.34.s1.02042.
Qiu, Ting, Yintao Lan, Zuwu Wei, Yanfen Zhang, Yanping Lin, Chenggong Tu, Guangjuan Mao, Lingmin Zhang, Bin Yang, and Jian Zhang. 2021. "In Vivo Multi-Scale Photoacoustic Imaging Guided Photothermal Therapy of Cervical Cancer Based on Customized Laser System and Targeted Nanoparticles." *International Journal of Nanomedicine* 16: 2879.

Shen, Z., X. Ma, and A. Wu. 2015. "Gd2O3 Nanocrystal-Based Autofluorescent Composite Nanoparticles as T1-Weighted Contrast Agents." *Journal of Controlled Release: Official Journal of the Controlled Release Society* 213 (September): e147–8.

Subramanian, A. P., S. Jaganathan, and E. Supriyanto. 2015. "Overview on in Vitro and in Vivo Investigations of Nanocomposite Based Cancer Diagnosis and Therapeutics." *RSC Advances*. https://doi.org/10.1039/C5RA11912J.

Suter, Evans K., H. L. Rutto, Omwoyo N. Wesley, and M. Banza. 2023. "Stabilized Bare Superparamagnetic Iron Oxide Nanoparticles: Synthesis and Characterization." *Journal of Nanoparticle Research: An Interdisciplinary Forum for Nanoscale Science and Technology*. https://doi.org/10.4028/p-f1ygDS.

Taherian, A., N. Esfandiari, and S. Rouhani. 2021. "Breast Cancer Drug Delivery by Novel Drug-Loaded Chitosan-Coated Magnetic Nanoparticles." *Cancer Nanotechnology*. https://doi.org/10.1186/s12645-021-00086-8.

Vangijzegem, Thomas, Valentin Lecomte, Indiana Ternad, Levy Van Leuven, Robert N. Muller, Dimitri Stanicki, and Sophie Laurent. 2023. "Superparamagnetic Iron Oxide Nanoparticles (SPION): From Fundamentals to State-of-the-Art Innovative Applications for Cancer Therapy." *Pharmaceutics* 15 (1). https://doi.org/10.3390/pharmaceutics15010236.

Vijayakumar, S., and S. Paulsi. 2013. "Gold Nanoparticles in Early Detection and Treatment of Cancer: Biodistribution and Toxicities T Review." *International Journal of Pharmaceutical Sciences Review and Research* 20(2/13): 80–8.

Vuong, Q. L., S. Van Doorslaer, J. L. Bridot, C. Argante, G. Alejandro, R. Hermann, S. Disch, C. Mattea, S. Stapf, and Y. Gossuin. 2012. "Paramagnetic Nanoparticles as Potential MRI Contrast Agents: Characterization, NMR Relaxation, Simulations and Theory." *Magma* 25 (6). https://doi.org/10.1007/s10334-012-0326-7.

Wallyn, J., N. Anton, D. Mertz, S. Begin-Colin, F. Perton, C. A. Serra, F. Franconi, et al. 2019. "Magnetite- and Iodine-Containing Nanoemulsion as a Dual Modal Contrast Agent for X-ray/Magnetic Resonance Imaging." *ACS Applied Materials & Interfaces* 11 (1). https://doi.org/10.1021/acsami.8b19517.

Wani, I. 2017. "Biomedical Applications of Gold Nanoparticles: Recent Advances and Future Prospects." https://doi.org/10.4018/978-1-5225-0610-2.CH004.

Wulandari, Anggita Dipika, SutriyoSutriyo, and Ratika Rahmasari. 2022. "Synthesis Conditions and Characterization of Superparamagnetic Iron Oxide Nanoparticles With Oleic Acid Stabilizer." *Journal of Advanced Pharmaceutical Technology & Research* 13 (2): 89.

Zhou, Z., R. Bai, Z. Wang, H. Bryant, L. Lang, H. Merkle, J. Munasinghe, et al. 2019. "An Albumin-Binding T1-T2 Dual-Modal MRI Contrast Agents for Improved Sensitivity and Accuracy in Tumor Imaging." *Bioconjugate Chemistry* 30 (6). https://doi.org/10.1021/acs.bioconjchem.9b00349.

Zhu, Hongming, He Zhu, Miao Tian, Dongying Wang, Jiaxing He, and Tianmin Xu. 2020. "DNA Methylation and Hydroxymethylation in Cervical Cancer: Diagnosis, Prognosis and Treatment." *Frontiers in Genetics* 11. https://doi.org/10.3389%2Ffgene.2020.00347.

7 Cancer Imaging Enhancement through Nanotechnology

Samjeet Singh Thakur and Bhagwati Prashad Sharma

ABBREVIATIONS

Acronym	Full Form
CT	computed tomography
XCT	X-ray computed tomography
PET	positron emission tomography
SPECT	single-photon emission computed tomography
MRI	magnetic resonance imaging
fMRI	functional magnetic resonance imaging
NMI	nuclear medicine imaging
DWI	diffusion-weighted imaging
SPIOs	superparamagnetic iron oxide nanoparticles
PEG	polyethylene glycol
PLGA	poly(lactic-co-glycolic acid)
PEI	polyethyleneimine
PVA	polyvinyl alcohol
ZnO	zinc oxide
C-Dot	quantum dot
Fe_2O_3	hematite
Fe_3O_4	magnetite
Au	gold
Bi	bismuth
Co	cobalt
Cu	copper
Fe	iron
Gd	gadolinium
I	iodine
Tc	technetium

7.1 INTRODUCTION

Cancer imaging (Chapman et al. 2013) refers to the use of various medical imaging techniques to visualize and detect cancer within the human body. The primary goal of cancer imaging is to identify the presence, location, size, and extent of tumors or cancerous lesions. It plays a critical role in cancer diagnosis, staging, treatment planning, and monitoring the response to treatment.

For the past few decades, nanotechnology in cancer treatment has involved the use of tiny particles and devices at the nanoscale to target and treat cancerous cells. These nanoscale tools can enhance the precision and effectiveness of therapies while minimizing damage to healthy tissue. Nanotechnology plays a pivotal role in enhancing cancer imaging by harnessing the unique properties of nanoscale materials (Zhang et al. 2019). By developing nanoscale contrast agents and

DOI: 10.1201/9781003463191-9

innovative imaging techniques, it has significantly improved the accuracy, sensitivity, and specificity of cancer diagnosis. Moreover, the ability to target and deliver these nanomaterials to tumor sites offers a promising avenue for early detection and precise monitoring of cancer, ultimately leading to more effective treatment strategies. Siddique and Chow, in 2020, reported that the integration of nanotechnology in cancer imaging stands as a beacon of progress in the quest for better diagnostics and outcomes in oncology. Cancer imaging plays a pivotal role in the early detection, staging, and monitoring of cancer, aiding in the planning of treatment and assessing treatment effectiveness (García-Figueiras et al. 2019). The key aspects of cancer imaging are early detection of tumor, diagnosis and staging, treatment planning, monitoring and follow-up, diverse modalities, minimally invasive techniques, advancements in technology, patient comfort, and personalized medicine.

Cancer imaging is a vital component of cancer care, assisting healthcare providers in diagnosing cancer, determining its stage, planning treatment strategies, and examining the effectiveness of the treatment (Dong et al. 2012; Li et al. 2018; Sun et al. 2018; Lin et al. 2019; Maleki, Rezazadeh, and Varmira 2021; Yu et al. 2021). Accurate and premature detection of cancer through imaging can significantly improve patient outcomes by allowing for timely intervention and targeted therapy. It is an interdisciplinary field that combines radiology, oncology, and various medical specialties to provide comprehensive cancer care. Cancer imaging is essential for many reasons in a modern world with growing population and pollution (Fass 2008).

Thus, early detection of cancerous cells is crucial for successful treatment and enhanced patient outcomes. Hunter, Hindocha, and Lee, in 2022, reported that many cancers are more treatable in their early stages, and imaging can help identify tumors or abnormal tissue growth before they become advanced, using machine learning and artificial intelligences.

Haldorsen et al. (2019) reported that accurate cancer staging is essential for determining the extent of the disease, which guides treatment decisions. Imaging helps in determining the size and visualization of the tumor, whether it has spread to lymph nodes in close proximity or it has metastasized to other parts of the body as well. Imaging provides critical information for treatment planning. It helps oncologists decide on the most appropriate treatment modality, such as surgery, chemotherapy, radiation therapy, immunotherapy, or targeted therapy.

Michalski and Chen (2011) described that imaging is used to monitor the effectiveness of cancer treatments. By tracking changes in tumor size and appearance, healthcare providers can adjust treatment strategies as needed to maximize their impact. For surgical procedures, imaging helps and guides the surgeon by providing real-time information about the location as well as size of tumors. It allows for more precise and minimally invasive surgical interventions. Imaging can guide in the precise collection of tissue samples for biopsy and also helping to authenticate the presence of carcinoma cells and determine its specific characteristics.

Hermans, in 2004, reported that some imaging techniques, such as MRI, can provide information about the aggressiveness of tumors, helping to tailor treatment approaches. After initial treatment, imaging is used to monitor for cancer recurrence. The early detection of recurrence can lead to prompt intervention. Cancer imaging is essential in clinical trials for evaluating new therapies and interventions. It allows researchers to assess treatment efficacy and safety. Cancer imaging can be valuable for patient education as it helps patients and their families understand the nature and extent of the disease, treatment options, and potential outcomes. By providing vital information for personalized treatment plans, cancer imaging can help minimize the side effects and complications associated with cancer treatments, ultimately improving the quality of patient's life. Cancer imaging contributes to population-level health by enabling early cancer screening programs and identifying high-risk individuals. This early detection can help reduce cancer-related mortality. Advanced imaging techniques, such as minimally invasive image-guided procedures, have reduced the invasiveness of cancer diagnosis and treatment, leading to shorter recovery times and less discomfort for patients.

Because nanotechnology offers cutting-edge molecular tools, it has completely changed the way cancer is diagnosed and treated. According to Augustine et al. (2021), early cancer diagnosis is made possible in diagnostics by highly sensitive imaging made possible by nanoscale agents.

Yao et al. (2020) reported that by delivering medications straight to cancer cells during therapy, nanoparticles serve as precise drug carriers and reduce adverse effects. By improving therapeutic efficacy and opening the door to individualized cancer care, this targeted strategy promises less-invasive and more-effective interventions.

Coccia and Wang, in 2015, reported that the potential of nanotechnology to revolutionize cancer treatment and open up new avenues for precision medicine and patient outcomes accounts for its significance.

7.2 IMPACT OF CANCER IN USA AND INDIA

Sathishkumar et al. (2023) reported in the *Indian Journal of Medical Research* the estimated cancer patient cases in India for the year 2022, as shown in Table 7.1, Figures 7.1 (A, B). The estimated total number of cancer cases was 14.6 lakhs, with a greater number of female cases (7.49 lakhs) estimated as compared to males (7.12 lakhs). The leading major sites with the highest cancer burden in both sexes were organs of the digestive system, breast, genitals, oral cavity and pharynx, and respiratory system. The major types of cancer in males and females in India as per reports are shown in Figures 7.1a and 7.1b.

TABLE 7.1
Report on Cancer Patients of India in 2022

Type of Cancer	Male	Female	Total
Oral cavity and pharynx-related cancer	145,844	52,594	198,438
Digestive system–related cancer	172,025	116,029	288,054
Esophagus-related cancer	34,272	21,300	55,572
Stomach–related cancer	34,353	18,353	52,706
Small intestine–related cancer	2,255	1,533	3,788
Colon-related cancer	21,595	16,512	38,107
Rectum-related cancer	22,985	15,767	38,752
Anus-, anal canal–related cancer	3,037	2,131	5,168
Liver and intra-hepatic bile duct–related cancer	28,020	11,306	39,326
Gallbladder and other biliary-related cancer	12,997	20,570	33,567
Pancreas-related cancer	12,511	8,557	21,068
Respiratory system–related cancer	108,848	34,214	143,062
Bone and joints-related cancer	8,426	6,087	14,513
Soft tissue	8,380	6,895	15,275
Skin-related cancer (excluding basal and squamous)	11,745	9,412	21,157
Breast-related cancer	5,649	216,108	221,757
Genital system–related cancer	54,625	163,694	218,319
Uterine cervix and corpus-related cancer	–	107,025	107,025
Ovary-related cancer	–	46,126	46,126
Vulva-related cancer	–	2,258	2258
Vaginal and other female genital–related cancers	–	7,961	7,961
Placenta-related cancer	–	324	324
Prostate-related cancer	43,691	–	43,691
Testicular and other male genital–related cancer	10,934	–	6,413
Urinary system–related cancer	34,942	11,861	46,803
Kidney and renal pelvis–related cancer	12,963	5,930	18,893
Ureter and other urinary organs–related cancer	456	218	674

(*Continued*)

TABLE 7.1 *(Continued)*
Report on Cancer Patients of India in 2022

Type of Cancer	Male	Female	Total
Eye and orbit-related cancer	1,326	977	2,303
Brain and other nervous system–related cancer	20,811	13,296	34,107
Endocrine system–related cancer	9682	27,847	37,529
Thyroid-related cancer	8,967	27,253	36,220
Adrenal gland–related cancer	715	594	1309
Lymphoma-related cancer	34,116	21,233	55,349
Malig Imn. Prol D–related cancer	58	50	108
Multiple myeloma–related cancer	11,261	8165	19,426
Leukemia-related cancer	33,604	21,969	55,573
Other unspecified primary sites–related cancer	50,892	38,870	89,762
All sites' cancer	**712,176**	**749,251**	**1,461,427**

Source: Data from Sathishkumar et al. (2023).

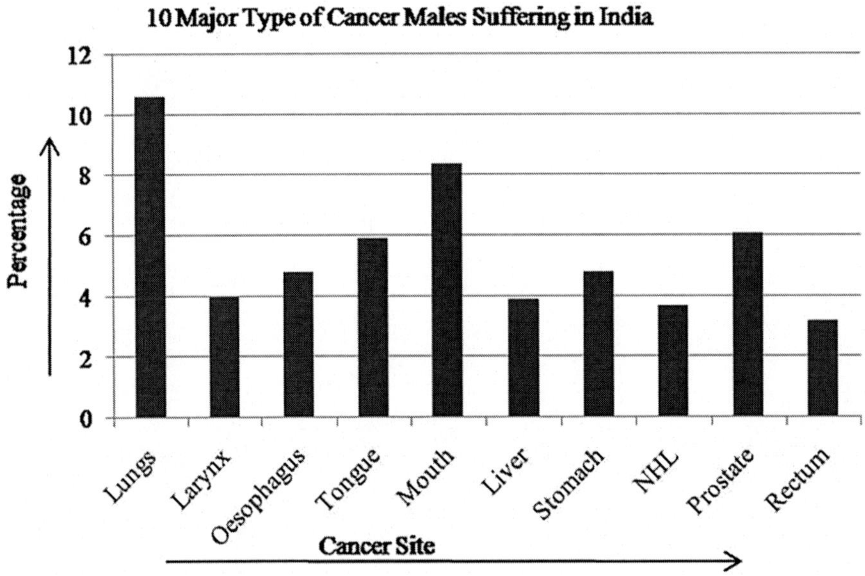

FIGURE 7.1A Ten major types of cancer, out of which lung cancer, mouth cancer, tongue cancer, and prostate cancer are the most common among Indian males. More than 10% of males are suffering from lung cancer, the reason being smoking; about 15% are suffering from mouth as well as tongue cancer, the reason being *gutkha tobacco*; and 6% are suffering from prostate cancer.

Source: Sathishkumar et al. (2023).

According to cancer data report compiled by Siegel et al. (2023) in *A Cancer Journal for Clinicians*, almost 2 million new cases of all types of cancer were diagnosed, and about 3% (0.6 million) of people died of cancer in the USA alone. All the data as reported in the same journal for different types of cancers in all sites for males and females are as shown in Table 7.2. The comparison of estimated deaths and estimated new cases in recent times is also shown in Figure 7.2 (A, B, C), which also shows the ten major types of cancer in males and females leading to deaths.

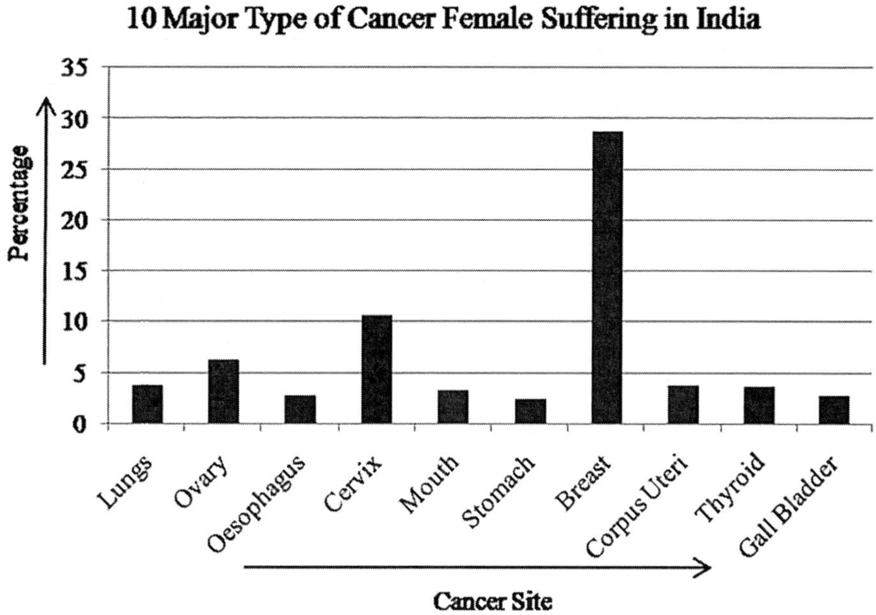

FIGURE 7.1B Ten major types of cancer, out of which breast cancer, ovarian cancer, and cervical cancer are the most common among Indian females. About 30% of females are suffering from breast cancer, 10% are suffering from cervical cancer, and 6% are suffering from ovarian cancer.

Source: Sathishkumar et al. (2023).

TABLE 7.2
Report on Cancer Patients in the USA in 2023

	Estimated Cases			Estimated Deaths		
Type of Cancer Site	**Female**	**Male**	**Total**	**Female**	**Male**	**Total**
Oral cavity– and pharynx-related cancer	15,250	39,290	54,540	3,440	8,140	11,580
Digestive-related cancer	153,860	194,980	348,840	72,660	99,350	172,010
Respiration-related cancer	125,140	131,150	256,290	61,160	71,170	132,330
Bones and joints cancer	1,810	2,160	3,970	940	1,200	2,140
Soft Tissue cancer	6,000	7,400	13,400	2,420	2,720	5,140
Skin cancer	42,120	62,810	104,930	3,990	8,480	12,470
Breast cancer	297,790	2,800	300,590	43,170	530	43,700
Genital-related cancer	114,810	299,540	414,350	34,020	35,640	69,660
Urinary system–related cancer	50,970	117,590	168,560	9,910	22,680	32,590
Eye and orbit cancer	1,590	1,900	3,490	190	240	430
Brain and other nervous system–related cancer	10,530	14,280	24,810	7,970	11,020	18,990
Endocrine system–related cancer	32,890	14,340	47,230	1,680	1,560	3,240
Lymphoma-related cancer	39,650	49,730	89,380	8,760	12,320	21,080
Myeloma-related cancer	15,870	19,860	35,730	5,590	7,000	12,590
Leukemia-related cancer	23,940	35,670	59,610	9,810	13,900	23,710
All sites	**948,000**	**1,010,310**	**1,958,310**	**287,740**	**322,080**	**609,820**

Source: Data from Siegel et al. (2023).

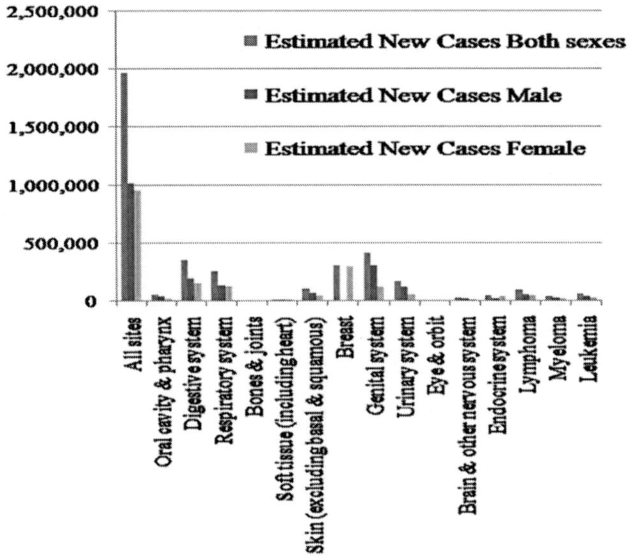

FIGURE 7.2A About 2 million new cases of cancer for both sexes were estimated for 2023 in the USA only. Most of the cases reported were related to digestive system, respiratory system, and genital systems for both sexes. For females, breast cancer was also the prime cause for new cases reported. Urinary tract–related cancer is another major type of factor causing cancer in males.

Source: Siegel et al. (2023).

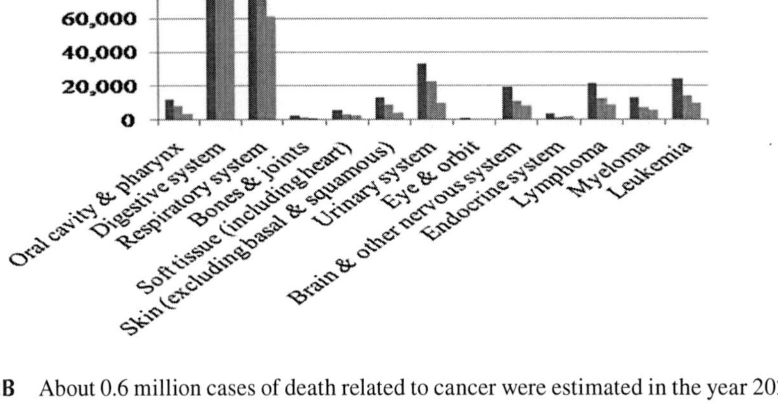

FIGURE 7.2B About 0.6 million cases of death related to cancer were estimated in the year 2023 in the USA alone. Most of the death cases reported due to cancer were related to the digestive system, the respiratory system, and genital cancer for both men and women. In females, the higher percentage of breast cancer cases was also the main reason for deaths. In males, urinary tract–related cancer also caused many deaths.

Source: Siegel et al. (2023).

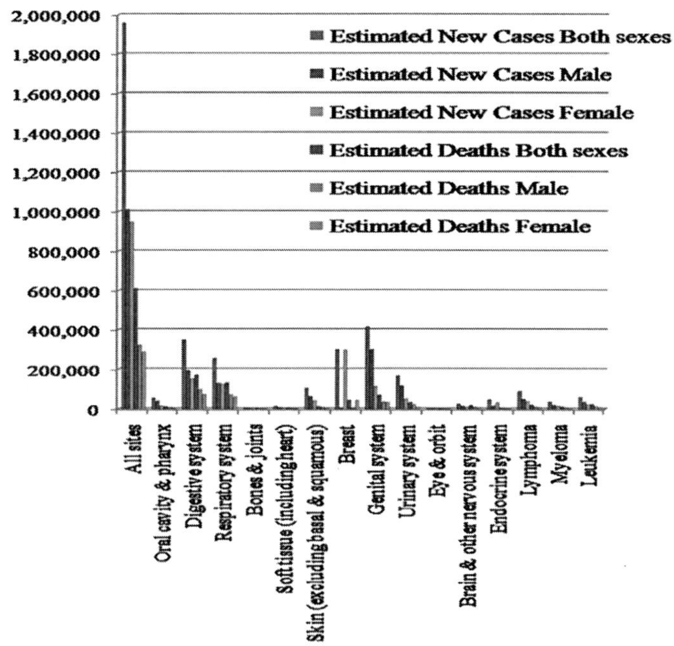

FIGURE 7.2C Comparison of estimated new cases and estimated deaths from cancer. Out of 2 million new cases of cancer reported, about 30% of patients die. Patients suffering from breast cancer, blood cancer (lymphoma, myeloma, and leukemia), and respiratory and digestive-related cancer have the least survival rates.

Source: Siegel et al. (2023).

Liu et al. (2021) have reported that metal ions play a crucial role in cancer imaging, particularly in the development of contrast agents for various imaging modalities. Nanotechnology-based polymers are being increasingly used in cancer imaging to enhance the accuracy and effectiveness of diagnostic methods. These nanoscale polymer structures (Elsabahy et al. 2015), often encapsulating contrast agents or imaging agents, offer several advantages in the field of cancer imaging, such as targeted delivery, enhanced contrast, prolonged circulation, reduced side effects, customizability, and biocompatibility. The incorporation of nano-polymers in cancer imaging represents a significant advancement in the field, offering improved targeting, enhanced contrast, and reduced side effects, all of which contribute to more accurate and safer cancer diagnostics. Cancer imaging enhancement through nanotechnology-based polymers (Toy et al. 2014) is a cutting-edge approach that leverages the unique properties of nanoscale materials to improve the accuracy and sensitivity of medical imaging in cancer diagnosis and monitoring. Herein in this chapter it is explored how nanotechnology has revolutionized cancer imaging by enhancing contrast, increasing specificity, and enabling targeted delivery of contrast agents. This innovative field holds great promise for improving cancer care and underscores the potential of nanotechnology in the realm of medical imaging

7.3 IMAGING MODALITIES IN THE DETECTION OF CANCER IMAGING

Alam et al. (2018) reported that various imaging modalities for cancer detection and confirmation encompass a range of techniques to visualize and characterize tumors. Several imaging modalities are commonly used in cancer imaging, as shown in Figure 7.3, and are explained in the following.

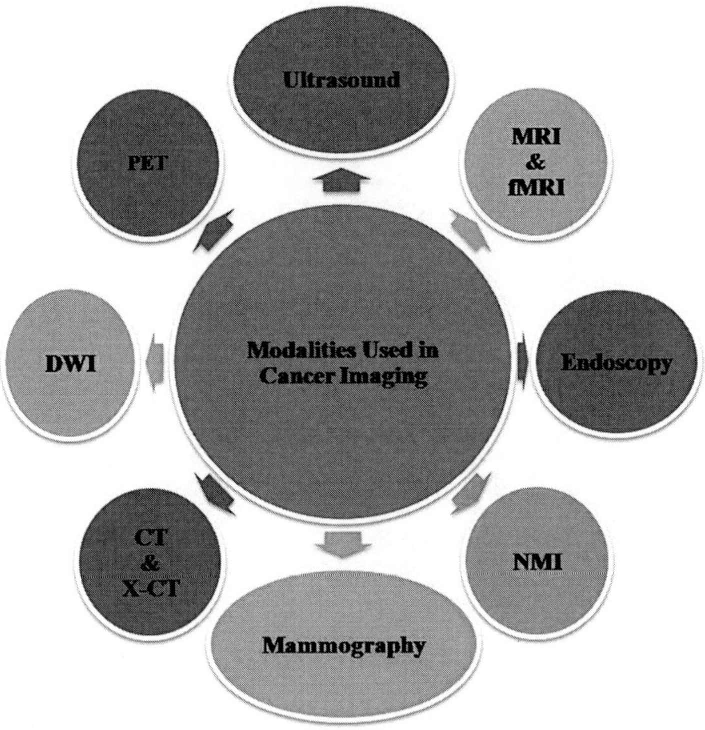

FIGURE 7.3 Different types of imaging modalities in cancer detection. The choice of imaging modality depends on factors such as the type of cancer, location, and the information needed for diagnosis and treatment planning. Usually, a combination of modalities can also be employed for a comprehensive assessment.

7.3.1 X-Ray-Based Computed Tomography (XCT)

XCT is based on the principle of X-rays for the structural imaging of tumors, etc. Traditional X-rays are useful for detecting solid tumors and assessing the variations in the bone density and are often used to screen lung cancer, bone metastases, and soft tissues (Gaikwad et al. 2018). Computed tomographic scans give detailed and cross-sectional images of the body under investigation, which are used to visualize internal structures, detect tumors, and assess their size and location. CT scans are valuable for staging cancer and guiding biopsies or surgeries.

7.3.2 Single-Photon Emission-Based Computed Tomography (SPECT)

Its principle is based upon the detection of gamma rays emitted by radiotracers. It is applied to visualize functional processes in tumors (Sano et al. 2019).

7.3.3 Magnetic Resonance Imaging Technique (MRI and fMRI)

It is based upon the principle of magnetic fields and radio waves for detailed soft tissue imaging. MRI uses powerful magnets and radio waves to create detailed images of soft tissues (Zhao et al. 2014; Cai et al. 2020; Schuerle et al. 2020). It is especially effective for visualizing brain tumors, breast cancer, prostate cancer, soft tissues, and cancers in various other body organ parts. On the other way, fMRI provides information about the functional activity of the brain, which is valuable for diagnosing brain tumors in regions responsible for language, motor function, or other important brain functions (Angelovski et al. 2014).

7.3.4 Ultrasound and Photoacoustic Imaging

Ultrasound is based upon the principle of sound waves for real-time imaging and is often used to evaluate tumors in the liver, pancreas, breast, and other abdominal organs (Zhang et al. 2022), and it can also help in guiding biopsies and assessing blood flow within the tumors. Photoacoustic imaging is based on the principle of detecting ultrasound signals generated by laser-induced photoacoustic effects (L. Li et al. 2022), and therefore, it is applied to visualize tumors with high resolution.

7.3.5 Positron Emission Tomography (PET)

It is based upon the principle where it detects gamma rays emitted by positron-emitting radiotracers. PET scans use a radioactive tracer to detect metabolic activity in tissues (Chen et al. 2023). Cancer cells are often more metabolically active than normal cells, making PET scans useful for detecting and staging cancer, as well as assessing treatment response.

7.3.6 Mammography

It is also based upon the principle of X-rays for breast imaging. Mammograms are specialized X-ray examinations or investigation of the breast tissue which are essential for premature detection of breast cancer (Salazar Berg and Blume 2008).

7.3.7 Endoscopy

It is based upon the principle of fiber optics and light for direct visualization of internal organs. It is used to identify tumors in the gastrointestinal and respiratory tracts. Endoscopic procedures involve inserting a thin flexible tube with a camera into the body's cavities to visualize and biopsy tissues, making it valuable for detecting cancers in the gastrointestinal tract and respiratory system (Ali et al. 2013; Muguruma et al. 2013).

7.3.8 Nuclear Medicine Imaging (NMI)

The principle of nuclear medicine imaging involves the use of radioactive tracers, or radiopharmaceuticals, to visualize and assess the functional and molecular processes within the body. This imaging technique is particularly valuable for studying physiological functions and identifying abnormalities at the cellular and molecular levels. Techniques such as bone scans, thyroid scans, and sentinel lymph node mapping utilize radioactive tracers to detect cancer cells or abnormalities within specific organs or tissues (Eary 1999).

7.3.9 Diffusion-Weighted Imaging (DWI)

It is a kind of MRI technique that provides information about the movement of water molecules within tissues (Afaq, Andreou, and Koh 2010). The principle of diffusion-weighted imaging is based on the random motion of water molecules, known as Brownian motion, and its sensitivity to barriers or restrictions within tissues. It measures the movement of water molecules in tissues and is often used to assess the cellular density of tumors. It can help in identifying and characterizing cancerous lesions.

7.3.10 Fluorescence Imaging

It is based on the principle of detecting emitted fluorescence after light excitation. It is very helpful in the location of tumors and assesses molecular processes (Miki et al. 2011; Pu et al. 2023).

Therefore, these imaging modalities offer diverse approaches for cancer detection, diagnosis, and monitoring, each with its unique strengths and applications. Integrating multiple modalities often provides a comprehensive view of the tumor's characteristics.

7.4 ROLE OF NANOTECHNOLOGY IN CANCER IMAGING

Nanotechnology plays a pivotal role in revolutionizing cancer imaging by enabling more precise, sensitive, and targeted approaches to detect and visualize cancer at the cellular and molecular dimensions (Zhang et al. 2019).

7.4.1 Nanoparticles of Metal Ions in Cancer Imaging

Metal ions are essential for cancer imaging, especially when it comes to creating contrast agents for different imaging modalities (Conde et al. 2012; Liu and Zhang 2012; Vinardell and Mitjans 2015; Sharma, Goyal, and Rath 2018). These contrast chemicals eventually aid in the distinction between healthy and malignant tissues by making tumors more visible. These are a few instances of how various metal ions are used for particular imaging methods.

7.4.1.1 Gadolinium (Gd) for Magnetic Resonance Imaging (MRI)

Gadolinium-based contrast agents are widely used in MRI. Gadolinium is a paramagnetic metal that shortens the relaxation times of nearby water protons, leading to increased signal intensity and improved contrast between different tissues. Gadolinium chelates, such as gadopentetate dimeglumine, are commonly used in clinical practice (Jung et al. 2012; Liu and Zhang 2012).

7.4.1.2 Iron (Fe) for Magnetic Resonance Imaging (MRI)

Iron oxide nanoparticles, such as superparamagnetic iron oxide (SPIO) and ultrasmall superparamagnetic iron oxide (USPIO), are used as contrast agents in MRI. These nanoparticles alter the magnetic properties of surrounding tissues, creating contrast in MR images (Lee et al. 2007; Jung et al. 2012; Rosen et al. 2012; Guo et al. 2021; Makela et al. 2022).

7.4.1.3 Iodine (I) for X-Ray and Computed Tomography (CT)

Iodine is usually used in contrast agents for X-ray and CT imaging. Such iodine-based agents absorb X-rays more strongly than surrounding tissues, leading to increased visibility in imaging. Examples include iohexol and iodixanol (Chuang et al. 2009; Lusic and Grinstaff 2013; Liu et al. 2019).

7.4.1.4 Gold (Au) for X-Ray and Photoacoustic Imaging

Gold nanoparticles are explored for their use in X-ray and photoacoustic imaging. They exhibit strong X-ray absorption and can convert absorbed light into heat, which makes them suitable for both imaging and therapeutic applications (Huang et al. 2011; Hajfathalian et al. 2018).

7.4.1.5 Copper (Cu) for Positron Emission Tomography (PET)

Copper radioisotopes, such as ^{64}Cu and ^{62}Cu, are used in PET imaging. These isotopes are incorporated into radiotracers that can be detected by PET scanners, providing information about metabolic activity in tissues (Shokeen and Anderson 2009; Hansen et al. 2015; Andreozzi et al. 2017).

7.4.1.6 Technetium (Tc) for Single-Photon Emission Computed Tomography (SPECT)

Technetium-99m (^^{99}mTc) is a commonly used radioisotope in SPECT imaging. It is incorporated into radiopharmaceuticals to visualize physiological processes and detect specific biomarkers associated with cancer (Pandit-Taskar et al. 2010; Lee and K-SPECT 2019).

7.4.1.7 Bismuth (Bi) for Computed Tomography (CT) and Photoacoustic Imaging

The potential of bismuth-based nanoparticles in CT and photoacoustic imaging has been studied and explored by Yu et al. in 2017 and H. Bi et al. in 2018. Strong X-ray attenuation and photoacoustic signal production are demonstrated by these nanoparticles.

7.4.1.8 Cobalt (Co) for Magnetic Resonance Imaging (MRI)

Kron et al. in 2006 and Bouchard et al. in 2009 have investigated the application of cobalt-based contrast agents in MRI. The relaxation periods of adjacent water protons can be influenced by cobalt ions, which can enhance contrast in magnetic resonance imaging.

Many types of metal ion nanoparticle can be used for the treatment of cancer, as reported in the literature by Pandit-Taskar et al. in 2010; Huang et al. in 2011; Lusic and Grinstaff in 2013; Vinardell and Mitjans in 2015; Hansen et al. in 2015; Andreozzi et al. in 2017; Yu et al. in 2017; D. Bi et al. in 2018; Hajfathalian et al. in 2018; Sharma et al. in 2018; Lee and K-SPECT in 2019; Liu et al. in 2019; Guo et al. in 2021; and Makela et al. in 2022. Figure 7.4 illustrates that their nature also depends upon shape, size, and kind of metal ion nanoparticles. These kinds of nanoparticles can be modified through the introduction of charge, functional groups, surface engineering, and targeting ligands. The metal ion nanoparticles are designed for cancer imaging techniques as they look like nano-hydrogels, dendrimers, carbon nanotubes, solid-lipid nanoparticles, drug–protein conjugates, and liposomes. Li, Nejadnik, and Daldrup-Link (2017) reported that the use of superparamagnetic iron oxide (SPIO) nanoparticles in cancer imaging has drawn attention, especially those coated with NanoTherm aminosilane or silica-gold nanoshells. These hybrid structures offer options for targeted imaging and potential therapeutic interventions by combining the special qualities of iron oxide for magnetic resonance imaging (MRI) with the functions of silica and gold. Superparamagnetism, or the ability to become strongly magnetic in the presence of an external magnetic field, is exhibited by SPIO nanoparticles, which makes them useful as contrast agents in magnetic resonance imaging. Tanaka et al. reported in 2010 that the addition of silica coating to SPIO nanoparticles improves their biocompatibility by shielding them from direct biological contact and lowering their potential for toxicity. It also offers a flexible surface modification platform that can be used to attach medicinal compounds, imaging agents, or targeting ligands. Contributing to the surface plasmon resonance are the gold nanoshells.

Zhang et al. reported in 2013 that glutathione-capped gold and iron oxide nanoparticles have been developed for a range of uses in cancer imaging, and due to their strong surface plasmon resonance, gold nanoshells are a great option for photothermal therapy. PEGylation improves stability and biocompatibility, whereas glucose-capped gold nanoparticles provide potential targeting of cancer cells over expressing glucose transporters (Ma, Sadoqi, and Shao 2012). Because of their unique optical properties and the stability that PEG imparts, carbon dots (C-Dots) with PEG-coated silicon dioxide offer a versatile platform that may be employed for imaging agents and maybe medication delivery. Chatterjee et al. reported in 2014 that for imaging and therapeutic applications, the multifunctional nanoparticles combine magnetic Fe_3O_4 nanoparticles, silica-gold nanoshells, and

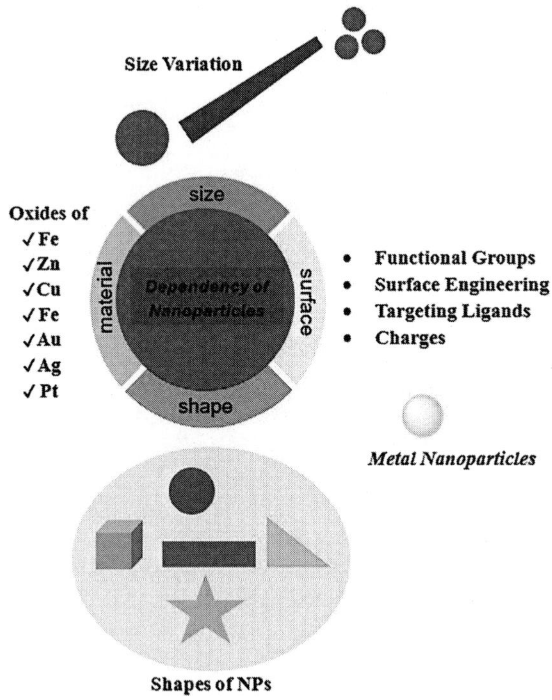

FIGURE 7.4 Pictorial representations show the dependence of cancer imaging on different parameters. In cancer imaging, the properties of metal ion nanoparticles, including size, shape, and the specific metal used, significantly influences their effectiveness. The dependence upon these factors is crucial for tailoring nanoparticles to enhance imaging outcome.

gold nanorods. Using PEG-coated silica-gold nanoshells as contrast agents provides stability and biocompatibility.

Majdalawieh et al. reported in 2014 that novel nanomaterials intended for cancer imaging applications include silver nanoshells with a carbon core and silver nanoparticles capped with polyvinyl pyrrolidone (PVP) encased in a polymer matrix. A carbon core and an exterior layer of silver make up the silver nanoshell structure. These nanoshells can be used for optical imaging because of the surface plasmon resonance produced by the silver layer, and photothermal therapy may be possible due to the carbon core's ability to absorb light and produce heat. Armentano et al. reviewed in 2010 that encapsulation within a polymeric matrix enhances the biocompatibility and stability of the silver nanoparticles and therefore the polymer matrix can offer additional stability and function as a platform for further cancer applications.

Platinum nanoparticles, cisplatin- and carboplatin-based drugs, oxaliplatin, nedaplatin (Yamada, Matthew, and Prow 2015; Fu et al. 2020) are all have wide applications in the ovarian cancer treatment. According to Wason and Zhao in 2013 and Pešić et al. in 2015, the polyvinyl alcohol–capped platinum nanoparticles, and lobaplatin, titanium dioxide, copper oxide, and cerium oxide nanoparticles, can also be used for the treatment of human lung cancer cells and ovarian cancer. ZnO nanoparticles also hold promise in the field of cancer imaging and treatment, offering a multifunctional platform with intrinsic fluorescence and therapeutic potential (Bisht and Rayamajhi 2016; Anjum et al. 2021). Table 7.3 summarizes the different types of metal ion nanoparticles used to detect cancer using different cancer imaging techniques.

Different nanoparticles have different surfaces and varied size to get bound through the strategic application of peptides, antibodies, ligands, genes, drugs, etc. The purpose of silver, gold, and platinum nanoparticles is quite old as well as innovative in fabricating multifunctional NPs, showcasing

TABLE 7.3
Metal-Based Nanoparticles in Cancer Imaging

S. No.	Type of Nanoparticles	Cancer Imaging Technique	References
1	Iron oxide and iron nanoparticles	Targeted cancer imaging; magnetic resonance imaging	Rosen et al. (2012); Guo et al. (2021); Makela et al. (2022)
2	Gadolinium and iron nanoparticles	Magnetic resonance imaging	Jung et al. (2012); Liu and Zhang (2012)
3	Gold-based nanoparticles	X-ray and photoacoustic imaging	Huang et al. (2011); Hajfathalian et al. (2018)
4	Silver-based nanoparticles	In vivo imaging	Haque et al. (2021)
5	Platinum-based nanoparticles	Magnetic resonance imaging	Chan et al. (2021)
6	Copper oxide nanoparticles	PET scanners	Shokeen and Anderson (2009); Hansen et al. (2015); Andreozzi et al. (2017)
7	Zinc oxide nanoparticles	Targeted optical imaging	Hong et al. (2011)
8	Technetium (Tc)	Single-photon emission computed tomography	Pandit-Taskar et al. (2010); Lee and K-SPECT (2019)
9	Bismuth-based nanoparticles	CT imaging and photoacoustic imaging	Yu et al. (2017); H. Bi et al. (2018)
10	Cobalt-based nanoparticles	Magnetic resonance imaging	Kron et al. (2006); Bouchard et al. (2009)

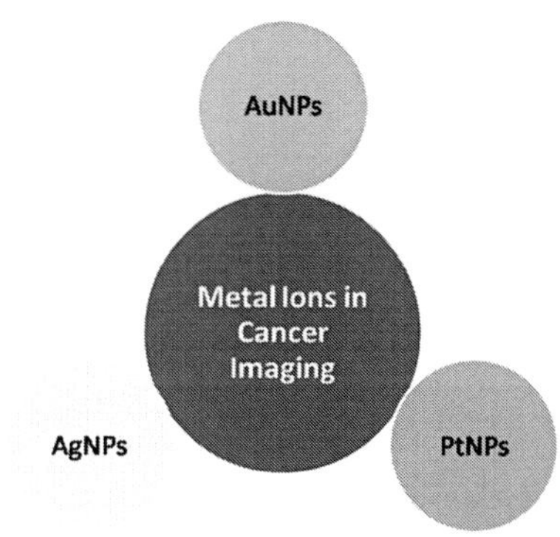

FIGURE 7.5 Silver nanoparticles (AgNPs), gold nanoparticles (AuNPs), and platinum nanoparticles (PtNPs) with biocompatible characteristics hold immense potential in cancer imaging applications. The biocompatibility of these nanoparticles is crucial for their safe administration in living organisms, allowing for targeted imaging of cancer cells and tissues.

their potential in theranostic applications, which integrate both therapeutic and diagnostic functionalities for advanced biomedical uses, as shown in Figure 7.5.

Silver nanoparticles (AgNPs) are promising agents in cancer imaging due to their unique optical properties, biocompatibility, and surface plasmon resonance characteristics, as shown in Figure 7.6. Pala et al. (2018) reported that functionalized silver nanoparticles are very useful for sensing, molecular imaging, and therapeutic applications. The silver nanoparticles serve as effective contrast agents in various imaging modalities, including surface plasmon resonance, optical and multimodal imaging, computed tomography (CT), targeted imaging, and photoacoustic imaging. AgNPs' strong

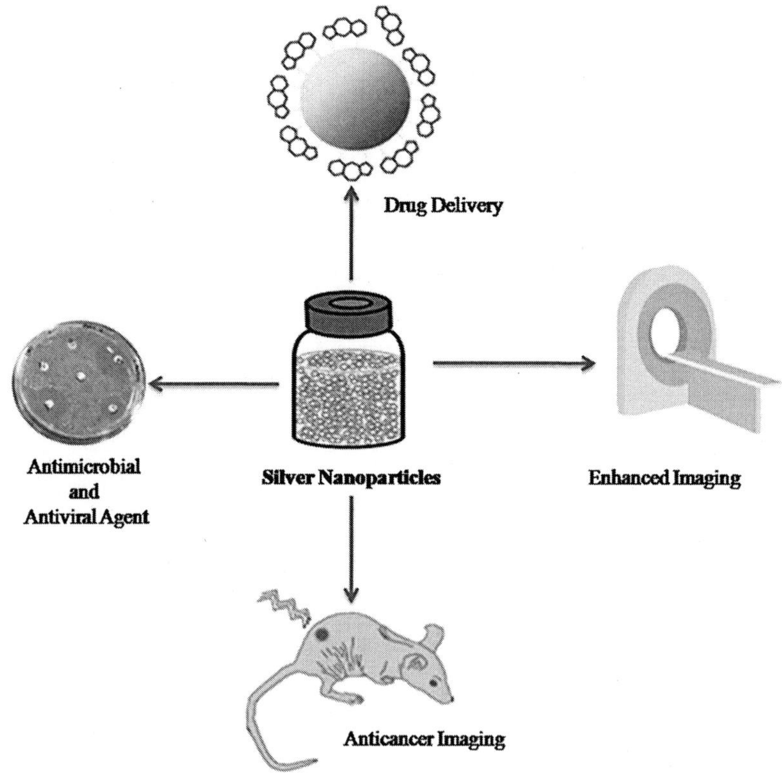

FIGURE 7.6 Silver nanoparticles (AgNPs) have emerged as promising agents in both drug delivery and imaging modalities, showcasing their versatility and potential in biomedical applications. The dual functionality of AgNPs in drug delivery and imaging underscores their potential in advancing precision medicine.

light absorption and scattering properties enhance imaging contrast, allowing for improved visualization of tumor tissues.

Bouché et al., in 2019, reported that gold nanoparticles are widely applied in recent advancements for the treatment of cancer using molecular imaging. With its adaptability in imaging modalities, ability to distribute drugs selectively, and potential for theranostic applications, gold nanoparticles (AuNPs) have enormous potential in cancer imaging and treatment. These nanoparticles will probably have a major impact on the development of precision medicine in oncology as research continues. Li and Chen, in 2015, reported that gold nanoparticles are ideal contrast agents for a variety of imaging techniques, such as optical and photoacoustic imaging, since they exhibit a significant surface plasmon resonance (SPR) in the visible and near-infrared ranges. Imaging contrast is improved by the SPR effect, which increases their capacity to absorb and scatter light.

Gold nanoparticles produce heat when subjected to laser radiation, which can be used for targeted cancer therapy as well as imaging. This phenomenon is known as localized hyperthermia. Several imaging modalities can be combined with gold nanoparticles to create multimodal imaging. For example, Cheheltani et al., in 2016, reported that AuNPs can be applied to both photoacoustic and computed tomography (CT) imaging, offering complementing data for precise tumor identification and characterization. Figure 7.7 illustrates how tunable forms and sizes of gold nanoshells and nanorods provide special optical features. Since tissue penetration is best in the near-infrared window, these nanoparticles have been investigated for improved imaging and therapy. Additionally, these AuNPs have demonstrated promise in in vivo tumor imaging. The enhanced permeability and

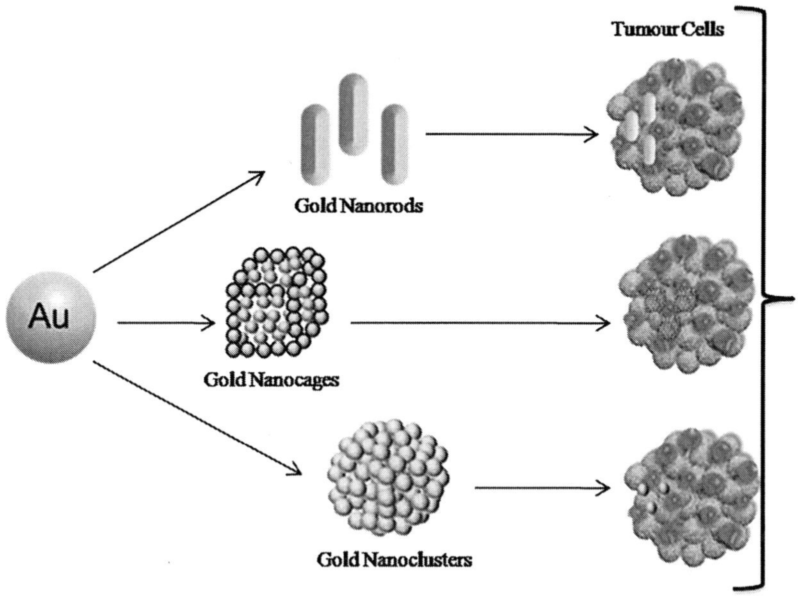

FIGURE 7.7 Gold nanoparticles (AuNPs) are widely applied in various forms, such as nanorods, nanocages, and nanoclusters, for their unique properties in cancer diagnostics and therapy. The specific binding of these AuNPs to tumor cell sites is facilitated by surface modifications and functionalization. The ability to precisely functionalize and tailor the surface properties of AuNPs allows researchers to design nanoparticles that can specifically recognize and bind to tumor cells. This targeted binding is crucial for improving the accuracy and efficiency of cancer diagnostics and therapeutic interventions.

retention (EPR) effect, which is their capacity to concentrate selectively in tumor tissues, makes it possible to image living species' tumors without intrusive procedures.

Jiang et al., in 2023, reported that the potential uses of platinum nanoparticles (PtNPs) as contrast agents in computed tomography (CT) imaging and other imaging modalities for cancer detection have drawn interest. Strong X-ray attenuation can be attained by the high atomic number of platinum, which results in increased contrast in CT images. This characteristic makes it easier to diagnose tumors accurately and enables thorough imaging of their tissues. PtNPs can be used to combine various imaging modalities for multimodal imaging. For example, they can be used as contrast agents for magnetic resonance imaging (MRI) and computed tomography (CT), which can enhance the accuracy of cancer detection by giving complementary information.

Figure 7.8 illustrates the PtNPs which have wide applications in photoacoustic and fluorescence imaging. T. Wang et al. in 2023 reviewed that PtNPs can be engineered to react to particular stimuli, including alterations in pH or redox conditions, in the tumor microenvironment. Because of its responsiveness, dynamic imaging can be performed, which offers insights into the tumor's physiological state and any treatment-related alterations. Q. Li et al. (2022) reported that photoacoustic imaging, which combines laser-induced ultrasound and optical imaging, can make use of platinum nanoparticles. Platinum nanoparticles are useful for observing malignancies because of their significant near-infrared absorbance, which enables high-resolution deep tissue imaging.

7.4.2 Role of Polymeric Nanoparticles in Cancer Imaging

Polymers are widely used in cancer imaging due to their versatility, biocompatibility, and ability to serve as carriers for contrast agents and imaging agents (Li, Pang, and Liu 2018). The pictorial representation of different type of polymeric nanoparticles used in cancer imaging is

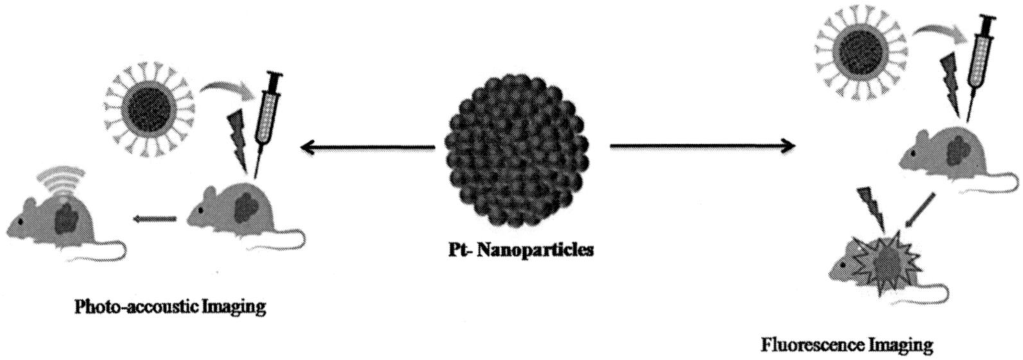

FIGURE 7.8 Platinum nanoparticles (PtNPs) exhibit unique properties that make them valuable in photo-acoustic and fluorescence imaging, contributing to advancements in cancer diagnostics. The dual capability of PtNPs in both photoacoustic and fluorescence imaging positions them as versatile contrast agents for non-invasive and real-time visualization of biological structures, including cancerous tissues.

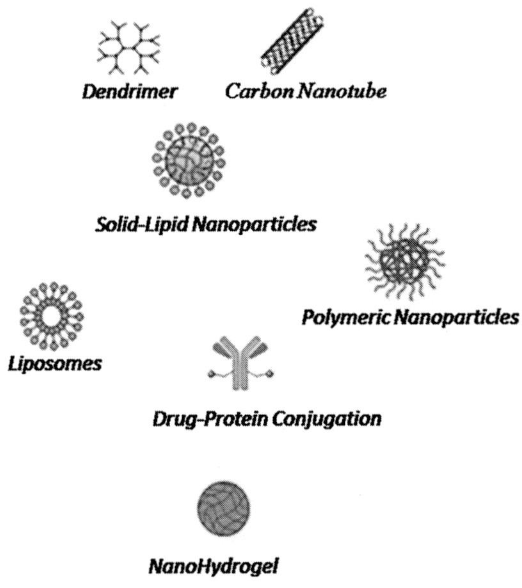

FIGURE 7.9 These depictions highlight the nanoscale size and structure of the particles, often resembling tiny spheres or capsules. These pictorial representations concisely capture the essential features of polymeric nanoparticles, aiding in conveying their use in cancer imaging in a visually accessible manner.

as shown in Figure 7.9. These polymers can enhance the performance and safety of imaging techniques (Haupt et al. 2020; Yin et al. 2020; Guo et al. 2022; Parveen et al. 2023). The choice of polymer depends on the specific imaging modality and application. Some polymers may be biopolymers, like dextran, chitosan, and hydrogels, which are usually biocompatible and biodegradable, whereas synthetic polymers, such as polyethylene glycol, poly(lactic-co-glycolic acid), polyethyleneimine, polyvinyl alcohol, polydopamine, etc., can also be used for cancer imaging in a controlled fashion.

7.4.2.1 Dextran

Dextran is a polysaccharide polymer that can be modified to create contrast agents for MRI (Predoi et al. 2023). Dextran-coated nanoparticles are used to enhance the imaging of tumor vasculature and angiogenesis.

7.4.2.2 Chitosan

Chitosan is a biocompatible and biodegradable polymer that can be used to formulate nanoparticles for targeted drug delivery and imaging (Herdiana et al. 2021; Kumar and Kumar 2023). It can be modified to enhance tumor-specific drug and contrast agent delivery.

7.4.2.3 Hydrogel Polymers

Hydrogel polymers can be used as drug delivery systems and carriers for imaging agents. They can be designed to release imaging agents slowly, providing sustained contrast enhancement for tumor imaging (Z. Wang et al. 2023).

7.4.2.4 Polymeric Micelles

Polymeric micelles are self-assembling nanoparticles formed from amphiphilic polymers.

They are used to encapsulate hydrophobic imaging agents and drugs (Movassaghian, Merkel, and Torchilin 2015). These micelles improve the solubility and delivery of imaging agents in cancer diagnostics and therapy (Oerlemans et al. 2010).

7.4.2.5 Polyethylene Glycol (PEG)

PEG is a biocompatible and hydrophilic polymer often used as a coating to improve the stability and circulation time of nanoparticles and contrast agents used in various imaging modalities, including MRI, CT, and ultrasound (Dabagh et al. 2023; Z. Wang et al. 2023).

7.4.2.6 Poly(Lactic-co-Glycolic Acid) (PLGA)

PLGA is a biodegradable polymer that can encapsulate imaging agents and drugs. It is commonly used in nanoparticle formulations for drug delivery and imaging in cancer diagnostics and therapy (Kim et al. 2019).

7.4.2.7 Polyethyleneimine (PEI)

PEI is used to coat nanoparticles and improve their cellular uptake. It is often used in combination with imaging agents for cancer imaging applications (Xia et al. 2009).

7.4.2.8 Polydopamine

Polydopamine is a versatile polymer used for surface modification of nanoparticles. It can improve the stability and biocompatibility of nanoparticles used in cancer imaging (D. Bi et al. 2018).

7.4.2.9 Polyvinyl Alcohol (PVA)

PVA is used as a stabilizer for nanoparticles and contrast agents in various imaging modalities. It helps prevent aggregation and enhances the circulation time of these agents (Mahmoudi et al. 2008).

Other various types of polymeric nanoparticles, such as polystyrene, polycaprolactone, and poly(l-lysine), can be designed and modified to encapsulate imaging agents for applications in cancer imaging (Joshi et al. 2019). Thus, various polymers are reported in the literature, in which they serve with different functions in cancer imaging, such as enhancing contrast, improving agent stability, enabling drug delivery, and targeting cancer-specific markers. The choice of polymer depends on the specific imaging technique, the desired properties of the imaging agent, and the goals of the imaging procedure. Researchers continue to develop and explore novel polymer-based systems to advance the field of cancer imaging and improve the accuracy and sensitivity of cancer diagnostics and treatment monitoring.

7.5 APPLICATIONS OF NANO-BASED POLYMERS IN CANCER IMAGING

By facilitating the speedy and susceptible detection of cancer-related molecules, nanotechnology allows the researchers to detect even in a smaller percentage of molecular changes (Kemp and Kwon 2021). Moreover, nanotechnology has the full potential to generate completely novel but effective therapeutic agents. Nano-based polymers have a wide range of applications in cancer imaging, enhancing the sensitivity and specificity of imaging modalities and enabling targeted delivery of imaging agents (Guo et al. 2022; Bhardwaj and Jangde 2023; Singh et al. 2023). Some key applications of nano-based polymers in cancer imaging include the following.

7.5.1 Improved Contrast Agents

According to O'Connor et al. (2011), nanoparticles can be engineered to enhance the contrast in various imaging modalities, such as MRI, CT, and ultrasound. They can carry contrast agents, making it easier to differentiate cancerous tissues from normal ones. For example, superparamagnetic iron oxide nanoparticles can enhance MRI contrast. Nano-based polymers are used to encapsulate or conjugate contrast agents, such as superparamagnetic nanoparticles for MRI, quantum dots for fluorescence imaging, or gold nanoparticles for CT imaging. These polymers enhance the stability and circulation time of the contrast agents, leading to improved imaging contrast and resolution (Hajfathalian et al. 2018; Cai et al. 2020; Schuerle et al. 2020; Dabagh et al. 2023).

7.5.2 Targeted Imaging

Polymer-based nanoparticles can be functionalized with ligands that specifically bind to cancer cell receptors or markers. This enables targeted imaging, allowing for the precise visualization of cancer cells while minimizing the impact on healthy tissues (Hong et al. 2011; Xu et al. 2022).

7.5.3 Enhanced Drug Delivery and Imaging

Polymer–drug conjugates and polymeric micelles can simultaneously carry imaging agents and therapeutic drugs. This approach allows for combined cancer therapy and imaging, enabling healthcare providers to monitor treatment effectiveness (Sahoo and Labhasetwar 2003).

7.5.4 Multimodal Imaging

Liang et al. 2023 reported that nanoparticles can carry multiple types of imaging agents, allowing for multimodal imaging. This means that one nanoparticle can be visualized using different imaging techniques, providing complementary information about the cancer site. Nano-based polymers can carry multiple imaging agents that are active in different modalities (e.g., MRI, fluorescence, and ultrasound). This enables multimodal imaging, providing complementary information for a more comprehensive assessment of tumors.

7.5.5 Theranostics

Theranostic nanoparticles serve a dual purpose by combining diagnostic and therapeutic capabilities. They can deliver drugs or therapies directly to cancer cells while simultaneously providing imaging to monitor the treatment's progress (Chan and Lin 2015; Kim et al. 2016; Kashyap et al.

2023). Polymer-based nanoparticles are employed in theranostics, which combine diagnostic and therapeutic capabilities. They can deliver therapeutic agents to cancer cells while also providing real-time imaging feedback on the treatment's effectiveness (Ma et al. 2017; Kashyap et al. 2023; Singh et al. 2023).

7.5.6 Personalized Medicine

By tailoring the surface properties and ligands of polymer-based nanoparticles to specific cancer cell receptors, nanotechnology allows for personalized cancer imaging and treatment. This approach considers the unique characteristics of each patient's cancer for more effective interventions (Lambin et al. 2017). By using nanoparticles to target specific genetic or molecular characteristics of a patient's cancer, nanotechnology can contribute to personalized medicine (Alghamdi et al. 2022). This approach tailors the treatment strategies based upon the unique attributes of each patient's cancer.

7.5.7 Minimally Invasive Procedures

Nanotechnology-based polymer systems, such as polymeric micelles, enable minimally invasive image-guided procedures. They can assist in tumor localization, targeted biopsies, and the assessment of treatment response, reducing the invasiveness of procedures (Blau et al. 2016). Nanoparticles can be used in minimally invasive procedures, such as image-guided biopsies, to precisely locate and extract cancerous tissues or cells for further analysis (Huang et al. 2023; Kataria et al. 2023).

7.5.8 Monitoring Treatment Response

Polymer-based nanoparticles can also be used to examine the response of cancer cells to treatment (Luk and Zhang 2014). This real-time monitoring can guide treatment adjustments and assess the effectiveness of therapies. Kashyap et al., in 2023, reported that nanotechnology enables real-time monitoring of cancer treatment. Nanoparticles can be used to track the delivery of therapeutic agents, monitor the response of cancer cells to treatment, and assess the effectiveness of therapy.

7.5.9 Lymph Node Mapping

In cancer surgeries, nanoparticles loaded with contrast agents can be used to map the lymphatic system, aiding in the identification of sentinel lymph nodes, which is particularly important in the staging and treatment of certain cancers (Jain et al. 2009).

7.5.10 Long Circulation Time

Nano-based polymers are designed to extend the circulation time of imaging agents, allowing for more precise and prolonged imaging of tumors. This is especially beneficial when using long-lived imaging agents or tracers (Claytor et al. 2014).

7.5.11 Radiosensitization

Some polymer-based nanoparticles are designed to increase the sensitivity of cancer cells by radiation therapy. They can be used in conjunction with radiotherapy and imaging to improve therapeutic outcomes in patients (Liu et al. 2018; Pan et al. 2022).

7.5.12 Early Detection

Liu et al. (2021) reported that nanoparticles can be designed to target specific biomarkers or proteins associated with cancer. These nanoparticles can be administered to patients, and their accumulation at the cancer site can be visualized using imaging techniques. This allows for early cancer detection, often before conventional methods can detect the disease. By enhancing the sensitivity of imaging modalities and allowing for earlier detection of cancer, nano-based polymers can improve the prognosis and treatment options for cancer patients (Lin et al. 2009; Liu et al. 2021; Pu et al. 2023).

7.5.13 Improved Specificity

Functionalized nanoparticles can be designed specifically to bind to the cancer cells or tissues, increasing the specificity of cancer imaging (Raj et al. 2021). Thus, it reduces false positives and improves the accuracy of cancer detection.

7.5.14 Improved Prognostic Information

Nanotechnology can provide detailed information about the size, location, and aggressiveness of tumors. This information can help healthcare providers make informed decisions about treatment options and prognostic assessments (Grigsby 2008; Schillaci et al. 2019).

7.5.15 In Vivo Imaging

Nanoparticles are often small enough to penetrate deep into tissues and reach cancer sites. This allows for in vivo imaging, where cancer detection and monitoring can occur within the living body, providing valuable insights into the disease's progression (Tong et al. 2010; Chan and Lin 2015).

7.5.16 Reduced Radiation Exposure

Some nanotechnology-based imaging techniques can reduce the need for high-energy ionizing radiation, which is particularly useful for patients who require repeated imaging procedures, such as those who suffer with cancer (Yu et al. 2009).

These applications of nano-based polymers in cancer imaging contribute to more accurate, targeted, and personalized approaches to the diagnosis, treatment, and monitoring of cancer. Researchers continue to explore and develop innovative polymer-based nanotechnologies to further advance cancer imaging and treatment.

7.6 SIDE EFFECTS OF NANOTECHNOLOGY IN CANCER IMAGING

The use of nano-polymers in cancer imaging is generally considered safe and well-tolerated, with minimal side effects. However, like any medical intervention, there can be some potential side effects and considerations associated with the use of nano-polymers in cancer imaging (Jin et al. 2020). Although these adverse effects are usually not severe and occur infrequently, healthcare practice should consider them. The following are some possible adverse effects to be aware of.

7.6.1 Allergic Reactions

According to Das et al. (2020), there are rare cases patients may exhibit allergic reactions to components of nano-polymers, such as polyethylene glycol (PEG). An allergic reaction typically appears as skin rash, itching, hives, swelling, and in more severe situations, breathing difficulty. Vigilant monitoring and thorough screening of patient histories can also help reduce this kind of danger (Plante et al. 2015).

7.6.2 Injection Site Reactions

Nano-polymers are often administered intravenously, like any injection, and can have localized reactions at the injection site. These reactions may include pain, discomfort, redness, and swelling. Proper administration techniques and monitoring can help manage all these reactions (Mudun et al. 2008).

7.6.3 Nonspecific Accumulation

In some cases, nano-polymers may accumulate in non-target tissues or organs, potentially leading to false-positive findings on imaging. This can be addressed by optimizing the design of nano-polymers to minimize off-target accumulation (Severin et al. 2015).

7.6.4 Renal Effects

In the case of some nanoparticles, such as those used in contrast agents for MRI or CT, there may be potential renal side effects. Kidney function should be evaluated, especially in patients with pre-existing kidney issues (Jiang et al. 2020).

7.6.5 Long-Term Effects

While nano-polymers are generally well-tolerated, their long-term effects in the body may not be fully understood. Continuous research is needed to review the safety and potential long-term consequences of their use (Jiang et al. 2020). It is important to remind that the overall benefits of using nano-polymers in cancer imaging typically outweigh the potential side effects. These side effects are generally rare and often manageable with appropriate patient screening, monitoring, and clinical care. Furthermore, ongoing research is aimed at improving the safety and efficacy of nano-polymers in cancer imaging, including efforts to minimize potential side effects. Before any medical procedure involving nano-polymers, patients should be informed about potential side effects, and healthcare providers should carefully consider the patient's medical history and overall health to minimize any risks. Additionally, research and clinical trials continue to advance our understanding of the safety and efficacy of nano-polymers in cancer imaging.

7.7 CONCLUSION AND FUTURE PROSPECTS

Hence, it is concluded that cancer imaging is a rapidly evolving field, and ongoing research and development continue to improve its capabilities in the fight against cancer. It has played a pivotal role in early detection, treatment planning, and monitoring, contributing to increased survival rates and better quality of life for cancer patients. Ultimately, it helps improve patient outcomes, increase the effectiveness of cancer treatments, and advance our understanding of the disease. Nanotechnology has significantly advanced the field of cancer imaging by offering more sensitive, precise, and personalized approaches for cancer detection, monitoring, and treatment. These innovations hold the potential to improve patient outcomes, reduce invasiveness in diagnostic procedures, and enhance our understanding of cancer at the molecular level. As nanotechnology continues to evolve, its role in cancer imaging is expected to expand further. Metal ions, when carefully incorporated into contrast agents or nanoparticles enable the visualization of tumors and aid in disease diagnosis and monitoring. The choice of metal ion depends upon the imaging modalities, the desired properties of contrast agents, and specific requirements of the imaging procedure. Ongoing research continues to explore metal-based novel contrast agents which further improve the specificity and sensitivity of cancer imaging. Hence, polymeric nanoparticles play a crucial role in cancer imaging by serving as versatile carriers for imaging agents. These nanoparticles, often biocompatible and biodegradable, enhance targeted delivery of contrast agents to tumor sites, improving imaging specificity. Their tunable properties, like size and surface characteristics, are also allowed for optimization in various imaging modalities. All in all, with the ability to encapsulate drugs and imaging agents simultaneously, polymeric nanoparticles contribute to theranostic applications, enabling personalized and effective cancer diagnostics and treatment monitoring.

Nanotechnology has a bright future ahead of it in cancer imaging, with many interesting possibilities suggested by ongoing research and development. Future directions and opportunities for nanotechnology are expected to include early and accurate tumor detection as targeted imaging agents, multimodal imaging to integrate imaging platforms, theranostics for combined imaging and therapy, customized nanoparticle designs in personalized medicine, enhanced intra-operative imaging through image-guided surgery, remote sensing and monitoring for implanting nanosensors, improved smart contrast agents for better visualization of tumor boundaries and microenvironments, integration of artificial intelligence for data analysis and interpretation, and clinical translation for large-scale clinical adoption. Although these opportunities seem bright, obstacles, including safety and regulatory approval, are needed to be addressed fairly.

REFERENCES

Afaq, Asim, Anna P. Andreou, and Dow-Mu Koh. 2010. "Diffusion-Weighted Magnetic Resonance Imaging for Tumour Response Assessment: Why, When and How?" *Cancer Imaging* 10 (1A): S179–88. https://doi.org/10.1102/1470-7330.2010.9032.

Alam, Israt S., Idan Steinberg, Ophir Vermesh, Nynke S. van den Berg, Eben L. Rosenthal, Gooitzen M. van Dam, Vasilis Ntziachristos, Sanjiv S. Gambhir, Sophie Hernot, and Stephan Rogalla. 2018. "Emerging Intraoperative Imaging Modalities to Improve Surgical Precision." *Molecular Imaging and Biology* 20: 705–15. https://doi.org/10.1007/s11307-018-1227-6.

Alghamdi, Maha Ali, Antonino N. Fallica, Nicola Virzì, Prashant Kesharwani, Valeria Pittalà, and Khaled Greish. 2022. "The Promise of Nanotechnology in Personalized Medicine." *Journal of Personalized Medicine* 12 (5): 673. https://doi.org/10.3390/jpm12050673.

Ali, Towhid, Peter L. Choyke, and Hisataka Kobayashi. 2013. "Endoscopic Molecular Imaging of Cancer." *Future Oncology* 9(10): 1501–13. https://doi.org/10.2217/fon.13.123.

Andreozzi, Erica M., Julia Baguña Torres, Kavitha Sunassee, Joel Dunn, Simon Walker-Samuel, Istvan Szanda, and Philip J. Blower. 2017 "Studies of Copper Trafficking in a Mouse Model of Alzheimer's Disease by Positron Emission Tomography: Comparison of ^{64}Cu Acetate and ^{64}CuGTSM." *Metallomics* 9 (11): 1622–33. https://doi.org/10.1039/c7mt00227k.

Angelovski, Goran, Sven Gottschalk, Milena Milošević, Jörn Engelmann, Gisela E. Hagberg, Pascal Kadjane, Pavle Andjus, and Nikos K. Logothetis. 2014. "Investigation of a Calcium-Responsive Contrast Agent in Cellular Model Systems: Feasibility for Use as a Smart Molecular Probe in Functional MRI." *ACS Chemical Neuroscience* 5 (5): 360–9. https://doi.org/10.1021/cn500049n.

Anjum, Sumaira, Mariam Hashim, Sara Asad Malik, Maha Khan, José M. Lorenzo, Bilal Haider Abbasi, and Christophe Hano. 2021. "Recent Advances in Zinc Oxide Nanoparticles (ZnO NPs) for Cancer Diagnosis, Target Drug Delivery, and Treatment." *Cancers* 13 (18): 4570. https://doi.org/10.3390/cancers13184570.

Armentano, Ilaria, Mariaserena Dottori, Elena Fortunati, Samantha Mattioli, and J. M. Kenny. 2010 "Biodegradable Polymer Matrix Nanocomposites for Tissue Engineering: A Review." *Polymer Degradation and Stability* 95 (11): 2126–46. https://doi.org/10.1016/j.polymdegradstab.2010.06.007.

Augustine, Robin, Abdulla Al Mamun, Anwarul Hasan, Shaheen Abdul Salam, Ramya Chandrasekaran, Rashid Ahmed, and Avnesh S. Thakor. 2021. "Imaging Cancer Cells With Nanostructures: Prospects of Nanotechnology Driven Non-Invasive Cancer Diagnosis." *Advances in Colloid and Interface Science* 294: 102457. https://doi.org/10.1016/j.cis.2021.102457.

Bhardwaj, Harish, and Rajendra Kumar Jangde. 2023. "Current Updated Review on Preparation of Polymeric Nanoparticles for Drug Delivery and Biomedical Applications." *Next Nanotechnology* 2: 100013. https://doi.org/10.1016/j.nxnano.2023.100013.

Bi, Dongdong, Lei Zhao, Runqi Yu, Haowen Li, Yifei Guo, Xiangtao Wang, and Meihua Han. 2018. "Surface Modification of Doxorubicin-Loaded Nanoparticles Based on Polydopamine With pH-Sensitive Property for Tumor Targeting Therapy." *Drug Delivery* 25 (1): 564–75. https://doi.org/10.1080/10717544.2018.1440447.

Bi, Huiting, Fei He, Yushan Dong, Dan Yang, Yunlu Dai, Liangge Xu, Ruichan Lv, Shili Gai, Piaoping Yang, and Jun Lin. 2018. "Bismuth Nanoparticles with 'Light' Property Served as a Multifunctional Probe for X-Ray Computed Tomography and Fluorescence Imaging." *Chemistry of Materials* 30 (10): 3301–7. https://doi.org/10.1021/acs.chemmater.8b00565.

Bisht, Gunjan, and Sagar Rayamajhi. 2016. "ZnO Nanoparticles: A Promising Anticancer Agent." *Nanobiomedicine* 3: 9. https://doi.org/10.5772/63437.

Blau, Rachel, Adva Krivitsky, Yana Epshtein, and Ronit Satchi-Fainaro. 2016. "Are Nanotheranostics and Nanodiagnostics-Guided Drug Delivery Stepping Stones Towards Precision Medicine?." *Drug Resistance Updates* 27: 39–58. https://doi.org/10.1016/j.drup.2016.06.003.

Bouchard, Louis-S., M. Sabieh Anwar, Gang L. Liu, Byron Hann, Z. Harry Xie, Joe W. Gray, Xueding Wang. 2009. Alexander Pines, and Fanqing Frank Chen. "Picomolar Sensitivity MRI and Photoacoustic Imaging of Cobalt Nanoparticles." *Proceedings of the National Academy of Sciences* 106 (11): 4085–9. https://doi.org/10.1073/pnas.081301910.

Bouché, Mathilde, Jessica C. Hsu, Yuxi C. Dong, Johoon Kim, Kimberly Taing, and David P. Cormode. 2019 "Recent Advances in Molecular Imaging With Gold Nanoparticles." *Bioconjugate Chemistry* 31 (2): 303–14. https://doi.org/10.1021/acs.bioconjchem.9b00669.

Cai, Yao, Yuqing Wang, Tongwei Zhang, and Yongxin Pan. 2020. "Gadolinium-Labeled Ferritin Nanoparticles as T1 Contrast Agents for Magnetic Resonance Imaging of Tumors." *ACS Applied Nano Materials* 3 (9): 8771–83. https://doi.org/10.1021/acsanm.0c01563.

Chan, Ming-Hsien, and Hsiu-Mei Lin. 2015. "Preparation and Identification of Multifunctional Mesoporous Silica Nanoparticles for In Vitro and In Vivo Dual-Mode Imaging, Theranostics, and Targeted Tracking." *Biomaterials* 46: 149–58. https://doi.org/10.1016/j.biomaterials.2014.12.034.

Chan, Ming-Hsien, Chih-Ning Lu, Yi-Lung Chung, Yu-Chan Chang, Chien-Hsiu Li, Chi-Long Chen, Da-Hua Wei, and Michael Hsiao. 2021. "Magnetically Guided Theranostics: Montmorillonite-Based Iron/Platinum Nanoparticles for Enhancing In Situ MRI Contrast and Hepatocellular Carcinoma Treatment." *Journal of Nanobiotechnology* 19 (308): 1–16. https://doi.org/10.1186/s12951-021-01052-7

Chapman, Sandra, Marina Dobrovolskaia, Keyvan Farahani, Andrew Goodwin, Amit Joshi, Hakho Lee, Thomas Meade, et al. 2013. "Nanoparticles for Cancer Imaging: The Good, The Bad, and The Promise." *Nano Today* 8 (5): 454–60. https://doi.org/10.1016/j.nantod.2013.06.001.

Chatterjee, Krishnendu, Sreerupa Sarkar, K. Jagajjanani Rao, and Santanu Paria. 2014 "Core/Shell Nanoparticles in Biomedical Applications." *Advances in Colloid and Interface Science* 209: 8–39. https://doi.org/10.1016/j.cis.2013.12.008.

Cheheltani, Rabee, Rami M. Ezzibdeh, Peter Chhour, Kumidini Pulaparthi, Johoon Kim, Martina Jurcova, Jessica C. Hsu, Cassidy Blundell, Harold I. Litt, Victor A. Ferrari, Harry R. Allcock, Chandra M. Sehgal, and David P. Cormode. 2016. "Tunable, Biodegradable Gold Nanoparticles as Contrast Agents for Computed Tomography and Photoacoustic Imaging." *Biomaterials* 102: 87–97. https://doi.org/10.1016/j.biomaterials.2016.06.015.

Chen, Liping, Haitian Fu, Huihui He, Kequan Lou, Qingbo Li, Jiacong Ye, Guokai Feng, and Chunjing Yu. 2023. "Automated Synthesis and Preclinical Evaluation of Optimized Integrin α6-Targeted Positron Emission Tomography Imaging of Pancreatic Cancer." *Molecular Pharmaceutics* 20 (8): 4277–84. https://doi.org/10.1021/acs.molpharmaceut.3c00321.

Chuang, Feng-Rong, Te-Chuan Chen, I-Kuan Wang, Chung-Hua Chuang, Hsueh-Wen Chang, Terry Ting-Yu Chiou, Yu-Fan Cheng, et al. 2009. "Comparison of Iodixanol and Iohexol in Patients Undergoing Intravenous Pyelography: A Prospective Controlled Study." *Renal Failure* 31 (3): 181–8. https://doi.org/10.1080/08860220802669636.

Claytor, Kevin, Thomas Theis, Yesu Feng, and Warren Warren. 2014. "Measuring Long-Lived $^{13}C_2$ State Lifetimes at Natural Abundance." *Journal of Magnetic Resonance* 239: 81–86. https://doi.org/10.1016/j.jmr.2013.12.009.

Coccia, Mario, and Lili Wang. 2015. "Path-Breaking Directions of Nanotechnology-Based Chemotherapy and Molecular Cancer Therapy." *Technological Forecasting and Social Change* 94: 155–69. https://doi.org/10.1016/j.techfore.2014.09.007

Conde, João, Gonçalo Doria, and Pedro Baptista. 2012. "Noble Metal Nanoparticles Applications in Cancer." *Journal of Drug Delivery* 12, Article ID 751075. https://doi.org/10.1155/2012/751075.

Dabagh, Shadab, Somayeh Asadi Haris, and Yavuz Nuri Ertas. 2023. "Engineered Polyethylene Glycol-Coated Zinc Ferrite Nanoparticles as a Novel Magnetic Resonance Imaging Contrast Agent." *ACS Biomaterials Science & Engineering* 9 (7): 4138–48. https://doi.org/10.1021/acsbiomaterials.3c00255.

Das, Sabya Sachi, Priyanshu Bharadwaj, Muhammad Bilal, Mahmood Barani, Abbas Rahdar, Pablo Taboada, Simona Bungau, and George Z. Kyzas. 2020 "Stimuli-Responsive Polymeric Nanocarriers for Drug Delivery, Imaging, and Theragnosis." *Polymers* 12 (6): 1397. https://doi.org/10.3390/polym 12061397

Dong, Ruijiao, Hongying Chen, Dali Wang, Yuanyuan Zhuang, Lijuan Zhu, Yue Su, Deyue Yan, and Xinyuan Zhu. 2012. Supramolecular Fluorescent Nanoparticles for Targeted Cancer Imaging. *ACS Macro Letters* 1 (10): 1208–11. https://doi.org/10.1021/mz300375c.

Eary, Janet F. 1999. "Nuclear Medicine in Cancer Diagnosis." *The Lancet* 354 (9181): 853–7. https://doi.org/10.1016/S0140-6736(99)80041-5.

Elsabahy, Mahmoud, Gyu Seong Heo, Soon-Mi Lim, Guorong Sun, and Karen L. Wooley. 2015. "Polymeric Nanostructures for Imaging and Therapy." *Chemical Reviews* 115 (19): 10967–1011. https://doi.org/10.1021/acs.chemrev.5b00135.

Fass, Leonard. 2008. "Imaging and Cancer: A Review." *Molecular Oncology* 2 (2): 115–52. https://doi.org/10.1016/j.molonc.2008.04.001.

Fu, Bei, Meng Dang, Jun Tao, Yanjun Li, and Yuxia Tang. 2020. "Mesoporous Platinum Nanoparticle-Based Nanoplatforms for Combined Chemo-Photothermal Breast Cancer Therapy." *Journal of Colloid and Interface Science* 570: 197–204. https://doi.org/10.1016/j.jcis.2020.02.051.

Gaikwad, Hanmant K., Darya Tsvirkun, Yael Ben-Nun, Emmanuelle Merquiol, Rachela Popovtzer, and Galia Blum. 2018. "Molecular Imaging of Cancer Using X-Ray Computed Tomography With Protease Targeted Iodinated Activity-Based Probes." 18 (3): 1582–91. https://doi.org/10.1021/acs.nanolett.7b03813.

García-Figueiras, Roberto, Sandra Baleato-González, Anwar R. Padhani, Antonio Luna-Alcalá, Juan Antonio Vallejo-Casas, Evis Sala, Joan C. Vilanova, Dow-Mu Koh, Michel Herranz-Carnero, and Herbert Alberto Vargas. 2019. "How Clinical Imaging Can Assess Cancer Biology." *Insights Into Imaging* 10: 1–35. https://doi.org/10.1186/s13244-019 0703-0.

Grigsby, Perry W. 2008. "The Prognostic Value of PET and PET/CT in Cervical Cancer." *Cancer Imaging* 8 (1): 146–55. https://doi.org/10.1102/1470-7330.2008.0022.

Guo, Kai, Nanyang Xiao, Yixuan Liu, Zhenming Wang, Judit Tóth, János Gyenis, Vijay Kumar Thakur, Ayako Oyane, and Quazi T. H. Shubhra. 2022. "Engineering Polymer Nanoparticles Using Cell Membrane Coating Technology and Their Application in Cancer Treatments: Opportunities and Challenges." *Nano Materials Science* 4 (4): 295–321. https://doi.org/10.1016/j.nanoms.2021.12.001.

Guo, Qianqian, Liwen Li, Shanshan Hou, Ziqiao Yuan, Chenhui Li, Wenzhou Zhang, Lufeng Zheng, and Xiaoman Li. 2021. "The Role of Iron in Cancer Progression." *Frontiers in Oncology* 11: 778492. https://doi.org/10.3389/fonc.2021.778492.

Hajfathalian, Maryam, Ahmad Amirshaghaghi, Pratap C. Naha, Peter Chhour, Jessica C. Hsu, Keely Douglas, Yuxi Dong, et al. 2018. "Wulff in a Cage Gold Nanoparticles as Contrast Agents for Computed Tomography and Photoacoustic Imaging." *Nanoscale* 10 (39): 18749–57. https://doi.org/10.1039/c8nr 05203d.

Haldorsen, Ingfrid S., Njål Lura, Jan Blaakær, Daniela Fischerova, and Henrica MJ Werner. 2019. "What is the Role of Imaging at Primary Diagnostic Work-Up in Uterine Cervical Cancer?" *Current Oncology Reports* 21 (9): 1–15. https://doi.org/10.1007/s11912-019-0824-0.

Hansen, Anders E., Anncatrine L. Petersen, Jonas R. Henriksen, Betina Boerresen, Palle Rasmussen, Dennis R. Elema, Per Munck af Rosenschöld, Annemarie T. Kristensen, Andreas Kjær, and Thomas L. Andresen. 2015. "Positron Emission Tomography Based Elucidation of the Enhanced Permeability and Retention Effect in Dogs With Cancer Using Copper-64 Liposomes." *ACS Nano* 9 (7): 6985–95. https://doi.org/10.1021/acsnano.5b01324.

Haque, Shagufta, Caroline Celine Norbert, Rajarshi Acharyya, Sudip Mukherjee, Muralidharan Kathirvel, and Chitta Ranjan Patra. 2021 "Biosynthesized Silver Nanoparticles for Cancer Therapy and In Vivo Bioimaging." *Cancers* 13 (23): 6114. https://doi.org/10.3390/cancers13236114.

Haupt, Karsten, Paulina X. Medina Rangel, and Bernadette Tse Sum Bui. 2020. "Molecularly Imprinted Polymers: Antibody Mimics for Bioimaging and Therapy." *Chemical Reviews* 120 (17): 9554–82. https://doi.org/10.1021/acs.chemrev.0c00428.

Herdiana, Yedi, Nasrul Wathoni, Shaharum Shamsuddin, and Muchtaridi Muchtaridi. 2022. "Drug Release Study of the Chitosan-Based Nanoparticles." *Heliyon* 8 (1): e08674. https://doi.org/10.1016/j.heliyon.2021.e08674.

Hermans, Robert. 2004. "Post-Treatment Imaging of Head and Neck Cancer." *Cancer Imaging* 4 (Spec No A): S6–15. https://doi.org/10.1102/1470-7330.2004.0007.

Hong, Hao, Jian Shi, Yunan Yang, Yin Zhang, Jonathan W. Engle, Robert J. Nickles, Xudong Wang, and Weibo Cai. 2011. "Cancer-Targeted Optical Imaging With Fluorescent Zinc Oxide Nanowires." *Nano Letters* 11 (9): 3744–50. https://doi.org/10.1021/nl201782m.

Huang, Guojia, Sihua Yang, Yi Yuan, and Da Xing. 2011. "Combining X-Ray and Photoacoustics for In Vivo Tumor Imaging With Gold Nanorods." *Applied Physics Letters* 99 (12): 123701. https://doi.org/10.1063/1.3643033.

Huang, Maohua, Ming Qi, Hongyan Yang, Zhi Peng, Shouguo Chen, Mingchao Liang, Youzhu Hu, Lijuan Deng, and Min Hu. 2023. "Noninvasive Strategies for the Treatment of Tiny Liver Cancer: Integrating Photothermal Therapy and Multimodality Imaging EpCAM-Guided Nanoparticles." *ACS Applied Materials & Interfaces* 15 (18): 21843–53. https://doi.org/10.1021/acsami.3c00211.

Hunter, Benjamin, Sumeet Hindocha, and Richard W. Lee. 2022. "The Role of Artificial Intelligence in Early Cancer Diagnosis." *Cancers* 14 (6): 1524. https://doi.org/10.3390/cancers14061524

Jain, Ratnesh, Prajakta Dandekar, and Vandana Patravale. 2009. "Diagnostic Nanocarriers for Sentinel Lymph Node Imaging." *Journal of Controlled Release* 138 (2): 90–102. https://doi.org/10.1016/j.jconrel.2009.05.010.

Jiang, Dawei, Zachary T. Rosenkrans, Dalong Ni, Jing Lin, Peng Huang, and Weibo Cai. 2020. "Nanomedicines for Renal Management: From Imaging to Treatment." *Accounts of Chemical Research* 53 (9): 1869–80. https://doi.org/10.1021/acs.accounts.0c00323.

Jiang, Zeyu, Meihua Zhang, Peifeng Li, Yin Wang, and Qinrui Fu. 2023 "Nanomaterial-Based CT Contrast Agents and Their Applications in Image-Guided Therapy." *Theranostics*13 (2): 483–509. https://doi.org/10.7150/thno.79625.

Jin, Cancan, Kankai Wang, Anthony Oppong-Gyebi, and Jiangnan Hu. 2020. "Application of Nanotechnology in Cancer Diagnosis and Therapy-a Mini-Review." *International Journal of Medical Sciences* 17 (18): 2964. https://doi.org/10.7150/ijms.49801

Joshi, Dheeraj Chandra, Sonashree Saxena, and Manickam Jayakannan. 2019. "Development of l-Lysine Based Biodegradable Polyurethanes and Their Dual-Responsive Amphiphilic Nanocarriers for Drug Delivery to Cancer Cells." *ACS Applied Polymer Materials* 1 (7): 1866–80. https://doi.org/10.1021/acsapm.9b00413.

Jung, Jongjin, Mi Ae Kim, Jee-Hyun Cho, Seung Jae Lee, Ilseung Yang, Janggeun Cho, Seong Keun Kim, Chulhyun Lee, and Joung Kyu Park. 2012. "Europium-Doped Gadolinium Sulfide Nanoparticles as a Dual-Mode Imaging Agent for T1-Weighted MR and Photoluminescence Imaging." *Biomaterials*33 (24): 5865–74. https://doi.org/10.1016/j.biomaterials.2012.04.059.e.

Kashyap, Brijendra Kumar, Virendra Vikram Singh, Manoj Kumar Solanki, Anil Kumar, Janne Ruokolainen, and Kavindra Kumar Kesari. 2023. "Smart Nanomaterials in Cancer Theranostics: Challenges and Opportunities." *ACS Omega* 8 (16): 14290–320. https://doi.org/10.1021/acsomega.2c07840.

Kataria, Swati, Jifa Qi, Ching-Wei Lin, Zhongming Li, Eric L. Dane, Archana Mahadevan Iyer, Jay Sacane, Darrell J. Irvine, and Angela M. Belcher. 2023. "Noninvasive In Vivo Imaging of T-Cells During Cancer Immunotherapy Using Rare-Earth Nanoparticles." *ACS Nano* 17 (18): 17908–19. https://doi.org/10.1021/acsnano.3c03882.

Kemp, Jessica A., and Young Jik Kwon. 2021. "Cancer Nanotechnology: Current Status and Perspectives." *Nano Convergence* 8 (1): 34. https://doi.org/10.1186/s40580-021-00282-7.

Kim, Inhye, Eun Hee Han, Jooyeon Ryu, Jin-Young Min, Hyungju Ahn, Young-Ho Chung, and Eunji Lee. 2016. "One-Dimensional Supramolecular Nanoplatforms for Theranostics Based on Co-Assembly of Peptide Amphiphiles." *Biomacromolecules* 17 (10): 3234–43. https://doi.org/10.1021/acs.biomac.6b00966.

Kim, Ki-Taek, Jae-Young Lee, Dae-Duk Kim, In-Soo Yoon, and Hyun-Jong Cho. 2019. "Recent Progress in the Development of Poly (Lactic-Co-Glycolic Acid)-Based Nanostructures for Cancer Imaging and Therapy." *Pharmaceutics* 11 (6): 280. https://doi.org/10.3390/pharmaceutics11060280.

Kron, Tomas, David Eyles, Schreiner L. John, and Jerry Battista. 2006 "Magnetic Resonance Imaging for Adaptive Cobalt Tomotherapy: A Proposal." *Journal of Medical Physics* 31 (4): 242–54. https://doi.org/10.4103/0971-6203.29194.

Kumar, Ashwini, and Awanish Kumar. 2023 "Chitosan-Based Drug Conjugated Nanocomposites: Advances and Innovation in Cancer Therapy." *Regenerative Engineering and Translational Medicine* 2013: 1–8. https://doi.org/10.1007/s40883-023-00310-4.

Lambin, Philippe, Ralph T. H. Leijenaar, Timo M. Deist, Jurgen Peerlings, Evelyn E. C. De Jong, Janita Van Timmeren, Sebastian Sanduleanu, et al. 2017. "Radiomics: The Bridge Between Medical Imaging and Personalized Medicine." *Nature Reviews Clinical Oncology* 14 (12): 749–62. https://doi.org/10.1038/nrclinonc.2017.141.

Lee, Haerim, Mi Kyung Yu, Sangjin Park, Sungmin Moon, Jung Jun Min, Yong Yeon Jeong, Hae-Won Kang, and Sangyong Jon. 2007. "Thermally Cross-Linked Superparamagnetic Iron Oxide Nanoparticles: Synthesis and Application as a Dual Imaging Probe for Cancer In Vivo." *Journal of the American Chemical Society* 129 (42): 12739–45. https://doi.org/10.1021/ja072210i.

Lee, Won Woo, and K-SPECT Group. 2019. "Clinical Applications of Technetium-99m Quantitative Single-Photon Emission Computed Tomography/Computed Tomography." *Nuclear Medicine and Molecular Imaging* 53 (3): 172–81. https://doi.org/10.1007/s13139-019-00588-9.

Li, Kai, Hossein Nejadnik, and Heike E. Daldrup-Link. 2017 "Next-Generation Superparamagnetic Iron Oxide Nanoparticles for Cancer Theranostics." *Drug Discovery Today* 22 (9): 1421–9. https://doi.org/10.1016/j.drudis.2017.04.008.

Li, Lanqing, Shiying Li, Zhijin Fan, Guojia Huang, Jianxin Tang, and Liming Nie. 2022. "Current Strategies of Photoacoustic Imaging Assisted Cancer Theragnostics Toward Clinical Studies." *ACS Photonics* 9 (8): 2555–78. https://doi.org/10.1021/acsphotonics.2c00440.

Li, Lei, Xin Pang, and Gang Liu. 2018. "Near-Infrared Light-Triggered Polymeric Nano-Micelles for Cancer Therapy and Imaging." *ACS Biomaterials Science & Engineering* 4 (6): 1928–41. https://doi.org/10.1021/acsbiomaterials.7b00648.

Li, Qingqing, Luntao Liu, Hongqi Huo, Lichao Su, Ying Wu, Hongxin Lin, Xiaoguang Ge, Jing Mu, Xuan Zhang, Liting Zheng, and Jibin Song. 2022. "Nanosized Janus AuNR-Pt Motor for Enhancing NIR-II Photoacoustic Imaging of Deep Tumor and Pt^{2+} Ion-Based Chemotherapy." *ACS Nano* 16 (5): 7947–60. https://doi.org/10.1021/acsnano.2c00732.

Li, Wanwan, and Xiaoyuan Chen. 2015. "Gold Nanoparticles for Photoacoustic Imaging." *Nanomedicine* 10 (2): 299–320. https://doi.org/10.2217/nnm.14.169.

Liang, Ranxi, Feize Li, Xijian Chen, Fuyuan Tan, Tu Lan, Jijun Yang, Jiali Liao, Yuanyou Yang, and Ning Liu. 2023. "Multimodal Imaging-Guided Strategy for Developing ^{177}Lu-Labeled Metal–Organic Framework Nanomedicine With Potential in Cancer Therapy." *ACS Applied Materials& Interfaces* 15 (39): 45713–24. https://doi.org/10.1021/acsami.3c11098.

Lin, Wenbin, Taeghwan Hyeon, Gregory M. Lanza, Miqin Zhang, and Thomas J. Meade. 2009. "Magnetic Nanoparticles for Early Detection of Cancer by Magnetic Resonance Imaging." *MRS Bulletin* 34 (6): 441–8. https://doi.org/10.1557/mrs2009.120.

Lin, Zhiqiang, Changrong Wang, Yang Li, Ridong Li, Lidong Gong, Yue Su, Zheng Zhai, et al. 2019. "Glutathione-Priming Nanoreactors Enable Fluorophore Core/Shell Transition for Precision Cancer Imaging." *ACS Applied Materials & Interfaces* 11 (37): 33667–75. https://doi.org/10.1021/acsami.9b11063.

Liu, Yan, Pengcheng Zhang, Feifei Li, Xiaodong Jin, Jin Li, Weiqiang Chen, and Qiang Li. 2018. "Metal-Based Nanoenhancers for Future Radiotherapy: Radiosensitizing and Synergistic Effects on Tumor Cells." *Theranostics* 8 (7): 1824. https://doi.org/10.7150/thno.22172.

Liu, Yang, Yinghui Wang, Shuyan Song, and Hongjie Zhang. 2021. "Cancer Therapeutic Strategies Based on Metal Ions." *Chemical Science* 12 (37): 12234–47. https://doi.org/10.1039/d1sc03516a.

Liu, Yijing, Pravin Bhattarai, Zhifei Dai, and Xiaoyuan Chen. 2019. "Photothermal Therapy and Photoacoustic Imaging via Nanotheranostics in Fighting Cancer." *Chemical Society Reviews* 48 (7): 2053–108. https://doi.org/10.1039/c8cs00618k.

Liu, Yongjun, and Na Zhang. 2012. "Gadolinium Loaded Nanoparticles in Theranostic Magnetic Resonance Imaging." *Biomaterials* 33 (21): 5363–75. https://doi.org/10.1016/j.biomaterials.2012.03.084.

Luk, Brian T., and Liangfang Zhang. 2014. "Current Advances in Polymer-Based Nanotheranostics for Cancer Treatment and Diagnosis." *ACS Applied Materials & Interfaces* 6 (24): 21859–421873. https://doi.org/10.1021/am5036225.

Lusic, Hrvoje, and Mark W. Grinstaff. 2013. "X-Ray-Computed Tomography Contrast Agents." *Chemical Reviews* 113 (3): 1641–66. https://doi.org/10.1021/cr200358s.

Ma, Ying, Mostafa Sadoqi, and Jun Shao. 2012. "Biodistribution of Indocyanine Green-Loaded Nanoparticles With Surface Modifications of PEG and Folic Acid." *International Journal of Pharmaceutics* 436 (1–2): 25–31. https://doi.org/10.1016/j.ijpharm.2012.06.007.

Ma, Ying-Yu, Ke-Tao Jin, Shi-Bing Wang, Hui-Ju Wang, Xiang-Min Tong, Dong-Sheng Huang, and Xiao-Zhou Mou. 2017. "Molecular Imaging of Cancer With Nanoparticle-Based Theranostic Probes." *Contrast Media & Molecular Imaging* 2017: 1026270. https://doi.org/10.1155/2017/1026270.

Mahmoudi, Morteza, Abdolreza Simchi, Mohammad Imani, Abbas S. Milani, and Pieter Stroeve. 2008. "Optimal Design and Characterization of Superparamagnetic Iron Oxide Nanoparticles Coated With Polyvinyl Alcohol for Targeted Delivery and Imaging." *The Journal of Physical Chemistry B*, 112 (46): 14470–81. https://doi.org/10.1021/jp803016n.

Majdalawieh, Amin, Marsha C. Kanan, Oussama El-Kadri, and Sofian M. Kanan. 2014. "Recent Advances in Gold and Silver Nanoparticles: Synthesis and Applications." *Journal of Nanoscience and Nanotechnology* 14 (7): 4757–80. https://doi.org/10.1166/jnn.2014.9526.

Makela, Ashley V., Melissa A. Schott, Olivia C. Sehl, Julia J. Gevaert, Paula J. Foster, and Christopher H. Contag. 2022. "Tracking the Fates of Iron-Labeled Tumor Cells In Vivo Using Magnetic Particle Imaging." *Nanoscale Advances* 4 (17): 3617–23. https://doi.org/10.1039/d2na00008c.

Maleki, Fariba, Farzaneh Rezazadeh, and Kambiz Varmira. 2021. "MUC1-Targeted Radiopharmaceuticals in Cancer Imaging and Therapy." *Molecular Pharmaceutics* 18 (5): 1842–61. https://doi.org/10.1021/acs.molpharmaceut.0c01249.

Michalski, Mark H., and Xiaoyuan Chen. 2011. "Molecular Imaging in Cancer Treatment." *European Journal of Nuclear Medicine and Molecular Imaging* 38: 358–77. https://doi.org/10.1007/s00259-010-1569-z

Miki, Koji, Akinori Kimura, Kazuaki Oride, Yoshiaki Kuramochi, Hideki Matsuoka, Hiroshi Harada, Masahiro Hiraoka, and Kouichi Ohe. 2011. "High-Contrast Fluorescence Imaging of Tumors In Vivo Using Nanoparticles of Amphiphilic Brush-Like Copolymers Produced by ROMP." *Angewandte Chemie International Edition* 50 (29), 6567–70. https://doi.org/10.1002/anie.201101005.

Movassaghian, Sara, Olivia M. Merkel, and Vladimir P. Torchilin. 2015. "Applications of Polymer Micelles for Imaging and Drug Delivery." *Wiley Interdisciplinary Reviews: Nanomedicine and Nanobiotechnology* 7 (5): 691–707. https://doi.org/10.1002/wnan.1332.

Mudun, Ayse, Yasemin Sanli, Vahit Ozmen, Cuneyt Turkmen, Sevda Ozel, Aylin Eroglu, Abdullah Igci, et al. 2008. "Comparison of Different Injection Sites of Radionuclide for Sentinel Lymph Node Detection in Breast Cancer: Single Institution Experience." *Clinical Nuclear Medicine* 33 (4): 262–7. https://doi.org/10.1097/RLU.0b013e3181662fc7.

Muguruma, Naoki, Hiroshi Miyamoto, Toshiya Okahisa, and Tetsuji Takayama. 2013. "Endoscopic Molecular Imaging: Status and Future Perspective." *Clinical Endoscopy* 46 (6): 603–10. https://doi.org/10.5946/ce.2013.46.6.603.

O'Connor, J. P. B., P. S. Tofts, K. A. Miles, L. M. Parkes, G. Thompson, and A. Jackson. 2011. "Dynamic Contrast-Enhanced Imaging Techniques: CT and MRI." *The British Journal of Radiology* 84 (2): S112–20. https://doi.org/10.1259/bjr/55166688.

Oerlemans, Chris, Wouter Bult, Mariska Bos, Gert Storm, J. Frank W. Nijsen, and Wim E. Hennink. 2010. "Polymeric Micelles in Anticancer Therapy: Targeting, Imaging and Triggered Release." *Pharmaceutical Research* 27: 2569–89. https://doi.org/10.1007/s11095-010-0233-4.

Pala, Rajasekharreddy, Yun Zeng, Subhaswaraj Pattnaik, Siddhardha Busi, Nedaa Alomari, Surya M. Nauli, and Gang Liu. 2018 "Functionalized Silver Nanoparticles for Sensing, Molecular Imaging and Therapeutic Applications." *Current Nanomedicine (Formerly: Recent Patents on Nanomedicine)* 8 (3): 234–50. https://doi.org/10.2174/2468187308666180508144919.

Pan, Yuanbo, Wei Tang, Wenpei Fan, Jianmin Zhang, and Xiaoyuan Chen. 2022. "Development of Nanotechnology-Mediated Precision Radiotherapy for Anti-Metastasis and Radioprotection." *Chemical Society Reviews* 51 (23): 9759–830. https://doi.org/10.1039/D1CS01145F.

Pandit-Taskar, Neeta, Mary L. Gemignani, Ashima Lyall, Steven M. Larson, Richard R. Barakat, and Nadeem R. Abu Rustum. 2010. "Single Photon Emission Computed Tomography SPECT-CT Improves Sentinel Node Detection and Localization in Cervical and Uterine Malignancy." *Gynecologic Oncology* 117 (1): 59–64. https://doi.org/10.1016/j.ygyno.2009.12.021.

Parveen, Shama, Pratishtha Gupta, Saurabh Kumar, and Monisha Banerjee. 2023. "Lipid Polymer Hybrid Nanoparticles as Potent Vehicles for Drug Delivery in Cancer Therapeutics." *Medicine in Drug Discovery* 2023: 100165. https://doi.org/10.1016/j.medidd.2023.100165.

Pešić, Milica, Ana Podolski-Renić, Sonja Stojković, Branko Matović, Danica Zmejkoski, Vesna Kojić, Gordana Bogdanović, et al. 2015. "Anti-Cancer Effects of Cerium Oxide Nanoparticles and Its Intracellular Redox Activity." *Chemico-Biological Interactions* 232: 85–93. https://doi.org/10.1016/j.cbi.2015.03.013.

Plante, Marie, Omar Touhami, Xuan-Bich Trinh, Marie-Claude Renaud, Alexandra Sebastianelli, Katherine Grondin, and Jean Gregoire. 2015. "Sentinel Node Mapping With Indocyanine Green and Endoscopic Near-Infrared Fluorescence Imaging in Endometrial Cancer. A Pilot Study and Review of the Literature." *Gynecologic Oncology* 137 (3): 443–7. https://doi.org/10.1016/j.ygyno.2015.03.004.

Predoi, Daniela, Mihaela Balas, Madalina Andreea Badea, Steluta Carmen Ciobanu, Nicolas Buton, and Anca Dinischiotu. 2023. "Dextran-Coated Iron Oxide Nanoparticles Loaded With 5-Fluorouracil for Drug-Delivery Applications." *Nanomaterials* 13(12): 1811. https://doi.org/10.3390/nano13121811.

Pu, Tao, Yawei Liu, Yuetian Pei, Jing Peng, Zehua Wang, Ming Du, Qiyu Liu, et al. 2023. "NIR-II Fluorescence Imaging for the Detection and Resection of Cancerous Foci and Lymph Nodes in Early-Stage Orthotopic and Advanced-Stage Metastatic Ovarian Cancer Models." *ACS Applied Materials & Interfaces* 15 (27): 32226–39. https://doi.org/10.1021/acsami.3c04949.

Raj, Sibi, Sartaj Khurana, Ramesh Choudhari, Kavindra Kumar Kesari, Mohammad Amjad Kamal, Neha Garg, Janne Ruokolainen, Bhudev C. Das, and Dhruv Kumar. 2021. "Specific Targeting Cancer Cells With Nanoparticles and Drug Delivery in Cancer Therapy." *Seminars in Cancer Biology* 69: 166–77. https://doi.org/10.1016/j.semcancer.2019.11.002.

Rosen, Joshua E., Lorena Chan, Dar-Bin Shieh, and Frank X. Gu. 2012. "Iron Oxide Nanoparticles for Targeted Cancer Imaging and Diagnostics." *Nanomedicine: Nanotechnology, Biology and Medicine* 8 (3): 275–90. https://doi.org/10.1016/j.nano.2011.08.017.

Sahoo, Sanjeeb K., and Vinod Labhasetwar. 2003. "Nanotech Approaches to Drug Delivery and Imaging." *Drug Discovery Today* 8 (24): 1112–20. https://doi.org/10.1016/S1359-6446(03)02903-9.

Salazar Berg, W. A., and J. Blume. 2008. "Combined Screening With Ultrasound and Mammography Compared to Mammography Alone in Women at Elevated Risk of Breast Cancer: Results of the First Year Screening ACRIN 6666." *JAMA* 299 (18): 2151–63. https://doi.org/10.1001/jama.299.18.2151.

Sano, Kohei, Ling Bao, Natsuka Suzuno, Kento Kannaka, Toshihide Yamasaki, Masayuki Munekane, and Takahiro Mukai. 2019. "Development of Cancer-Targeted Single Photon Emission Computed Tomography/Fluorescence Dual Imaging Probe Based on Polyoxazoline." *ACS Applied Polymer Materials* 1 (5): 953–8. https://doi.org/10.1021/acsapm.8b00238.

Sathishkumar, Krishnan, Meesha Chaturvedi, Priyanka Das, S. Stephen, and Prashant Mathur. 2023. "Cancer Incidence Estimates for 2022 & Projection for 2025: Result From National Cancer Registry Programme, India." *Indian Journal of Medical Research*. https://doi.org/10.4103/ijmr.ijmr_1821_22

Schillaci, Orazio, Manuel Scimeca, Nicola Toschi, Rita Bonfiglio, Nicoletta Urbano, and Elena Bonanno. 2019. "Combining Diagnostic Imaging and Pathology for Improving Diagnosis and Prognosis of Cancer." *Contrast Media & Molecular Imaging* 2019: 9429761. https://doi.org/10.1155/2019/9429761.

Schuerle, Simone, Maiko Furubayashi, Ava P. Soleimany, Tinotenda Gwisai, Wei Huang, Christopher Voigt, and Sangeeta N. Bhatia. 2020. "Genetic Encoding of Targeted Magnetic Resonance Imaging Contrast Agents for Tumor Imaging." *ACS Synthetic Biology* 9 (2): 392–401. https://doi.org/10.1021/acssynbio.9b00416.

Severin, Gregory W., Jesper T. Jørgensen, Stefan Wiehr, Anna-Maria Rolle, Anders E. Hansen, Andreas Maurer, Mike Hasenberg, Bernd Pichler, Andreas Kjaer, and Andreas I. Jensen. 2015. "The Impact of Weakly Bound ^{89}Zr on Preclinical Studies: Non-Specific Accumulation in Solid Tumors and Aspergillus Infection." *Nuclear Medicine and Biology* 42 (4): 360–8. https://doi.org/10.1016/j.nucmedbio.2014.11.005.

Sharma, Ankush, Amit K. Goyal, and Goutam Rath. 2018. "Recent Advances in Metal Nanoparticles in Cancer Therapy." *Journal of Drug Targeting* 26 (8): 617–32. https://doi.org/10.1080/1061186x.2017.1400553.

Shokeen, Monica, and Carolyn J. Anderson. 2009 "Molecular Imaging of Cancer With Copper-64 Radiopharmaceuticals and Positron Emission Tomography (PET)." *Accounts of Chemical Research* 42 (7): 832–41. https://doi.org/10.1021/ar800255q.

Siddique, Sarkar, and James C. L. Chow. 2020 "Application of Nanomaterials in Biomedical Imaging and Cancer Therapy." *Nanomaterials* 10 (9): 1700. https://doi.org/10.3390/nano10091700.

Siegel, Rebecca L., Kimberly D. Miller, and Ahmedin Jemal. 2023. "Cancer Statistics." *A Cancer Journal of Clinicians* 73 (1): 17–48. https://doi.org/10.3322/caac.21763.

Singh, Nem, Jungryun Kim, Jaewon Kim, Kyungwoo Lee, Zehra Zunbul, Injun Lee, Eunji Kim, Sung-Gil Chi, and Jong Seung Kim. 2023. "Covalent Organic Framework Nanomedicines: Biocompatibility for Advanced Nanocarriers and Cancer Theranostics Applications." *Bioactive Materials* 21: 358–80. https://doi.org/10.1016/j.bioactmat.2022.08.016.

Sun, Haotian, Lingyue Yan, Kevin A. Carter, Jiaqi Zhang, Julia S. Caserto, Jonathan F. Lovell, Yun Wu, and Chong Cheng. 2018. "Zwitterionic Cross-Linked Biodegradable Nanocapsules for Cancer Imaging." *Langmuir*35 (5): 1440–9. https://doi.org/10.1021/acs.langmuir.8b01633.

Tanaka, Kazuo, Asako Narita, Narufumi Kitamura, Wataru Uchiyama, Masahito Morita, Toshiro Inubushi, and Yoshiki Chujo. 2010. "Preparation for Highly Sensitive MRI Contrast Agents Using Core/Shell Type Nanoparticles Consisting of Multiple SPIO Cores With Thin Silica Coating." *Langmuir* 26 (14): 11759–62. https://doi.org/10.1021/la1015077.

Tong, Rong, Virginia J. Coyle, Li Tang, Anne M. Barger, Timothy M. Fan, and Jianjun Cheng. 2010 "Polylactide Nanoparticles Containing Stably Incorporated Cyanine Dyes for In Vitro and In Vivo Imaging Applications." *Microscopy Research and Technique* 73 (9): 901–9. https://doi.org/10.1002/jemt.20824.

Toy, Randall, Lisa Bauer, Christopher Hoimes, Ketan B. Ghaghada, and Efstathios Karathanasis. 2014. "Targeted Nanotechnology for Cancer Imaging." *Advanced Drug Delivery Reviews* 76: 79–97. https://doi.org/10.1016/j.addr.2014.08.002.

Vinardell, Maria Pilar, and Montserrat Mitjans. 2015. "Antitumor Activities of Metal Oxide Nanoparticles." *Nanomaterials* 5 (2): 1004–21. https://doi.org/10.3390/nano5021004.

Wang, Tianshuai, Chen Wu, Yanggen Hu, Yan Zhang, and Junkai Ma. 2023 "Stimuli-Responsive Nanocarrier Delivery Systems for Pt-Based Antitumor Complexes: A Review." *RSC Advances* 13 (24): 16488–511. https://doi.org/10.1039/D3RA00866E.

Wang, Zihan, Qinzhou Ye, Sheng Yu, and Behnam Akhavan. 2023. "Poly Ethylene Glycol (PEG)-Based Hydrogels for Drug Delivery in Cancer Therapy." *Advanced Healthcare Materials* 2300105. https://doi.org/10.1002/adhm.202300105.

Wason, Melissa S., and Jihe Zhao. 2013. "Cerium Oxide Nanoparticles: Potential Applications for Cancer and Other Diseases." *American Journal of Translational Research* 5 (2): 126. PMID: 23573358; PMCID: PMC3612509.

Xia, Tian, Michael Kovochich, Monty Liong, Huan Meng, Sanaz Kabehie, Saji George, Jeffrey I. Zink, and Andre E. Nel. 2009. "Polyethyleneimine Coating Enhances the Cellular Uptake of Mesoporous Silica Nanoparticles and Allows Safe Delivery of siRNA and DNA Constructs." *ACS Nano* 3 (10): 3273–86. https://doi.org/10.1021/nn900918w.

Xu, Jia-Jie, Wan-Chen Zhang, Ya-Wen Guo, Xiao-Yi Chen, and You-Ni Zhang. 2022. "Metal Nanoparticles as a Promising Technology in Targeted Cancer Treatment." *Drug Delivery* 29 (1): 664–78. https://doi.org/10.1080/10717544.2022.2039804.

Yamada, Miko, Matthew Foote, and Tarl W. Prow. 2015 "Therapeutic Gold, Silver, and Platinum Nanoparticles." *Wiley Interdisciplinary Reviews: Nanomedicine and Nanobiotechnology* 7 (3): 428–45. https://doi.org/10.1002/wnan.1322.

Yao, Yihan, Yunxiang Zhou, Lihong Liu, Yanyan Xu, Qiang Chen, Yali Wang, Shijie Wu, Yongchuan Deng, Jianmin Zhang, and Anwen Shao. 2020. "Nanoparticle-Based Drug Delivery in Cancer Therapy and Its Role in Overcoming Drug Resistance." *Frontiers in Molecular Biosciences* 7: 193. https://doi.org/10.3389/fmolb.2020.00193.

Yin, Hua-Qing, Pei-Pei Cao, Xin-Yao Wang, Yu-Hao Li, and Xue-Bo Yin. 2020. "Computed Tomography Imaging-Guided Tandem Catalysis-Enhanced Photodynamic Therapy With Gold Nanoparticle Functional Covalent Organic Polymers." *ACS Applied Bio Materials* 3 (4): 2534–42. https://doi.org/10.1021/acsabm.0c00244.

Yu, Lifeng, Xin Liu, Shuai Leng, James M. Kofler, Juan C. Ramirez-Giraldo, Mingliang Qu, Jodie Christner, Joel G. Fletcher, and Cynthia H. McCollough. 2009. "Radiation Dose Reduction in Computed Tomography: Techniques and Future Perspective." *Imaging in Medicine* 1 (1): 65–84. https://doi.org/10.2217/iim.09.5.

Yu, Xujiang, Ang Li, Chengzhi Zhao, Kai Yang, Xiaoyuan Chen, and Wanwan Li. 2017. "Ultrasmall Semimetal Nanoparticles of Bismuth for Dual-Modal Computed Tomography/Photoacoustic Imaging and Synergistic Thermoradiotherapy." *ACS Nano* 11 (4): 3990–4001. https://doi.org/10.1021/acsnano.7b00476.

Yu, Xujiang, Xinyi Liu, Kai Yang, Xiaoyuan Chen, and Wanwan Li. 2021. "Pnictogen Semimetal (Sb, Bi)-Based Nanomaterials for Cancer Imaging and Therapy: A Materials Perspective. *ACS Nano* 15 (2): 2038–67. https://doi.org/10.1021/acsnano.0c07899.

Zhang, Chunlei, Zhijun Zhou, Qirong Qian, Guo Gao, Chao Li, Lili Feng, Qing Wang, and Daxiang Cui. 2013 "Glutathione-Capped FluorescentGold Nanoclusters for Dual-Modal Fluorescence/X-Ray Computed Tomography Imaging." *Journal of Materials Chemistry B* 1(38): 5045–53. https://doi.org/10.1039/C3TB20784F.

Zhang, Ge, Hua-Rong Ye, Yao Sun, and Zhen-Zhong Guo. 2022. "Ultrasound Molecular Imaging and Its Applications in Cancer Diagnosis and Therapy." *ACS Sensors* 7 (10): 2857–64. https://doi.org/10.1021/acssensors.2c01468.

Zhang, Ye, Maoyu Li, Xiaomei Gao, Yongheng Chen, and Ting Liu. 2019. “Nanotechnology in Cancer Diagnosis: Progress, Challenges and Opportunities.” *Journal of Hematology & Oncology* 12 (1): 1–13. https://doi.org/10.1186/s13045-019-0833-3.

Zhao, Zilong, Huanhuan Fan, Gaofeng Zhou, Huarong Bai, Hao Liang, Ruowen Wang, Xiaobing Zhang, and Weihong Tan. 2014. “Activatable Fluorescence/MRI Bimodal Platform for Tumor Cell Imaging *via* MnO_2 Nanosheet–Aptamer Nanoprobe.” *Journal of the American Chemical Society* 136 (32): 11220–3. https://doi.org/10.1021/ja5029364.

8 Cancer Detection
Nanodevices at the Forefront of Early Diagnosis

Arshiya Sood, Ishant Arora, and Neelam Thakur

ABBREVIATIONS

Acronym	Full Form
AuNPs	gold nanoparticles
CNTs	carbon nanotubes
CT	computed tomography
EPR	enhanced permeability and retention
MRI	magnetic resonance imaging
MWTs	multi-walled nanotubes
NP	Nanoparticles
PET	positron emission tomography
QDs	quantum dots
SERS	surface-enhanced Raman scattering
SWNTs	single-walled nanotubes
WHO	World Health Organization

8.1 INTRODUCTION

Cancer is a fatal disease; cells multiply uncontrollably and metastasize (spread) from their original site to other parts of the body. To mitigate the transmission of disease and reduce fatalities, timely identification and treatment of cancers are imperative. It was predicted that there would be 18.1 million newly diagnosed cases and 9.6 million deaths by 2018 due to cancer (Bray et al. 2018). More than 10.3 million people will lose their lives due to cancer in 2020, according to the World Health Organization (WHO) (Sung et al. 2021). The number of cancer-related deaths is projected to rise by 32% by 2040 compared to 2020, according to experts. This is largely attributable to the aging population.

Factors contributing to high cancer rates in developing nations include air and water pollution, radiation exposure, sedentary lifestyles, poor dietary choices, bacterial infections, and other environmental hazards. Any one of these factors has the potential to harm oncogenes, the cancer-causing genes found inside host cells (Parsa 2012). Common imaging techniques, including X-rays, magnetic resonance imaging (MRI), computed tomography (CT scan), endoscopy, and ultrasounds, can only spot cancer when there is already an obvious change in the tissue. The imaging methods help in the morphological study of tissues (histopathology) or cells (cytology) which may have grown and metastasized (Kim, Jeong, and Jon 2010). Moreover, existing imaging technologies cannot distinguish between benign and malignant tumors. Furthermore, cytology and histopathology are inadequate on their own to diagnose cancer in its early stages. That is

DOI: 10.1201/9781003463191-10

why it is important to work on methods of early cancer detection, before the disease has spread. The cancer cells can only be detected with the help of tools such as cantilevers, nanosized tubes, pores, dendrimers, nanoshells, etc., among which dendrimers are utilized for diagnostic procedures, while nanoshells for the eradication of the cancer cell (Agrawal and Awasthi 2023). Some of the factors, such as inheritance, that contribute to rise in cancer proliferation are also utilized to help in the early identification of cancer.

Nanotechnology is being refined to create more nanoscale materials with applications in biological systems in tandem with the expansion of modern biology and medicine (Alrushaid et al. 2023). The study of biosystems can benefit greatly from the application of nanoscale ideas and methods. Nanotechnology in cancer care demonstrates promising outcome across drug delivery, gene therapy, detection and diagnostic drugs, biomarkers, mapping, targeted therapy, and molecular imaging, reflecting encouraging results (Hu et al. 2016). At the atomic and molecular levels, the field of nanotechnology seeks to discover medicinally useful compounds with desirable characteristics.

The modifying composition of nanoparticles involves utilizing diverse starting materials, such as biological and supramolecular scales (1–100 nm). Utilizing nanotechnology, nanomaterials such as gold nanoparticles, quantum dots have been crafted for molecular diagnosis of cancer, showing advancement in precision and sensitivity (L. Huang et al. 2017) (Figure 8.1). Nanomaterials, with their active and passive targeting, have long been utilized for effective and targeted drug delivery in medicinal prospects. The sensitivity of the medications used to treat tumors sometimes results now in development (Wu et al. 2018). For accurate cancer detection, these devices not only recognize circulating tumor cells and human DNA but also detect a range of cancer-related proteins, like exosomes, highlighting their versatility in identifying diverse cancer biomarkers (Jia et al. 2017). Nanoparticles play a crucial role in medicine, leveraging their quantum properties for enhanced adsorption, facilitating the transport of probes, proteins,

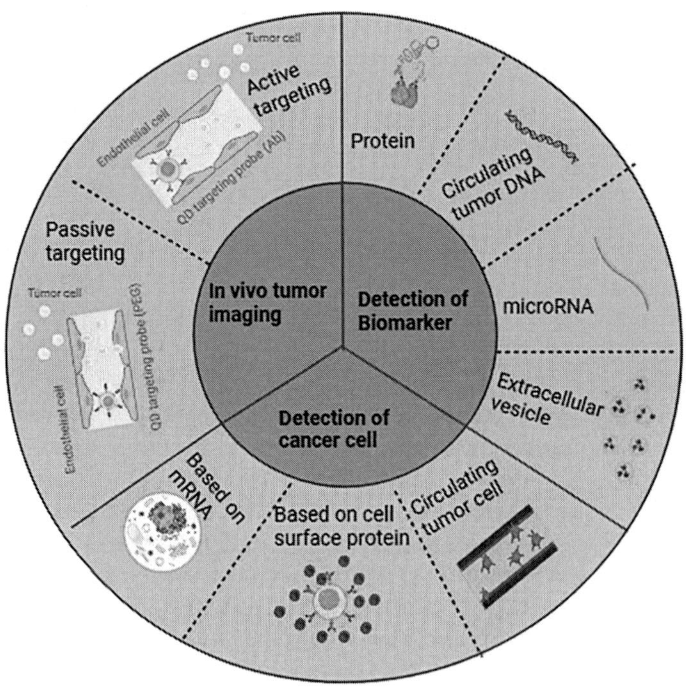

FIGURE 8.1 Application of nanotechnology in diagnosis of cancer. This diagram depicts the detection of cancer cells, cancer biomarkers, and aiding in in vivo imaging for the early detection of cancer.

and drugs in various dextran, phospholipids, lipids, chitosan, lactic acid, and chemicals like silica, carbon, or metals (Saadh and Jadullah 2021).

8.2 STRATEGIES FOR DETECTING CANCER USING NANOTECHNOLOGY

Nanotechnology has recently shown promise in confirming cancer imaging on molecular, cellular, and tissue levels (Garrigue et al. 2018). Nanotechnology has the capability to explore the tumor's environment. It is possible to detect tumor-associated, fibroblast-activated protein on their cell membranes by the pH response to fluorescent nanoprobes (Ji et al. 2013). Nanoparticles can be designed to specifically target cancer cells or tissues. When combined with imaging techniques like MRI, CT scans, or PET scans, these nanoparticles enhance contrast, making it easier to detect tumors. Nanosized sensors can detect specific biomarkers indicative of cancer, and these sensors can be engineered to recognize unique molecular signatures, providing early detection and precise diagnosis. Nanotechnology enables the development of nanoscale devices for analyzing circulating tumor cells or cell-free DNA in the blood. This approach, known as liquid biopsy, allows for non-invasive cancer detection and monitoring. It can serve a dual purpose by not only detecting cancer but also delivering therapeutic agents directly to the tumor site. This approach, called theranostics, combines diagnostics and therapy in a single nanoscale system. Nanotechnology enhances existing imaging methods by improving resolution and sensitivity. Techniques like photoacoustic imaging and quantum dot–based imaging offer more precise visualization of tumors. Next, this chapter will look over various spatial and temporal methods that are based on nanotechnology that can be used to monitor dynamic cellular events in tumors and correctly track living cells.

8.2.1 Cancer Biomarkers Detection

Cancer biomarkers, identifiable biological molecules present in the body fluids, accompany blood, saliva, and urine, which serve as vital indicators during surveillance, signaling the potential presence of cancer cells in the body (Harshita and Kailasa 2023). The secreted proteins or proteins on the surface of cells, carbohydrates like glucose or fructose, and nucleic acids like deoxyribonucleic acid (DNA) and ribonucleic acid (RNA) are the biomarkers used for cancer theragnostic as they are released by the body or cancer cells (Figure 8.2).

The level of these biomarkers can be measured to help in assessing the cancer at earlier stages or to track the tumor repetition and for the success of treatment (Chevillet et al. 2014). Albumin and immunoglobulins are examples of high-molecular-weight proteins that would typically be excluded from protein profiling assays. The problem is that when these proteins are removed, the biomarkers of interest with low-molecular-weight proteins attached to them are also removed (Conti et al. 2019). Nowadays, mesoporous silica particles, hydrogel nanoparticles, and carbon nanotubes (CNTs) have electric charge and functional biomolecules on their surfaces, which make them competitors with the carrier proteins (Shi et al. 2021). Raising the sensitivity of mass spectrometry is another way to enhance nanocarrier screening. The exceptional thermal and optical characteristics of carbon nanotubes facilitate the analyte's absorption and ionization while reducing or eliminating the impact of matrix ions on the energy transfer efficiency of the analyte. Lab-on-chip microfluidics devices made possible by nanotechnology could be employed for immuno-screening or for studying the characteristics of tumor cell (Shah et al. 2022). One promising technology is lab-on-a-chip, which uses QDs made up of cadmium selenide (CdSe) core coated with a zinc sulfide (ZnS) shell bound to the antibodies of carcinoembryonic antigen, cancer antigen 125, and Her-2/Neu. It allows for elevated performance of multiplexed protein detection (Jokerst et al. 2009). The fact is that cells of various sizes can differentiate amongst tumor cells. These cells were found on surfaces that are just nanometer broad (Bakshi et al. 2019). It goes without saying that nanotechnology-based biomarker screening still produces some false-positive and false-negative results, so there is a pressing need to enhance sensitivity without sacrificing specificity.

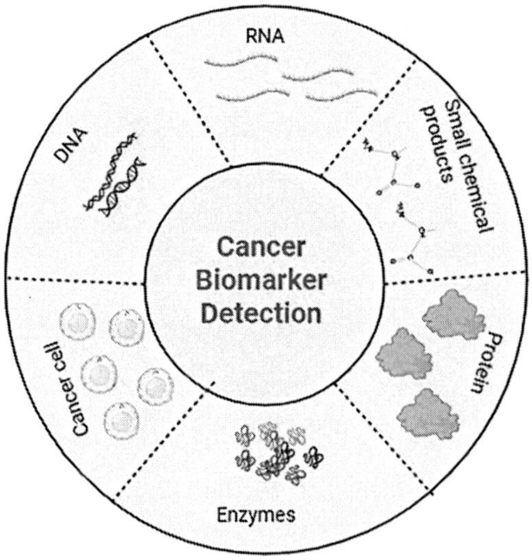

FIGURE 8.2 Detection of different biomarkers of cancer. This figure shows the schematic representation of various biomarkers that aid in early detection of cancer. The level of these biomarkers is measured to help in assessing the cancer at earlier stages or to track tumor repetition.

8.2.2 Cancer Cells Detection

Nanoparticles have the ability to adsorb and transport other molecules, making them useful in medical applications, and these substances include probes, proteins, and medicines. Nanoparticles may be made up of biological materials like lipids, phospholipids, dextran, lactic acid, chitosan, and chemicals (carbon, metals, and polymers). Several types of these particles are employed now for molecular imaging and have seen considerable interest over the past several decades as a means of aiding in the diagnosis and monitoring of cancer (Dessale, Mengistu, and Mengist 2022). Advancements in portability and biocompatibility have propelled their integration, positioning them at the forefront of recent cancer research endeavors.

Nanoparticles can be used to detect illness by binding to cells that have been damaged. Chemotherapy medications can also be delivered using nanoparticles which target cancer cells while sparing healthy tissue (Jin et al. 2020). Biological studies and clinical uses of cancer therapies use in vivo and in vitro models, medical equipment for diagnosis, analysis, physical therapy, and medication administration (Zhou et al. 2020). The primary method to detect cancer cells is by the binding of nanoparticle probes with moieties (such as proteins, short peptides, antibodies, or oligonucleotide aptamers) and to the markers present on the surface or those that enter the cell and analyze their genetic content (Table 8.1). Materials such as nanowires are one-dimensional, and nanotubes are two-dimensional, while particles, such as quantum dots (very small pieces of semiconductor material), precipitates, colloids, and other similar materials, are known as nanoscale materials in three dimensions (Subramani and Mehta 2017). Contrast agents are made of nanoparticles for diagnostic imaging. Layers, like thin films or surface coatings, are materials with one nanoscale dimension and two additional dimensions of extension, and this class includes some of the capabilities found in computer chips.

Nanoparticle probes commonly engaged in cancer diagnostics include quantum dots (QDs), polymer dots (PDs), and gold nanoparticles (AuNPs), nanotubes, and dendrimers, which are shown in Figure 8.3.

TABLE 8.1
Cancer Cell Detection with Nanotechnology

Nanoparticles	Probe Used	Kind of Cancer	References
Gold nanoparticle	Aptamer/antibody	Breast/leukemia	Zhang et al. (2014)
Quantum dots	Aptamer	Leukemia	Pang et al. (2018)
Polymer dots	Antibody	Breast	Liu et al. (2020)
Upconversion NPs	Antibody	Breast	He et al. (2021)
Carbon nanotube	Antibody	Liver	Ahmadian et al. (2022)
Magnetic nanoparticle	Antibody	Colon/breast/liver/lung	Maffei (2022)

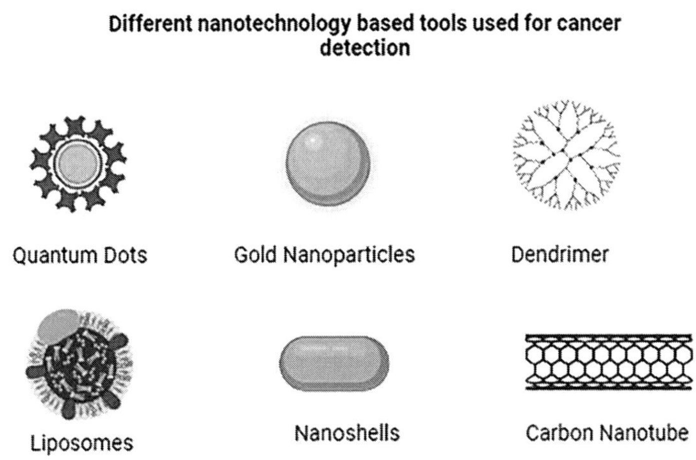

FIGURE 8.3 Nanotechnology tools used for cancer detection. This diagram illustrates the array of nanotechnology tools used for detection of cancer cells, including quantum dots (QDs), liposomes, gold nanoparticles (AuNPs), nanotubes, and dendrimers.

8.3 NANOTECHNOLOGY-BASED TOOLS USED FOR CANCER DETECTION

8.3.1 Quantum Dots (QDs)

QDs are semiconductor nanocrystals with sizes ranging from 2 nm to 10 nm. They have an electron property that is between the mass of a semiconductor and that of a discrete atom, according to the ratio of the height of surface to their volume (Fang et al. 2017). QD immunostaining is superior than standard immunochemical techniques when dealing with low levels of protein expression and/or low context. QD immunostaining has the ability to aid in the identification of many tumor biomarkers in a heterogeneous tumor sample, such as a cell protein (Kaur et al. 2022). The size of the Q dots deduces the wavelength or the color of visible light they emit. Researchers can create quantum dots that attach to certain disease-related DNA sequences (Liang et al. 2021). Light excitation of the quantum dots causes them to produce their own barcodes, or labels, revealing the cancer-related DNA sequences. They have an in vivo application that dispenses with the requirement for invasive biopsies (Vinduska et al. 2021). Quantum dots emit a powerful ultraviolet light when exposed to cancer cells. It is possible to coat them with a substance that causes the dots to bind to the target

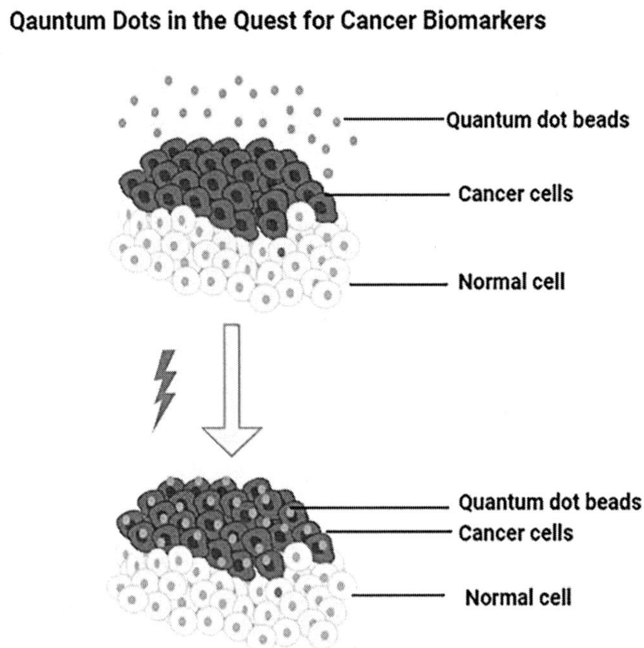

FIGURE 8.4 Quantum dots in the quest for cancer biomarkers. This figure demonstrates the role of quantum dots in detection of cancer by attaching them to specific molecules that target cancer cells. These emit distinct fluorescent signal, enabling precise imaging of the targeted cell.

molecule, as shown in Figure 8.4. One way to see tumors is by the use of quantum dots, which attach to proteins found in cancer cells (Subramani and Mehta 2017).

8.3.2 Nanobots

The robots known as nanobots are approximately 50–100 nm broad and designed to perform a single, narrow task. The term "medical nanorobot" refers to autonomous nanostructures that can carry out a medical procedure by means of an engine or the conversion of various forms of energy into mechanical forces (Soto et al. 2020). Nanorobots, because of their small size, are able to engage directly with cells and even permeate them, granting unimpeded entry to the machinery within cells (Lenaghan et al. 2013; Soto and Chrostowski 2018). Nanorobots are miniature machines with remarkable capabilities. They can transport various cargos, such as drugs, genes, or sensing molecules, and perform diagnostic and therapeutic tasks. Additionally, nanorobots can be aimed at specific locations, like tumors or disease sites, and can be powered either actively or passively. The former allows them to draw power from outside sources, such as near-infrared light, ultrasound, or magnetic fields, while the latter allows them to harness the medium and blood flow route already present in biological systems (Li et al. 2017; Martel 2017; Kim et al. 2018). Researchers in the field of nanobiotechnology have developed microchips that incorporate biological molecules into their surface. When the molecules identify symptoms of an illness, the chip is programmed to send out an electrical impulse signal. It is now possible to inject specialized sensor nanobots into the bloodstream subcutaneously, allowing them to monitor blood contents and alert doctors to potential illnesses. They can also be utilized for the purpose of tracking blood sugar levels. One benefit of employing such nanobots is their portability and low production cost (Stiepel et al. 2023). Introductory nanorobots (e.g., computational genes) have potential applications in nanomedicine for the detection and repair of injuries and infections. Scientists have established rigorous requirements for the core components of nanorobots to guarantee that they can successfully eradicate oncogenic cells present inside the body. The advancement and extensive use of medical nanorobots are still in their preliminary phases, which is worth mentioning. The components of nanobots include the shell, power source, sensor, actuators, payload, and communication. Their designated use and significance in safety, efficiency, and scalability will determine the precise structure and composition of these devices, shown in Tables 8.2 and 8.3 (Suhail et al. 2022).

8.3.3 Nanoshells

Nanoshells are composed of a thin gold metal shell around a dielectric core that is between 10 and 300 nm in size. These convert electrical energy mediated by plasma into light energy, and they can be optically controlled in a diverse way utilizing UV infrared emission or absorption arrays (Aminolroayaei et al. 2023). Although their huge sizes restrict their applications, nanoshells are

TABLE 8.2
Components of Medical Nanorobots

Sr. No.	Component	Descriptive Structure
1	Shell	A nanorobot's performance and safety are greatly affected by its shell construction. Some examples of such designs are spherical and smooth shells, which minimize friction and the risk of tissue damage. When it comes to nanorobots, a rough and irregular shell design can improve their ability to connect to tumor tissues or cancer cells. For various uses, the shell's dimensions, shape, and surface characteristics can be fine-tuned.
2	Power source	The performance, stability, and safety of the nanorobot are significantly affected by how its power source is integrated into its design. Both internal and external attachments to the surface are viable options for housing the power source. To get peak performance, it is important to think about the power source's size and location.
3	Sensor	An array of sensors can be built within a nanorobot's shell or attached to its surface. The necessary information for optimal functioning and the intended application will determine the type and quantity of sensors that are required. The sensors on a nanorobot made for imaging could pick up on things like light or local oxygen levels, whereas sensors on a nanorobot made for drug delivery could pick up on things like pH levels, glutathione concentrations, and so on.
4	Actuators	It is possible to incorporate actuators into a nanorobot's shell or to attach them to its surface. The actions needed for efficient functioning will determine the kind and quantity of actuators required. An example of an actuator would be a mechanism that allows a nanorobot to either manipulate tissues or remove detritus; another example would be a mechanism that allows a nanorobot to administer medications in response to targeted local signals.
5	Payload	Both internal and external attachments are viable options for medical nanorobot payload integration. The envisioned use and the necessity for efficacy and safety will determine the type and quantity of payloads that are necessary. For example, nanorobots can carry therapeutic agents or medications in their payloads when they are designed for drug delivery, and imaging agents or contrast agents when they are designed for imaging.
6	Communication	Various methods exist for achieving communication, including physical connections, electromagnetic wave signals, and wireless signals. What kind of communication is needed and how far it needs to go depend on the application and how much control and coordination are needed. One type of nanorobot can communicate with a computer to send pictures, while another type of nanorobot may manage the release of medications by exchanging messages with other nanorobots.

TABLE 8.3
Examples of Medical Nanorobots

Sr. No.	Nanorobot Types	Characteristics	References
1	Microbivores	• For nanomedical applications, the nanorobot has a flat and spheroidal shape. • Its main axis has a diameter of 3.4 μm, and its minor axis has a diameter of 2.0 μm. • Its phagocytic power is over 80 times more proficient than that of other macrophages.	Gandhi and Joshi (2020)
2	Pharmacyte	• It measures 1–2 μm in diameter • To guarantee the accuracy of the targeting system, molecular markers or chemotactic sensors are employed. • Once the tasks are completed, they can be removed or restored using centrifuge and apheresis.	Mani et al. (2021)
3	Microchips	• Microchips on nanorobots can provide current impulses when the molecules detect disease. • Easy operation and low production costs are two advantages.	Stans (2021)
4	Respirocyte	• A nanorobot that functions similarly to an artificial red blood cell in terms of carrying oxygen. • Generation of power is accomplished by means of endogenous serum glucose.	Kumar et al. (2021)
5	Clottocytes	• Artificial mechanical platelets, which they possess, have the biological function of hemostasis "instantly." • In addition, they carry chemicals that aid in blood clotting.	Javaid (2021)
6	Chromallocytes	• In order to determine the current state of affairs, the restoration machine will initially examine the cellular substances, actions, and works. • These maintenance devices can overhaul the entire cell.	Sapra et al. (2021)

appealing due to the absence of heavy metal toxicity in their imaging. Nanoshells focus infrared light's destructive heat on cancer cells while sparing healthy tissue. In cancer detection, nanoshells are primarily employed in a technique known as surface-enhanced Raman scattering (SERS). This method leverages the ability of nanoshells to greatly enhance the Raman signals of molecules in their vicinity, enabling highly sensitive molecular detection (Siddique and Chow 2020). Nanoshells have the characteristics of nano-beads that have been coated with gold. Scientists may tailor the beads' absorption to a desired wavelength by adjusting their thickness (Kasi et al. 2023). Nanoshells absorb light, which causes cells to become overheated and die. It is now possible to attach nanoshells to antibodies that target cancer cells. After guiding these nanoshells to their cancerous target, researchers plan to employ near-infrared light (Guan and Wang 2021). Light-absorbing nanoshells have successfully eradicated cancer cells without hurting the surrounding healthy tissue.

The design of nanoshells plays a pivotal role in their function. By adjusting the size and composition of the core and shell, scientists can tune the optical properties of these nanostructures to interact with specific wavelengths of light. This ability to precisely control the interaction with light forms the basis of their application in cancer detection (Agrawal et al. 2011; Billingsley, Riley, and Day 2017). When utilized in SERS-based detection, nanoshells are functionalized with targeting agents—such as antibodies or peptides—that recognize and bind to cancer-specific biomarkers or antigens. Upon encountering these targeted molecules, the nanoshells amplify the Raman signals emitted by these molecules, generating distinct spectral fingerprints that can be detected and analyzed (You et al. 2020). The specificity of this approach allows for the identification of cancer biomarkers at extremely low concentrations, facilitating early-stage detection with high sensitivity. This is crucial in the clinical management of cancer, as early detection significantly improves treatment outcomes and patient prognosis. Furthermore, the adaptability of nanoshells allows for multiplexed detection, enabling the simultaneous identification of multiple biomarkers associated with different types or stages of cancer (Shetty and Chandra 2022). This capability holds immense promise in developing comprehensive diagnostic platforms for various cancer types, aiding in personalized treatment strategies. Another facet where nanoshells excel is in their potential for non-invasive imaging techniques, such as photoacoustic imaging. When exposed to light, nanoshells generate heat, leading to the emission of ultrasound waves detectable by imaging devices (Kang et al. 2021; Shetty and Chandra 2022). This feature allows for the visualization of tumors and their precise localization within the body, facilitating accurate diagnosis and monitoring of cancer progression.

Moreover, nanoshells hold promise in theranostics—a field integrating therapy and diagnostics. They can be designed not only for detection but also for delivering therapeutic agents directly to cancer cells (Siddique and Chow 2020; Suhito, Koo, and Kim 2021). By loading these nanoshells with drugs or other therapeutic molecules and guiding them to the tumor site using targeting agents, they offer a potential avenue for targeted cancer therapy while simultaneously enabling real-time monitoring of treatment efficacy.

8.3.4 Carbon Nanotubes (CNTs)

Carbon nanotubes are cylindrical nanostructures composed of carbon atoms that exhibit exceptional electrical, optical, and mechanical properties, making them versatile tools for various biomedical applications, including cancer detection (Jiameng Wang, Wen, and Yan 2021). They are roughly half the diameter of a DNA molecule and aid in the detection of DNA alterations that are linked to cancer (Lisik and Krokosz 2021). Functionalized CNTs can be modified with specific biomolecules, such as antibodies, peptides, or DNA strands, capable of selectively binding to cancer-related biomarkers or antigens. When these modified CNTs come into contact with targeted biomolecules present in biological samples, such as blood or tissue, the binding interactions cause measurable changes in the electrical or optical properties of the nanotubes (Suhito, Koo, and Kim 2021). This alteration can be detected and quantified, providing information about the presence and concentration of the cancer-specific molecules. The high surface area and electrical conductivity of carbon nanotubes contribute to their sensitivity in detecting biomolecular interactions at very low concentrations, enabling the detection of cancer biomarkers with high accuracy and precision. Moreover, carbon nanotubes hold promise in imaging techniques for cancer diagnostics. They can be used as contrast agents in imaging modalities like photoacoustic imaging, where their unique optical properties allow them to absorb light and convert it into ultrasound signals. This technique enables the visualization of tumors with high resolution, aiding in the localization and characterization of cancerous tissues (Choi, Kwak, and Park 2010; Jiameng Wang, Wen, and Yan 2021). Nanotubes are also employed in damaged bones to provide a scaffolding upon which new bone may form. The characteristics of nanotubes include the identification of mutated genes and localize the mutations throughout the genome. It finds and binds to individual DNA mutations and to determine the actual DNA structure. Disease prognosis will benefit greatly from these methods (Brar et al. 2021). These are classified into single-walled (SWNTs) and multi-walled (MWNTs) types according to their atomic structure and diameter, respectively. Unlike MWNTs, which are made up of concentric layers of graphene, SWNTs are made up of a single layer of graphene arranged in a cylinder shape (SamadiPakchin et al. 2020). Carbon nanotubes are an excellent contender for widespread biomedical applications due to their attributes: surface area, physical durability, metal characteristics, electrical and thermal conductivity (Vijayan et al. 2022).

Moreover, carbon nanotubes can selectively target tumor cells by absorbing light in the near-infrared (NIR) range, inducing a thermal effect that causes the nanotubes to heat up. Additionally, natural carbon nanotubes serve as effective carriers for delivering various therapeutic compounds into live cells and enable the non-intrusive permeation of biofilms (Shkodra et al. 2021). To treat cancer, carbon nanotubes are used to build medications like paclitaxel, which may then be given in vitro and in vivo.

8.3.5 Dendrimers

Dendrimers are nanocarriers characterized by a spherical polymer core adorned with regularly arranged branches. Dendritic macromolecules have a greater propensity to adopt a spherical shape as their diameter increases (Svenson and Tomalia 2012). Two common approaches to dendrimer synthesis are the divergent and convergence methods. In the former, dendrimers expand outward from the nucleus, while in the latter, they contract inward from the periphery and eventually reach the nucleus (Mendes, Pan, and Torchilin 2017). Poly2,2-bis(hydroxymethyl) propionicacid, polylysine, melamine, polyglycerin, polyacrylamide, and polyglycerol succinic acid are the variety of ingredients which form the dendrimers (Martos-Maldonado et al. 2020). By increasing their production or altering their surface groups, it is possible to regulate the chemical composition and characteristics of these dendritic macromolecules, including charge, hydrogen bond capacity, and alkalinity. Covalent attachment of anticancer medications to dendritic peripheral groups typically results in the formation of dendritic drug conjugates (Sherje et al. 2018). So each dendritic molecule can bind to many drug molecules, and the therapeutic molecules released can be modulated in part by the type of attachment. Dendritic macromolecules have the potential to be used as nanoscale carriers due to their physicochemical and biological characteristics, which include their charge, multiligand groups, lipid bilayer interactions, size, cytotoxicity, internalization, plasma retention time, biological allocations, and filtration (Garrigue et al. 2018). Moreover, multiple investigations have demonstrated that cancer cells expressing abundant folate receptors are capable of assembling dendritic molecules coupled to folate into foils (Reddy and Bhargava 2019). Dendrimers have a number of benefits, one of which is their DNA-binding capability; for example, DNA–polyamidoamine is a potent killer of cancer cells that express the folate receptor (Jiang et al. 2018).

8.3.6 Colloidal Gold Nanoparticle (AuNPs)

AuNPs are an effective contrast agent because of their high atomic number, excellent biocompatibility, and tiny size. There are active and passive mechanisms by which AuNPs target cells, according to the research. Gathering gold nanoparticles enhances visualization due to the permeability tension impact in tumor tissues that regulates the principle of passive targeting (Sakthi Devi et al. 2022). However, to achieve targeted delivery of medicines to tumor cells using AuNPs, specific medication aimed at the tumor, like EGFR monoclonal antibodies, is coupled with AuNPs for precise location. At energies more than 80 keV, gold's mass attenuation rate is greater than that of other elements, such as iodine, suggesting that gold nanoparticles have a better chance of success (Jayanti and Prabhatkumar 2020). Blended AuNPs with hepatocellular carcinoma cells are discovered by means of X-ray imaging, noticing that the hepatocellular carcinoma clusters in the nanocomposite group were more robust than the hepatocellular carcinoma cells present alone (X. Huang, O'connor, and Kwizera 2017). The discovery has significant ramifications for early detection because the method can detect cancers as little as a few millimeters in diameter (Medici et al. 2021).

8.3.7 Liposomes

Nanoscale spheres made of water-phase nuclei and phospholipid bilayer membranes, either naturally occurring or artificially produced, are known as liposomes, and they have been the subject of extensive research. The amphiphilicity of phospholipids facilitates the spontaneous formation of liposomes, where hydrophilic medications settle into the monolayer liposome while hydrophobic drugs develop prior to the multilayer liposome (Bozzuto and Molinari 2015; Nanotechnology-Based

Targeted Drug Delivery Systems for Lung Cancer 2019). By switching them from an acidic to a neutral buffer, certain medications could be loaded into liposomes. Even though neutral medications can be delivered in liposomes, their release from the inside is not as rapid since they are not very keen for acidic surroundings (Mukherjee et al. 2022). Liposomes, which are formed by combining saturated medicines with organic solvents, are another method of drug delivery. The enhanced permeability and retention (EPR) effect allows vesicles of around 4,000 kDa or 500 nm in size to pass across tumor-invading blood channel gaps. They can endocytose into tumor cells, merge with those cells, and then release medicines into the intercellular spaces (Omidi 2011). Evidence suggests that liposome size influences half-life. Liposomes as small as 100 nm have an easier time penetrating tumors and remaining there for extended periods of time, but larger liposomes have a shorter half-life due to their rapid clearance by the mononuclear phagocyte system (D. E. Wang et al. 2020). To guarantee active targeting and drug delivery to the tumor, antibodies coupled to liposomes first target tumor-specific antigens. Because of their many advantageous pharmacokinetic properties, several liposomal medications have recently gained clinical approval (Tsukada et al. 2018).

8.3.8 Cantilevers

Cantilevers, often employed in atomic force microscopy (AFM), are used in cancer detection through a method called microcantilever-based sensing. These tiny beams can detect biomolecular interactions at a nanoscale level. When modified with specific receptors or antibodies, they can identify cancer markers or antigens present in a sample, causing mechanical deflection in the cantilever, which is then translated into a measurable signal, aiding in cancer diagnosis (Damborska et al. 2017). These cantilevers, often made from materials like silicon or polymers, possess exceptional sensitivity due to their nanoscale dimensions. To enable cancer detection, these cantilevers are modified with specific receptors or antibodies. These biological elements serve as recognition sites for the targeted biomarkers or antigens associated with cancer cells. When a sample containing these substances comes into contact with the modified cantilever, a series of molecular interactions occurs, leading to the bending or deflection of the cantilever, as shown in Figure 8.5 (Elmi and Elmi 2018). This mechanical bending is incredibly small, often in the range of nanometers, but it is precisely these minute alterations that hold significant diagnostic potential. The change in the cantilever's structure or position is then translated into an electrical or optical signal using various detection methods, such as piezoelectric sensors, interferometry, or optical readouts (Kurmendra and

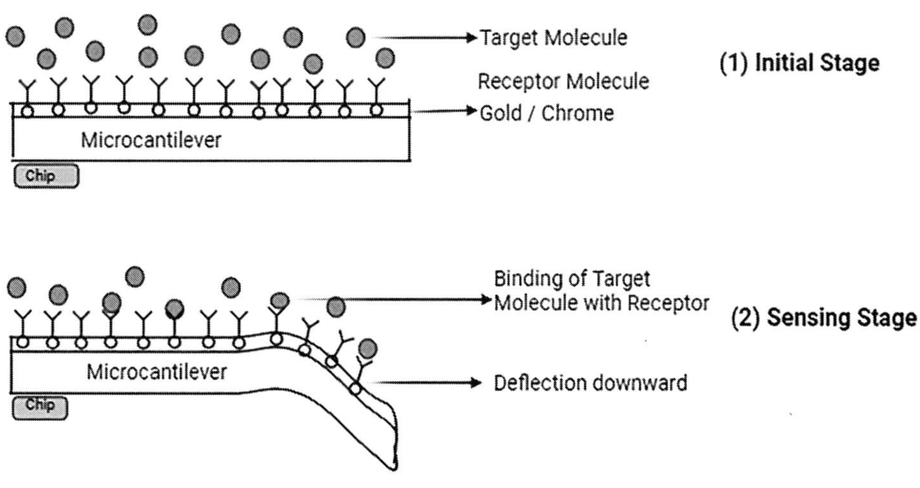

FIGURE 8.5 Cancer detection by using cantilever. This diagram illustrates the role of microcantilever in cancer detection by emphasizing its ability to bend downwards in response to specific biomolecular interaction.

Kumar 2019; Jingjing Wang et al. 2020). The sensitivity and specificity of cantilever-based sensing make it an invaluable tool in cancer detection. The ability to identify specific biomarkers or antigens associated with cancer cells provides crucial insights into the presence and progression of the disease (Lakshman et al. 2021). Early detection is a cornerstone in effective cancer management, and cantilever-based sensing offers a promising avenue for detecting cancer at its nascent stages.

8.4 FUTURE PROSPECTS

Over the years, nanotechnology has demonstrated great potential in cancer diagnosis. Nanomaterials have helped advance cancer detection and treatment with their enhanced pharmacokinetic and pharmacodynamic characteristics. Because of their specificity, nanoparticles enable the targeted delivery of drugs to diseased organs with little systemic toxicity. Nevertheless, similar to other treatment approaches, nanotechnology does have some toxicities and has a few problems associated with its use, such as systemic and specific organ toxicities, which hinder its clinical applicability. Drug delivery, maximizing their efficacy while minimizing their drawbacks, requires greater developments in light of nanotechnology's constraints. An enhanced insight on how the physicochemical properties of nanomaterials are used will lead to secure advancement and more efficient cancer diagnostic and therapeutic compounds. We aim to summarize the benefits and drawbacks of nanotechnology in meeting cancer clinical needs. Furthermore, nanotechnology possesses the capacity to treat a diversity of diseased conditions, and further developments in the field may open up new avenues for treatment. Ischemic stroke and rheumatoid arthritis are two examples of conditions that can necessitate the localized administration of an appropriate pharmacologic agent.

8.5 CONCLUSION

Over the past decade, extensive efforts have been dedicated to developing nanotechnology-based cancer diagnostic tests. Several NP-based assays showcase an improvement in selectivity, sensitivity, and overall capabilities in cancer diagnostics, surpassing the capabilities of conventional methods and even introducing entirely new functionalities. Due to these innovations, cancer patients will have a better chance of survival due to earlier detection. Furthermore, these advancements have the potential to track how cancer is responding to treatment, which could lead to more effective cancer treatment tactics. Cancer diagnostics powered by nanotechnology has made significant strides in the past decade, and our knowledge of the subject has expanded substantially. Researchers, engineers, and physicians are working closely together, and nanotechnology-based cancer diagnostics could soon be available in clinics, despite a limited number of NP-based tests that have proceeded to clinical trials. Nanotechnology offers promising avenues for enhancing cancer diagnostics and survival rates by virtue of its high stability, specificity, and ability to conduct multiple measurements simultaneously.

REFERENCES

Agrawal, Ajay, and Aishwary Awasthi. 2023. "A Review on Nano Devices." *AIP Conference Proceedings* 2427. https://doi.org/10.1063/5.0101587.

Agrawal, Ojas, Rutali Brahme, Supriya Shidhaye, and Morse Faria. 2011. "Nanotechnology in Cancer: A Clinical Review." *Journal of Applied Pharmaceutical Science* 01 (03).

Ahmadian, Elham, Dawid Janas, Aziz Eftekhari, and Najme Zare. 2022. "Application of Carbon Nanotubes in Sensing/Monitoring of Pancreas and Liver Cancer." *Chemosphere* 302. https://doi.org/10.1016/j.chemosphere.2022.134826.

Alrushaid, Noor, Firdos Alam Khan, Ebtesam Abdullah Al-Suhaimi, and Abdelhamid Elaissari. 2023. "Nanotechnology in Cancer Diagnosis and Treatment." *Pharmaceutics*. https://doi.org/10.3390/pharmaceutics15031025.

Aminolroayaei, Fahimeh, Daryoush Shahbazi-Gahrouei, Mahboubeh Rostami, Seyed Hossein Hejazi, and Amin Farzadniya. 2023. "Chitosan–Imidazolium Core–Shell Nanoparticles of Gd-Mn-Mo Polyoxometalate as Novel Potential MRI Nano-Agent for Breast Cancer Detection." *Micromachines* 14 (4). https://doi.org/10.3390/mi14040741.

Bakshi, Saira, Andrey Zakharchenko, SergiyMinko, Dmitry M. Kolpashchikov, and Evgeny Katz. 2019. "Towards Nanomaterials for Cancer Theranostics: A System of Dna-Modified Magnetic Nanoparticles for Detection and Suppression of Rna Marker in Cancer Cells." *Magnetochemistry* 5 (2). https://doi.org/10.3390/magnetochemistry5020024.

Billingsley, Margaret M., Rachel S. Riley, and Emily S. Day. 2017. "Antibody-Nanoparticle Conjugates to Enhance the Sensitivity of ELISA-Based Detection Methods." *PLoS One* 12 (5). https://doi.org/10.1371/journal.pone.0177592.

Bozzuto, Giuseppina, and Agnese Molinari. 2015. "Liposomes as Nanomedical Devices." *International Journal of Nanomedicine*. https://doi.org/10.2147/IJN.S68861.

Brar, Basanti, Koushlesh Ranjan, Ankur Palria, Rajesh Kumar, Mayukh Ghosh, Sweety Sihag, and Prasad Minakshi. 2021. "Nanotechnology in Colorectal Cancer for Precision Diagnosis and Therapy." *Frontiers in Nanotechnology*. https://doi.org/10.3389/fnano.2021.699266.

Bray, Freddie, Jacques Ferlay, Isabelle Soerjomataram, Rebecca L. Siegel, Lindsey A. Torre, and Ahmedin Jemal. 2018. "Global Cancer Statistics 2018: GLOBOCAN Estimates of Incidence and Mortality Worldwide for 36 Cancers in 185 Countries." *CA: A Cancer Journal for Clinicians* 68 (6): 394–424. https://doi.org/10.3322/caac.21492.

Chevillet, John R., Inyoul Lee, Hilary A. Briggs, Yuqing He, and Kai Wang. 2014. "Issues and Prospects of MicroRNA-Based Biomarkers in Blood and Other Body Fluids." *Molecules*. https://doi.org/10.3390/molecules19056080.

Choi, Young Eun, Ju Won Kwak, and Joon Won Park. 2010. "Nanotechnology for Early Cancer Detection." *Sensors*. https://doi.org/10.3390/s100100428.

Conti, Amalia, Alessandra Luchini, Gastone Castellani, Enrico Giampieri, Laura Pazzaglia, Serena Pollino, Giovanna Magagnoli, et al. 2019. "Abstract 421: Potential Biomarkers for Monitoring Therapy With Denosumab in Patients Affected by Giant Cell Tumor of Bone." *Cancer Research* 79 (13_Supplement). https://doi.org/10.1158/1538-7445.am2019-421.

Damborska, Dominika, Tomas Bertok, Erika Dosekova, Alena Holazova, Lenka Lorencova, Peter Kasak, and Jan Tkac. 2017. "Nanomaterial-Based Biosensors for Detection of Prostate Specific Antigen." *Microchimica Acta*. https://doi.org/10.1007/s00604-017-2410-1.

Dessale, Mesfin, Getachew Mengistu, and Hylemariam Mihiretie Mengist. 2022. "Nanotechnology: A Promising Approach for Cancer Diagnosis, Therapeutics and Theragnosis." *International Journal of Nanomedicine*. https://doi.org/10.2147/IJN.S378074.

Elmi, Soheila, and Zahra Elmi. 2018. "Improving the Sensitivity and Accuracy of Microcantilever Biosensors by a Truss Structure Within Air Medium." *Turkish Journal of Electrical Engineering and Computer Sciences* 26 (5). https://doi.org/10.3906/elk-1708-353.

Fang, Min, Ming Chen, Lulu Liu, and Yan Li. 2017. "Applications of Quantum Dots in Cancer Detection and Diagnosis: A Review." *Journal of Biomedical Nanotechnology*. https://doi.org/10.1166/jbn.2017.2334.

Gandhi, Mamta, and Preeti Nigam Joshi. 2020. "Nanorobots for in Vivo Monitoring: The Future of Nano-Implantable Devices." *Nanobiomaterial Engineering: Concepts and Their Applications in Biomedicine and Diagnostics*. https://doi.org/10.1007/978-981-32-9840-8_12.

Garrigue, Philippe, Jingjie Tang, Ling Ding, Ahlem Bouhlel, Aura Tintaru, Erik Laurini, Yuanyu Huang, et al. 2018. "Self-Assembling Supramolecular Dendrimer Nanosystem for PET Imaging of Tumors." *Proceedings of the National Academy of Sciences of the United States of America* 115 (45). https://doi.org/10.1073/pnas.1812938115.

Guan, Qingwen, and Min Wang. 2021. "Core-Shell Structured Theranostics." *Nano LIFE* 11 (04). https://doi.org/10.1142/s179398442141004x.

Harshita, Hui Fen Wu, and Suresh Kumar Kailasa. 2023. "Recent Advances in Nanomaterials-Based Optical Sensors for Detection of Various Biomarkers (Inorganic Species, Organic and Biomolecules)." *Luminescence* 38 (7). https://doi.org/10.1002/bio.4353.

He, Lu, Fan He, Yanting Feng, Xu Wang, Yongxin Li, Yonghui Tian, Aihua Gao, et al. 2021. "Hybridized Nanolayer Modified Ω-Shaped Fiber-Optic Synergistically Enhances Localized Surface Plasma Resonance for Ultrasensitive Cytosensor and Efficient Photothermal Therapy." *Biosensors and Bioelectronics* 194. https://doi.org/10.1016/j.bios.2021.113599.

Hu, Jiangnan, Weijie Huang, Shengwei Huang, Qichuan Zhu Ge, Kunlin Jin, and Yiping Zhao. 2016. "Magnetically Active Fe3O4 Nanorods Loaded With Tissue Plasminogen Activator for Enhanced Thrombolysis." *Nano Research* 9 (9). https://doi.org/10.1007/s12274-016-1152-4.

Huang, Lijie, Jiangnan Hu, Shengwei Huang, Brian Wang, Felix Siaw-Debrah, Mark Nyanzu, Yu Zhang, and Qichuan Zhuge. 2017. "Nanomaterial Applications for Neurological Diseases and Central Nervous System Injury." *Progress in Neurobiology*. https://doi.org/10.1016/j.pneurobio.2017.07.003.

Huang, Xiaohua, Ryan O'connor, and Elyahb Allie Kwizera. 2017. "Gold Nanoparticle Based Platforms for Circulating Cancer Marker Detection." *Nanotheranostics*. https://doi.org/10.7150/ntno.18216.

Javaid, Adeel. 2021. "Medical Nanorobots: Our New Healthcare Defense." *Academia Letters*. https://doi.org/10.20935/al1629.

Jayanti, Mishra, and Sahoo Prabhatkumar. 2020. "Gold Nanoparticles: Potential Nanomaterial for Application in Detection and Drug Delivery." *International Journal of Pharma and Bio Sciences* 11 (2). https://doi.org/10.22376/ijpbs.2020.11.2.p46-58.

Ji, Tianjiao, Ying Zhao, Jing Wang, Xin Zheng, Yanhua Tian, Yuliang Zhao, and Guangjun Nie. 2013. "Tumor Fibroblast Specific Activation of a Hybrid Ferritin Nanocage-Based Optical Probe for Tumor Microenvironment Imaging." *Small* 9 (14). https://doi.org/10.1002/smll.201300600.

Jia, Shiyu, Rui Zhang, Ziyang Li, and Jinming Li. 2017. "Clinical and Biological Significance of Circulating Tumor Cells, Circulating Tumor DNA, and Exosomes as Biomarkers in Colorectal Cancer." *Oncotarget*. https://doi.org/10.18632/oncotarget.17184.

Jiang, Lei, Sensen Zhou, Xiaoke Zhang, Wei Wu, and Xiqun Jiang. 2018. "Dendrimer-Based Nanoparticles in Cancer Chemotherapy and Gene Therapy." *Science China Materials*. https://doi.org/10.1007/s40843-018-9242-3.

Jin, Cancan, Kankai Wang, Anthony Oppong-Gyebi, and Jiangnan Hu. 2020. "Application of Nanotechnology in Cancer Diagnosis and Therapy—A Mini-Review." *International Journal of Medical Sciences* 17 (18). https://doi.org/10.7150/ijms.49801.

Jokerst, Jesse V., Archana Raamanathan, Nicolaos Christodoulides, Pierre N. Floriano, Amanda A. Pollard, Glennon W. Simmons, Jorge Wong, et al. 2009. "Nano-Bio-Chips for High Performance Multiplexed Protein Detection: Determinations of Cancer Biomarkers in Serum and Saliva Using Quantum Dot Bioconjugate Labels." *Biosensors and Bioelectronics* 24 (12). https://doi.org/10.1016/j.bios.2009.05.026.

Kang, Xun, Tao Sun, Liang Zhang, Chunyu Zhou, Zhongsheng Xu, Mengmeng Du, Shilin Xiao, Yun Liu, Mingfu Gong, and Dong Zhang. 2021. "Synergistic Theranostics of Magnetic Resonance Imaging and Photothermal Therapy of Breast Cancer Based on the Janus Nanostructures Fe3o4-Aushell-Peg." *International Journal of Nanomedicine* 16. https://doi.org/10.2147/IJN.S322894.

Kasi, Phanindra Babu, Venkata Ramana Mallela, Filip Ambrozkiewicz, Andriy Trailin, Václav Liška, and Kari Hemminki. 2023. "Theranostics Nanomedicine Applications for Colorectal Cancer and Metastasis: Recent Advances." *International Journal of Molecular Sciences*. https://doi.org/10.3390/ijms24097922.

Kaur, Simran, Anshika Srivastava, Vidushi Aggarwal, and Bansi D. Malhotra. 2022. "Applications of Carbon Quantum Dots in Cancer Detection and Therapy." *Advances in Transdisciplinary Engineering* 27. https://doi.org/10.3233/ATDE220759.

Kim, Dongkyu, Yong Yeon Jeong, and Sangyong Jon. 2010. "A Drug-Loaded Aptamer—Gold Nanoparticle Bioconjugate for Combined Ct Imaging and Therapy of Prostate Cancer." *ACS Nano* 4 (7). https://doi.org/10.1021/nn901877h.

Kim, Kwanoh, Jianhe Guo, Zexi Liang, and Donglei Fan. 2018. "Artificial Micro/Nanomachines for Bioapplications: Biochemical Delivery and Diagnostic Sensing." *Advanced Functional Materials* 28 (25). https://doi.org/10.1002/adfm.201705867.

Kumar, Jagatheesa Perumal Senthil, Ramakrishnan Sankaranarayanan, Jesudoss Angela Jennifa Sujana, and Navasingh Rajesh Jesudoss Hynes. 2021. "Advantages and Disadvantages of Nanodevices." *Nanomedicine Manufacturing and Applications*. https://doi.org/10.1016/B978-0-12-820773-4.00015-9.

Kurmendra, and Rajesh Kumar. 2019. "MEMS Based Cantilever Biosensors for Cancer Detection Using Potential Bio-Markers Present in VOCs: A Survey." *Microsystem Technologies*. https://doi.org/10.1007/s00542-019-04326-1.

Lakshman, K., Siddharth B. Dabhade, Y. S. Rode, Avinash Pawar, S. Deshmukh, and Ranjan Maheshwari. 2021. "Early Detection of Cancer Using Nano-Fabrication Technology MEMS Cantilever Sensor." *SSRN Electronic Journal*. https://doi.org/10.2139/ssrn.3851193.

Lenaghan, Scott C., Yongzhong Wang, Ning Xi, Toshio Fukuda, Tzyhjong Tarn, William R. Hamel, and Mingjun Zhang. 2013. "Grand Challenges in Bioengineered Nanorobotics for Cancer Therapy." *IEEE Transactions on Biomedical Engineering* 60 (3). https://doi.org/10.1109/TBME.2013.2244599.

Li, Jinxing, Berta Esteban Fernández De Ávila, Wei Gao, Liangfang Zhang, and Joseph Wang. 2017. "Micro/Nanorobots for Biomedicine: Delivery, Surgery, Sensing, and Detoxification." *Science Robotics*. https://doi.org/10.1126/scirobotics.aam6431.

Liang, Zhengyan, Muhammad Babar Khawar, Jingyan Liang, and Haibo Sun. 2021. "Bio-Conjugated Quantum Dots for Cancer Research: Detection and Imaging." *Frontiers in Oncology*. https://doi.org/10.3389/fonc.2021.749970.

Lisik, Katarzyna, and Anita Krokosz. 2021. "Application of Carbon Nanoparticles in Oncology and Regenerative Medicine." *International Journal of Molecular Sciences*. https://doi.org/10.3390/ijms22158341.

Liu, Meng Xian, Shuai Chen, Na Ding, Yong Liang Yu, and Jian Hua Wang. 2020. "A Carbon-Based Polymer Dot Sensor for Breast Cancer Detection Using Peripheral Blood Immunocytes." *Chemical Communications* 56 (20). https://doi.org/10.1039/c9cc10016d.

Maffei, Massimo E. 2022. "Magnetic Fields and Cancer: Epidemiology, Cellular Biology, and Theranostics." *International Journal of Molecular Sciences* 23 (3). https://doi.org/10.3390/ijms23031339.

Mani, Shubhangi A., Shivani Sachdeva, Amit Mani, Hiral R. Vora, Sonali S. Gholap, and Jasleen Kaur Sodhi. 2021. "Nano-Robotics: The Future of Health and Dental Care." *IP International Journal of Periodontology and Implantology* 6 (1). https://doi.org/10.18231/j.ijpi.2021.002.

Martel, Sylvain. 2017. "Beyond Imaging: Macro-A Nd Microscale Medical Robots Actuated by Clinical MRI Scanners." *Science Robotics* 2 (3). https://doi.org/10.1126/scirobotics.aam8119.

Martos-Maldonado, Manuel C., Indalecio Quesada-Soriano, Luis García-Fuentes, and Antonio Vargas-Berenguel. 2020. "Multivalent Lactose–Ferrocene Conjugates Based on Poly (Amido Amine) Dendrimers and Gold Nanoparticles as Electrochemical Probes for Sensing Galectin-3." *Nanomaterials* 10 (2). https://doi.org/10.3390/nano10020203.

Medici, Serenella, Massimiliano Peana, Donatella Coradduzza, and Maria Antonietta Zoroddu. 2021. "Gold Nanoparticles and Cancer: Detection, Diagnosis and Therapy." *Seminars in Cancer Biology* 76. https://doi.org/10.1016/j.semcancer.2021.06.017.

Mendes, Livia Palmerston, Jiayi Pan, and Vladimir P. Torchilin. 2017. "Dendrimers as Nanocarriers for Nucleic Acid and Drug Delivery in Cancer Therapy." *Molecules*. https://doi.org/10.3390/molecules22091401.

Mukherjee, Anubhab, Bharti Bisht, Suman Dutta, and Manash K. Paul. 2022. "Current Advances in the Use of Exosomes, Liposomes, and Bioengineered Hybrid Nanovesicles in Cancer Detection and Therapy." *Acta Pharmacologica Sinica*. https://doi.org/10.1038/s41401-022-00902-w.

Nanotechnology-Based Targeted Drug Delivery Systems for Lung Cancer. 2019. *Nanotechnology-Based Targeted Drug Delivery Systems for Lung Cancer*. https://doi.org/10.1016/c2017-0-03894-6.

Omidi, Yadollah. 2011. "Smart Multifunctional Theranostics: Simultaneous Diagnosis and Therapy of Cancer." *BioImpacts*. https://doi.org/10.5681/bi.2011.019.

Pang, Xuehui, Cheng Cui, Minhui Su, Yaoguang Wang, Qin Wei, and Weihong Tan. 2018. "Construction of Self-Powered Cytosensing Device Based on ZnO Nanodisks@g-C3N4 Quantum Dots and Application in the Detection of CCRF-CEM Cells." *Nano Energy* 46. https://doi.org/10.1016/j.nanoen.2018.01.018.

Parsa, N. 2012. "Environmental Factors Inducing Human Cancers." *Iranian Journal of Public Health*.

Reddy, T. Srinivasa, and Suresh K. Bhargava. 2019. "Design of Dendrimer Based Prodrugs." *Pharmaceutical Applications of Dendrimers*. https://doi.org/10.1016/B978-0-12-814527-2.00008-1.

Saadh, Mohamed J., and Roaa K. Jadullah. 2021. "Nanotechnology in Drug Delivery." *Pharmacologyonline* 3. https://doi.org/10.17148/ijarcce.2016.55255.

Sakthi Devi, R., Agnishwar Girigoswami, M. Siddharth, and Koyeli Girigoswami. 2022. "Applications of Gold and Silver Nanoparticles in Theranostics." *Applied Biochemistry and Biotechnology*. https://doi.org/10.1007/s12010-022-03963-z.

Samadi Pakchin, Parvin, Marziyeh Fathi, Hossein Ghanbari, Reza Saber, and Yadollah Omidi. 2020. "A Novel Electrochemical Immunosensor for Ultrasensitive Detection of CA125 in Ovarian Cancer." *Biosensors and Bioelectronics* 153. https://doi.org/10.1016/j.bios.2020.112029.

Sapra, Varun, Luxmi Sapra, Jasminder Kaur Sandhu, and Gunjan Chhabra. 2021. "Biomedical Diagnostics Through Nanocomputing." *Nanotechnology*. https://doi.org/10.1201/9781003120261-13.

Shah, Nimit, Ritesh K. Shukla, Ashish Badiye, and Neeti Kapoor. 2022. "Nano-Biosensors for Biochemical Analysis." *Nanobioanalytical Approaches to Medical Diagnostics*. https://doi.org/10.1016/B978-0-323-85147-3.00005-0.

Sherje, Atul P., Mrunal Jadhav, Bhushan R. Dravyakar, and Darshana Kadam. 2018. "Dendrimers: A Versatile Nanocarrier for Drug Delivery and Targeting." *International Journal of Pharmaceutics*. https://doi.org/10.1016/j.ijpharm.2018.07.030.

Shetty, Aishwarya, and Sudeshna Chandra. 2022. "Engineered Hybrid Nanoparticles for Multimodal Medical Imaging and Diagnosis." *Nanomaterials for Cancer Detection Using Imaging Techniques and Their Clinical Applications*. https://doi.org/10.1007/978-3-031-09636-5_12.

Shi, Zhiao, Bo Wen, Qiang Gao, and Bing Zhang. 2021. "Feature Selection Methods for Protein Biomarker Discovery From Proteomics or Multiomics Data." *Molecular and Cellular Proteomics* 20. https://doi.org/10.1016/J.MCPRO.2021.100083.

Shkodra, Bajramshahe, Mattia Petrelli, Martina Aurora Costa Angeli, Denis Garoli, Nako Nakatsuka, Paolo Lugli, and Luisa Petti. 2021. "Electrolyte-Gated Carbon Nanotube Field-Effect Transistor-Based Biosensors: Principles and Applications." *Applied Physics Reviews*. https://doi.org/10.1063/5.0058591.

Siddique, Sarkar, and James C. L. Chow. 2020. "Application of Nanomaterials in Biomedical Imaging and Cancer Therapy." *Nanomaterials*. https://doi.org/10.3390/nano10091700.

Soto, Fernando, and Robert Chrostowski. 2018. "Frontiers of Medical Micro/Nanorobotics: In Vivo Applications and Commercialization Perspectives Toward Clinical Uses." *Frontiers in Bioengineering and Biotechnology*. https://doi.org/10.3389/fbioe.2018.00170.

Soto, Fernando, Jie Wang, Rajib Ahmed, and Utkan Demirci. 2020. "Medical Micro/Nanorobots in Precision Medicine." *Advanced Science*. https://doi.org/10.1002/advs.202002203.

Stans, J. 2021. "Injection Site Sarcomas in Other Species Than the Domestic Cat." *Journal of the Hellenic Veterinary Medical Society* 72 (3). https://doi.org/10.12681/JHVMS.28480.

Stiepel, Rebeca T., Eliza Duggan, Cole J. Batty, and Kristy M. Ainslie. 2023. "Micro and Nanotechnologies: The Little Formulations That Could." *Bioengineering and Translational Medicine*. https://doi.org/10.1002/btm2.10421.

Subramani, Karthikeyan, and Manjula Mehta. 2017. "Nanodiagnostics in Microbiology and Dentistry." *Emerging Nanotechnologies in Dentistry*. https://doi.org/10.1016/B978-0-12-812291-4.00019-4.

Suhail, Muhammad, Arshad Khan, Muhammad Abdur Rahim, Abid Naeem, Muhammad Fahad, Syed Faisal Badshah, Abdul Jabar, and Ashok Kumar Janakiraman. 2022. "Micro and Nanorobot-Based Drug Delivery: An Overview." *Journal of Drug Targeting*. https://doi.org/10.1080/1061186X.2021.1999962.

Suhito, Intan Rosalina, Kyeong Mo Koo, and Tae Hyung Kim. 2021. "Recent Advances in Electrochemical Sensors for the Detection of Biomolecules and Whole Cells." *Biomedicines*. https://doi.org/10.3390/biomedicines9010015.

Sung, Hyuna, Jacques Ferlay, Rebecca L. Siegel, Mathieu Laversanne, Isabelle Soerjomataram, Ahmedin Jemal, and Freddie Bray. 2021. "Global Cancer Statistics 2020: GLOBOCAN Estimates of Incidence and Mortality Worldwide for 36 Cancers in 185 Countries." *CA: A Cancer Journal for Clinicians* 71 (3): 209–49. https://doi.org/10.3322/caac.21660.

Svenson, Sönke, and Donald A. Tomalia. 2012. "Dendrimers in Biomedical Applications-Reflections on the Field." *Advanced Drug Delivery Reviews*. https://doi.org/10.1016/j.addr.2012.09.030.

Tsukada, Yusuke, Aiko Sasai, Hiroyuki Tsujimoto, Hiromitsu Yamamoto, and Yoshiaki Kawashima. 2018. "PLGA Nanosphere Technology for Novel Nanomedicine and Functional Cosmetics." *Nanoparticle Technology Handbook*. https://doi.org/10.1016/B978-0-444-64110-6.00018-4.

Vijayan, Varsha M., Lavanya Jothi, Ravi Sankar Arunagirinathan, and Gomathi Nageswaran. 2022. "Recent Advances in the Electrochemical Sensing of Lung Cancer Biomarkers." *Biosensors and Bioelectronics: X* 12. https://doi.org/10.1016/j.biosx.2022.100235.

Vinduska, Vojtech, Caleb Edward Gallops, Ryan O'connor, Yongmei Wang, and Xiaohua Huang. 2021. "Exosomal Surface Protein Detection With Quantum Dots and Immunomagnetic Capture for Cancer Detection." *Nanomaterials* 11 (7). https://doi.org/10.3390/nano11071853.

Wang, Dong En, Xiaohua Gao, Shangqi You, Meng Chen, Li Ren, Wujin Sun, Hui Yang, and Huiyun Xu. 2020. "Aptamer-Functionalized Polydiacetylene Liposomes Act as a Fluorescent Sensor for Sensitive Detection of MUC1 and Targeted Imaging of Cancer Cells." *Sensors and Actuators, B: Chemical* 309. https://doi.org/10.1016/j.snb.2020.127778.

Wang, Jiameng, Jia Wen, and Hongyuan Yan. 2021. "Recent Applications of Carbon Nanomaterials for MicroRNA Electrochemical Sensing." *Chemistry—An Asian Journal*. https://doi.org/10.1002/asia.202001260.

Wang, Jingjing, Li Zhang, Houyong Cao, Yinfang Zhu, Jinling Yang, and Erdan Gu. 2020. "Characterization Method of Biological Functionalization Process of Silicon Surface Based on Cantilever Biosensor." *Integrated Ferroelectrics* 208 (1). https://doi.org/10.1080/10584587.2020.1728731.

Wu, Xuan, Tingyu Xiao, Zhang Luo, Rongxiang He, Yiping Cao, ZhenzhongGuo, Weiying Zhang, and Yong Chen. 2018. "A Micro-/Nano-Chip and Quantum Dots-Based 3D Cytosensor for Quantitative Analysis of Circulating Tumor Cells." *Journal of Nanobiotechnology* 16 (1). https://doi.org/10.1186/s12951-018-0390-x.

You, Qing, Kaiyue Zhang, Jingyi Liu, Changliang Liu, Huayi Wang, Mengting Wang, Siyuan Ye, et al. 2020. "Persistent Regulation of Tumor Hypoxia Microenvironment via a Bioinspired Pt-Based Oxygen Nanogenerator for Multimodal Imaging-Guided Synergistic Phototherapy." *Advanced Science* 7 (17). https://doi.org/10.1002/advs.201903341.

Zhang, Yuan, Beibei Chen, Man He, Bin Yang, Jing Zhang, and Bin Hu. 2014. "Immunomagnetic Separation Combined With Inductively Coupled Plasma Mass Spectrometry for the Detection of Tumor Cells Using Gold Nanoparticle Labeling." *Analytical Chemistry* 86 (16). https://doi.org/10.1021/ac500964s.

Zhou, Yun, Ziye Dong, Hermella Andarge, Wei Li, and Dimitri Pappas. 2020. "Nanoparticle Modification of Microfluidic Cell Separation for Cancer Cell Detection and Isolation." *Analyst* 145 (1). https://doi.org/10.1039/c9an01719d.

Part III

Nanoparticles in Cancer Therapy

9 Conventional Methods of Cancer Therapy

Priyanka Chambial, Prudhvi Lal Bhukya, Vidushi Bahl, and Neelam Thakur

ABBREVIATIONS

Acronym	Full Form
EBRT	external beam radiation therapy
IMRT	intensity-modulated radiation treatment
IGRT	image-guided radiotherapy
IV	intravenous
NCI	National Cancer Institute
MTAs	microtubule-targeted agents
SERMs	selective estrogen receptor modulators
FDA	Food and Drug Administration
TILs	tumor-infiltrating lymphocytes
VEGF	vascular endothelial growth factor

9.1 INTRODUCTION

Cancer is an inheritable disorder caused by genetic mutations. Cancer cells proliferate uncontrollably due to gene abnormalities originating from a single cell, resulting in an aberrant cell cycle and the acquisition of traits associated with uncontrolled cell division (Mattiuzzi and Lippi 2019). Through the accumulation of numerous mutations, benign cancer cells undergo a transformation into malignant cells, leading to the invasion of surrounding tissues. This process is known as metastasis. The expenses associated with cancer diagnosis and treatment have experienced a substantial rise, resulting in a substantial financial strain on both the global economy and the affected individuals and their families (Miller et al. 2016).

Conventional cancer therapies consist of many methods that aim to specifically target and eradicate cancer cells (Johnson et al. 2018). Common conventional cancer treatments include surgery, chemotherapy, radiation therapy, hormone therapy, immunotherapy, targeted therapy, and an integrated approach that blends conventional procedures with alternative medicines (Citron et al. 2003). The optimal traditional approaches for treating cancer often involve the surgical removal of tumors, followed by the administration of radiation using X-rays or chemotherapy. Among these options, surgery is the most efficacious when the disease is in its early stages (Demaria, Golden, and Formenti 2015). Radiation therapy possesses the capacity to inflict harm onto healthy cells, organs, and tissues. Chemotherapy, although efficacious in diminishing rates of disease and mortality, induces harm to healthy cells, especially those undergoing rapid division and development. The treatment for cancer is tailored to the specific type of cancer, the stage of the disease, the rate at which it is advancing, the overall health of the patient, and how they respond to therapy (Baskar et al. 2012).

DOI: 10.1201/9781003463191-12

TABLE 9.1
An Analysis of Traditional Approaches for the Management of Cancer

Cancer Treatment	Advantages	Drawbacks	References
Radiotherapy	It exerts a substantial impact on malignancies in their early and middle stages. Localized therapy. The local side effects are quite benign.	Radiation therapy causes non-selective destruction of both the targeted area and surrounding healthy cells. The doctor's skill is subject to demands.	Markman (2003)
Surgery	Significant likelihood of recuperation. Easily accessible.	Significant incidence of local recurrence and metastasis. Not feasible for all forms of cancer. Characterized by the tendency to spread aggressively and intrude upon other areas or systems.	Vanneman and Dranoff (2012)
Chemotherapy	It exerts a substantial impact on malignancies in the early and intermediate stages. Systemic therapy.	Chemotherapy invariably results in toxic side effects. Chemotherapy exhibits minimal efficacy in people with drug-resistant cancer.	Willers et al. (2013)
Immunotherapy	Prolonged efficacy.	Some patients may have a range of nonspecific harmful and side effects following usage, and in certain cases, hyperprogressive illness may arise, hastening the death of individuals.	Baudino (2015)
Targeted therapy	Inhibit or deactivate signals that stimulate the proliferation and division of cancer cells. Inhibit cellular longevity beyond the typical lifespan.	Typical symptoms encompass skin rashes, diarrhea, hypertension, and complications related to blood coagulation or wound recovery. Certain specific therapeutic medications have the potential to cause damage to a developing fetus.	Tohme, Simmons, and Tsung (2017)

Unsurprisingly, conventional treatment approaches exhibit numerous drawbacks, such as the presence of toxic side effects that can result in substantial harm to healthy tissue, unavoidable off-target effects, considerable psychological distress for patients due to treatment-related pain, and the potential for cancer recurrence due to incomplete surgical removal (Spranger 2016) (Table 9.1).

9.2 TYPES OF CONVENTIONAL CANCER TREATMENT

9.2.1 Surgery

Surgery is essential in the management of cancer, particularly when the tumor is confined to a specific area and has not metastasized to other regions of the body. The objective of surgical intervention is to excise the tumor and adjacent tissues in order to inhibit the dissemination of cancerous cells (Hughes, Scheele, and Sugarbaker 1989). The efficacy of surgical intervention in cancer treatment depends on several factors, including the stage of the disease, the kind and location of the tumor, and the overall health of the patient. Surgery is often combined with other therapy techniques to offer complete cancer care (Coffey et al. 2003).

Surgery, the most ancient method of cancer therapy, is the primary intervention that provides cancer patients with a significantly elevated likelihood of being completely cured from non-metastatic

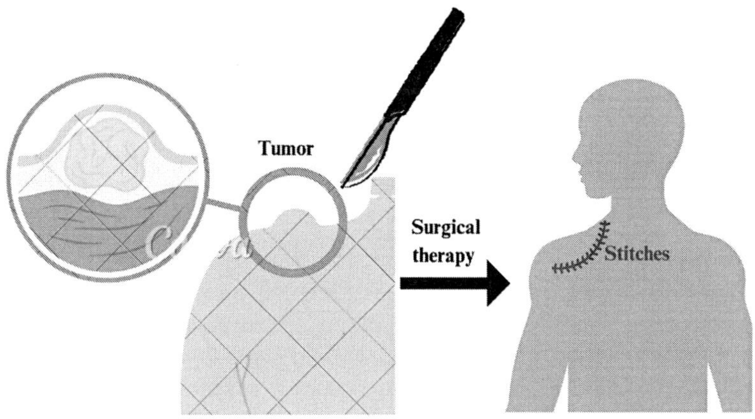

FIGURE 9.1A Illustration of surgical method. Cancer cells are removed by surgery.

tumors, especially when the disease is identified in its first phase and paired with other therapeutic approaches. However, the feasibility of doing surgery to excise the tumor necessitates additional evaluation of the malignant tissue, including tumor imaging and biopsy (Clarke et al. 2005). Complete surgical removal is the preferred therapy and the most efficient approach for local primary tumors (Figure 9.1A).

Regrettably, relying solely on surgery as a treatment method exhibits a significantly elevated incidence of local recurrence and metastatic complications. Abundant empirical evidence and clinical data indicate that surgical and postoperative inflammation may contribute to the recurrence and spread of cancer. Surgery elicits alterations in both the target tissue and cancer cells, promoting the infiltration and spread of cancer. The surgical procedure can induce both systemic and local inflammatory reactions, which have been seen to enhance the development rate of micrometastases based on clinical evidence (Janicke et al. 1992). Combining surgery with radiation and chemotherapy can effectively diminish the presence of tiny remaining cancer cells, hence minimizing the likelihood of cancer recurrence.

Various surgical procedures are beneficial for those diagnosed with cancer. Certain surgical procedures are employed in conjunction with other modalities of therapy. There are several types of procedures, such as the following.

9.2.1.1 Curative Surgery

Curative surgery entails the extraction of the malignant tumor or growth from the body. Surgeons employ curative surgery when the malignant tumor is confined to a particular region of the body (Singletary et al. 2003). This form of therapy is commonly regarded as the main course of treatment. Nevertheless, alternative forms of cancer therapy, such as radiation, might be administered prior to or following the surgical procedure (Ohlsson et al. 1995).

9.2.1.2 Prophylactic and Diagnostic Surgery

Preventive surgery is the removal of non-cancerous tissue that has the potential to grow into a malignant tumor. For instance, the presence of polyps in the colon may be seen as tissue that has the potential to develop into cancer (Scheuer et al. 2002). In order to avoid this, surgical intervention may be undertaken to eliminate them. Diagnostic surgery is employed to ascertain the malignancy of cells. Diagnostic surgery entails the extraction of a tissue sample for the purpose of further examination and assessment, often conducted by a pathologist in a laboratory setting. Tissue samples are utilized to validate a diagnosis, ascertain the specific kind of cancer, or establish the stage of the malignancy (Jayakar et al. 2014).

9.2.1.3 Surgical Staging

This surgical procedure is conducted to ascertain the exact extent of cancer or disease within the body. Laparoscopy, a minimally invasive surgical technique, involves the insertion of a slender tube equipped with a lens or camera through a small incision. This treatment allows for the internal examination of the body and the collection of tissue samples. It serves as an illustrative example of a surgical staging process (Orr, Orr, and Taylor 1996).

9.2.1.4 Debulking

This surgery refers to a surgical procedure aimed at removing a significant portion of a tumor or mass in order to reduce its size and alleviate symptoms. Debulking surgery entails the removal of a portion, but not the entirety, of a malignant tumor (Van Der Burg et al. 1995). It is employed in specific circumstances where excising a whole tumor may result in harm to an organ or the overall body. Other forms of cancer treatment, such as chemotherapy and radiation, may be employed after debulking surgery is completed. Surgical intervention aims at providing relief from symptoms and improving the quality of life, rather than curing the underlying condition (Melamed et al. 2017).

9.2.1.5 Palliative Surgery

This is employed to address cancer in its later stages. While it may not be effective in curing cancer, it serves the purpose of alleviating discomfort or addressing other issues that may have arisen from cancer or its treatment. Supportive surgery, similar to palliative surgery, does not aim to cure cancer. Instead, it enhances the efficacy of other cancer therapies. An instance of supportive surgery involves the placement of a catheter to facilitate the administration of chemotherapy (Hallissey et al. 1988).

9.2.1.6 Reconstructive Surgery

Restorative surgery is occasionally employed as a subsequent procedure following curative or other procedures in order to modify or reinstate an individual's physical appearance or the functionality of a certain body component. Women diagnosed with breast cancer may require breast reconstruction surgery to restore the anatomical form of the damaged breast. Oral cancer curative surgery can result in alterations to the morphology and aesthetic of an individual's oral cavity. Restorative surgery can be conducted to mitigate these consequences (Carpentier et al. 1980).

9.2.1.7 Cryosurgery

Cryotherapy is a medical practice that utilizes extremely low temperatures to eliminate aberrant or damaged tissue. Cryotherapy is utilized to eliminate cancer cells by exposing them to exceedingly low temperatures (Babaian et al. 2008). Cryosurgery is mostly utilized for the treatment of skin and cervical cancer. The utilization of liquid nitrogen differs based on the specific location of the tumor. If the tumor is external, liquid nitrogen is directly applied to the skin (Kuflik and Gage 1991). If the tumor is internal, a cryoprobe is put into the body to make contact with the tumor, and then liquid nitrogen is used (El-Aziz, Nafea, and El-Hafiz 2019). The efficacy of cryosurgery as a surgical intervention for various cancer types is now under evaluation.

9.2.1.8 Laser Surgery and Electrosurgery

Laser ablation is a method that uses concentrated beams of light energy to eliminate minute cancerous growths while preserving adjacent tissue, diminish or eradicate tumors, or activate medications to exterminate cancer cells (Ansarin et al. 2009). Laser surgery is a highly accurate medical method that may effectively treat hard-to-access parts of the body, such as the skin, cervix, rectum, and larynx. Electrosurgery is occasionally used as a treatment for both skin cancer and mouth cancer. Electrotherapy employs electrical current to eradicate cancerous cells (Pellegrino et al. 2008). *Microscopically controlled surgery* refers to a surgical procedure that is performed using a microscope to provide precise visualization and manipulation of tissues at a microscopic level. This surgical procedure is beneficial in cases where cancer impacts sensitive areas of the body, such as the ocular region (Sheridan and Dawber 2000). The process involves the removal and microscopic examination of skin layers until the absence of malignant cells is confirmed.

9.2.2 Radiotherapy

Radiation therapy, sometimes referred to as *radiotherapy*, is a cancer treatment that utilizes significant doses of radiation to eradicate cancer cells and diminish the size of tumors (Figure 9.1B). At lower levels of exposure, radiation is utilized in X-ray imaging to visualize the internal structures of your body, such as your teeth or fractured bones (Mayles, Nahum, and Rosenwald 2007). Radiation treatment employs ionizing radiation beams of high intensity to eradicate cancer cells and reduce the size of tumors. This focused therapy can be used as the main method of treatment or in combination with other methods, such as chemotherapy or surgery (Joiner and Van Der Kogel 2009). The efficacy of radiation therapy depends on the particular kind of cancer, the exact tumor site, and the dosage and duration of radiation treatment. Although radiation therapy can result in transient adverse effects, such as tiredness and skin irritation, it has demonstrated efficacy as a therapeutic modality for several cancer patients (Delaney et al. 2005). The two primary forms of radiation therapy are external beam radiation therapy and internal radiation therapy. Both variants function by eradicating the DNA of a cancerous cell. In the absence of DNA instructions stimulating their proliferation, cancer cells undergo apoptosis and tumors regress (Chen and Kuo 2017).

9.2.2.1 External Beam Radiation Therapy (EBRT)

EBRT is a medical treatment that uses high-energy beams of radiation to target and destroy cancer cells. EBRT is the predominant kind of radiotherapy. EBRT involves the use of a machine that precisely targets and delivers beams of high-energy radiation to the tumor (Figure 9.2A). The energy might manifest as X-rays (most prevalent), electrons, or protons. Accuracy is crucial when it comes to EBRT (Golding and Shrimpton 2002).

EBRT encompasses many modalities:

3D conformal radiation treatment uses CT images and computer software to generate a three-dimensional representation of the tumor. The equipment uses the model as a reference to precisely aim radiation beams toward the cancerous area, while minimizing exposure to healthy tissue (Shepard et al. 1999).

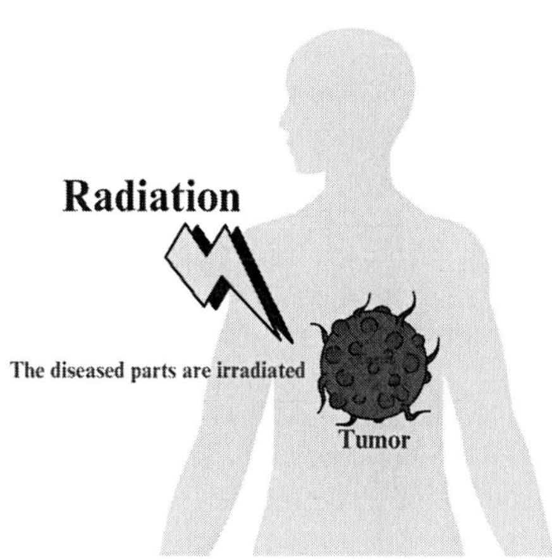

FIGURE 9.1B Illustration of radiation therapy. In radiation therapy, the diseased parts are irradiated by the radiations, hence results in the cancer eradication.

Intensity-modulated radiation treatment (IMRT) is a more sophisticated iteration of radiation therapy. IMRT employs several radiation beams that modulate the strength of the treatment. It administers a greater amount of radiation to the tumor while minimizing exposure to healthy tissue (Timmerman et al. 2010). Arc-based radiotherapy is a kind of IMRT. It projects energy beams with different levels of intensity in a circular arc-shaped trajectory. This technique provides radiation at a higher rate compared to conventional IMRT. Volumetric modulated arc treatment and tomotherapy are two types of arc-based radiation techniques (Cox, Stetz, and Pajak 1995).

Image-guided radiotherapy (IGRT) is a type of EBRT where the radiation equipment acquires a low-dose X-ray or small CT scan prior to each treatment. This picture facilitates the alignment of the treatment site, leading to enhanced accuracy in the administration of radiation. Particle treatment employs proton radiation therapy instead of photon radiation therapy (X-rays). Protons have the ability to administer an equivalent amount of radiation to the tumor while minimizing radiation exposure to healthy tissues, especially in certain individuals (Bradley et al. 2015; Clarke et al. 2005).

9.2.2.2 Internal Radiation Therapy

Brachytherapy is an alternative term for internal radiation therapy. Implants can have either a permanent or temporary nature. Hospitalization may be necessary for this therapy (Han et al. 2013). Brachytherapy involves the placement of radioactive sources directly within the body, in close proximity to cancerous cells (Figure 9.2B). It is used to address minor tumors located in the head, neck, breast, cervix, uterus, or prostate (Taylor et al. 2015). Brachytherapy involves the insertion of a solid radioactive source, commonly referred to as a "seed," either inside or next to a tumor (Hilaris and Martini 1979). The source emits radiation within a localized region with the intention of eliminating cancerous cells. Certain implants administer sustained, minimal dosages for extended durations, typically spanning weeks. Some individuals may provide large quantities for shorter durations (minutes). Certain implants utilized in brachytherapy have a transitory nature. Some substances remain permanently within your body. Ultimately, they cease emitting radiation (Skowronek 2017).

Systemic treatment administers intravenous radioactive substances to target and eradicate cancerous cells circulating in the bloodstream (Wolpin and Mayer 2008). Certain forms can be ingested. Alternatively, in the case of other individuals, the administration of the injection will be done intravenously (Figure 9.2C). Therapeutic options include radionuclide treatment, namely, radioimmunotherapy. Radioimmunotherapy employs a radioactive protein that selectively identifies and binds to particular cancer cells, subsequently emitting radiation to eliminate them (Howell, De Aguiar Ribeiro, and Swindell 1992).

Delivery of interim brachytherapy form of radiation treatment can be achieved via needle, catheter, or specialized applicators. The duration of radiation retention in the body ranges from a few minutes to a few days. The duration of internal radiation treatment for most individuals is typically limited to a few minutes. Occasionally, extended durations of internal radiation treatment may be administered (Strnad et al. 2004). If such is the case, individuals remain in a secluded chamber to minimize the risk of radiation exposure to others.

It is widely recognized that radiation therapy might marginally increase the likelihood of developing a secondary cancer. It is a potential adverse consequence of therapy that clinicians must consider while evaluating the advantages and disadvantages of each treatment (Zeléfsky et al. 2002). In general, the likelihood of developing a second cancer as a result of these therapies is minimal and is surpassed by the advantages of treating the initial cancer. Nevertheless, it is crucial to acknowledge that the risk is not entirely nonexistent. Each situation is unique, and it is essential for individuals to actively participate in determining the most suitable therapy for themselves (Waks and Winer 2019). This is only one of the numerous factors contributing to

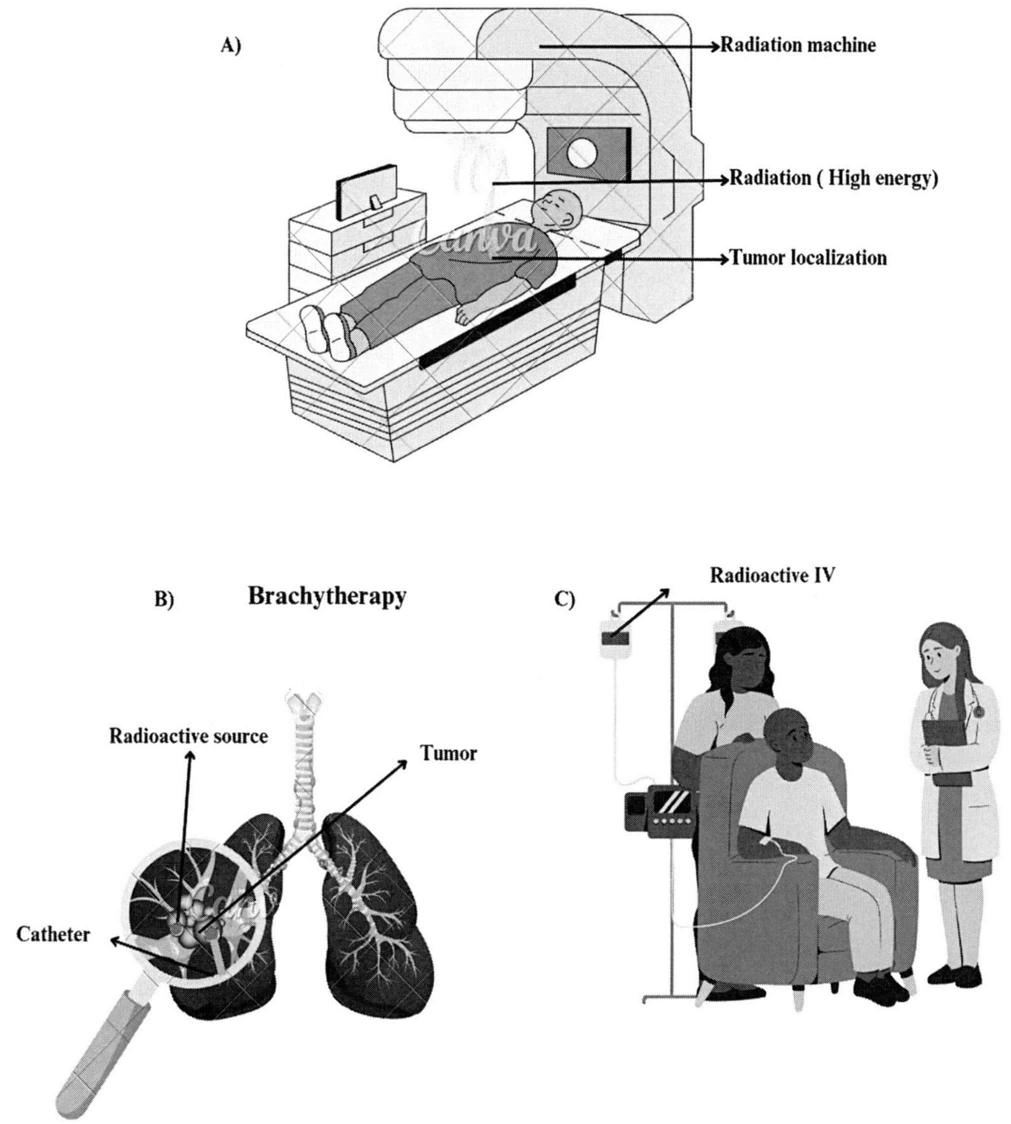

FIGURE 9.2 The figure illustrates the various forms of radiation treatment. External beam radiation treatment uses an external equipment to provide radiation, whereas internal radiation therapy utilizes implants or medications to deliver radiation inside the body.

the need for personalized decision-making. The risk varies based on the location of the radiation therapy within the body.

9.2.3 Chemotherapy

The utilization of nitrogen mustards and antifolate medicines marked the commencement of the chemotherapy era in the 1940s. Chemotherapy employs cytotoxic medications to eradicate cancerous cells. These medications also affect healthy cells, resulting in various side effects, such as nausea, fatigue, decreased hemoglobin levels, and an elevated susceptibility to infections

(Fischer et al. 2004). However, the majority of the adverse effects tend to ameliorate once the therapy is finished. Healthy cells often undergo self-repair, in contrast to malignant cells. Chemotherapy is provided as a main treatment or in conjunction with other medicines to reduce the likelihood of cancer recurrence. Additionally, it may be used to reduce the size of a cancerous tumor prior to undergoing surgery or radiation. It is sometimes employed in conjunction with radiation treatment (chemoradiation) (Creech et al. 1958). Additionally, it can be employed to alleviate symptoms and manage the proliferation of malignancy. The selection of chemotherapy for the patient will be contingent upon the specific form of cancer, the likelihood of its recurrence, and the extent of its metastasis. Tests are necessary for certain individuals undergoing chemotherapy in order to assess the effectiveness of the treatment on the malignancy. Chemotherapy is often administered either via intravenous injection or infusion or orally in the form of pills. Occasionally, it is administered intrathecally or intravesically, depending on the specific cancer type (Schirrmacher 2018).

The chemical compounds employed in cancer therapy exhibit a wide range of structures and mechanisms of action. These categories encompass hormones, hormone antagonists, natural products, alkylating compounds, antimetabolite analogs, and other agents targeting specific molecular targets (Figure 9.3). Targeted treatment originated from the significant progress in science and technology that coincided with the identification of novel chemotherapeutic drugs (Abbas and Rehman 2018). The replacement of cytotoxic medicines by new therapies seems improbable in the near future, notwithstanding the notable efficacy of targeted therapy pharmaceuticals in treating specific types of cancer. However, clinical trials have demonstrated that the combination of conventional cytotoxic medicines and targeted compounds can be highly effective. These chemotherapeutic agents can be divided (Table 9.2) into the following categories.

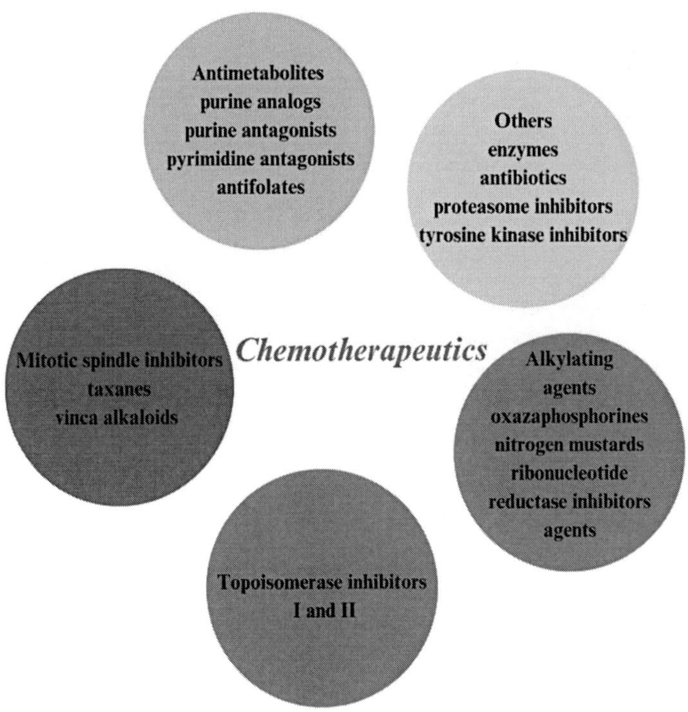

FIGURE 9.3 Classification of commonly used chemotherapeutics in cancer treatment.

TABLE 9.2
Different Classes of Chemotherapeutics Along with Their Mechanism of Action

Class	Action Mechanism	Primary Toxicity	Drug	Reference
Antibiotics	Disrupt DNA replication by generating free radicals and inserting between nucleotides	Variable	Bleomycin	Hawkins et al. (1996)
Alkylating agents	Cross-link DNA either inter-strand, intrastrand, or to proteins; inhibit transcription, stop replication	Nephrotoxicity Alopecia	Cyclophosphamide	Larsen, Escargueil, and Składanowski (2003)
Antimetabolites	Inhibit the enzymes necessary for DNA synthesis	Dermatologic, hepatotoxicity	Methotrexate	J. Chen and Stubbe (2005)
Topoisomerase inhibitors	Suppress the activity of topoisomerase, leading to the formation of breaks in the DNA strands	Myelosuppression	Etoposide	Scagliotti and Selvaggi (2006)
Plant (vinca) alkaloids	Inhibit microtubule assembly	Myelosuppression	Vincristine	Ramesha et al. (2013)

9.2.3.1 Alkylating Agents

Genotoxic chemicals known as alkylating agents attach specifically to DNA, interfering with transcription and replication to ultimately produce mutations. The structure and function of nucleic acids undergo alterations as a consequence. Hence, the objective of utilizing these medications is to impair the DNA of cancer cells to a degree that triggers apoptosis (Ralhan and Kaur 2007). Alkylating agents are categorized into many subcategories, including nitrogen mustards, other forms of alkylating chemicals such as nitrosoureas and triazenes, and platinum complexes. The first success of nitrogen mustards in clinical trials marked them as the first successful anticancer treatments. Subsequently, its derivatives, such as cyclophosphamide, have remained widely used as potent antitumor drugs (Kelland 2007). *Cyclophosphamide* is a nitrogen mustard derivative that has been chemically modified to enhance its selectivity for cancer cells (Arnold, Bourseaux, and Brock 1958).

9.2.3.2 Nitrosoureas and Triazenes

The National Cancer Institute (NCI) was the site of nitrosourea production. Because of their hydrophobic characteristics, medications in this class can penetrate the blood–brain barrier. This important feature makes them highly valuable for treating brain tumors and non-Hodgkin's lymphoma (Wasserman, Slavik, and Carter 1975). Triazenes are a family of alkylating drugs that include dacarbazine and temozolomide. These chemicals have significant therapeutic relevance and have comparable physical, chemical, anticancer, and mutagenic properties. Triazene compounds demonstrate low toxicity and exceptional pharmacokinetic characteristics.

9.2.3.3 Platinum Compounds

The efficacy of platinum complexes in treating human cancer patients was demonstrated in the 1970s (Desoise 2004). Subsequently, over 3,000 variations of platinum have been created and examined in laboratory conditions to assess their effectiveness against cancer cells (Dhar et al. 2008). Currently, there are six platinum compounds that are utilized in therapeutic settings: cisplatin (since 1978), carboplatin, oxaliplatin, nedaplatin, lobaplatin, etc. Platinum–DNA adducts are primarily responsible for the cytotoxic effects of platinum compounds (Rosenberg, Van Camp, and Krigas 1965).

9.2.3.4 Antimetabolites

Antimetabolites are a class of drugs that interfere with the normal functioning of metabolites in the body. Antimetabolites are cytotoxic substances that are currently recognized as crucial in cancer treatment. These chemicals have a similar structure to natural metabolites, which are essential for the correct metabolic processes that take place in cells (Parker 2009). Their mechanism of action includes the inclusion of nucleic acids and the competition with enzymes responsible for crucial biosynthetic activities for the binding sites. This hinders their normal functioning, therefore initiating the apoptotic process. The antimetabolites may be classified into four classes based on their function and structure: pyrimidine analogs, purine analogs, and folic acid analogs (Asuncion 2014). Analogues of folic acid are aminopterin and methotrexate. Aminopterin was the initial medicine used to provide temporary treatment for acute lymphoblastic leukemia in children (Muscaritoli et al. 2006). Subsequently, methotrexate, a different antifolate drug, has shown effectiveness in treating cancer. Currently, this category of medications is essential for cancer treatment due to its multifaceted mode of action. Due to the fact that mammalian cells are unable to produce reduced folate derivatives on their own, it is necessary for them to be obtained from external sources, such as food and dietary supplements (Farber and Lk 1948).

9.2.3.5 Agents That Specifically Target Microtubules

Microtubules are a fundamental component of the cytoskeleton. Microtubule-associated proteins and α–β-tubulin heterodimers join together to form these constantly changing structures. Microtubules play a crucial role in several biological processes, including protein trafficking, mitosis, and cell structure preservation (Mukhtar, Adhami, and Mukhtar 2014). Chemotherapy for cancer can be enhanced by drugs that modify microtubules due to their pivotal function in mitosis. On the other hand, microtubule-targeted agents, also known as MTAs, are a class of anticancer medications that are often employed for the treatment of solid tumors and hematological cancers (Zelnak 2007). MTA are potent substances that primarily belong to two main groups: microtubule-stabilizing medications (such as taxanes and epothilones) and microtubule-destabilizing drugs (such as vinca alkaloids). Vinblastine and vincristine, two vinca alkaloids that received initial clinical approval in the late 1960s, were the pioneering natural anticancer medicines (Evans et al. 1963).

9.2.3.6 Derivatives of Camptothecin

The fruit, bark, and wood of the Asian tree known as *Camptotheca acuminate* contain the pentacyclic quinoline alkaloid known as camptothecin. Only topotecan and irinotecan have been granted permission for clinical usage, despite the fact that alternative camptothecin molecules have been produced (Wall et al. 1966). Currently, irinotecan and topotecan, which are two analogs that are more soluble and less toxic, are being utilized to effectively treat various types of malignancies. Topotecan is frequently used in treatment regimens for cervical and ovarian cancers. For the treatment of colorectal cancer that has spread to other parts of the body, the prodrug irinotecan is utilized (Pommier 2006).

9.2.3.7 Epipodophyllotoxins

The isolation of podophyllotoxin occurred in 1880; however, its structure remained undiscovered until 1951. Because of its toxicity, podophyllotoxin was not used in clinical practice, despite the fact that it was demonstrated to be effective against cancer. Teniposide and etoposide are two analogues of it that have been authorized for therapeutic usage (Mirault, Boucher, and Tremblay 2006). Etoposide is mostly employed in the treatment of lung and testicular malignancies. However, it also has applications in the treatment of soft-tissue sarcomas, gastric cancer, acute nonlymphocytic leukemia, as well as both Hodgkin's and non-Hodgkin's lymphomas. Teniposide has proven beneficial in the treatment of pediatric leukemias and lymphomas (Lucas et al. 2010).

9.2.3.8 Antibiotics

Antibiotics like doxorubicin, epirubicin, idarubicin, etc. are often used as chemotherapeutic drugs to treat different types of malignancies. Daunorubicin and idarubicin have superior efficacy in the treatment of acute leukemias. Doxorubicin and epirubicin exhibit superior efficacy against solid cancers. Doxorubicin plays a crucial role in the treatment of several types of cancer, including non-Hodgkin's lymphomas, sarcoma, thyroid, ovarian, and pediatric malignancies. Epirubicin, an epimer of doxorubicin, is suggested for inclusion in breast cancer therapy (Cortes and Coronado 2007). Anthracenediones are a significant adjunct antibacterial chemotherapeutic drug. Mitoxantrone is the most powerful anthracenedione molecule, which has been approved for treating prostate cancer (Trifilio et al. 2012). In the 1960s, scientists successfully extracted a group of glycopeptide antibiotics known as bleomycins from *Streptomyces verticillis*. Bleomycin has antineoplastic activity against germcell tumors, Kaposi's sarcoma, cervical cancer, testicular tumors, head and neck malignancies, and some types of lymphoma (J. Chen and Stubbe 2005).

9.2.4 Hormonal Therapy

Hormones are endogenous molecules that are spontaneously produced inside the body. They exert their influence on cell division and activity by functioning as chemical messengers. The endocrine system comprises many organs and glands that collectively synthesize hormones. Hormonal treatments function by altering the production or activity of certain hormones inside the body (Collins, Blake, and Crosignani 2005). These treatments are often used for prostate and breast cancer. Various hormone therapy will be delivered based on the specific type of cancer being treated. There are several types of hormonal treatment available. Typically, they are supplied by injections or pills (Abe et al. 2005). The adverse effects may vary depending on the individual drug. General side effects encompass symptoms such as fatigue, headaches, nausea, and muscular or joint problems. Hormones and their associated compounds are described in what follows.

Glucocorticoids, which are the primary stress hormones, are responsible for controlling a variety of biological processes, such as the immune response, bone formation, and survival of cells. Additionally, they contribute to the regulation of homeostasis (Obradović et al. 2019). Glucocorticoids like prednisone and dexamethasone are commonly used to treat leukemias and lymphomas because of their impact on apoptosis and the advancement of the cell cycle. Moreover, their ability to mitigate the cytotoxic effects of other therapeutic interventions renders them valuable as adjunctive therapy for solid tumors. Furthermore, apart from their effectiveness in treating the malignancy, they help alleviate symptoms such as edema, electrolyte imbalance, pain, nausea, and vomiting (Lin and Wang 2016).

Progestational drugs, such as megestrol and megestrol acetate, are employed to control endometrial cancer after it has been treated with radiation and surgery. Additionally, they are used as a secondary treatment in chemotherapy for hormone-dependent metastatic breast cancer (Gottesman 2002).

Anti-estrogens and anti-androgens inhibit the activation of receptor signaling pathways that are commonly seen in cancer cells. This results in the inhibition of cancer cell proliferation (Heldring et al.). Fulvestrant, an anti-estrogen, was FDA-approved in 2002 for the treatment of hormone receptor positive metastatic breast cancer in postmenopausal women who have demonstrated resistance to prior tamoxifen therapy. The information is sourced from the US Food and Drug Administration database in 2012.

Selective estrogen receptor modulators (SERMs) are chemicals that have tissue-selective effects. Depending on their location of action, they can have agonistic effects on bone, brain, and the cardiovascular system, antagonistic effects on the brain and breast, and mixed effects on the uterus (Van Weelden et al. 2019). Currently, the FDA has granted approval for toremifene, tamoxifen, and raloxifen as SERMs. It is used to treat osteoporosis and to reduce the possibility of getting invasive breast cancer in women who have osteoporosis or who are at a higher risk of developing invasive breast cancer (Gelmann 1996). Raloxifen is also used to treat osteoporosis. Toremifene is the standard treatment for postmenopausal women who have been diagnosed with metastatic breast cancer. The information is sourced from the US Food and Drug Administration database in 2011. Tamoxifen is employed as an adjunctive therapy for breast cancer that has spread to the lymph nodes and other parts of the body. In addition, tamoxifen has demonstrated prophylactic advantages for women with a high susceptibility to breast cancer, as documented in the US FDA database in 2005.

9.2.5 Targeted Therapy

Targeted treatments, sometimes referred to as *biological therapies*, possess the capacity to enhance the immune system, hinder the growth of cancer cells, or alleviate treatment-induced adverse effects. Targeted therapies encompass many treatments, such as vaccines, angiogenesis inhibitors, monoclonal antibodies, and cancer growth inhibitors (Perez-Herrero and Fernandez-Medarde 2015).

Angiogenesis inhibitors are a type of anticancer treatment which work to prevent the production of blood vessels that supply food for the growth of tumors. Angiogenesis is the formation of new blood vessels. During this process, the endothelial cells that form a lining on the inner wall of blood arteries undergo migration, proliferation, and differentiation. The angiogenesis process is regulated by chemical signals within the body (Carmeliet and Jain 2000). The surface receptors of healthy endothelial cells selectively attach to certain signals, such as vascular endothelial growth factor (VEGF). Endothelial cells initiate signals that promote the proliferation and viability of nascent blood vessels. Angiogenesis inhibitors, a distinct category of chemical signals, impede the formation of new blood vessels (Folkman 1995). Angiogenesis inhibitors impede several phases of blood vessel formation through distinct mechanisms.

Several of them are monoclonal antibodies that selectively identify and attach to VEGF. These drugs are unable to activate the VEGF receptor when VEGF is bound to them. To hinder their activities, supplementary angiogenesis inhibitors bind to VEGF and/or its receptor, as well as to other receptors on endothelial cells and to other proteins involved in subsequent signaling cascades. Specific monoclonal antibodies facilitate the recognition and elimination of cancer cells by the immune system in a more efficient manner (Carmeliet 2005). Rituximab exemplifies this phenomenon by specifically binding to the CD20 protein found on B cells and select cancer cells, therefore stimulating the immune system to eliminate them. Some angiogenesis inhibitors possess immunomodulatory properties and can either stimulate or depress the immune system while also exhibiting antiangiogenic effects (Ramjiawan, Griffioen, and Duda 2017).

Approved angiogenesis inhibitors include axitinib, bevacizumab, lenalidomide, cabozantinib, mesylateeverolimus, and lenvatinib. Angiogenesis inhibitors can be used either alone (monotherapy) or in conjunction with other anticancer drugs (El-Kenawi and El-Remessy 2013).

Cancer growth blockers, commonly referred to as cancer growth inhibitors, are a type of targeted cancer treatments. Cancer growth inhibitors function by obstructing the growth factors responsible for the propagation of cancerous cells. These medicines function by inhibiting the signaling pathways that cancer cells utilize for proliferation. Cancer cells often exhibit heightened sensitivity when exposed to growth stimuli. Hence, by obstructing the proliferation and division of certain malignancies, we can effectively halt their growth (Hirsch et al. 2009). Scientists are now developing a wide range of inhibitors targeting different groups of growth factors. Examples of tyrosine kinase inhibitors include axitinib and dasatinib, whereas proteasome inhibitors such as carfilzomib and ixazomib are also used in cancer research (Cancer Research UK).

The administration of human papillomavirus (HPV) and hepatitis B immunizations can effectively prevent several types of malignancies, including liver cancer. The HPV vaccine does not provide a remedy for pre-existing diseases or infections; instead, it serves as a preventive measure against future HPV infections (Saraiya et al. 2015). The ideal approach is to provide the HPV vaccination before any encounter to the HPV virus. The suggested age range for administering this is often between 11 and 12 years old; however, it can be administered as early as 9 years old. It is recommended for those up to the age of 26 who have not yet been vaccinated (Gillison, Chaturvedi, and Lowy 2008).

9.2.6 Immunotherapy

Immunotherapy is a form of cancer treatment that enhances the ability of your immune system to combat cancer. The immune system aids in the body's defense against infections and many disorders. It consists of leukocytes and the lymphatic system's organs and tissues. Immunotherapy is a form of biological treatment (Graham and Unger 2018). Biological therapy, often known as immunotherapy, employs therapeutic agents derived from live organisms to combat cancer. The immune system, in its regular operation, identifies and eliminates anomalous cells, so possibly impeding or restraining the development of several malignancies. Immune cells can occasionally be seen within and in the vicinity of malignancies (Restifo, Dudley, and Rosenberg 2012). Tumor-infiltrating lymphocytes, often known as TILs, indicate an immune system response to the tumor. Individuals with malignancies that possess TILs often experience superior outcomes compared to individuals whose tumors lack TILs. While the immune system has the ability to impede or decelerate the progression of cancer, cancer cells possess mechanisms to evade eradication by the immune system (Kirkwood et al. 2012).

Various forms of immunotherapy function through distinct mechanisms. Certain immunotherapies aid in the inhibition or deceleration of cancer cell proliferation by bolstering the immune system. Additional individuals assist the immune system in eradicating cancerous cells or inhibiting the dissemination of malignancy to different bodily regions. Various forms of immunotherapy encompass monoclonal antibodies and immune checkpoint inhibitors, T cell therapy, and vaccines (Yang and Rosenberg 2016). The specific immunotherapy modality, dosage, and treatment regimen recommended by the physician are contingent upon several factors. These factors may encompass the cancer's classification, dimensions, location, and metastasis. Age, overall health, body weight, and potential adverse reactions are other significant factors to consider.

Utilizing dendritic cell–based (DC) vaccination, immunotherapy has been authorized as a method to exploit the patient's immune system in eradicating tumor cells in metastatic hormone-refractory cancer (Leen, Rooney, and Foster 2007). Dendritic cell treatment elicits antitumor reactions by inducing dendritic cells to display tumor antigens to lymphocytes, therefore stimulating and preparing them to eliminate additional cells that exhibit the antigen (Figure 9.3). Dendritic cells serve as antigen-presenting cells within the immune system of mammals. Cancer antigen targeting is facilitated in cancer therapy.

Nonspecific immunotherapies, also known as nonspecific immunomodulating drugs, aid in the eradication of cancer cells by enhancing the activity of your immune system. Various types of nonspecific immunotherapies function through distinct mechanisms.

9.2.6.1 Cytokines

The immune system relies heavily on cytokines as an essential component. These proteins function as messengers between cells, triggering the activation of the immune system (Conlon, Miljković, and Waldmann 2019). Two categories of cytokines are employed in the treatment of cancer (Kirkwood and Ernstoff 1984).

Interferon alpha (Roferon-A [2a], Intron A [2b], Alferon [2a]) is the prevailing kind of interferon employed in cancer therapy. Interferon can be utilized in the treatment of several forms of cancer. Possible adverse effects of interferon therapy encompass flu-like symptoms, heightened susceptibility to infection, dermatological rashes, and alopecia (Dunn, Koebel, and Schreiber 2006).

9.2.6.2 Interleukins

Interleukins are a class of proteins that facilitate cell-to-cell communication by transmitting signals. Additionally, they stimulate an immunological response. Lab-manufactured interleukin-2 (IL-2) can effectively cure kidney cancer. Typical adverse effects of IL-2 therapy encompass increased body weight and hypotension. Additionally, certain individuals may have symptoms like those of the flu (Briukhovetska et al. 2021).

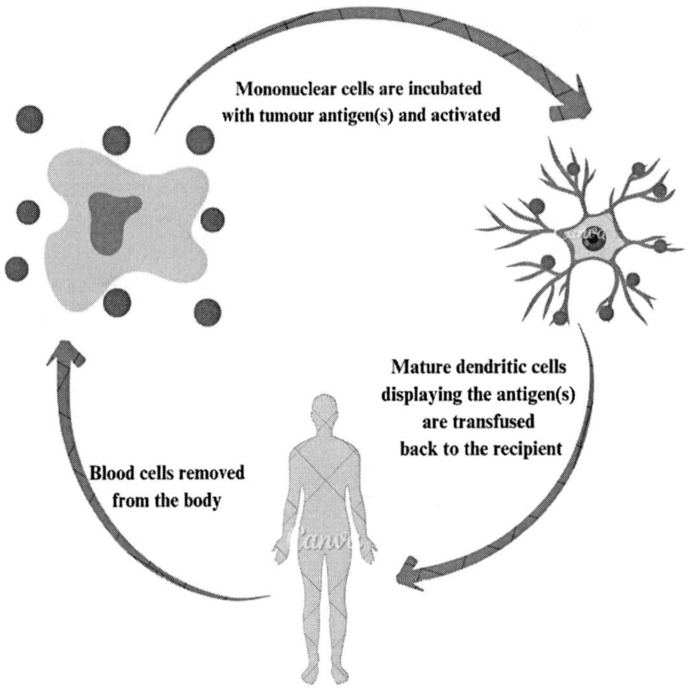

FIGURE 9.4 Dendritic cell therapy. The process involves extracting blood cells from the body, subjecting them to incubation with cancer antigen(s), and subsequently activating them. The mature dendritic cells are subsequently reintroduced into the original cancer-afflicted donor in order to provoke an immunological response.

Immunotherapy may have adverse consequences, mostly due to the immune system's heightened activity against both cancerous cells and healthy cells and tissues in the body.

9.3 INTEGRATIVE APPROACH: MERGING TRADITIONAL TECHNIQUES WITH ALTERNATIVE THERAPIES

The field of medical science is in a perpetual state of development, with continuing study consistently revealing novel discoveries and breakthroughs in traditional cancer therapies (Carter and Comis 1975). Scientists and researchers are investigating new methods of therapy, such as targeted immunotherapies, customized medicine, and gene treatments. These innovations seek to enhance the effectiveness of treatment, reduce adverse effects, and ultimately improve patient outcomes. The future of cancer treatment is quite promising, as we persist in deciphering the intricacies of this ailment. The integrated approach to cancer therapy merges traditional modalities with alternative therapies to offer a comprehensive and all-encompassing approach to patient care (Tascilar et al. 2006). This approach acknowledges the significance of attending to the patient's bodily, emotional, and spiritual requirements. Alternative therapies, such as acupuncture, massage, and herbal therapy, can enhance conventional treatments, enhance the quality of life, and decrease adverse effects associated with treatment. Nevertheless, it is crucial to get advice from healthcare specialists to guarantee the safety and effectiveness of these alternative medicines. The primary goal of alternative cancer therapy is to expedite the rate of recovery and effectiveness, while also offering psychological solace for the entirety of the cancer treatment procedure (Perros et al. 2014).

One of the most important aspects of cancer treatment is the integration of a wide variety of therapeutic approaches, with the specific goal of addressing pathways that promote cancer or those that protect cell integrity. In spite of the fact that monotherapy continues to be a common treatment choice for a number of different forms of cancer, it is generally seen as being less effective when compared to the combination therapy method. The integration of many therapeutic interventions to particularly address cancer-promoting or cell-maintaining pathways is a fundamental aspect of cancer treatment. While the monotherapy technique remains a prevalent treatment option for several types of cancer, it is typically considered less efficacious compared to the combination therapy approach. Traditional monotherapy approaches indiscriminately attack actively dividing cells, resulting in the elimination of both healthy and malignant cells. Chemotherapy poses a danger to patients because to its toxicity, resulting in many side effects. Additionally, it significantly weakens the immune system by impacting bone marrow cells, making the patient more vulnerable to contracting infections from their environment (Stub et al. 2018). While combination therapy may have toxic effects when one of the medicines employed is chemotherapeutic, the overall toxicity is much reduced due to the targeting of several pathways. Ultimately, this operates in a synergistic or additive fashion, resulting in a reduced therapeutic dose for each particular medicine.

9.4 DRAWBACKS OF CONVENTIONAL CANCER TREATMENT

Conventional chemotherapy largely functions by disrupting the process of DNA synthesis and mitosis, resulting in the death of cancer cells that are actively proliferating and dividing. The drugs exhibit nonselectivity and have the potential to damage healthy normal tissues, resulting in significant unwanted and undesired side effects, such as decreased appetite and nausea. There is a clear correlation between the adverse effects of chemotherapy medications on normal tissues and organs and the high rates of morbidity and death that are reported in cancer patients (Parkin et al. 2001). Moreover, due to the limited ability of these medications to reach tumor tissues, larger amounts are necessary, resulting in heightened toxicity in healthy cells and a greater likelihood of developing resistance to several treatments.

Excessive administration of chemotherapy might result in significant adverse consequences in individuals. Hence, it is crucial to use caution while determining the optimal dose. In the early 1950s, many methods were authorized for estimating personalized chemotherapeutic dose, including the use of body surface area formulas and mathematical calculations based on the patient's weight and height (Corrie 2008). The efficacy of chemotherapeutic drugs is influenced by the concentration of the medication in the patient's circulation, which is determined by several variables, such as metabolism, the state of cancer, interactions between the drug and its target, as well as the physiological and genetic status of the patient (Chakraborty and Rahman 2016). Currently, researchers are endeavoring to develop a formula that enables individual patients to attain the most favorable systemic medication exposure, hence maximizing treatment effectiveness while minimizing harmful consequences.

Side effects mostly arise from the chemotherapy's detrimental impact on the healthy cells responsible for maintaining the body's function and appearance. Various adverse effects manifest based on the characteristics of the medication. For instance, alkylating drugs and antimetabolites exert their effects by directly impairing DNA, therefore inhibiting the replication of cancer cells. Consequently, these treatments might result in lasting harm to the bone marrow, ultimately increasing the risk of developing acute leukemia (Partridge, Burstein, and Winer 2001). Anthracyclines, likewise, are a class of antitumor antibiotics that disrupt the activity of enzymes responsible for DNA replication. These medications are effective at all stages of the cellular division process. An important factor to consider while administering these medications is that prolonged high-dose use might result in irreversible cardiac damage. Therefore, these medications are frequently subject to lifetime dosage restrictions. Similarly, some plant alkaloids and other chemicals produced from natural sources are frequently recognized as mitotic inhibitors. They have the ability to halt mitosis or hinder enzymes responsible for synthesizing essential proteins required for regular cell replication (Burstein 2000). These medications are recognized for their capacity to induce peripheral nerve injury, which may serve as a limiting factor for the dosage due to their adverse effect. Similarly, topoisomerase inhibitors, which induce DNA damage in cancer cells, elicit adverse effects, such as manifestations of hypersensitivity reactions, including rapid heart rate, pruritus or urticaria, facial or hand edema, oral or throat swelling or tingling, chest constriction, and wheezing. Cytotoxic medications possess significant potency, although may give rise to several undesirable adverse reactions. Given that cytotoxic medications primarily function by eliminating cells during their divisional phases, regardless of whether they are healthy or cancerous cells, safeguarding normal cells is crucial during cancer treatment (Aslam et al. 2014).

Acute radiation damage mostly affects cells that are quickly dividing, such as the epithelial surfaces of the skin or digestive system. Radiation causes harm to stem cells, resulting in tissue loss during the natural process of cell turnover (Gilman and Philips 1946). However, the ability of stem cells to adequately replace the lost tissue is compromised due to the damage caused by radiation. This leads to a disruption in the defensive barrier, typically occurring in the skin, oral mucosa, and gastrointestinal system, particularly within one to five years after the conclusion of radiation (Bentzen 2006). As a result, the stem cells undergo compensatory hyperplasia, leading to recovery. Consequently, the symptoms subside within a span of a few weeks. *Consequential late effects* refer to lesions that result from acute damage that does not fully heal and continues to exist in the late phase (Al-Mefty et al. 1990). These effects are typically observed in treatment plans that combine chemotherapy with radiation, when tissues are unable to heal because of the simultaneous toxic effects of chemotherapy.

9.5 ROLE OF NANOTECHNOLOGY IN OVERCOMING THE LIMITATIONS

Traditional therapy approaches provide small challenges, although they exhibit significant adverse effects and unfavorable outcomes in clinical settings. Therefore, there is a need for efficient methods to promptly identify and treat cancer (Milewska et al. 2021). Currently, a wide variety of nanoparticles has captured the attention of researchers as potentially valuable tools for diagnostic tools and medical devices. Due to their intrinsic physicochemical features and customizable surface modification, they can overcome some limitations and achieve the desired diagnostic and therapeutic effects. Nanotechnology is an exceptional discipline that has completely transformed the field and is leading to the development of novel cancer therapies (Chaturvedi et al. 2019). It facilitates more accurate diagnosis with reduced use of dangerous chemicals and is establishing current treatment protocols. Nanotechnology greatly enhances clinical practice in the areas of cancer diagnosis, treatment, and care. Biomaterials possessing unique (bio)physicochemical characteristics have demonstrated the capacity to enhance cellular activity and potentially address illnesses, restore biological processes, or regenerate tissues (Kim, Lee, and Chen 2013).

Nanotechnology has enhanced the precision of drug targeting and the capacity to distribute drugs effectively, improved the availability of drugs in biological systems, increased the sensitivity of diagnostic imaging for detecting biomarkers, and optimized the efficiency of drug delivery. Nanomedicine employs a diverse range of nanoparticles and materials which are selected based on their specific application. The liposomes, dendrimers, polymers, carbon nanotubes, quantum dots, and nanoshells are among the most commonly utilized (Shi et al. 2010).

The three fundamental modalities for cancer treatment are chemotherapy, radiation, and surgery. These procedures are designed to eliminate all cancer cells while minimizing any unintended impact on other types of cells. The majority of medications exhibit significant side effects as a result of their limited target selectivity. However, the development of resistance to existing medications has become a significant barrier in cancer chemotherapy, enabling cancer cells to multiply regardless of the specific chemotherapy treatment being used (Aliosmanoglu 2012). Nanotechnology-based medicinal treatments are a solution to this problem. These therapies will demonstrate significant potential in overcoming resistance, with the majority of nano-based medications currently undergoing clinical evaluation. Nanoparticle-based drug delivery techniques have shown several advantages in cancer treatment, such as favorable pharmacokinetics, precise tumor cell targeting, less side effects, and reduced drug resistance (Zhao et al. 2018).

9.6 CONCLUSION AND FUTURE PROSPECTS

Traditional chemotherapeutic agents exhibit significant adverse effects, such as immune system and organ damage, primarily affecting rapidly dividing cells. These effects arise from their nonselective targeting, poor solubility, and inability to penetrate the central region of tumors. Consequently, treatment efficacy is compromised, necessitating lower doses and resulting in reduced survival rates. Nanotechnology enables targeted and selective access to cancer cells, enhancing medication localization and cellular absorption. Nanoparticles may be engineered to specifically identify malignant cells and deliver drugs with precision, while minimizing any contact with healthy cells. Nanoparticles address the constraints of traditional cancer therapy and surmount multidrug resistance. Furthermore, with the discovery and examination of novel multidrug resistance pathways, there is a growing emphasis on the intensive investigation of nanoparticles. The development of nanoformulations has opened up new possibilities for cancer treatment, with a range of therapeutic applications.

The efficacy and longevity of traditional cancer therapies are contingent upon several elements, such as the specific type and stage of cancer, the patient's general well-being, and the treatment's reaction. While many types of cancer exhibit high remission rates with traditional therapies, others may have lower rates of recovery. The measurement of survival rates commonly uses the concept of five-year survival, which denotes the proportion of patients who remain alive for a period of five years or more following their diagnosis. It is crucial to acknowledge that these rates are always changing as medical research progresses. So there is a need of methods that can enhance the survival rate in cancer patients.

The field of medical science is in a perpetual state of development, with continuing study consistently revealing novel discoveries and breakthroughs in traditional cancer therapies. Scientists and researchers are investigating new methods of therapy, such as targeted immunotherapies, customized medicine, and gene treatments. The purpose of these improvements is to enhance the effectiveness of treatment, reduce the occurrence of adverse effects, and eventually improve the results for patients. The future of cancer treatment has immense potential as we persist in deciphering the intricacies of this ailment. To summarize, traditional approaches to cancer therapy have been crucial in fighting against this widespread illness. Surgery, chemotherapy, radiation treatment, hormone therapy, immunotherapy, targeted therapy, and the integrative approach have all demonstrated effectiveness in various situations. Nevertheless, the efficacy of these therapies fluctuates based on the specific type and stage of cancer, as well as unique patient characteristics. Healthcare practitioners must customize treatment regimens to suit the individual requirements of each patient and diligently track their progress. The future of cancer therapy appears auspicious due to continuous research and technological progress, instilling optimism in patients and their families.

REFERENCES

Abbas, Zaigham, and Sakina Rehman. 2018. *An Overview of Cancer Treatment Modalities*. InTech eBooks. https://doi.org/10.5772/intechopen.76558.

Abe, Osahiko, Rikiya Abe, Kohji Enomoto, K. Kikuchi, Hiroki Koyama, Hiroko Masuda, Yasuo Nomura, et al. 2005. "Effects of Chemotherapy and Hormonal Therapy for Early Breast Cancer on Recurrence and 15-Year Survival: An Overview of the Randomised Trials." *The Lancet* 365 (9472): 1687–717. https://doi.org/10.1016/s0140-6736(05)66544-0.

Aliosmanoglu, Akin. 2012. "Nanotechnology in Cancer Treatment." *Journal of Nanomedicine & Biotherapeutic Discovery* 2 (4). https://doi.org/10.4172/2155-983x.1000107.

Al-Mefty, Ossama, Jane E. Kersh, A. Routh, and Robert R. Smith. 1990. "The Long-Term Side Effects of Radiation Therapy for Benign Brain Tumors in Adults." *Journal of Neurosurgery* 73 (4): 502–12. https://doi.org/10.3171/jns.1990.73.4.0502.

Ansarin, Mohssen, Luigi Santoro, Augusto Cattaneo, Maria Massaro, Luca Calabrese, Gioacchino Giugliano, Fausto Maffini, Angelo Ostuni, and Fausto Chiesa. 2009. "Laser Surgery for Early Glottic Cancer." *Archives of Otolaryngology-Head & Neck Surgery* 135 (4): 385. https://doi.org/10.1001/archoto.2009.10.

Arnold, Herbert, Friedrich Bourseaux, and N. Brock. 1958. "Chemotherapeutic Action of a Cyclic Nitrogen Mustard Phosphamide Ester (B 518-ASTA) in Experimental Tumours of the Rat." *Nature* 181 (4613): 931. https://doi.org/10.1038/181931a0.

Aslam, Muhammad Shahbaz, Sidra Naveed, Aftab Ahmed, Zaigham Abbas, Iram Gull, and Makshoof Athar. 2014. "Side Effects of Chemotherapy in Cancer Patients and Evaluation of Patients Opinion About Starvation Based Differential Chemotherapy." *Journal of Cancer Therapy* 5 (8): 817–22. https://doi.org/10.4236/jct.2014.58089.

Asuncion, Malyn May. 2014. "Antimetabolite Treatment for Pancreatic Cancer." *Chemotherapy* 3 (3). https://doi.org/10.4172/2167-7700.1000137.

Babaian, R. Joseph, Bryan J. Donnelly, Duke Bahn, John G. Baust, Martin Dineen, D. S. Ellis, Aaron E. Katz, et al. 2008. "Best Practice Statement on Cryosurgery for the Treatment of Localized Prostate Cancer." *The Journal of Urology* 180 (5): 1993–2004. https://doi.org/10.1016/j.juro.2008.07.108.

Baskar, Rajamanickam, Kuo Ann Lee, Reuben J. Yeo, and Kheng Wei Yeoh. 2012. "Cancer and Radiation Therapy: Current Advances and Future Directions." *International Journal of Medical Sciences* 9 (3): 193–9. https://doi.org/10.7150/ijms.3635.

Baudino, Troy A. 2015. "Targeted Cancer Therapy: The next Generation of Cancer Treatment." Current *Drug Discovery Technologies* 12 (1): 3–20. https://doi.org/10.2174/1570163812666150602144310.

Bentzen, Søren M. 2006. "Preventing or Reducing Late Side Effects of Radiation Therapy: Radiobiology Meets Molecular Pathology." *Nature Reviews Cancer* 6 (9): 702–13. https://doi.org/10.1038/nrc1950.

Bradley, Jeffrey D., Rebecca Paulus, Ritsuko Komaki, Gregory A. Masters, George R. Blumenschein, Steven E. Schild, Jeffrey A. Bogart, et al. 2015. "Standard-Dose versus High-Dose Conformal Radiotherapy with Concurrent and Consolidation Carboplatin plus Paclitaxel with or without Cetuximab for Patients with Stage IIIA or IIIB Non-Small-Cell Lung Cancer (RTOG 0617): A Randomised, Two-by-Two Factorial Phase 3 Study." *The Lancet Oncology* 16 (2): 187–99. https://doi.org/10.1016/s1470-2045(14)71207-0.

Briukhovetska, Daria, Janina Dörr, Stefan Endres, Peter Libby, Charles A. Dinarello, and Sebastian Kobold. 2021. "Interleukins in Cancer: From Biology to Therapy." *Nature Reviews Cancer* 21 (8): 481–99. https://doi.org/10.1038/s41568-021-00363-z.

Burstein, Harold J. 2000. "Side Effects of Chemotherapy." *Journal of Clinical Oncology* 18 (3): 693. https://doi.org/10.1200/jco.2000.18.3.693.

Carmeliet, Peter. 2005. "VEGF as a Key Mediator of Angiogenesis in Cancer." *Oncology* 69 (Suppl. 3): 4–10. https://doi.org/10.1159/000088478.

Carmeliet, Peter, and Rakesh K. Jain. 2000. "Angiogenesis in Cancer and Other Diseases." *Nature* 407 (6801): 249–57. https://doi.org/10.1038/35025220.

Carpentier, Alain, Sylvain Chauvaud, Jean-Noël Fabiani, A. Deloche, J. Relland, A. Lessana, C. D'Allaines, P. Blondeau, A. Piwnica, and C. Dubost. 1980. "Reconstructive Surgery of Mitral Valve Incompetence." *The Journal of Thoracic and Cardiovascular Surgery* 79 (3): 338–48. https://doi.org/10.1016/s0022-5223(19)37942-5.

Carter, Stephen K., and Robert L. Comis. 1975. "The Integration of Chemotherapy into a Combined Modality Approach for Cancer Treatment." *Cancer Treatment Reviews* 2 (3): 193–214. https://doi.org/10.1016/s0305-7372(75)80003-x.

Chakraborty, Sajib, and Taibur Rahman. 2016. "The Difficulties in Cancer Treatment." *Ecancermedicalscience* (December). https://doi.org/10.3332/ecancer.2012.ed16.

Chaturvedi, Vivek K., Anshuman Singh, Vinay Kumar Singh, and Mohan Singh. 2019. "Cancer Nanotechnology: A New Revolution for Cancer Diagnosis and Therapy." *Current Drug Metabolism* 20 (6): 416–29. https://doi.org/10.2174/1389200219666180918111528.

Chen, Helen H. W., and M. Tien Kuo. 2017. "Improving Radiotherapy in Cancer Treatment: Promises and Challenges." *Oncotarget* 8 (37): 62742–58. https://doi.org/10.18632/oncotarget.18409.

Chen, Jingyang, and JoAnne Stubbe. 2005. "Bleomycins: Towards Better Therapeutics." *Nature Reviews Cancer* 5 (2): 102–12. https://doi.org/10.1038/nrc1547.

Citron, Marc L., Donald A. Berry, Constance Cirrincione, Clifford A. Hudis, Eric P. Winer, William J. Gradishar, Nancy E. Davidson, et al. 2003. "Randomized Trial of Dose-Dense Versus Conventionally

Scheduled and Sequential Versus Concurrent Combination Chemotherapy as Postoperative Adjuvant Treatment of Node-Positive Primary Breast Cancer: First Report of Intergroup Trial C9741/Cancer and Leukemia Group B Trial 9741." *Journal of Clinical Oncology* 21 (8): 1431–9. https://doi.org/10.1200/jco.2003.09.081.

Clarke, Mike, Rory Collins, Sarah C. Darby, Christina Davies, P. Elphinstone, Vaughan Evans, Jon Godwin, et al. 2005. "Effects of Radiotherapy and of Differences in the Extent of Surgery for Early Breast Cancer on Local Recurrence and 15-Year Survival: An Overview of the Randomised Trials." *The Lancet* 366 (9503): 2087–106. https://doi.org/10.1016/s0140-6736(05)67887-7.

Coffey, J. Calvin, J. H. Wang, Myles Smith, David Bouchier-Hayes, Thomas G. Cotter, and H. P. Redmond. 2003. "Excisional Surgery for Cancer Cure: Therapy at a Cost." *The Lancet Oncology* 4 (12): 760–8. https://doi.org/10.1016/s1470-2045(03)01282-8.

Collins, John A., Jennifer Blake, and Pier Giorgio Crosignani. 2005. "Breast Cancer Risk with Postmenopausal Hormonal Treatment." *Human Reproduction Update* 11 (6): 545–60. https://doi.org/10.1093/humupd/dmi028.

Conlon, Kevin C., Miloš D. Miljković, and Thomas A. Waldmann. 2019. "Cytokines in the Treatment of Cancer." *Journal of Interferon and Cytokine Research* 39 (1): 6–21. https://doi.org/10.1089/jir.2018.0019.

Corrie, Pippa. 2008. "Cytotoxic Chemotherapy: Clinical Aspects." *Medicine* 36 (1): 24–8. https://doi.org/10.1016/j.mpmed.2007.10.012.

Cortés, Javier, and Cyntia Coronado. 2007. "Role of Anthracyclines in the Era of Targeted Therapy." *Cardiovascular Toxicology* 7 (2): 56–60. https://doi.org/10.1007/s12012-007-0015-3.

Cox, James D., Jo Ann Stetz, and Thomas F. Pajak. 1995. "Toxicity Criteria of the Radiation Therapy Oncology Group (RTOG) and the European Organization for Research and Treatment of Cancer (EORTC)." *International Journal of Radiation Oncology Biology Physics* 31 (5): 1341–6. https://doi.org/10.1016/0360-3016(95)00060-c.

Creech, Oscar, Edward T. Krementz, Robert F. Ryan, and J. N. Winblad. 1958. "Chemotherapy of Cancer." *Annals of Surgery* 148 (4): 616–32. https://doi.org/10.1097/00000658-195810000-00009.

Delaney, Geoff P., Susannah Jacob, C. Featherstone, and Michael Bartoň. 2005. "The Role of Radiotherapy in Cancer Treatment." *Cancer* 104 (6): 1129–37. https://doi.org/10.1002/cncr.21324.

Demaria, Sandra, Encouse B. Golden, and Silvia C. Formenti. 2015. "Role of Local Radiation Therapy in Cancer Immunotherapy." *JAMA Oncology* 1 (9): 1325. https://doi.org/10.1001/jamaoncol.2015.2756.

Desoize, B. 2004. "Metals and Metal Compounds in Cancer Treatment." *PubMed* 24 (3a): 1529–44. https://pubmed.ncbi.nlm.nih.gov/15274320.

Dhar, Shanta, Frank Gu, Robert Langer, Omid C. Farokhzad, and Stephen J. Lippard. 2008. "Targeted Delivery of Cisplatin to Prostate Cancer Cells by Aptamer Functionalized Pt(IV) Prodrug-PLGA-PEG Nanoparticles." *Proceedings of the National Academy of Sciences of the United States of America* 105 (45): 17356–61. https://doi.org/10.1073/pnas.0809154105.

Dunn, Gavin P., Catherine M. Koebel, and Robert D. Schreiber. 2006. "Interferons, Immunity and Cancer Immunoediting." *Nature Reviews Immunology* 6 (11): 836–48. https://doi.org/10.1038/nri1961.

El-Aziz, Ahmed Shawky Abd, Mohammed A. Nafea, and Abd El-Hafiz Hosny. 2019. "Surgical Reconstruction after Excision of Pilonidal Sinus with Modified Limberg Transposition Flap." *The Egyptian Journal of Hospital Medicine* 77 (4): 5392–8. https://doi.org/10.21608/ejhm.2019.58014.

El-Kenawi, Asmaa, and Azza B. El-Remessy. 2013. "Angiogenesis Inhibitors in Cancer Therapy: Mechanistic Perspective on Classification and Treatment Rationales." *British Journal of Pharmacology* 170 (4): 712–29. https://doi.org/10.1111/bph.12344.

Evans, Audrey E., Sidney Farber, S. Brunet, and Pacita J. Mariano. 1963. "Vincristine in the Treatment of Acute Leukemia in Children." *Cancer* 16 (10): 1302–6. https://doi.org/10.1002/1097-0142(196310)16:10.

Farber, Sidney, and Diamond Lk. 1948. "Temporary Remissions in Acute Leukemia in Children Produced by Folic Acid Antagonist, 4-Aminopteroyl-Glutamic Acid (Aminopterin)." *The New England Journal of Medicine* 238 (23): 787–93. https://doi.org/10.1056/nejm194806032382301.

Fischer, David, M. K. Tish Knobf, Henry J. Durivage, and Nancy J. Beaulieu. 2004. "The Cancer Chemotherapy Handbook." *International Journal of Gynecological Cancer* 14 (1): 181. https://doi.org/10.1111/j.1525-1438.2004.014000.x.

Folkman, Judah. 1995. "Angiogenesis in Cancer, Vascular, Rheumatoid and Other Disease." *Nature Medicine* 1 (1): 27–30. https://doi.org/10.1038/nm0195-27.

Gelmann, Edward P. 1996. "Tamoxifen Induction of Apoptosis in Estrogen Receptor-Negative Cancers: New Tricks for an Old Dog?" *JNCI: Journal of the National Cancer Institute* 88 (5): 224–6. https://doi.org/10.1093/jnci/88.5.224.

Gillison, Maura L., Anil K. Chaturvedi, and Douglas R. Lowy. 2008. "HPV Prophylactic Vaccines and the Potential Prevention of Noncervical Cancers in Both Men and Women." *Cancer* 113 (S10): 3036–46. https://doi.org/10.1002/cncr.23764.

Gilman, Alfred G., and Frederick S. Philips. 1946. "The Biological Actions and Therapeutic Applications of the B-Chloroethyl Amines and Sulfides." *Science* 103 (2675): 409–36. https://doi.org/10.1126/science.103.2675.409.

Golding, Stephen J., and Paul Shrimpton. 2002. "Radiation Dose in CT: Are We Meeting the Challenge?" *British Journal of Radiology* 75 (889): 1–4. https://doi.org/10.1259/bjr.75.889.750001.

Gottesman, Michael M. 2002. "Mechanisms of Cancer Drug Resistance." *Annual Review of Medicine* 53 (1): 615–27. https://doi.org/10.1146/annurev.med.53.082901.103929.

Graham, Kaitlin, and Evan C. Unger. 2018. "Overcoming Tumor Hypoxia as a Barrier to Radiotherapy, Chemotherapy and Immunotherapy in Cancer Treatment." *International Journal of Nanomedicine* 13 (October): 6049–58. https://doi.org/10.2147/ijn.s140462.

Hallissey, M. T., W. H. Allum, J. W. L. Fielding, and Claudia Roginski. 1988. "Palliative Surgery for Gastric Cancer." *Cancer* 62 (2): 440–4. https://doi.org/10.1002/1097-0142(19880715)62:2.

Han, Kathy, Michael Milosevic, Anthony Fyles, Melania Pintilie, and Akila Viswanathan. 2013. "Trends in the Utilization of Brachytherapy in Cervical Cancer in the United States." *International Journal of Radiation Oncology Biology Physics* 87 (1): 111–19. https://doi.org/10.1016/j.ijrobp.2013.05.033.

Hawkins, Michael M., Lisa Wilson, Hazel S. Burton, Michael H. N. Potok, D. Winter, H. B. Marsden, and Marilyn Stovall. 1996. "Radiotherapy, Alkylating Agents, and Risk of Bone Cancer after Childhood Cancer." *JNCI: Journal of the National Cancer Institute* 88 (5): 270–8. https://doi.org/10.1093/jnci/88.5.270.

Hilaris, Basil S., and Nael Martini. 1979. "Interstitial Brachytherapy in Cancer of the Lung: A 20 Year Experience." *International Journal of Radiation Oncology Biology Physics* 5 (11–12): 1951–6. https://doi.org/10.1016/0360-3016(79)90944-1.

Hirsch, Heather A., Dimitrios Iliopoulos, Philip N. Tsichlis, and Kevin Struhl. 2009. "Metformin Selectively Targets Cancer Stem Cells, and Acts Together with Chemotherapy to Block Tumor Growth and Prolong Remission." *Cancer Research* 69 (19): 7507–11. https://doi.org/10.1158/0008-5472.can-09-2994.

Howell, Anthony, Gustavo Calado De Aguiar Ribeiro, and Ric Swindell. 1992. "Systemic Treatment of Early Breast Cancer by Hormonal, Cytotoxic, or Immune Therapy." *The Lancet* 339 (8785): 71–85. https://doi.org/10.1016/0140-6736(92)90997-h.

Hughes, Kevin S., J. Scheele, and Paul H. Sugarbaker. 1989. "Surgery for Colorectal Cancer Metastatic to the Liver: Optimizing the Results of Treatment." *Surgical Clinics of North America* 69 (2): 339–59. https://doi.org/10.1016/s0039-6109(16)44790-0.

Jänicke, F., A. Search Holscher, Walther Kuhn, R. Von Hugo, L. Pache, J. R. Siewert, and Henner Graef. 1992. "Radical Surgical Procedure Improves Survival Time in Patients with Recurrent Ovarian Cancer." *Cancer* 70 (8): 2129–36. https://doi.org/10.1002/1097-0142(19921015)70:8.

Jayakar, Prasanna, William D. Gaillard, Manjari Tripathi, Mark H. Libenson, Gary W. Mathern, and J. Helen Cross. 2014. "Diagnostic Test Utilization in Evaluation for Resective Epilepsy Surgery in Children." *Epilepsia* 55 (4): 507–18. https://doi.org/10.1111/epi.12544.

Johnson, Skyler B., Henry S. Park, Cary P. Gross, and James B. Yu. 2018. "Complementary Medicine, Refusal of Conventional Cancer Therapy, and Survival among Patients with Curable Cancers." *JAMA Oncology* 4 (10): 1375. https://doi.org/10.1001/jamaoncol.2018.2487.

Joiner, Michael C., and Albert J. Van Der Kogel. 2009. *Basic Clinical Radiobiology*. CRC Press eBooks. https://doi.org/10.1201/b15450.

Kèlland, Lloyd R. 2007. "The Resurgence of Platinum-Based Cancer Chemotherapy." *Nature Reviews Cancer* 7 (8): 573–84. https://doi.org/10.1038/nrc2167.

Kim, Tae Hyung, Seulki Lee, and Xiaoyuan Chen. 2013. "Nanotheranostics for Personalized Medicine." *Expert Review of Molecular Diagnostics* 13 (3): 257–69. https://doi.org/10.1586/erm.13.15.

Kirkwood, John M., Lisa H. Butterfield, Ahmad A. Tarhini, Hassane M. Zarour, Paweł Kaliński, and Soldano Ferrone. 2012. "Immunotherapy of Cancer in 2012." *CA: A Cancer Journal for Clinicians* 62 (5): 309–35. https://doi.org/10.3322/caac.20132.

Kirkwood, John M., and Marc S. Ernstoff. 1984. "Interferons in the Treatment of Human Cancer." *Journal of Clinical Oncology* 2 (4): 336–52. https://doi.org/10.1200/jco.1984.2.4.336.

Kuflik, Emanuel G., and Andrew A. Gage. 1991. "The Five-Year Cure Rate Achieved by Cryosurgery for Skin Cancer." *Journal of the American Academy of Dermatology* 24 (6): 1002–4. https://doi.org/10.1016/0190-9622(91)70160-4.

Larsen, Annette K., Alexandre E. Escargueil, and Andrzej Składanowski. 2003. "Catalytic Topoisomerase II Inhibitors in Cancer Therapy." *Pharmacology & Therapeutics* 99 (2): 167–81. https://doi.org/10.1016/s0163-7258(03)00058-5.

Leen, Ann M., Cliona M. Rooney, and Aaron E. Foster. 2007. "Improving T Cell Therapy for Cancer." *Annual Review of Immunology* 25 (1): 243–65. https://doi.org/10.1146/annurev.immunol.25.022106.141527.

Lin, Kai-Ti, and Lu-Hai Wang. 2016. "New Dimension of Glucocorticoids in Cancer Treatment." *Steroids* 111 (July): 84–8. https://doi.org/10.1016/j.steroids.2016.02.019.

Lucas, David M., Patrick C. Still, Lynette Bueno Pérez, Michael R. Grever, and A. Douglas Kinghorn. 2010. "Potential of Plant-Derived Natural Products in the Treatment of Leukemia and Lymphoma." *Current Drug Targets* 11 (7): 812–22. https://doi.org/10.2174/138945010791320809.

Markman, Maurie. 2003. "Cancer Medicine 6." *Cancer* 98 (11): 2521. https://doi.org/10.1002/cncr.11824.

Mattiuzzi, Camilla, and Giuseppe Lippi. 2019. "Current Cancer Epidemiology." *Journal of Epidemiology and Global Health* 9 (4): 217. https://doi.org/10.2991/jegh.k.191008.001.

Mayles, Philip, A. Nahum, and Jean-Claude Rosenwald. 2007. *Handbook of Radiotherapy Physics*. CRC Press eBooks. https://doi.org/10.1201/9781420012026.

Melamed, Alexander, Roni Nitecki, David M. Boruta, Marcela G. Del Carmen, Rachel M. Clark, Whitfield B. Growdon, Annekathryn Goodman, John O. Schorge, and J. Alejandro Rauh-Hain. 2017. "Laparoscopy Compared with Laparotomy for Debulking Ovarian Cancer after Neoadjuvant Chemotherapy." *Obstetrics & Gynecology* 129 (5): 861–9. https://doi.org/10.1097/aog.0000000000001851.

Milewska, Sylwia, Katarzyna Niemirowicz-Laskowska, Gabriela Siemiaszko, Piotr Nowicki, Agnieszka Z. Wilczewska, and Halina Car. 2021. "Current Trends and Challenges in Pharmacoeconomic Aspects of Nanocarriers as Drug Delivery Systems for Cancer Treatment." *International Journal of Nanomedicine* 16 (September): 6593–644. https://doi.org/10.2147/ijn.s323831.

Miller, Kimberly D., Rebecca L. Siegel, Chun Chieh Lin, Angela B. Mariotto, Joan L. Kramer, Julia H. Rowland, Kevin Stein, Rick Alteri, and Ahmedin Jemal. 2016. "Cancer Treatment and Survivorship Statistics, 2016." *CA: A Cancer Journal for Clinicians* 66 (4): 271–89. https://doi.org/10.3322/caac.21349.

Mirault, Marc-Edouard, P. Boucher, and Alain Tremblay. 2006. "Nucleotide-Resolution Mapping of Topoisomerase-Mediated and Apoptotic DNA Strand Scissions at or near an MLL Translocation Hotspot." *The American Journal of Human Genetics* 79 (5): 779–91. https://doi.org/10.1086/507791.

Mukhtar, Eiman, Vaqar M. Adhami, and Hasan Mukhtar. 2014. "Targeting Microtubules by Natural Agents for Cancer Therapy." *Molecular Cancer Therapeutics* 13 (2): 275–84. https://doi.org/10.1158/1535-7163.mct-13-0791.

Muscaritoli, Maurizio, Maurizio Bossola, Zaira Aversa, Rocco Domenico Alfonso Bellantone, and Filippo Rossi Fanelli. 2006. "Prevention and Treatment of Cancer Cachexia: New Insights into an Old Problem." *European Journal of Cancer* 42 (1): 31–41. https://doi.org/10.1016/j.ejca.2005.07.026.

Obradović, Milan, Baptiste Hamelin, Nenad Manevski, Joana Couto, Atul Sethi, Marie-May Coissieux, Simone Münst, et al. 2019. "Glucocorticoids Promote Breast Cancer Metastasis." *Nature* 567 (7749): 540–4. https://doi.org/10.1038/s41586-019-1019-4.

Ohlsson, Björn, U. Breland, Henrik Ekberg, Hans Graffner, and Karl-Göran Tranberg. 1995. "Follow-Up After Curative Surgery for Colorectal Carcinoma." *Diseases of the Colon & Rectum* 38 (6): 619–26. https://doi.org/10.1007/bf02054122.

Orr, James W., Pamela F. Orr, and Peyton T. Taylor. 1996. "Surgical Staging Endometrial Cancer." *Clinical Obstetrics and Gynecology* 39 (3): 656–68. https://doi.org/10.1097/00003081-199609000-00014.

Parker, William B. 2009. "Enzymology of Purine and Pyrimidine Antimetabolites Used in the Treatment of Cancer." *Chemical Reviews* 109 (7): 2880–93. https://doi.org/10.1021/cr900028p.

Parkin, D. Maxwell, Freddie Bray, Jacques Ferlay, and Paola Pisani. 2001. "Estimating the World Cancer Burden: Globocan 2000." *International Journal of Cancer* 94 (2): 153–6. https://doi.org/10.1002/ijc.1440.

Partridge, Ann H., Harold J. Burstein, and Eric P. Winer. 2001. "Side Effects of Chemotherapy and Combined Chemohormonal Therapy in Women with Early-Stage Breast Cancer." *Journal of the National Cancer Institute Monographs* 2001 (30): 135–42. https://doi.org/10.1093/oxfordjournals.jncimonographs.a003451.

Pellegrino, A., Robert Fruscio, Andrea Maneo, Silvia Corso, Marco Battistello, Valentina Chiappa, and M. Stomati. 2008. "Harmonic Scalpel versus Conventional Electrosurgery in the Treatment of Vulvar Cancer." *International Journal of Gynecology & Obstetrics* 103 (2): 185–8. https://doi.org/10.1016/j.ijgo.2008.07.004.

Pérez-Herrero, Edgar, and Alberto Fernández-Medarde. 2015. "Advanced Targeted Therapies in Cancer: Drug Nanocarriers, the Future of Chemotherapy." *European Journal of Pharmaceutics and Biopharmaceutics* 93 (June): 52–79. https://doi.org/10.1016/j.ejpb.2015.03.018.

Perros, Petros, Kristien Boelaert, Steve Colley, Carol Evans, Rhordi M. Evans, Georgina Gerrard Ba, Jackie Gilbert, et al. 2014. "Guidelines for the Management of Thyroid Cancer." *Clinical Endocrinology* 81 (s1): 1–122. https://doi.org/10.1111/cen.12515.

Pommier, Yves. 2006. "Topoisomerase I Inhibitors: Camptothecins and Beyond." *Nature Reviews Cancer* 6 (10): 789–802. https://doi.org/10.1038/nrc1977.

Ralhan, Ranju, and Jasbir Kaur. 2007. "Alkylating Agents and Cancer Therapy." *Expert Opinion on Therapeutic Patents* 17 (9): 1061–75. https://doi.org/10.1517/13543776.17.9.1061.

Ramesha, B. T., H. K. Suma, Senthilkumar Umapathy, V. Priti, G. Ravikanth, R. Vasudeva, T. R. Santhosh Kumar, K. N. Ganeshaiah, and R. Uma Shaanker. 2013. "New Plant Sources of the Anti-Cancer Alkaloid, Camptothecine from the Icacinaceae Taxa, India." *Phytomedicine* 20 (6): 521–7. https://doi.org/10.1016/j.phymed.2012.12.003.

Ramjiawan, Rakesh R., Arjan W. Griffioen, and Dan G. Duda. 2017. "Anti-Angiogenesis for Cancer Revisited: Is There a Role for Combinations with Immunotherapy?" *Angiogenesis* 20 (2): 185–204. https://doi.org/10.1007/s10456-017-9552-y.

Restifo, Nicholas P., Mark E. Dudley, and Steven A. Rosenberg. 2012. "Adoptive Immunotherapy for Cancer: Harnessing the T Cell Response." *Nature Reviews Immunology* 12 (4): 269–81. https://doi.org/10.1038/nri3191.

Rosenberg, Barnett, Loretta Van Camp, and Thomas Krigas. 1965. "Inhibition of Cell Division in Escherichia Coli by Electrolysis Products from a Platinum Electrode." *Nature* 205 (4972): 698–9. https://doi.org/10.1038/205698a0.

Saraiya, Mona, Elizabeth R. Unger, Trevor Thompson, Charles F. Lynch, Brenda Y. Hernandez, Cancan Lyu, Martin Steinau, et al. 2015. "US Assessment of HPV Types in Cancers: Implications for Current and 9-Valent HPV Vaccines." *JNCI: Journal of the National Cancer Institute* 107 (6). https://doi.org/10.1093/jnci/djv086.

Scagliotti, Giorgio V., and Giovanni Selvaggi. 2006. "Antimetabolites and Cancer: Emerging Data with a Focus on Antifolates." *Expert Opinion on Therapeutic Patents* 16 (2): 189–200. https://doi.org/10.1517/13543776.16.2.189.

Scheuer, Lauren, Noah D. Kauff, Mark E. Robson, Bridget B. Kelly, Richard R. Barakat, Jaya M. Satagopan, Nathan A. Ellis, et al. 2002. "Outcome of Preventive Surgery and Screening for Breast and Ovarian Cancer in BRCA Mutation Carriers." *Journal of Clinical Oncology* 20 (5): 1260–8. https://doi.org/10.1200/jco.2002.20.5.1260.

Schirrmacher, Volker. 2018. "From Chemotherapy to Biological Therapy: A Review of Novel Concepts to Reduce the Side Effects of Systemic Cancer Treatment (Review)." *International Journal of Oncology* 54 (2): 407–19. https://doi.org/10.3892/ijo.2018.4661.

Shepard, David, Michael C. Ferris, G. Olivera, and Thomas Rockwell Mackie. 1999. "Optimizing the Delivery of Radiation Therapy to Cancer Patients." *Siam Review* 41 (4): 721–44. https://doi.org/10.1137/s0036144598342032.

Sheridan, Adam T., and R. P. R. Dawber. 2000. "Curettage, Electrosurgery and Skin Cancer." *Australasian Journal of Dermatology* 41 (1): 19–30. https://doi.org/10.1046/j.1440-0960.2000.00383.x.

Shi, Jinjun, Alexander R. Votruba, Omid C. Farokhzad, and Robert Langer. 2010. "Nanotechnology in Drug Delivery and Tissue Engineering: From Discovery to Applications." *Nano Letters* 10 (9): 3223–30. https://doi.org/10.1021/nl102184c.

Singletary, S. Eva, Garrett L. Walsh, Jean-Nicolas Vauthey, Steven A. Curley, Raymond Sawaya, Kristin L. Weber, Funda Meric, and Gabriel N. Hortobágyi. 2003. "A Role for Curative Surgery in the Treatment of Selected Patients with Metastatic Breast Cancer." *Oncologist* 8 (3): 241–51. https://doi.org/10.1634/theoncologist.8-3-241.

Skowronek, Janusz. 2017. "Current Status of Brachytherapy in Cancer Treatment—Short Overview." *Journal of Contemporary Brachytherapy* 9 (6): 581–9. https://doi.org/10.5114/jcb.2017.72607.

Spranger, Stefani. 2016. "Mechanisms of Tumor Escape in the Context of the T-Cell-Inflamed and the Non-T-Cell-Inflamed Tumor Microenvironment." *International Immunology* 28 (8): 383–91. https://doi.org/10.1093/intimm/dxw014.

Strnad, Vratislav, Oliver J. Ott, Richard Pötter, Guido Hildebrandt, J. Hammer, Alexandra Resch, Michael Lotter, S. Ackermann, Matthias W. Beckmann, and Rolf Sauer. 2004. "Interstitial Brachytherapy Alone after Breast Conserving Surgery: Interim Results of a German-Austrian Multicenter Phase II Trial." *Brachytherapy* 3 (3): 115–19. https://doi.org/10.1016/j.brachy.2004.08.003.

Stub, Trine, Sara A. Quandt, Thomas A. Arcury, Joanne C. Sandberg, and Agnete Egilsdatter Kristoffersen. 2018. "Conventional and Complementary Cancer Treatments: Where Do Conventional and Complementary

Providers Seek Information About These Modalities?" *BMC Health Services Research* 18 (1). https://doi.org/10.1186/s12913-018-3674-9.

Tascilar, Metin, Floris A. De Jong, Jaap Verweij, and Ron H. J. Mathijssen. 2006. "Complementary and Alternative Medicine during Cancer Treatment: Beyond Innocence." *Oncologist* 11 (7): 732–41. https://doi.org/10.1634/theoncologist.11-7-732.

Taylor, Carolyn, Zhe Wang, Elizabeth Macaulay, Reshma Jagsi, F. Duane, and Sarah C. Darby. 2015. "Exposure of the Heart in Breast Cancer Radiation Therapy: A Systematic Review of Heart Doses Published During 2003 to 2013." *International Journal of Radiation Oncology Biology Physics* 93 (4): 845–53. https://doi.org/10.1016/j.ijrobp.2015.07.2292.

Timmerman, Robert, Rebecca Paulus, James M. Galvin, J. Michalski, William L. Straube, Jeffrey D. Bradley, Achilles J. Fakiris, et al. 2010. "Stereotactic Body Radiation Therapy for Inoperable Early Stage Lung Cancer." *JAMA* 303 (11): 1070. https://doi.org/10.1001/jama.2010.261.

Tohme, Samer, Richard L. Simmons, and Allan Tsung. 2017. "Surgery for Cancer: A Trigger for Metastases." *Cancer Research* 77 (7): 1548–52. https://doi.org/10.1158/0008-5472.can-16-1536.

Trifilio, Steven, Alfred Rademaker, Diane Newman, Katherine Coyle, Katrin M. Carlson-Leuer, Jayesh Mehta, Jessica K. Altman, Olga Frankfurt, and Martin S. Tallman. 2012. "Mitoxantrone and Etoposide with or without Intermediate Dose Cytarabine for the Treatment of Primary Induction Failure or Relapsed Acute Myeloid Leukemia." *Leukemia Research* 36 (4): 394–6. https://doi.org/10.1016/j.leukres.2011.10.027.

Van Der Burg, M. E. L., M. Van Lent, Marc Buyse, A. Kobierska, Nicoletta Colombo, G. Favalli, Ángel J. Lacave, Mario Nardi, Josette Rénard, and Sërgio Pecorelli. 1995. "The Effect of Debulking Surgery after Induction Chemotherapy on the Prognosis in Advanced Epithelial Ovarian Cancer." *The New England Journal of Medicine* 332 (10): 629–34. https://doi.org/10.1056/nejm199503093321002.

Vanneman, Matthew W., and Glenn Dranoff. 2012. "Combining Immunotherapy and Targeted Therapies in Cancer Treatment." *Nature Reviews Cancer* 12 (4): 237–51. https://doi.org/10.1038/nrc3237.

Van Weelden, Willem Jan, Leon F. A. G. Massuger, Enitec, Johanna M. A. Pijnenborg, and Andrea Romano. 2019. "Anti-Estrogen Treatment in Endometrial Cancer: A Systematic Review." *Frontiers in Oncology* 9 (May). https://doi.org/10.3389/fonc.2019.00359.

Waks, Adrienne G., and Eric P. Winer. 2019. "Breast Cancer Treatment." *JAMA* 321 (3): 288. https://doi.org/10.1001/jama.2018.19323.

Wall, Monroe E., Mansukh Wani, Clarence Cook, Kh Palmer, A. T. McPhail, and G. A. Sim. 1966. "Plant Antitumor Agents. I. The Isolation and Structure of Camptothecin, a Novel Alkaloidal Leukemia and Tumor Inhibitor from Camptotheca Acuminata1,2." *Journal of the American Chemical Society* 88 (16): 3888–90. https://doi.org/10.1021/ja00968a057.

Wasserman, Todd H., Milan Slavik, and Stephen K. Carter. 1975. "Clinical Comparison of the Nitrosoureas." *Cancer* 36 (4): 1258–68. https://doi.org/10.1002/1097-0142(197510)36:4.

Willers, Henning, Christopher G. Azzoli, Wil L. Santivasi, and Fang Xia. 2013. "Basic Mechanisms of Therapeutic Resistance to Radiation and Chemotherapy in Lung Cancer." *The Cancer Journal* 19 (3): 200–7. https://doi.org/10.1097/ppo.0b013e318292e4e3.

Wolpin, Brian M., and Robert J. Mayer. 2008. "Systemic Treatment of Colorectal Cancer." *Gastroenterology* 134 (5): 1296–310.e1. https://doi.org/10.1053/j.gastro.2008.02.098.

Yang, James Chih-Hsin, and Steven A. Rosenberg. 2016. "Adoptive T-Cell Therapy for Cancer." *Advances in Immunology*: 279–94. https://doi.org/10.1016/bs.ai.2015.12.006.

Zeléfsky, Michael J., Zvi Fuks, Margie Hunt, Yoshiya Yamada, C. Marion, C. Clifton Ling, H. Amols, Ennapadam Venkatraman, and Steven A. Leibel. 2002. "High-Dose Intensity Modulated Radiation Therapy for Prostate Cancer: Early Toxicity and Biochemical Outcome in 772 Patients." *International Journal of Radiation Oncology Biology Physics* 53 (5): 1111–16. https://doi.org/10.1016/s0360-3016(02)02857-2.

Zelnak, Amelia. 2007. "Clinical Pharmacology and Use of Microtubule-Targeting Agents in Cancer Therapy." *Methods in Molecular Medicine*: 209–34. https://doi.org/10.1007/978-1-59745-442-1_15.

Zhao, Chenyang, Rui Cheng, Zhe Yang, and Zhongmin Tian. 2018. "Nanotechnology for Cancer Therapy Based on Chemotherapy." *Molecules* 23 (4): 826. https://doi.org/10.3390/molecules23040826.

10 Exploring the Nanoparticles in Cancer Treatment

Priyanka Chambial, Dr. Christy Thomas, and Neelam Thakur

ABBREVIATIONS

Acronym	Full Form
NPs	nanoparticles
EPR	enhanced permeability and retention effect
TME	tumor microenvironment
MRI	magnetic resonance imaging
FDA	Food and Drug Administration
MNPs	magnetic nanoparticles
FA	folic acid
PSMA	prostate-specific membrane antigen
PtNPs	platinum nanoparticles
NSCLC	non–small cell lung cancer
PNPs	polymeric nanoparticles
QDs	quantum dots

10.1 INTRODUCTION

Cancer death and incidence rates are both expanding worldwide. GLOBOCAN 2022 predicts that between 2022 and 2040, the number of cancer cases in India will increase from 1.08 million to 2.08 million (Sung et al. 2021). In 2022, the United States experienced 609,360 fatalities due to cancer, with an estimated 1.9 million new cancer cases anticipated to be diagnosed during that year (Siegel et al. 2022). While oncology is currently the most visible and early adopter of nanotechnology in the medical field, it is expected that other fields will benefit in the future. *Nanotechnology* refers to the process of creating products at the atomic and molecular levels (Alenazi 2016). The field of nanotechnology has shown considerable promise in drug delivery, gene therapy, and biomarker imaging for the treatment of cancer. Different types of nanoparticles and their properties are shown in Figure 10.1. To detect cancer at its molecular level, scientists use quantum dots (QDs) and gold nanoparticles (Misra, Acharya, and Sahoo 2010). These nanoparticles are at the center of molecular diagnostic approaches, such as the detection of biomarkers, that allow for rapid and accurate tumor diagnosis (Morales and Grodzinski 2023). Nanotechnology has changed the face of cancer research by facilitating the rapid and precise identification of chemicals and molecular abnormalities linked to cancer (J. Zhang, Chen, and Chen 2024). The high surface-to-volume ratio of nanoparticles is one of their main benefits since it increases their interactions with their intended molecules. Coating nanoparticles with chemicals like polyethylene glycol (PEG), fluorescent probes, andaptamers can improve their functionality. These coatings have a variety of functions, including enhanced targeting, increased stability, and cancer cell detection and imaging. This improves the bioassay's sensitivity and specificity (Jin et al. 2020).

DOI: 10.1201/9781003463191-13

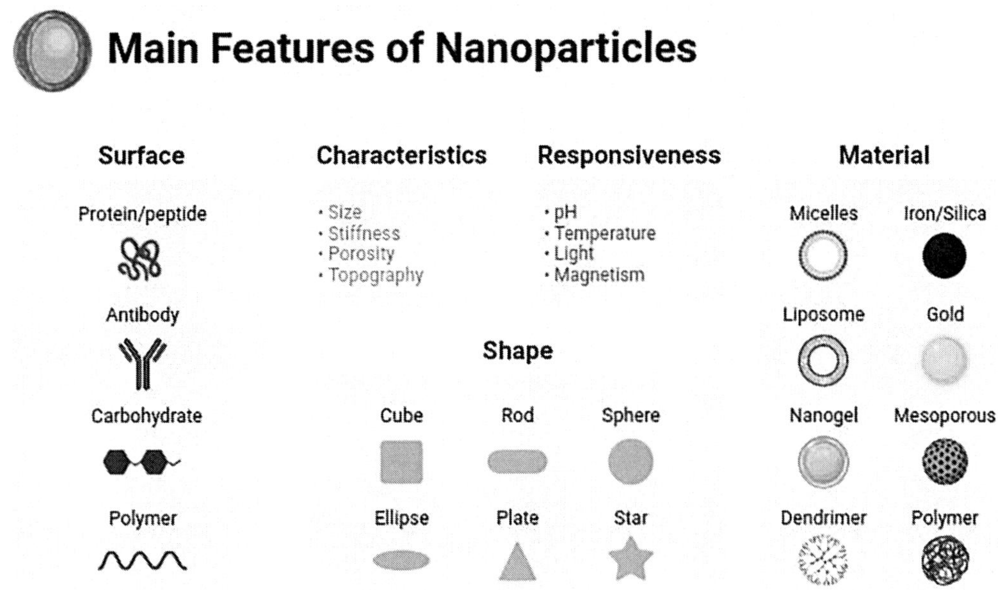

FIGURE 10.1 Different characteristics, shapes, and properties of nanoparticles (NPs) in cancer treatment. Nanoparticles have different shapes, such as sphere, rod, cube, star, etc., and possess different properties. They are stimuli-responsive.

Chemotherapy, gene therapy, radiation, and immunotherapy are all examples of nanoparticle-based approaches to cancer treatment. Since chemotherapy is supplied directly to cancer cells, it is more effective and has fewer adverse effects than other cancer treatments. Enhanced permeability and retention effect (EPR) is often achieved through the use of passive targeting (B. Kumar et al. 2018).

Nanotechnology has enormous applications as nanomedicine in clinical settings. Some of them available for cancer treatment using nanotechnology are mentioned in Table 10.1. This review describes several types of nanoparticles used to treat cancer: (1) Nanoshells and gold nanoparticles (AuNSs) are two examples of how nanoscience could be used to solve biological issues (Mundekkad and Cho 2022). (2) QDs are semiconductor nanocrystals with exceptional physical features (Naik et al. 2022). Their ability to penetrate tissues deeply is due to their surface plasmon resonance, which may be adjusted to the near-infrared. Significant progress has been made in in vivo and cellular molecular imaging using quantum dot–based probes (Zhao et al. 2016). The use of quantum dot–based technologies to cure cancer has been shown to have promise, according to research. (3) Dendrimers are one-of-a-kind nanostructures because of their spherical three-dimensional nature, nanometric size range, and monodisperse unimicellar character. To avoid unwanted side effects, powerful medications like doxorubicin have been delivered via dendrimers (Martins, LaGrow, and Prior 2022). (4) Liposomal nanoparticles are nanostructures that target cancer cells by attaching ligands to their surfaces. The lipid bilayers of liposomal nanoparticles can encapsulate medications, making them more stable and resistant to breakdown. When applied to cancer treatment, liposomal nanoparticles have demonstrated encouraging results thus far (Nsairat et al. 2022). Therapeutic and diagnostic compounds can be designed to target cancer cells in particular. Liposomes significantly improve medication solubility. They shield the drug from pH changes and extend the half-life of the drug in the body (Yao et al. 2020). It is common practice to use medications like irinotecan,

TABLE 10.1
Currently Available Cancer Treatments That Use Nanotechnology

Product Name	Formulation	Indication	Approval	References
Eligard	Leuprolide acetate	Prostate cancer	USA (2004)	Stinchcombe et al. (2007)
Abraxane	Albumin-bound paclitaxel	Pancreatic cancer	USA (2005)	Stinchcombe et al. (2007)
Lipusu	Liposomal paclitaxel	Breast and cell lung cancer	China (2006)	Q. Zhang, Huang, and Gao (2009)
Oncaspar	L-asparaginase conjugate	Acute lymphoblastic leukemia	USA (2006)	Lin et al. (2016)
NanoTherm	Iron oxide NPs	Brain tumors	Europe (2011)	Lin et al. (2016)
ONIVYDE	Liposomal irinotecan	Advanced pancreatic cancer	US (2015)	Blair (2018)
Genexal PM	Paclitaxel micelles	Breast cancer	Korea (2007)	Blair (2018)
Cyclosert	Cyclodextrin	Solid tumors	USA (2017)	Farjadian et al. (2019)
Apealea	Paclitaxel micellar	Ovarian, peritoneal, and fallopian tube cancer	Europe (2018)	Salvioni et al. (2019)
Hensify	Hafnium oxide NPs	Locally advanced soft tissue sarcoma	Europe (2019)	Salvioni et al. (2019)
Paclical	Paclitaxel NPs	Ovarian cancer	Phase III completed	Jin et al. (2020)
AstraZeneca	Durvalumab	Biliary tract cancer/ gastrointestinal cancer	Trials	Tokunaga et al. (2021)

paclitaxel, daunorubicin, cytarabine, and mitoxantrone while employing liposome delivery. (5) Carbon nanotubes, which are burned graphite cylinders with hollow interiors, have distinct features that make them interesting candidates for biomolecule and drug delivery transporters (Bozzuto and Molinari 2015).

10.2 EFFECTIVENESS OF NANOPARTICLES IN CANCER TREATMENT OVER CONVENTIONAL APPROACHES, CONVENTIONAL CANCER TREATMENTS

Conventional chemotherapy has some limitations, both in terms of efficiency and unwanted effects, due to cytotoxicity and unequal dispersion. Therefore, cautious dosing is required for effective cancer cell destruction without substantially increasing toxicity. Many barriers stand between the medicine and its intended recipient. Chemotherapy is typically used as a first line of defense against tumors. DNA damage is an unfortunate side effect of conventional chemotherapeutic drugs, such as antimetabolites, topoisomerase inhibitors, alkylating agents, mitotic inhibitors, and antibiotics (Miller, Samec, and Alexander-Bryant 2021). Although traditional chemotherapies are highly effective, patients are harmed by their lack of specificity. Although they kill some cancer cells, conventional chemotherapies kill many healthy cells in the process (Figure 10.2) and have a much greater negative impact on the patient's health. There are many different inhibitors out there aimed at targeting the enzymes in these signaling pathways. Protein synthesis and glucose metabolism are both influenced by hyperactivation of the phosphoinositide 3-kinase (PI3K) and the mammalian

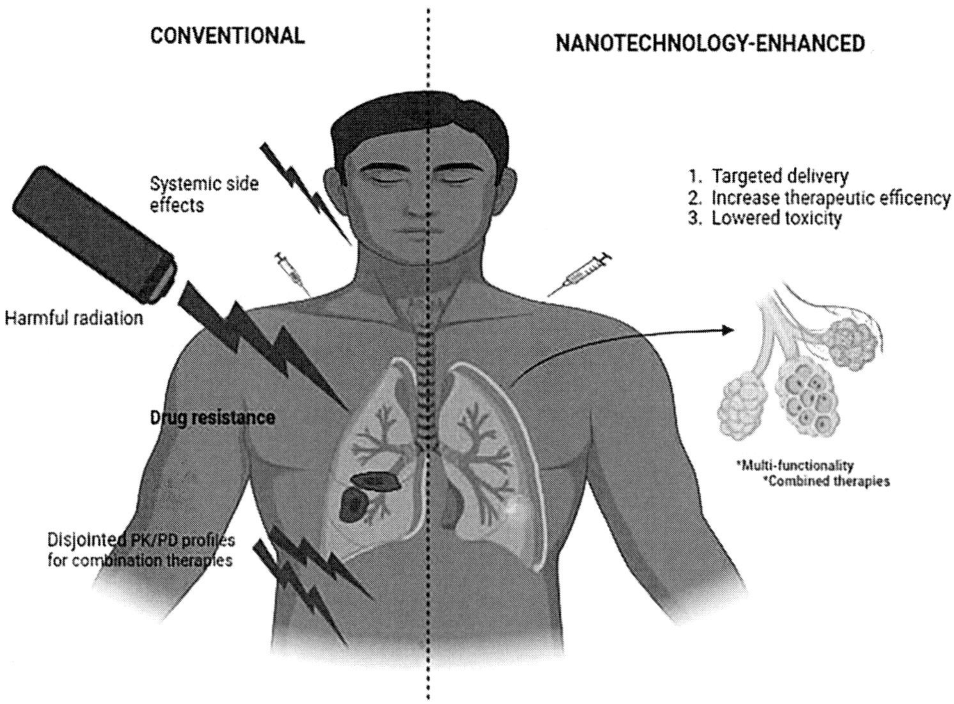

FIGURE 10.2 Compared to traditional anticancer medications, radiation therapy, diagnostics, and imaging, nanotechnology offers many benefits. Nanomedicines can reduce systemic toxicity while boosting therapeutic effectiveness at the target site by using tailored delivery. Certain nanomaterials have inherent physicochemical characteristics that improve bioimaging, localize radiation therapy, enable multimodal treatments, and make early diagnosis and medication resistance possible.

Source: Bashraheel, Domling, and Goda (2020).

target of the rapamycin pathway (Navya et al. 2019). The RAS/RAF/MEK/ERK pathway plays a crucial role in the initiation of cell division, proliferation, and development, making mutations in this system a common finding in a wide variety of malignancies (Duffy et al. 2014). The FDA of the United States has approved sotorasib as the first medicine to target KRAS (Kirsten rat sarcoma virus oncogene homolog). His-RAS (Ha-ras tagged with histidine) protein mutations are frequently linked to human malignancies (M. Chen et al. 2010).

10.3 IMPROVED CANCER TREATMENT USING NANOTECHNOLOGY

Active or passive targeting using NPs increases medication concentrations inside cells while decreasing off-target toxicity (Calixto et al. 2016). To initiate and control medication release, the NPs might be designed to react to changes in pH or temperature (Wells et al. 2019). Medication can be delivered to the TME, despite its acidic environment, using a pH-sensitive drug delivery strategy. NPs are carriers; therefore, they protect their payload from deterioration, which makes the drug more stable. Large quantities of medications can be stored inside without fear of chemical change. The abnormal pathophysiology of tumors includes things like leaky blood vessels, too much new blood vessel growth (angiogenesis), and blocked lymphatic vessels (Georgakopoulou, Stebbing, and Scully 2018). Because of these characteristics, the NPs can be directed to tumors. Oral, nasal, intravenous, and other routes of administration are all viable options for nanoparticles. NPs are easily absorbed by cells due to their high surface-area-to-volume ratio. According to studies, NPs are far more effective than microparticles.

10.4 NANOPARTICLES IN CANCER TREATMENT

10.4.1 Nanoliposomes

Liposomes exhibit several favorable characteristics, such as being compatible with living organisms and capable of undergoing natural degradation. These attributes render them well-suited for utilization in many biological applications (Sell et al. 2023). Liposomes consist of naturally occurring phospholipids that closely resemble the lipid bilayers present in cell membranes. Liposomes possess a high degree of similarity that enables them to effectively interact with biological systems, hence reducing the likelihood of unfavorable responses. In addition, liposomes may be readily altered to improve their durability, selectively target particular cells or tissues, and regulate the release of drugs. In general, liposomes are regarded as harmless and non-toxic, exhibiting little immune response, which renders them highly promising for treatment purposes (Al-Jamal and Kostarelos 2011). Researchers have applied pH-responsive liposomes for treating glioma tumor cells. The work employed tumor-specific, pH-sensitive peptides and liposomes to develop a system that reacts to the acidic pH of gliomas, leading to the liberation of the medication doxorubicin (Olusanya et al. 2018). The liposome-based theranostic system has been investigated for both imaging and medication delivery applications. Researchers devised a device in which a pharmacologically active substance was enclosed, enabling the visualization of its distribution inside the body in real time by magnetic resonance imaging (MRI). The liposome-based method exhibited superior efficacy and an extended duration of circulation in vivo, in comparison to a commercially available MRI contrast agent. In addition, liposomes have the benefit of encapsulating both polar and non-polar chemotherapeutic medicines, allowing for synergistic treatment through extended release and less toxicity, as shown in Figure 10.3 (Ren et al. 2016).

10.4.1.1 Nanoemulsions

Nanoemulsions are a captivating collection of structures that possess favorable qualities, rendering them highly suitable for cancer treatment. An important characteristic of them is their increased surface area, which facilitates greater interactions and more effective drug delivery. In addition, nanoemulsions have a prolonged half-life in circulation, which means that the medications they

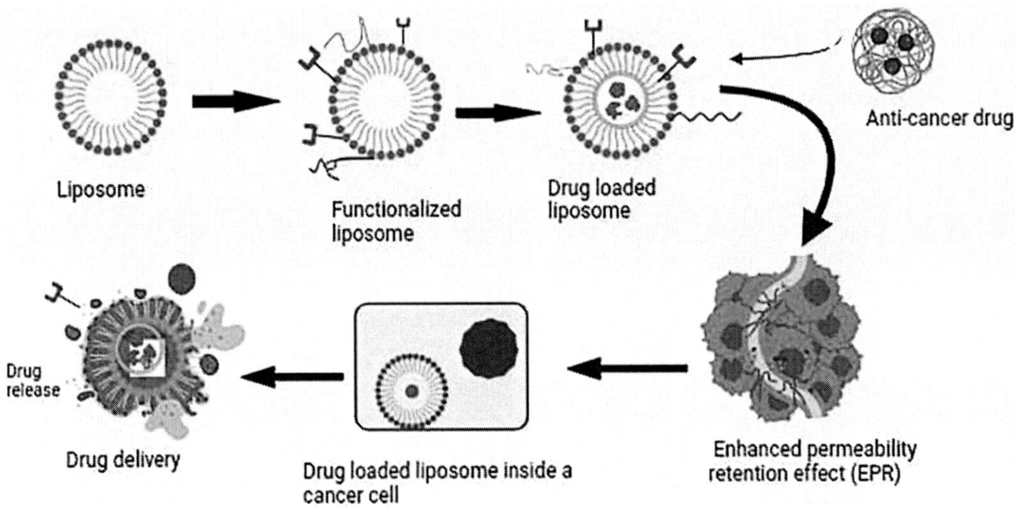

FIGURE 10.3 An illustration of liposome-based drug delivery for cancer treatment. There are three ways to locate cancer locations: (1) smart nanocarriers containing anticancer drugs, (2) targeting mechanisms, and (3) stimulation strategies to release payloads at previously localized cancer cell sites.

contain stay in the body for a longer time (V. Kumar, Sangwan, and Dureja 2022). Furthermore, these structures include distinct targeting abilities, enabling accurate administration of medication to the intended locations inside the body. In addition, nanoemulsions have a surface charge that enhances their stability and enables them to interact effectively with biological systems. Furthermore, they possess imaging capabilities, allowing for the observation and tracking of medication distribution inside the body. Nanoemulsions may also be altered to create heterogeneous emulsions, which provide possibilities for the precise release of medications (Mohite et al. 2023). The emulsions have a droplet size of around 100 nm, which guarantees the ideal dispersion of the medicine. Nanoemulsions are composed of oil, water, and an emulsifier, making them a flexible system for encapsulating pharmaceuticals that have low solubility in water. The hydrophobic property of pharmaceuticals provides protection against degradation and improves their stability. By enclosing medications within nanoemulsions, it is possible to greatly extend the duration of their presence in the bloodstream, resulting in a continuous release of the drug and prolonged therapeutic benefits (Ganta et al. 2014).

Researchers created lipid nanoemulsions that included paclitaxel in a separate research investigation. The nanoemulsions were especially engineered to attach to lipoprotein receptors, leading to reduced drug toxicity and improved antitumoral effectiveness (Khatri, Lohani, and Gandhi 2013). This specific delivery mechanism shows potential in enhancing the efficacy of paclitaxel in the treatment of cancer. The research carried out by researchers showcased the effectiveness of a nanoemulsion in reversing the growth of colon cancer cells (HT-29). The researchers noted that this formulation resulted in a reduction in the levels of tumoral markers. The change in gene expression was followed by programmed cell death, suggesting the potential of the nanoemulsion in cancer treatment (Sanchez-Lopez et al. 2019).

10.4.2 Polymeric Nanoparticles (PNPs)

Polymeric nanoparticles are being recognized as very promising vehicles for cancer therapy, owing to their distinctive characteristics and adaptable qualities. The nanoparticles consist of polymers that are both biocompatible and biodegradable (Gref et al. 1994). They have the ability to encapsulate therapeutic medicines and transport them directly to tumor locations. A significant benefit of PNPs is their capacity to safeguard pharmaceuticals against degradation and improve their stability, so enabling regulated and prolonged release. The polymeric matrix may be customized to regulate the release kinetics, guaranteeing an extended therapeutic impact while reducing adverse reactions (Parveen and Sahoo 2008).

In addition, PNPs have the capacity to enhance the solubility of medications that are not easily soluble in water, hence improving their bioavailability and therapeutic effectiveness. Nanoparticles have the ability to contain a diverse array of medications, such as chemotherapeutic agents, gene treatments, and immunotherapies. Furthermore, these nanoparticles have the capability to undergo surface functionalization by attaching targeting ligands, such as antibodies or peptides, which enables them to selectively identify and attach to cancer cells. By employing this active targeting strategy, it becomes possible to achieve specific medication distribution, hence minimizing unintended consequences and enhancing therapeutic efficacy (Vilos et al. 2013).

PNPs have the capacity for combination treatment. The nanoparticles have the capability to encapsulate many medications simultaneously, which enables the occurrence of synergistic effects and the ability to overcome drug resistance. Moreover, the nanoparticles may be manipulated to react to particular stimuli, such as pH, temperature, or enzymes, allowing for controlled medication release at the location of the tumor (Afsharzadeh et al. 2017). PNPs can be supplied by several ways, such as intravenous, oral, topical, or other routes, depending on the individual cancer type and therapy approach. PNPs have significant potential in cancer treatment since they enhance drug transport, improve therapeutic effectiveness, minimize adverse effects, and enable customized and focused treatments. Continuous study and progress in nanoparticle engineering will further broaden their use in the domain of cancer (Karlsson, Vaughan, and Green 2018).

Folic acid and PLGA nanoparticle conjugation with chitosan as the carrier was investigated for the treatment of prostate cancer (C. Zhang et al. 2010). The chemical was subjected to in vitro testing after being loaded with bicalutamide. For the sake of comparison, we also synthesized and subjected unfunctionalized PLGA nanoparticles to the identical conditions. The functionalized nanoparticles outperformed the unfunctionalized ones in terms of efficiency, because of their modified surface and targeted delivery system (Dhas, Ige, and Kudarha 2015). Doxorubicin was loaded into folic acid–poly(3-hydroxybutyrate-co-3-hydroxyoctanoate), and the drug encapsulation performance was over 80%.

10.4.3 Quantum Dots (QDs)

Quantum dots are nanocrystals made of semiconducting materials. The charge carriers inside these nanocrystals are restricted to three dimensions, resulting in observable quantum size effects in their optical characteristics (Sant 2012). These inorganic nanoparticles have been synthesized using many chemical processes. However, the ones based on colloidal synthesis have significant benefits for nanomedicines, particularly in terms of their convenient biofunctionalization, specifically for bioimaging diagnostics. QDs are notable biomarkers because of their photoluminescence, which is dependent on their size, as well as their narrow and adjustable emission bands, and significant shift (Juzenas et al. 2008).

Moreover, the detection of size-dependent photoluminescence in quantum dots when exposed to radiation using a solitary light source renders these particles appropriate for multiplexing techniques in analysis (Derivery et al. 2017). The initial research on colloidal quantum dots mostly focused on synthesizing materials containing cadmium using hot injection techniques. These materials may then be further modified with biomolecules. Presently, there are other options to hazardous quantum dots that include cadmium which have garnered attention for their potential use in bioimaging. These alternatives include zincsulfide–coated indium phosphide quantum dots and other forms of fluorescent nanoparticles, such as silica nanocomposites (Mangeolle et al. 2019).

10.4.4 Gold Nanoparticles (AuNPs)

Gold nanoparticles have become a potential technique in the field of cancer therapy. They have the potential to be utilized for precise administration of drugs to cancer cells and as agents that generate heat to kill tumor cells. AuNPs possess a compact size that enables them to infiltrate tumor tissue to a significant extent. Moreover, their capacity to attach to proteins and medicines renders them very efficient carriers for transporting therapeutic substances (Zhou et al. 2015). Moreover, gold nanoparticles exhibit excellent biocompatibility, rendering them very appropriate for utilization in medical contexts. Current research is dedicated to investigating the potential of gold nanoparticles, namely, gold nanorods, in battling several forms of cancer, including breast, colon, lung, prostate, pancreatic, and oral cancer. Extensive research is being conducted on AuNPs due to their potential application in cancer treatment (Sztandera, Gorzkiewicz, and Klajnert-Maculewicz 2018). These nanoparticles have demonstrated favorable outcomes as vehicles for drugs, agents that generate heat from light, substances that enhance contrast in medical imaging, and substances that increase the sensitivity of tumors to radiation (Shukla et al. 2005). AuNPs have been discovered to increase the responsiveness of cancer cells to radiation in laboratory experiments conducted on animals, both within and outside the body, using various amounts of energy. Multiple studies have shown the amplified radiation effects produced by the utilization of gold nanoparticles in conjunction with radiation treatment (Amendola et al. 2017). AuNPs are now being extensively studied for their potential application in cancer therapy, as evidenced by the ongoing clinical studies.

Due to their immunogenicity, low toxicity, remarkable biocompatibility, and great endurance, AuNPs have garnered a great deal of research into their application as drug delivery scaffolds. Covalent attachment of chemotherapeutics, oligonucleotides, and proteins to the surface of AuNPs has shown promise, making them promising delivery vehicles (Perera et al. 2021). SMI#9, a Rad6 inhibitor implicated in DNA damage resistance, mitochondrial stability, and post-replicative DNA repair, has been shown in recent research to be enabled by AuNPs, to which the small molecule inhibitor is bound (Fan et al. 2020). When combined with tumor necrosis factor (TRAIL), AuNPs may induce mitochondrial damage through the connected dynamin-related protein 1 (Drpl) pathway, leading to apoptosis and autophagy (Taggart et al. 2014).

10.4.5 Iron Oxide Nanoparticles

Iron oxide nanoparticles (IONPs) are a promising nanomaterial for cancer therapy. The NPs possess distinctive magnetic characteristics that can be utilized for both diagnostic and therapeutic applications. IONPs can be utilized as contrast agents in cancer diagnostics, specifically for MRI, to generate precise and comprehensive pictures of tumor localization and development (Bayda et al. 2018). IONPs in cancer therapy can function as hyperthermia agents, exhibiting the ability to produce heat upon exposure to an alternating magnetic field. The process of targeted heating can be employed to specifically eliminate cancerous cells while preserving unaffected tissue. In addition, IONPs have the capability to be loaded with anticancer medications and directed towards tumor locations, facilitating precise drug administration and reducing the occurrence of general adverse effects (Han et al. 2019).

Studies have demonstrated the potential of IONPs in treating many forms of cancer, such as breast, lung, liver, and brain cancer. Ongoing clinical trials are being conducted to better investigate the safety and effectiveness of IONPs in the treatment of cancer (Hosseinkazemi et al. 2022). Nevertheless, further investigation is required to enhance the characteristics of these substances, refine the methods of directing them to specific targets, and guarantee their compatibility with living organisms over extended periods of time. Thus, IONPs present a hopeful opportunity for enhancing cancer treatment (Han et al. 2019).

Therapeutic applications for spherical IONPs include magnetic tumor heating in the brain and radiotherapy or chemotherapy for prostate cancer (Sadhukhan et al. 2019). The multimodal drug transport and imaging capabilities of IONPs in the treatment of cancer have led to their widespread application in biomedicine. Unfortunately, issues with their biological safety and therapeutic efficacy slowed their development and translation into clinical use (Yang and Yu 2016). Heating magnetite in an alternating magnetic field can be used for hyperthermia, as an imaging contrast material, or as a theranostic for breast cancer (Figure 10.4). Another extensively studied use is the utilization of magnetic NPs in hyperthermia therapy. In this therapy, these nanoparticles are subjected to alternating magnetic fields, generally with frequencies ranging from around 100 to 300 kHz. As a result of magnetic hysteresis loss, heat is generated by these systems. Hyperthermia can elevate the temperature of cancerous tissues to a range of 41–46°C, leading to many outcomes, such as necrosis, apoptosis, protein denaturation, and immune system responses. However, the primary objective is to achieve genuine selectivity for tumoral tissue, while minimizing damage to adjacent healthy tissues. At present, a number of iron oxide nanoparticles, such as NanoTherm® and ThermoDox, have received approval for utilization in hyperthermia-based cancer treatment.

10.4.5.1 Platinum Nanoparticles

Platinum nanoparticles have many applications in the field of medicine. Research has demonstrated that platinum nanoparticles (PtNPs) have inherent anticancer properties due to their antioxidant capacities, leading to a suppressive impact on tumor development (Chang et al. 2018). Moreover, the use of ligands that are attached to functionalized metal PtNPs has resulted in enhanced tumor targeting. Additionally, PtNPs have played a crucial role in facilitating superior drug release and enhancing the effectiveness of drug delivery. Nevertheless, new research has documented the harmful consequences of nanoplatinum, mostly attributed to the size of the

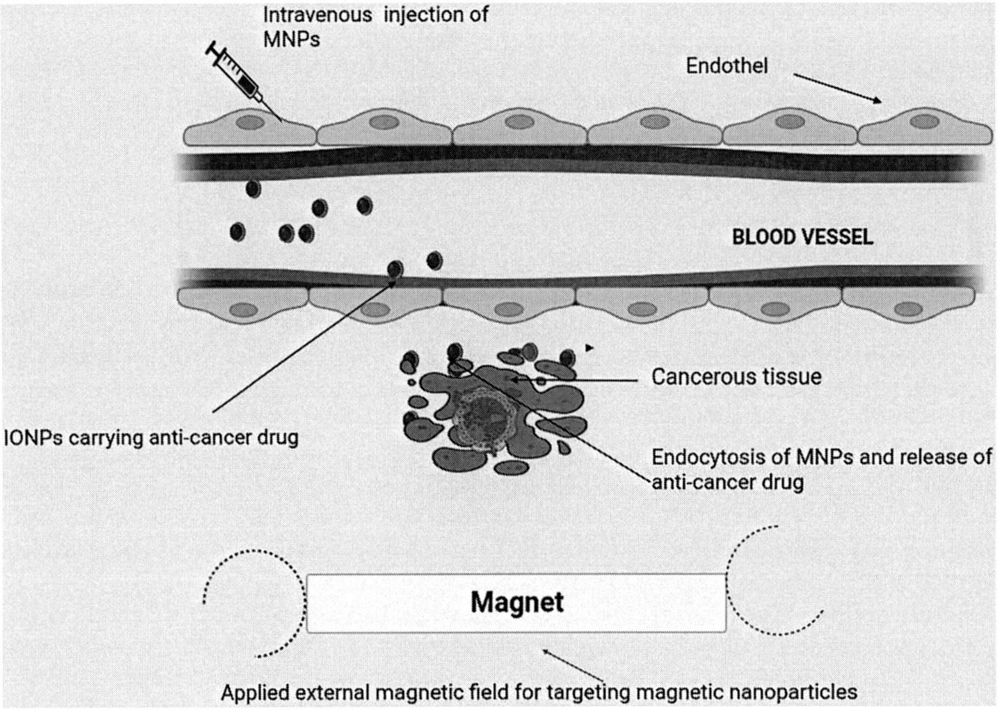

FIGURE 10.4 Targeted drug delivery presentation for an agent that uses iron oxide nanoparticles (FeONPs) to treat cancer. FeONPs can be conjugated with many chemotherapeutic drugs to reduce their toxicity by increasing targeted drug delivery efficiency against tumor cells. Higher temperatures have been demonstrated to affect tumoral cells and decrease the sensitivity of tumors to radiation.

TABLE 10.2
Utilization of Platinum-Based Nanoparticles in Several Forms of Cancer Treatment

Cancer	Nanoparticle	Application	Result	Reference
Colon cells	PtNPs	Enhancing the imaging of colon cancer cells by the use of microscopy pictures	The death rate of cancer cells rose to 62% in an in vitro setting.	Gao et al. (2018)
Glioblastoma cells	Ag-Pt nanoparticles	Cancer cell treatment	There were no harmful effects observed in healthy cells when tested in a laboratory setting (in vitro).	Gurunathan et al. (2020)
Colon cells	Pt/MgO	Induced apoptosis in colon cells	Colon cancer cells have a decrease in the expression of Bcl2. Increased expression of Bax and p53 in cancer cells cultured in a laboratory setting.	Depciuch et al. (2020)
Breast cancer line	Biogenic PtNPs	Antimicrobial agent	Potential antibacterial and anticancer properties.	Ruiz et al. (2020)
Neuroblastoma cancer	PtNPs	Cell death	PtNPs caused cancer cell death by apoptosis, and oxidative DNA damage under laboratory conditions.	Wang et al. (2022)

Source: Alrushaid et al. (2023).

nanoparticles. These nanoparticles have been found to concentrate in vital organs and tissues (Alrushaid et al. 2023). The utilization of platinum-based nanoparticles in cancer treatment is demonstrated in Table 10.2.

10.5 SMART NANOMATERIALS IN CANCER TREATMENT

Nanomaterials with high intelligence have demonstrated significant promise in transforming cancer therapy. These nanomaterials are engineered to react to certain stimuli, such as pH, temperature, light, or enzymes, enabling precise and regulated administration of drugs to cancer cells (Prasanna et al. 2018). In addition, nanomaterials, such as carbon nanotubes and QDs, have been investigated for their potential applications in cancer imaging and photodynamic treatment. These materials may be altered to specifically focus on cancer cells and produce reactive oxygen species upon light exposure, resulting in the eradication of tumors (Sun et al. 2023). Smart nanomaterials have the benefit of augmenting medication delivery, minimizing adverse effects, and promoting therapy effectiveness in individuals with cancer. However, further study is required to enhance their design, comprehend their long-term safety, and guarantee their implementation in clinical practice (Li et al. 2010). However, the realm of intelligent nanomaterials has significant potential in enhancing individualized and precise cancer treatments. Some of the smart nanomaterials are described in what follow.

10.5.1 Dendrimers

Dendrimers, due to their distinctive structure and characteristics, have encouraging prospects in the field of cancer treatment. Their symmetrical structure, which is arranged in a radial manner, is both compact and efficient. The presence of functional groups on the outer layer enables drug conjugation and targeting, while the inner layer enhances drug encapsulation efficiency and facilitates controlled release mechanisms (Wolinsky and Grinstaff 2008). Dendrimers possess adjustable attributes that render them very adaptable in the process of synthesis, facilitating the creation of targeted molecules with predetermined characteristics.

Dendrimers have been employed to tackle issues such as the inadequate ability of anticancer medications to dissolve in water. The water solubility of medications can be significantly increased by incorporating them with dendritic molecules, hence enhancing their efficacy within the body. In addition, dendrimers have the ability to surmount obstacles such as the blood–brain barrier, therefore facilitating the transportation of drugs to the central nervous system (García-Gallego et al. 2017). Polylysine dendrimers can function as biodegradable vehicles for cytotoxic medicines in solid tumors.

Moreover, dendrimers have the ability to surmount drug resistance and toxicity, as well as regulate drug release. This renders them highly suitable as intelligent nanoparticles for cancer treatment. Their nanoscale uniformity, extensive branching, solubility in water, presence of internal cavities, ability to bind to several targets, and compatibility with biological systems make them promising candidates for use as active ingredients in pharmaceutical formulations (Santos, Veiga, and Figueiras 2019). In general, dendrimers show great potential in boosting drug delivery, minimizing toxicity, and improving the effectiveness of anticancer therapies. Researchers developed a carbosilane dendrimer that improves compatibility with lipophilic cargo and boosts nanoscale structures. This is achieved because the carbosilane scaffolds are very stable, inert, and lipophilic (Cheng et al. 2011). Furthermore, the heightened growth of dendrites might result in the medication producing supplementary effects. Drug distribution into the central nervous system is challenging due to the presence of the blood–brain barrier. Nevertheless, this can be accomplished by conjugating the medication with a polyamidoamine dendrimer in order to surmount the blood–brain barrier (Kaminskas et al. 2011). Polylysine dendrimers have the capacity to function as biodegradable vehicles, facilitating the transportation of cytotoxic medications to solid tumors (Ambekar, Choudhary, and Kandasubramanian 2020). Dendrimers are effective in overcoming medication resistance, toxicity, and controlling drug release in capsules. This makes them highly suitable as intelligent nanoparticles for cancer therapy.

10.5.2 Micelles

Polymer micelles possess a distinct configuration comprising of a core area that is colloidally stable and a corona region that is hydrophilic. This configuration enables them to enhance the water solubility of hydrophobic substances, rendering them appropriate for medication delivery purposes (Owen, Chan, and Shoichet 2012). Through the physical encapsulation of hydrophobic pharmaceuticals within their core, polymer micelles have the ability to improve drug solubility, regulate release rates, and safeguard medications against degradation caused by pH or temperature (H. Wang et al. 2019).

Moreover, progress in synthetic chemistry has facilitated the chemical conjugation of medicines to the central structure of micelles, resulting in the creation of intelligent polymer micelles. Micelles may be engineered to have precise molecular targeting and sensitive drug release mechanisms, enabling precise and regulated drug delivery. Polymer micelles have several benefits in drug delivery, such as enhanced solubility, regulated release, and drug protection, which make them a very promising tool in the fields of biomedicine and nanocarrier applications (Sosnik, Carcaboso, and Chiappetta 2008).

Typically, nanoscale vesicles that have been changed on their surface are used to transport small compounds with antitumor properties, such as paclitaxel. Multiple studies have demonstrated that micelles have EPR effects, which result in their selective accumulation in the vascular beds of solid tumors with increased vascular permeability. Micellar solubilization enhances the stability and bioavailability of medicines that are insoluble or nearly insoluble (Guan, Rizzello, and Battaglia 2015). Alterations in pH can lead to the reconstitution of certain micellar structures, hence facilitating the release of drugs. The pH disparity between healthy tissue/blood and the extracellular environment of the tumor is inherent, and it has been extensively employed in drug delivery methods that provide sustained release. One example is the use of a pH-sensitive micellar system that targets the transferrin receptor. This technology may be employed as intelligent nanoparticles to address the issue of multidrug resistance and minimize the adverse effects of the treatment (M. Li et al. 2019). The ultimate goal is to obtain precise delivery of the treatment to tumors. The incorporation of folate-modified, pH-sensitive micelles with the antitumor medicine doxorubicin can significantly decrease the overall toxicity of doxorubicin, minimize harm to the heart and lung tissues, and enhance its effectiveness in combating tumors. The stimulation-reactive nanodrug delivery system utilizes pH-sensitive and thermosensitive polymer micelles to exploit the acidic conditions of solid tumors and photothermally induced hyperthermia. This allows for precise control of drug release, making it highly suitable for chemo-photothermal therapy (Xinru et al. 2015). Micellar solubilizers are amphiphilic compounds that possess minimal toxicity and excellent biocompatibility. Moreover, they hold significant promise as intelligent nanoparticles for delivering drugs to the eye. Micellar eye drops are highly biodegradable and biocompatible substances that effectively address issues related to ocular irritation and toxicity. Ginsenosides Rb1 micelle is an innovative method of delivering pharmaceuticals to the eyes, which effectively enhances the absorption of diclofenac and other medications. The antioxidant activity of myricetin may be greatly enhanced in vitro by using Polyoxyl 15 hydroxystearate micelle. Additionally, the membrane permeability for optical transport of myricetin can be accelerated with the use of this micelle (Hou et al. 2019).

10.5.3 Cell Membrane Nanoparticles

Nanoparticles composed of cell membranes. Traditional nanoparticles still encounter several challenges, such as rapid clearance from the bloodstream, easy identification by the immune system, and limited accumulation at the desired target location. Cell membrane coating has gained recognition as a feasible method for addressing the restrictions caused by the abundance of proteins on cell membrane surfaces (Zhen, Cheng, and Pu 2018). Cell membrane–coated nanoparticles (CMCNPs) are biomimetic nanoparticles consisting of a nanoparticle core enveloped by a cell-derived membrane. The membrane can be derived from different cell sources, such as cancer cells, stem cells, platelets, or white blood cells. These nanoparticles are utilized in the development of therapeutic devices. The conventional approach to produce CMCNPs involves extracting the plasma membrane from various cell sources and integrating core nanoparticles into membrane vesicles (R. Li et al. 2018). The unique characteristics of their tailored nanomaterials and sophisticated intelligent nanoparticles for cancer treatment have lately garnered significant attention. An example of effective creation is the development of platelet membrane–coated nanoparticles (Hu et al. 2011). These nanoparticles contain Dox inside their inner structure and are coated with tumor necrosis factor (TNF)–related apoptosis-inducing ligand (TRAIL) on their outer membrane. The findings from an animal model, where a tumor was implanted under the skin and a site of metastasis was present, showed that nanoparticles coated with platelet membranes had the most potent anticancer effects (Wei et al. 2016).

10.5.3.1 Protein Nanoparticles

Proteins are found not only in soy, milk, and grains but also in egg white, bovine serum, and human serum. Protein-based nanoparticles have several advantages, such as easy production, a large capacity to bind various drugs, lack of toxicity, absence of immune response, compatibility with living organisms, ability to break down naturally, and extended presence in the bloodstream (L. Sun et al. 2018).

Protein nanoparticle surfaces possess functional groups that facilitate the binding of certain ligands and other surface modifications, therefore transforming them into intelligent nanoparticles (Z. Fan et al. 2016). Albumin is one of the most important proteins in plasma and has been employed in different therapeutic applications over the past few decades. When tested on neuroblastoma cell lines, it was shown that human serum albumin nanoparticles loaded with dox exhibited more potent in vitro anticancer effects compared to the pure drug (M. Sun et al. 2020). Observation has been made of the effective targeting of human prostate cancer cell lines utilizing bovine serum albumin nanoparticles loaded with PTX. These nanoparticles are produced using a dissolving procedure and are adorned with folic acid (Iglesias 2009). Protein nanoparticles utilize beneficial, reversible binding to transport hydrophobic chemicals naturally. This enables the compounds to move through body fluids and be released at the cell surface. Moreover, protein has the ability to engage with the glycoprotein receptor and enhance the process of transcytosis for molecules that are attached to albumin (Hawkins, Soon-Shiong, and Desai 2008). Abraxane, a medicine approved by the FDA, is the first commercially available medication that has shown significant effectiveness in treating metastatic breast cancer. Abraxane has a diameter of around 130 nm.

10.6 BIOENGINEERED NANOPARTICLES IN CANCER TREATMENT

The area of nanomedicine involves the development of nanoscale materials with specific features that can be utilized to improve the effectiveness of cancer therapy. Nanoscale materials have the potential to serve as carriers for cancer drugs, facilitate cancer diagnosis, and enable medication targeting using imaging techniques (Rai et al. 2021).

10.6.1 Co-Encapsulation of Icotinib and Doxorubicin (DOX) in Energy-Dispersive Spectrometry (EDS) NPs for the Treatment of Lung Cancer

The majority of patients with non–small cell lung cancer (NSCLC) have an excessive expression of the epidermal growth factor receptor (EGFR), making it a critical target for therapeutic interventions (Singh and Jadhav 2018). Despite the development of many chemotherapeutic drugs as EGFR inhibitors, they have finally shown resistance to inhibiting EGFR. Thus, it was determined that the treatment of NSCLC was ineffective when using chemotherapy with a single medication. Combining several treatment modalities in combination chemotherapy has the potential to target many processes and pathways, which might be advantageous for treating cancer (Pusuluri et al. 2019). Researchers enhanced the effectiveness of DOX by optimizing its combination with three distinct EGFR inhibitors (erlotinib, apatinib, and icotinib) to treat A549, NCI-H1975, and PC9 cancer cells (K. Li et al. 2020). Prior studies have indicated that the combination of erlotinib and DOX exhibits a synergistic impact in several breast cancer cell lines. The combination of apatinib and DOX has demonstrated a synergistic benefit in the treatment of soft tissue sarcomas. It has been observed that the combination of icotinib with chemotherapeutic drugs can enhance the survival rates of patients with NSCLC (Han et al. 2017).

The study determined that the most effective combination of drugs was icotinib and DOX. These drugs were co-encapsulated using hyaluronic acid and cationic amphipathic starch to create EDS nanoparticles. Both in vivo and in vitro investigations demonstrated the high efficacy of targeted administration using EDS nanoparticles, resulting in improved drug accumulation within tumor cells (Kim, Lee, and Kim 2021). The in vivo toxicity was reduced as a result of the decrease in nonspecific accumulation in healthy tissues. The combined impact of DOX and icotinib was effectively augmented to demonstrate the inhibition of NSCLC (Hou et al. 2015).

10.6.2 Glutathione and Iron Redox Couple Reaction for the Purpose of Ferroptosis Therapy in Breast Cancer Treatment

Ferroptosis is the process in which there is an increase in the concentration of harmful lipid peroxide (LPO), which is dependent on iron and disrupts the balance of cellular redox homeostasis, potentially leading to the death of cancer cells. The Fenton reaction occurs when hydrogen peroxide in tumor cells reacts with iron, resulting in the production of reactive oxygen species. This process leads to the buildup of LPO (Wang et al. 2020). However, in areas affected by tumors, there is an inadequate quantity of naturally occurring hydrogen peroxide, which prevents the iron-mediated process from occurring. Thus, an LPO generator that is not dependent on the Fenton reaction might efficiently facilitate ferroptosis treatment, where lipid peroxidation can take place without the presence of hydrogen peroxide through the iron redox pair (Fe^{3+}/Fe^{2+}) (Dayem et al. 2016).

The redox interaction between unsaturated lipids and oxygen necessitates electron transport, facilitated by the presence of both Fe^{2+} and Fe^{3+}. Glutathione in tumor cells can convert Fe^{3+} to Fe^{2+} by the use of several reductive agents (Lien et al. 2016). Recently, researchers created glutathione and iron redox couples specifically for ferroptosis treatment that does not rely on the Fenton reaction. In this study, a lipid peroxide generator was employed to promote ferroptosis. The generator had a tiny particle size, resulting in enhanced tumor formation and permeability. An additional advantage of utilizing a lipid peroxide generator was discovered in both in vivo and in vitro models, demonstrating its ability to inhibit tumor growth without exhibiting any adverse consequences (He et al. 2020).

10.6.3 Utilizing Amino Acid-Modified Gold Nanoparticles for Photothermal Therapy (PTT) in Skin Cancer Treatment

Gold nanoparticles have been engineered with targeting agents like antibodies and peptides to prevent unintended targeting and to deliver tumor-specific treatments (Her, Jaffray, and Allen 2017). This method improves the specificity of targeting tumors. Nevertheless, the use of this technology in real-world scenarios remains difficult due to the exorbitant expenses, rapid elimination by the immune system, and inherent instability of proteins inside biological systems (Haume et al.

2016). Previous observations have indicated that a limited number of nanoparticles, which have been altered with targeting proteins, are able to successfully reach the specific location of the tumor, leading to a lack of precision in targeting. Off-targeting might have detrimental effects on healthy tissues. To address this problem, the in situ construction of tiny gold nanoparticles as photothermal agents might offer targeted treatment with reduced harm to healthy tissues and organs. Light-dependent gold nanoparticles have been synthesized by the aggregation of dimerized molecules. In order to perform PTT, modified amino acid gold nanoparticles were synthesized and carefully assembled at the tumor site (Li et al. 2023). In this study, the intracellular enzyme (transglutaminase, TGase) catalyzed the polymerization of amino acids on the surface of gold nanoparticles to achieve PTT control. In order to avoid unwanted triggering of normal cell polymerization, a pH-responsive zwitterion surface was developed because TGase is abundant in tumor cells (Carneiro and Barbosa 2016).

10.7 PASSIVE AND ACTIVE TARGETING

The capability of nanocarriers to target cancer cells and boost treatment efficacy is one of the most important aspects of these delivery systems. Tumor cells exhibit many abnormalities compared to healthy cells, such as an increased number of proliferating endothelial cells, increased vascular tortuosity, and the absence of pericytes (Niculescu and Grumezescu 2022). The best particles for extravasation of tumor microvasculature are those with a diameter of less than 200 nm due to the inverse relationship between particle extravasation and size. The lymphatic system of the tumor is also abnormal, causing fluid retention within the tumor and high interstitial pressure due to the outward flow of interstitial fluid (Maeda et al. 2000). This could result in tumor metastasis and prevent nanocarriers from extravasating from the microvasculature into the tumor stroma. Due to the poor removability of nanocarriers from the stroma, the absence of a functional lymphatic system also causes their retention in the stroma. The accumulation of higher concentrations of nanocarriers in tumors than in plasma and other tissues, coupled with the leaky microvasculature, enhances the EPR effect, resulting in "passive" cancer targeting (Shi et al. 2020). When drugs are released from nanocarriers, there is a correspondingly larger intratumoral drug concentration, which increases tumor cytotoxicity. By adding ligands like antibodies, aptamers to the surface of these nanocarriers, which bind to tumor-specific antigens in the tumor microenvironment, it is possible to further modify them for "active" cancer targeting (Wilhelm et al. 2016).

10.7.1 Passive Targeting

Passive targeting becomes an effective method for the deposition of nanovectors in tumors because of the tumor microenvironment's peculiar characteristics that are absent in normal tissues. Maeda and Matsumura's discovery of the EPR phenomenon is important to the practice of passive targeting (Maeda 2001). NPs and other macromolecules are particularly susceptible to this process, which leads to their preferential accumulation in malignant tissues. The blood arteries in a tumor release macromolecule-like NPs. This accumulation is caused by the fast and inadequate angiogenesis that occurs with tumor growth (Bazak et al. 2014). Taking into account all these details, it is clear that passive targeting provides substantial benefits for delivering therapeutic chemicals to malignant tissues and promises effective treatment options. Due to impaired lymphatic drainage, cancer patients are more likely to retain NPs, which facilitates the delivery of their cargo to malignant cells. It is through these mechanisms that the EPR effect is generated; this effect is a driving force in passive targeting (Danhier, Feron, and Préat 2010). We may manipulate passive targeting by adjusting the shape, size, and surface properties of these nanoparticles. An important drawback of passive targeting, however, is that it may not be able to distinguish between healthy and diseased tissue, in contrast to chemotherapy. Scientists first found that tumors tended to collect certain macromolecules over 30 years. Tumor accumulation was first shown for the therapeutic macromolecule poly(styrene-co-maleic acid)-NeoCarzinoStatin (SMANCS) that non-covalently binds albumin in the circulation (Byrne, Betancourt, and Brannon-Peppas 2008).

10.7.2 Active Targeting

To increase the delivery system's specificity, active targeting often makes use of a robust interaction, like a ligand receptor or other molecular recognition. This results in less pharmaceutical localization outside of blood vessels and fewer unwelcome nonspecific interactions. Tumor cells that have overexpressed in certain receptors, such as folate, on their surface can be actively targeted (Maeda 2001). Polymeric micelles are an example of a nanosystem where surface chemistries can be tweaked to improve selectivity (Ghosh and Biswas 2021). Active targeting nanoparticles, which have targeting ligands attached to their surfaces, make cancer drugs more selective for the diseased cell. Advantages of actively targeted nanoparticles include increased dispersion across target tissues, enhanced internalization into target cells, accumulation on circulating cancer cells, and translocation over semipermeable barriers due to the nanoparticles' ability to bind to and enter the cells of their intended targets. As opposed to NPs that rely merely on the permeability of blood arteries and passive diffusion, they are actively targeted (Shen et al. 2011). Unfortunately, it is possible that passive targeting cannot tell the difference between normal and malignant tissue. However, active targeting allows for more targeted delivery of therapeutic medications to cancer cells. Although therapeutic medication accumulation is enhanced in tumor cells, cellular components can nevertheless obstruct the release of these treatments. Active targeting techniques increase the delivery of NPs to cancer cells by recognizing and binding to tumor-specific antigens and growth factor receptors, such as EGFR, death receptor complexes, folate ligand, and transferrin (Cho et al. 2008).

10.8 CONCLUSION AND FUTURE PROSPECTS

The utilization of nanomedicines in cancer therapy has revolutionized the field due to their distinctive characteristics at the nanoscale and their ability to effectively reach the targeted site of action. This brief overview focuses on the significant advancements in utilizing nanoparticle-based strategies for cancer therapy during the past decade. Specifically, this study has examined the utilization of nanoliposomes, polymeric nanoparticles, nanoemulsions, quantum dots, gold nanoparticles, iron oxide nanoparticles, etc. The advent of nanotechnology has facilitated the targeted delivery of small molecules for cancer treatment, enabling their direct administration to the specific location of the disease. The unique characteristics of nanoparticles provide them with a highly promising novel approach for the delivery of therapeutic agents in the treatment of cancer. Improved pharmacokinetics, biocompatibility, tumor targeting, and stability are only some of the benefits of NP-based drug delivery systems over conventional drugs. New possibilities for treating and diagnosing cancer have arisen thanks to the incorporation of nanoparticles, which have improved qualities. Passive or active nanostructures can be employed to transport drugs to regions that are inaccessible through the body's circulatory or digestive systems. Further investigation is necessary to establish efficacious treatment regimens, which include exploring the potential for improved homogeneity and release characteristics in materials. In the future of cancer treatment, drug delivery systems will require the integration of several tasks, such as detection, diagnosis, and therapy. To do so, we need to design combination medicines that have shown promise in clinical translation and tackle several obstacles. The future of cancer therapy is poised to change dramatically as nanotechnology continues to improve.

REFERENCES

Afsharzadeh, Maryam, Maryam Hashemi, Ahad Mokhtarzadeh, Khalil Abnous, and Mohammad Ramezani. 2017. "Recent Advances in Co-Delivery Systems Based on Polymeric Nanoparticle for Cancer Treatment." *Artificial Cells Nanomedicine and Biotechnology* 46 (6): 1095–110. https://doi.org/10.1080/21691401.2017.1376675.

Alenazi, Mashal. 2016. "Nanotechnology in Drugs Delivery." *International Journal of Advanced Research in Computer and Communication Engineering* 5 (5): 1052–4. https://doi.org/10.17148/ijarcce.2016.55255.

Al-Jamal, Wafa' T., and Kostas Kostarelos. 2011. "Liposomes: From a Clinically Established Drug Delivery System to a Nanoparticle Platform for Theranostic Nanomedicine." *Accounts of Chemical Research* 44 (10): 1094–104. https://doi.org/10.1021/ar200105p.

Alrushaid, Noor, Firdos Alam Khan, Ebtesam A. Al-Suhaimi, and Abdelhamid ElaïSsari. 2023. "Nanotechnology in Cancer Diagnosis and Treatment." *Pharmaceutics* 15 (3): 1025. https://doi.org/10.3390/pharmaceutics 15031025.

Ambekar, Rushikesh S., Maya Choudhary, and Balasubramanian Kandasubramanian. 2020. "Recent Advances in Dendrimer-Based Nanoplatform for Cancer Treatment: A Review." *European Polymer Journal* 126 (March): 109546. https://doi.org/10.1016/j.eurpolymj.2020.109546.

Amendola, Vincenzo, Roberto Pilot, Marco Frasconi, Onofrio M. Maragò, and Maria Antonia Iatì. 2017. "Surface Plasmon Resonance in Gold Nanoparticles: A Review." *Journal of Physics: Condensed Matter* 29 (20): 203002. https://doi.org/10.1088/1361-648x/aa60f3.

Bashraheel, Sara S., Alexander Dömlingł, and Sayed K. Goda. 2020. "Update on Targeted Cancer Therapies, Single or in Combination, and Their Fine Tuning for Precision Medicine." *Biomedicine & Pharmacotherapy* 125 (May): 110009. https://doi.org/10.1016/j.biopha.2020.110009.

Bayda, Samer, Mohamad Hadla, Stefano Palazzolo, Pietro Riello, Giuseppe Corona, Giuseppe Toffoli, and Flavio Rizzolio. 2018. "Inorganic Nanoparticles for Cancer Therapy: A Transition from Lab to Clinic." *Current Medicinal Chemistry* 25 (34): 4269–303. https://doi.org/10.2174/0929867325666171229141156.

Bazak, Remon, M. Houri, Samar El Achy, Wael K. A. Hussein, and Tamer Refaat. 2014. "Passive Targeting of Nanoparticles to Cancer: A Comprehensive Review of the Literature." *Molecular and Clinical Oncology* 2 (6): 904–8. https://doi.org/10.3892/mco.2014.356.

Blair, Hannah A. 2018. "Daunorubicin/Cytarabine Liposome: A Review in Acute Myeloid Leukaemia." *Drugs* 78 (18): 1903–10. https://doi.org/10.1007/s40265-018-1022-3.

Bozzuto, Giuseppina, and Agnese Molinari. 2015. "Liposomes as Nanomedical Devices." *International Journal of Nanomedicine* (February): 975. https://doi.org/10.2147/ijn.s68861.

Byrne, James D., Tania Betancourt, and Lisa Brannon-Peppas. 2008. "Active Targeting Schemes for Nanoparticle Systems in Cancer Therapeutics." *Advanced Drug Delivery Reviews* 60 (15): 1615–26. https://doi.org/10.1016/j.addr.2008.08.005.

Calixto, Giovana Maria Fioramonti, Jéssica Bernegossi, Laura Marise De Freitas, Carla Raquel Fontana, and Marlus Chorilli. 2016. "Nanotechnology-Based Drug Delivery Systems for Photodynamic Therapy of Cancer: A Review." *Molecules* 21 (3): 342. https://doi.org/10.3390/molecules21030342.

Carneiro, María Fernanda Hornos, and Fernando Barbosa. 2016. "Gold Nanoparticles: A Critical Review of Therapeutic Applications and Toxicological Aspects." *Journal of Toxicology & Environmental Health Part B: Critical Reviews* 19 (3–4): 129–48. https://doi.org/10.1080/10937404.2016.1168762.

Chang, Yu, Binbin Ding, Xinyang Zhang, Xiaoran Deng, Kerong Deng, Ziyong Cheng, Bengang Xing, DayongJin, Ping'an Ma, and Jun Lin. 2018. "Targeted Iron Nanoparticles with Platinum-(IV) Prodrugs and Anti-EZH2 siRNA Show Great Synergy in Combating Drug Resistance in Vitro and in Vivo." *Biomaterials* 155 (February): 112–23. https://doi.org/10.1016/j.biomaterials.2017.11.014.

Chen, Mao, Li Xin Qiu, Ruyi Liao, Fang Du, Hong Ding, Wan Chun Yang, Jin Li, and Qing Chen. 2010. "KRAS Mutations and Resistance to EGFR-TKIs Treatment in Patients with Non-Small Cell Lung Cancer: A Meta-Analysis of 22 Studies." *Lung Cancer* 69 (3): 272–8. https://doi.org/10.1016/j.lungcan.2009.11.020.

Cheng, Yiyun, Libo Zhao, Yiwen Li, and Tongwen Xu. 2011. "Design of Biocompatible Dendrimers for Cancer Diagnosis and Therapy: Current Status and Future Perspectives." *Chemical Society Reviews* 40 (5): 2673. https://doi.org/10.1039/c0cs00097c.

Cho, Kwangjae, Xu Wang, Shuming Nie, Zhuo Georgia Chen, and Dong M. Shin. 2008. "Therapeutic Nanoparticles for Drug Delivery in Cancer." *Clinical Cancer Research* 14 (5): 1310–16. https://doi.org/10.1158/1078-0432.ccr-07-1441.

Danhier, Fabienne, Olivier Feron, and Véronique Préat. 2010. "To Exploit the Tumor Microenvironment: Passive and Active Tumor Targeting of Nanocarriers for Anti-Cancer Drug Delivery." *Journal of Controlled Release* 148 (2): 135–46. https://doi.org/10.1016/j.jconrel.2010.08.027.

Dayem, Ahmed Abdal, Hye Yeon Choi, Gwang-Mo Yang, Kyeongseok Kim, Subbroto Kumar Saha, and Ssang-Goo Cho. 2016. "The Anti-Cancer Effect of Polyphenols against Breast Cancer and Cancer Stem Cells: Molecular Mechanisms." *Nutrients* 8 (9): 581. https://doi.org/10.3390/nu8090581.

Depciuch, Joanna, Małgorzata Stec, Bartosz Klębowski, A. Maximenko, Elżbieta Drzymała, Jarosław Baran, and Magdalena Parlińska-Wojtan. 2020. "Size Effect of Platinum Nanoparticles in Simulated Anticancer

Photothermal Therapy." *Photodiagnosis and Photodynamic Therapy* 29 (March): 101594. https://doi.org/10.1016/j.pdpdt.2019.101594.

Derivery, Emmanuel, Eline Bartolami, Stefan Matile, and Marcos González-Gaitán. 2017. "Efficient Delivery of Quantum Dots into the Cytosol of Cells Using Cell-Penetrating Poly(Disulfide)s." *Journal of the American Chemical Society* 139 (30): 10172–5. https://doi.org/10.1021/jacs.7b02952.

Dhas, Namdev, Pradum Pundlikrao Ige, and Ritu Kudarha. 2015. "Design, Optimization and in-Vitro Study of Folic Acid Conjugated-Chitosan Functionalized PLGA Nanoparticle for Delivery of Bicalutamide in Prostate Cancer." *Powder Technology* 283 (October): 234–45. https://doi.org/10.1016/j.powtec.2015.04.053.

Duffy, Alison, Jackson Le, Edward A. Sausville, and Ashkan Emadi. 2014. "Autophagy Modulation: A Target for Cancer Treatment Development." *Cancer Chemotherapy and Pharmacology* 75 (3): 439–47. https://doi.org/10.1007/s00280-014-2637-z.

Fan, Miao, Han Ye, Shutao Gao, Hongyuan Yan, Lingzhi Cao, Zhenhua Li, Xing-Jie Liang, and Jinchao Zhang. 2020. "Ultrasmall Gold Nanoparticles in Cancer Diagnosis and Therapy." *Theranostics* 10 (11): 4944–57. https://doi.org/10.7150/thno.42471.

Fan, Zhen, Leming Sun, Yujian Huang, Yongzhong Wang, and Mingjun Zhang. 2016. "Bioinspired Fluorescent Dipeptide Nanoparticles for Targeted Cancer Cell Imaging and Real-Time Monitoring of Drug Release." *Nature Nanotechnology* 11 (4): 388–94. https://doi.org/10.1038/nnano.2015.312.

Farjadian, Fatemeh, Amir Ghasemi, Omid Gohari, Mahdi Karimi, and Michael R. Hamblin. 2019. "Nanopharmaceuticals and Nanomedicines Currently on the Market: Challenges and Opportunities." *Nanomedicine* 14 (1): 93–126. https://doi.org/10.2217/nnm-2018-0120.

Ganta, Srinivas, Meghna Talekar, Amit Singh, Timothy P. Coleman, and Mansoor M. Amiji. 2014. "Nanoemulsions in Translational Research—Opportunities and Challenges in Targeted Cancer Therapy." *AAPS PharmSciTech* 15 (3): 694–708. https://doi.org/10.1208/s12249-014-0088-9.

Gao, Tao, Zhi Jun, Chaoli Mu, Shiyu Gu, Xiao Jianping, Jie Yang, Zhaoxia Wang, and Yang Xiang. 2018. "One-Step Detection for Two Serological Biomarker Species to Improve the Diagnostic Accuracy of Hepatocellular Carcinoma." *Talanta* 178 (February): 89–93. https://doi.org/10.1016/j.talanta.2017.09.011.

García-Gallego, Sandra, Gianluigi Franci, Annarita Falanga, Rafael Gómez, Veronica Folliero, Stefania Galdiero, Francisco De La Mata, and Massimiliano Galdiero. 2017. "Function Oriented Molecular Design: Dendrimers as Novel Antimicrobials." *Molecules* 22 (10): 1581. https://doi.org/10.3390/molecules22101581.

Georgakopoulou, Eleni, Justin Stebbing, and Crispian Scully. 2018. "Targeted Cancer Therapies." *Journal of the American Dental Association* 149 (2): 100–11. https://doi.org/10.1016/j.adaj.2017.08.046.

Ghosh, Balaram, and Swati Biswas. 2021. "Polymeric Micelles in Cancer Therapy: State of the Art." *Journal of Controlled Release* 332 (April): 127–47. https://doi.org/10.1016/j.jconrel.2021.02.016.

Gref, Ruxandra, Yoshiharu Minamitake, Maria Teresa Peracchia, Vladimir S. Trubetskoy, Vladimir P. Torchilin, and Robert Langer. 1994. "Biodegradable Long-Circulating Polymeric Nanospheres." *Science* 263 (5153): 1600–3. https://doi.org/10.1126/science.8128245.

Guan, Lijuan, Loris Rizzello, and Giuseppe Battaglia. 2015. "Polymersomes and Their Applications in Cancer Delivery and Therapy." *Nanomedicine* 10 (17): 2757–80. https://doi.org/10.2217/nnm.15.110.

Gurunathan, Sangiliyandi, M. Jeyaraj, Min-Hee Kang, and Jin-Hoi Kim. 2020. "Anticancer Properties of Platinum Nanoparticles and Retinoic Acid: Combination Therapy for the Treatment of Human Neuroblastoma Cancer." *International Journal of Molecular Sciences* 21 (18): 6792. https://doi.org/10.3390/ijms21186792.

Han, Cuiping, Aiwei Zhang, Ying Kong, Naitong Yu, Ting Xie, Binru Dou, Ké Li, Yong Wang, Jingjing Li, and Kai Xu. 2019. "Multifunctional Iron Oxide-Carbon Hybrid Nanoparticles for Targeted Fluorescent/MR Dual-Modal Imaging and Detection of Breast Cancer Cells." *Analytica Chimica Acta* 1067 (August): 115–28. https://doi.org/10.1016/j.aca.2019.03.054.

Han, Tao, Yuting Luan, Ying Xu, Xiaodan Yang, Jing Li, Ran Liu, Qing Li, and Zhendong Zheng. 2017. "Successful Treatment of Advanced Pancreatic Liposarcoma With Apatinib: A Case Report and Literature Review." *Cancer Biology & Therapy* 18 (9): 635–39. https://doi.org/10.1080/15384047.2017.1345394.

Haume, Kaspar, Soraia Rosa, Sophie Grellet, Małgorzata A. Śmiałek, Karl T. Butterworth, Andrey V. Solov'yov, Kevin M. Prise, Jon P. Golding, and Nigel J. Mason. 2016. "Gold Nanoparticles for Cancer Radiotherapy: A Review." *Cancer Nanotechnology* 7 (1). https://doi.org/10.1186/s12645-016-0021-x.

Hawkins, Michael, Patrick Soon-Shiong, and Neil Desai. 2008. "Protein Nanoparticles as Drug Carriers in Clinical Medicine." *Advanced Drug Delivery Reviews* 60 (8): 876–85. https://doi.org/10.1016/j.addr.2007.08.044.

He, Yujing, Xiaoying Li, Xing Liu, Xing Wan, Xiaoai Chang, and Hu-Lin Jiang. 2020. "Fenton Reaction-Independent Ferroptosis Therapy via Glutathione and Iron Redox Couple Sequentially Triggered Lipid Peroxide Generator." *Biomaterials* 241 (May): 119911. https://doi.org/10.1016/j.biomaterials.2020.119911.

Her, Sohyoung, David A. Jaffray, and Christine Allen. 2017. "Gold Nanoparticles for Applications in Cancer Radiotherapy: Mechanisms and Recent Advancements." *Advanced Drug Delivery Reviews* 109 (January): 84–101. https://doi.org/10.1016/j.addr.2015.12.012.

Hosseinkazemi, Hessam, Saeed Samani, Andrew O'Neill, Mahdieh Soezi, Mohsen Moghoofei, Mohammad H. Azhdari, Farzaneh Aavani, Abolfazl Nazbar, Saeed Heidari Keshel, and Mohammad Doroudian. 2022. "Applications of Iron Oxide Nanoparticles Against Breast Cancer." *Journal of Nanomaterials* 2022 (May): 1–12. https://doi.org/10.1155/2022/6493458.

Hou, Shuguang, Jiangyue Wu, Xu Li, and Hong Shu. 2015. "Practical, Regulatory and Clinical Considerations for Development of Inhalation Drug Products." *Asian Journal of Pharmaceutical Sciences* 10 (6): 490–500. https://doi.org/10.1016/j.ajps.2015.08.008.

Hou, Yuzhen, Fan Zhang, Jie Lan, Feilong Sun, Jun Li, Mengshuang Li, Kaichao Song, and Xianggen Wu. 2019. "Ultra-Small Micelles Based on Polyoxyl 15 Hydroxystearate for Ocular Delivery of Myricetin: Optimization, in Vitro, and in Vivo Evaluation." *Drug Delivery* 26 (1): 158–67. https://doi.org/10.1080/10717544.2019.1568624.

Hu, Che Ming Jack, Li Zhang, Santosh Aryal, Connie Cheung, Ronnie H. Fang, and Liangfang Zhang. 2011. "Erythrocyte Membrane-Camouflaged Polymeric Nanoparticles as a Biomimetic Delivery Platform." *Proceedings of the National Academy of Sciences of the United States of America* 108 (27): 10980–5. https://doi.org/10.1073/pnas.1106634108.

Iglesias, J. 2009. "Nab-Paclitaxel (Abraxane®): An Albumin-Bound Cytotoxic Exploiting Natural Delivery Mechanisms into Tumors." *Breast Cancer Research* 11 (S1). https://doi.org/10.1186/bcr2282.

Jin, Cancan, Kankai Wang, Anthony Oppong-Gyebi, and Jiangnan Hu. 2020. "Application of Nanotechnology in Cancer Diagnosis and Therapy—A Mini-Review." *International Journal of Medical Sciences* 17 (18): 2964–73. https://doi.org/10.7150/ijms.49801.

Juzenas, Petras, Wei Chen, Ya Ping Sun, Manuel a. N. Coelho, Roman Generalov, Natalia Generalova, and Ingeborg Lie Christensen. 2008. "Quantum Dots and Nanoparticles for Photodynamic and Radiation Therapies of Cancer." *Advanced Drug Delivery Reviews* 60 (15): 1600–14. https://doi.org/10.1016/j.addr.2008.08.004.

Kaminskas, Lisa M., Brian D. Kelly, Victoria M. McLeod, Gian Sberna, David J. Owen, Ben J. Boyd, and Christopher John Porter. 2011. "Characterisation and Tumour Targeting of PEGylated Polylysine Dendrimers Bearing Doxorubicin via a pH Labile Linker." *Journal of Controlled Release* 152 (2): 241–8. https://doi.org/10.1016/j.jconrel.2011.02.005.

Karlsson, Johan, Hannah J. Vaughan, and Jordan J. Green. 2018. "Biodegradable Polymeric Nanoparticles for Therapeutic Cancer Treatments." *Annual Review of Chemical and Biomolecular Engineering* 9 (1): 105–27. https://doi.org/10.1146/annurev-chembioeng-060817-084055.

Khatri, Smriti, Pratyush Lohani, and Shweta Gandhi. 2013. "Nanoemulsions in Cancer Therapy." *Indo Global Journal of Pharmaceutical Sciences* 3 (2): 124–33. https://doi.org/10.35652/igjps.2013.14.

Kim, Seong-Ryong, Hyun Jung Lee, and Dalyong Kim. 2021. "Consistent Response on Challenge and Rechallenge of Liposomal Irinotecan in a Patient with Metastatic Pancreatic Adenocarcinoma Previously Treated with Gemcitabine Plus Nab-Paclitaxel: A Case Report." *Case Reports in Oncology* 14 (3): 1882–8. https://doi.org/10.1159/000521315.

Kumar, Bhupinder, Sandeep Singh, Ira Skvortsova, and Vinod Kumar. 2018. "Promising Targets in Anti-Cancer Drug Development: Recent Updates." *Current Medicinal Chemistry* 24 (42). https://doi.org/10.2174/0929867324666170331123648.

Kumar, Virender, Vandana Sangwan, and Harish Dureja. 2022. "Nanoemulsion for Delivery of Anticancer Drugs." *TMR Cancer—Cancer Advances* 5: e22016. https://doi.org/10.53388/2022522016.

Li, Ké, Wenbin Zhan, Min Jia, Yufeng Zhao, Yingguang Liu, Rajiv Kumar Jha, and Liansuo Zhou. 2020. "Dual Loading of Nanoparticles with Doxorubicin and Icotinib for the Synergistic Suppression of Non-Small Cell Lung Cancer." *International Journal of Medical Sciences* 17 (3): 390–402. https://doi.org/10.7150/ijms.39172.

Li, Mengshuang, Jie Lan, Xuefei Li, Xia Meng, Hui Wang, Fan Zhang, Xiaohong Lü, Zengfang Zhuang, and Xianggen Wu. 2019. "Novel Ultra-Small Micelles Based on Ginsenoside Rb1: A Potential Nanoplatform for Ocular Drug Delivery." *Drug Delivery* 26 (1): 481–9. https://doi.org/10.1080/10717544.2019.1600077.

Li, Qian, Xizheng Wu, Shengdong Mu, Chao He, Xiancheng Ren, Xingguang Luo, Mohsen Adeli, Xianglong Han, Lang Ma, and Qian Li. 2023. "Microenvironment Restruction of Emerging 2D Materials and Their Roles in Therapeutic and Diagnostic Nano-Bio-Platforms." *Advanced Science* 10 (20). https://doi.org/10.1002/advs.202207759.

Li, Ruixiang, Yuwei He, Shuya Zhang, Jing Qin, and Jianxin Wang. 2018. "Cell Membrane-Based Nanoparticles: A New Biomimetic Platform for Tumor Diagnosis and Treatment." *Acta Pharmaceutica Sinica B* 8 (1): 14–22. https://doi.org/10.1016/j.apsb.2017.11.009.

Li, Xiaohui, Cheng Zhang, Laurent Le Guyader, and Chunying Chen. 2010. " 'Smart' Nanomaterials for Cancer Therapy." *Science China Chemistry* 53 (11): 2241–9. https://doi.org/10.1007/s11426-010-4122-9.

Li, Xinru, Xiucong Yang, Zhiqiang Lin, Dan Wang, Mei Dong, Bing He, Xiaoyou Wang, Xueqing Wang, Qiang Zhang, and Wei Gao. 2015. "A Folate Modified pH Sensitive Targeted Polymeric Micelle Alleviated Systemic Toxicity of Doxorubicin (DOX) in Multi-Drug Resistant Tumor Bearing Mice." *European Journal of Pharmaceutical Sciences* 76 (August): 95–101. https://doi.org/10.1016/j.ejps.2015.04.018.

Lien, Evan C., Costas A. Lyssiotis, Ashish Juvekar, Hai Hu, John M. Asara, Lewis C. Cantley, and Alex Toker. 2016. "Glutathione Biosynthesis Is a Metabolic Vulnerability in PI(3)K/Akt-Driven Breast Cancer." *Nature Cell Biology* 18 (5): 572–8. https://doi.org/10.1038/ncb3341.

Maeda, Hiroshi. 2001. "The Enhanced Permeability and Retention (EPR) Effect in Tumor Vasculature: The Key Role of Tumor-Selective Macromolecular Drug Targeting." *Advances in Enzyme Regulation* 41 (1): 189–207. https://doi.org/10.1016/s0065-2571(00)00013-3.

Maeda, Hiroshi. 2012. "Macromolecular Therapeutics in Cancer Treatment: The EPR Effect and Beyond." *Journal of Controlled Release* 164 (2): 138–44. https://doi.org/10.1016/j.jconrel.2012.04.038.

Maeda, Hiroshi, Jun Wu, Tomohiro Sawa, Yasuhiro Matsumura, and Kentaro Hori. 2000. "Tumor Vascular Permeability and the EPR Effect in Macromolecular Therapeutics: A Review." *Journal of Controlled Release* 65 (1–2): 271–84. https://doi.org/10.1016/s0168-3659(99)00248-5.

Mangeolle, Tristan, Ilya Yakavets, Nicolas Lequeux, Thomas Pons, Lina Bezdetnaya, and Frédéric Marchal. 2019. "The Targeting Ability of Fluorescent Quantum Dots to the Folate Receptor Rich Tumors." *Photodiagnosis and Photodynamic Therapy* 26 (June): 150–6. https://doi.org/10.1016/j.pdpdt.2019.03.010.

Martins, Catarina S. M., Alec P. LaGrow, and João A. V. Prior. 2022. "Quantum Dots for Cancer-Related mIRNA Monitoring." *ACS Sensors* 7 (5): 1269–99. https://doi.org/10.1021/acssensors.2c00149.

Miller, Emily, Timothy Samec, and Angela Alexander-Bryant. 2021. "Nanoparticle Delivery Systems to Combat Drug Resistance in Ovarian Cancer." *Nanomedicine: Nanotechnology, Biology and Medicine* 31 (January): 102309. https://doi.org/10.1016/j.nano.2020.102309.

Misra, Ranjita, Sarbari Acharya, and Sanjeeb K. Sahoo. 2010. "Cancer Nanotechnology: Application of Nanotechnology in Cancer Therapy." *Drug Discovery Today* 15 (19–20): 842–50. https://doi.org/10.1016/j.drudis.2010.08.006.

Mohite, Popat, Tanavirsing Rajput, Ramdas Pandhare, Adinath Sangale, Sudarshan Singh, and Bhupendra G. Prajapati. 2023. "Nanoemulsion in Management of Colorectal Cancer: Challenges and Future Prospects." *Nanomanufacturing* 3 (2): 139–66. https://doi.org/10.3390/nanomanufacturing3020010.

Morales, Carolina Salvador, and Piotr Grodzinski. 2023. "Current Landscape of Treating Different Cancers Using Nanomedicines: Trends and Perspectives." *Wiley Interdisciplinary Reviews. Nanomedicine and Nanobiotechnology* 16 (1). https://doi.org/10.1002/wnan.1927.

Mundekkad, Deepa, and William C. Cho. 2022. "Nanoparticles in Clinical Translation for Cancer Therapy." *International Journal of Molecular Sciences* 23 (3): 1685. https://doi.org/10.3390/ijms23031685.

Naik, Kaustubh, Shilpi Chaudhary, Lei Ye, and Avanish Singh Parmar. 2022. "A Strategic Review on Carbon Quantum Dots for Cancer-Diagnostics and Treatment." *Frontiers in Bioengineering and Biotechnology* 10 (May). https://doi.org/10.3389/fbioe.2022.882100.

Navya, P. N., Anubhav Kaphle, Sangly P. Srinivas, Suresh K. Bhargava, Vincent M. Rotello, and Hemant Kumar Daima. 2019. "Current Trends and Challenges in Cancer Management and Therapy Using Designer Nanomaterials." *Nano Convergence* 6 (1). https://doi.org/10.1186/s40580-019-0193-2.

Niculescu, Adelina-Gabriela, and Alexandru Mihai Grumezescu. 2022. "Novel Tumor-Targeting Nanoparticles for Cancer Treatment—A Review." *International Journal of Molecular Sciences* 23 (9): 5253. https://doi.org/10.3390/ijms23095253.

Nsairat, Hamdi, Dima Khater, Usama Sayed, Fadwa Odeh, Abeer Al Bawab, and Walhan Alshaer. 2022. "Liposomes: Structure, Composition, Types, and Clinical Applications." *Heliyon* 8 (5): e09394. https://doi.org/10.1016/j.heliyon.2022.e09394.

Olusanya, Temidayo, Hayat Ahmad, Madu Daniel Ibegbu, James R. Smith, and Amal Elkordy. 2018. "Liposomal Drug Delivery Systems and Anticancer Drugs." *Molecules* 23 (4): 907. https://doi.org/10.3390/molecules23040907.

Owen, Shawn C., Dianna P. Y. Chan, and Molly S. Shoichet. 2012. "Polymeric Micelle Stability." *Nano Today* 7 (1): 53–65. https://doi.org/10.1016/j.nantod.2012.01.002.
Parveen, Suphiya, and Sanjeeb K. Sahoo. 2008. "Polymeric Nanoparticles for Cancer Therapy." *Journal of Drug Targeting* 16 (2): 108–23. https://doi.org/10.1080/10611860701794353.
Perera, Y. Randika, Joanna Xiuzhu Xu, Dhanush L. Amarasekara, Alex C. Hughes, Ibraheem Abbood, and Nicholas C. Fitzkee. 2021. "Understanding the Adsorption of Peptides and Proteins onto PEGylated Gold Nanoparticles." *Molecules* 26 (19): 5788. https://doi.org/10.3390/molecules26195788.
Prasanna, Akshatha, R. Pooja, V. Suchithra, Akhil Ravikumar, Praveen Kumar Gupta, and Vidya Niranjan. 2018. "Smart Drug Delivery Systems for Cancer Treatment Using Nanomaterials." *Materials Today: Proceedings* 5 (10): 21047–54. https://doi.org/10.1016/j.matpr.2018.06.498.
Pusuluri, Anusha, Vinu Krishnan, Debra Wu, C. Wyatt Shields, Lily Li-Wen Wang, and Samir Mitragotri. 2019. "Role of Synergy and Immunostimulation in Design of Chemotherapy Combinations: An Analysis of Doxorubicin and Camptothecin." *Bioengineering & Translational Medicine* 4 (2). https://doi.org/10.1002/btm2.10129.
Rai, Ayushi, Saba Noor, Shahnawaz Ahmad, Mohamed F. Alajmi, Afzal Hussain, Hashim Abbas, and Gulam Mustafa Hasan. 2021. "Recent Advances and Implication of Bioengineered Nanomaterials in Cancer Theranostics." *Medicina-Lithuania* 57 (2): 91. https://doi.org/10.3390/medicina57020091.
Ren, Lili, Shizhen Chen, Haidong Li, Zhiying Zhang, Jiahao Zhong, Maili Liu, and Xin Zhou. 2016. "MRI-Guided Liposomes for Targeted Tandem Chemotherapy and Therapeutic Response Prediction." *Acta Biomaterialia* 35 (April): 260–8. https://doi.org/10.1016/j.actbio.2016.02.011.
Ruiz, Aida López, Caterina Bartomeu Garcia, Sandra Navarro Gallón, and Thomas J Webster. 2020. "Novel Silver-Platinum Nanoparticles for Anticancer and Antimicrobial Applications." *International Journal of Nanomedicine* 15 (January): 169–79. https://doi.org/10.2147/ijn.s176737.
Sadhukhan, Pritam, Mousumi Kundu, Sharmistha Chatterjee, Noyel Ghosh, Prasenjit Manna, Joydeep Das, and Parames C. Sil. 2019. "Targeted Delivery of Quercetin via pH-Responsive Zinc Oxide Nanoparticles for Breast Cancer Therapy." *Materials Science and Engineering: C* 100 (July): 129–40. https://doi.org/10.1016/j.msec.2019.02.096.
Salvioni, Lucia, Maria Antonietta Rizzuto, Jessica Bertolini, Laura Pandolfi, Miriam Colombo, and Davide Prosperi. 2019. "Thirty Years of Cancer Nanomedicine: Success, Frustration, and Hope." *Cancers* 11 (12): 1855. https://doi.org/10.3390/cancers11121855.
Sánchez-López, Elena, Mariana Guerra, João Dias-Ferreira, Ana López-Machado, Miren Ettcheto, Marta Espina, Antoni Camins, María L. García, and Eliana B. Souto. 2019. "Current Applications of Nanoemulsions in Cancer Therapeutics." *Nanomaterials* 9 (6): 821. https://doi.org/10.3390/nano9060821.
Sant, Sudhindra B. 2012. "Nanoparticles: From Theory to Applications." *Materials and Manufacturing Processes* 27 (12): 1462–63. https://doi.org/10.1080/10426914.2012.663137.
Santos, Ana Isabel, Francisco Veiga, and Ana Figueiras. 2019. "Dendrimers as Pharmaceutical Excipients: Synthesis, Properties, Toxicity and Biomedical Applications." *Materials* 13 (1): 65. https://doi.org/10.3390/ma13010065.
Sell, Manfred, Ana Rita Lopes, Maria Escudeiro, Bruno Esteves, Ana R. Monteiro, Tito Trindade, and Luísa Cruz-Lopes. 2023. "Application of Nanoparticles in Cancer Treatment: A Concise Review." *Nanomaterials* 13 (21): 2887. https://doi.org/10.3390/nano13212887.
Shen, Zheyu, Yan Li, Kazuhiro Kohama, Brian K. O'Neill, and Jingxiu Bi. 2011. "Improved Drug Targeting of Cancer Cells by Utilizing Actively Targetable Folic Acid-Conjugated Albumin Nanospheres." *Pharmacological Research* 63 (1): 51–8. https://doi.org/10.1016/j.phrs.2010.10.012.
Shi, Yang, Roy Van Der Meel, Xiaoyuan Chen, and Twan Lammers. 2020. "The EPR Effect and Beyond: Strategies to Improve Tumor Targeting and Cancer Nanomedicine Treatment Efficacy." *Theranostics* 10 (17): 7921–4. https://doi.org/10.7150/thno.49577.
Shukla, Ravi, Vipul Bansal, Minakshi Chaudhary, Atanu Basu, Ramesh Bhonde, and Murali Sastry. 2005. "Biocompatibility of Gold Nanoparticles and Their Endocytotic Fate Inside the Cellular Compartment: A Microscopic Overview." *Langmuir* 21 (23): 10644–54. https://doi.org/10.1021/la0513712.
Siegel, Rebecca L., Kimberly D. Miller, Hannah Fuchs, and AhmedinJemal. 2022. "Cancer Statistics, 2022." *CA: A Cancer Journal for Clinicians* 72 (1): 7–33. https://doi.org/10.3322/caac.21708.
Singh, Mahaveer, and Hemant R. Jadhav. 2018. "Targeting Non-Small Cell Lung Cancer with Small-Molecule EGFR Tyrosine Kinase Inhibitors." *Drug Discovery Today* 23 (3): 745–53. https://doi.org/10.1016/j.drudis.2017.10.004.
Sosnik, Alejandro, Ángel M. Carcaboso, and Diego Andrés Chiappetta. 2008. "Polymeric Nanocarriers: New Endeavors for the Optimization of the Technological Aspects of Drugs." *Recent Patents on Biomedical Engineering* 1 (1): 43–59. https://doi.org/10.2174/1874764710801010043.

Stinchcombe, Thomas E., Mark A. Socinski, Christine M. Walko, Bert H. O'Neil, Frances A. Collichio, Anastasia Ivanova, Hua Mao, et al. 2007. "Phase I and Pharmacokinetic Trial of Carboplatin and Albumin-Bound Paclitaxel, ABI-007 (Abraxane®) on Three Treatment Schedules in Patients with Solid Tumors." *Cancer Chemotherapy and Pharmacology* 60 (5): 759–66. https://doi.org/10.1007/s00280-007-0423-x.

Sun, Leming, Zhen Fan, Tao Yue, Jun Yin, Jianzhong Fu, and Mingjun Zhang. 2018. "Additive Nanomanufacturing of Lab-on-a-Chip Fluorescent Peptide Nanoparticle Arrays for Alzheimer's Disease Diagnosis." *Bio-Design and Manufacturing* 1 (3): 182–94. https://doi.org/10.1007/s42242-018-0019-9.

Sun, Leming, Hongmei Li, Yanqi Ye, Lei Yang, Rehmat Islam, Siyu Tan, Rongsheng Tong, Yang-Bao Miao, and Lulu Cai. 2023. "Smart Nanoparticles for Cancer Therapy." *Signal Transduction and Targeted Therapy* 8 (1). https://doi.org/10.1038/s41392-023-01642-x.

Sun, Min, Howard Hu, Limin Sun, and Zhen Fan. 2020. "The Application of Biomacromolecules to Improve Oral Absorption by Enhanced Intestinal Permeability: A Mini-Review." *Chinese Chemical Letters* 31 (7): 1729–36. https://doi.org/10.1016/j.cclet.2020.02.035.

Sung, Hyuna, Jacques Ferlay, Rebecca L. Siegel, Mathieu Laversanne, Isabelle Soerjomataram, Ahmedin Jemal, and Freddie Bray. 2021. "Global Cancer Statistics 2020: GLOBOCAN Estimates of Incidence and Mortality Worldwide for 36 Cancers in 185 Countries." *CA: A Cancer Journal for Clinicians* 71 (3): 209–49. https://doi.org/10.3322/caac.21660.

Sztandera, Krzysztof, Michał Gorzkiewicz, and Barbara Klajnert-Maculewicz. 2018. "Gold Nanoparticles in Cancer Treatment." *Molecular Pharmaceutics* 16 (1): 1–23. https://doi.org/10.1021/acs.molpharmaceut.8b00810.

Taggart, Laura E., S. J. McMahon, Frederick Currell, Kevin M. Prise, and Karl T. Butterworth. 2014. "The Role of Mitochondrial Function in Gold Nanoparticle Mediated Radiosensitisation." *Cancer Nanotechnology* 5 (1). https://doi.org/10.1186/s12645-014-0005-7.

Tokunaga, Hideki, Mikio Mikami, Satoru Nagase, Yoichi Kobayashi, Tsutomu Tabata, Masanori Kaneuchi, Toyomi Satoh, et al. 2021. "The 2020 Japan Society of Gynecologic Oncology Guidelines for the Treatment of Ovarian Cancer, Fallopian Tube Cancer, and Primary Peritoneal Cancer." *Journal of Gynecologic Oncology* 32 (2). https://doi.org/10.3802/jgo.2021.32.e49.

Vilos, Cristián, Francisco Álvarez Morales, Paula Solar, Natalia Herrera, Fernando González-Nilo, Daniel Aguayo, Hegaly Mendoza, et al. 2013. "Paclitaxel-PHBV Nanoparticles and Their Toxicity to Endometrial and Primary Ovarian Cancer Cells." *Biomaterials* 34 (16): 4098–108. https://doi.org/10.1016/j.biomaterials.2013.02.034.

Wang, Haili, Shenggang Ding, Ze Zhang, Long-Hai Wang, and Ye-Zi You. 2019. "Cationic Micelle: A Promising Nanocarrier for Gene Delivery with High Transfection Efficiency." *The Journal of Gene Medicine* 21 (7). https://doi.org/10.1002/jgm.3101.

Wang, Li, Xianrang Song, Miao Yu, LiminNiu, Yajing Zhao, Yulong Tang, Baibing Zheng, and Li Xie. 2022. "Serum Exosomal miR-377-3p and miR-381-3p as Diagnostic Biomarkers in Colorectal Cancer." *Future Oncology* 18 (7): 793–805. https://doi.org/10.2217/fon-2021-1130.

Wang, Xiaowei, Yuhan Qiu, Mengyan Wang, Conghui Zhang, Tianshu Zhang, Huimin Zhou, Wenxia Zhao, Wei Zhao, Guimin Xia, and Rong-Guang Shao. 2020. "Endocytosis and Organelle Targeting of Nanomedicines in Cancer Therapy." *International Journal of Nanomedicine* 15 (November): 9447–67. https://doi.org/10.2147/ijn.s274289.

Wei, Xiaoli, Jie Gao, Ronnie H. Fang, Brian T. Luk, Ashley V. Kroll, Diana Dehaini, Jiarong Zhou, et al. 2016. "Nanoparticles Camouflaged in Platelet Membrane Coating as an Antibody Decoy for the Treatment of Immune Thrombocytopenia." *Biomaterials* 111 (December): 116–23. https://doi.org/10.1016/j.biomaterials.2016.10.003.

Wells, Carlos M., Michael A. Harris, Landon Choi, Vishnu Priya Murali, Fernanda D. Guerra, and Jessica Amber Jennings. 2019. "Stimuli-Responsive Drug Release from Smart Polymers." *Journal of Functional Biomaterials* 10 (3): 34. https://doi.org/10.3390/jfb10030034.

Wilhelm, Stefan, Anthony J. Tavares, Qing Dai, Seiichi Ohta, Julie Audet, Harold F. Dvorak, and Warren C. W. Chan. 2016. "Analysis of Nanoparticle Delivery to Tumours." *Nature Reviews Materials* 1 (5). https://doi.org/10.1038/natrevmats.2016.14.

Wolinsky, Jesse B., and Mark W. Grinstaff. 2008. "Therapeutic and Diagnostic Applications of Dendrimers for Cancer Treatment☆." *Advanced Drug Delivery Reviews* 60 (9): 1037–55. https://doi.org/10.1016/j.addr.2008.02.012.

Yang, Yannan, and Chengzhong Yu. 2016. "Advances in Silica Based Nanoparticles for Targeted Cancer Therapy." *Nanomedicine: Nanotechnology, Biology and Medicine* 12 (2): 317–32. https://doi.org/10.1016/j.nano.2015.10.018.

Yao, Yihan, Yunxiang Zhou, Lihong Liu, Yanyan Xu, Qiang Chen, Yali Wang, Shijie Wu, Yongchuan Deng, Jianmin Zhang, and Anwen Shao. 2020. "Nanoparticle-Based Drug Delivery in Cancer Therapy and Its Role in Overcoming Drug Resistance." *Frontiers in Molecular Biosciences* 7 (August). https://doi.org/10.3389/fmolb.2020.00193.

Zhang, Chan, Zhao Li, Yuefeng Dong, Xiaoyan Zhang, Ji Lin, and Zhang Chen. 2010. "Folate-Mediated Poly(3-Hydroxybutyrate-Co-3-Hydroxyoctanoate) Nanoparticles for Targeting Drug Delivery." *European Journal of Pharmaceutics and Biopharmaceutics* 76 (1): 10–16. https://doi.org/10.1016/j.ejpb.2010.05.005.

Zhang, Jiajie, Zhong Chen, and Qi Chen. 2024. "Advanced Nano-Drug Delivery Systems in the Treatment of Ischemic Stroke." *Molecules/Molecules Online/Molecules Annual* 29 (8): 1848. https://doi.org/10.3390/molecules29081848.

Zhang, Qian, Xin-En Huang, and Lili Gao. 2009. "A Clinical Study on the Premedication of Paclitaxel Liposome in the Treatment of Solid Tumors." *Biomedicine & Pharmacotherapy* 63 (8): 603–7. https://doi.org/10.1016/j.biopha.2008.10.001.

Zhao, Mei-Xia, Bingjie Zhu, Wenqian Yao, and Di-Feng Chen. 2016. "Therapeutic Effect of Quantum Dots for Cancer Treatment." *RSC Advances* 6 (114): 113791–5. https://doi.org/10.1039/c6ra24063a.

Zhen, Xu, Penghui Cheng, and Kanyi Pu. 2018. "Recent Advances in Cell Membrane–Camouflaged Nanoparticles for Cancer Phototherapy." *Small* 15 (1). https://doi.org/10.1002/smll.201804105.

Zhou, Wen, Xia Gao, Dingbin Liu, and Xiaoyuan Chen. 2015. "Gold Nanoparticles for in Vitro Diagnostics." *Chemical Reviews* 115 (19): 10575–636. https://doi.org/10.1021/acs.chemrev.5b00100.

11 Lipid-Based Nanoparticles to Diagnose and Cure Cancer

Anju Singh and Kamal Kishor Thakur

ABBREVIATIONS

Acronym	Full Form
LBNP	lipid-based nanoparticle
MRI	magnetic resonance imaging
PDT	photodynamic therapy
SLN	solid nanoparticles
LNP	lipid nanoparticles
PC	phosphatidylcholine
PE	phosphatidylethanolamine
PG	phosphatidylglycerol
PS	phosphatidylserine
PI	phosphatidylinositol
ULV	unilamellar vesicles
SUV	small unilamellar vesicles
LUV	large unilamellar vesicles
DOPE	dioleoylphosphatidylethanolamine
DOTAP	1, 2-dioleoyl-3-trimethylammoniumpropane
SNALP	stabilized nucleic acid lipid particles
PEG	polyethylene glycol
LDC	lipid–drug conjugates
NLC	nanostructured lipid carriers
TNBC	triple-negative breast cancer cells
CMC	critical micelle concentration
HPH	high-pressure homogenization
DLS	dynamic light scattering
ZP	zetapotential
SAXS	Small angle X-ray scattering
TLD	1-talidox
PPE	palmar–plantar erythrodysesthesia
LTLD	lyso-thermosensitive liposomal doxorubicin
RAF	radiofrequency ablation
TfR	transferrin
EPHARNA	EphA2-siRNA
CLL	chronic lymphocytic leukemia
DOX	doxorubicin
VPF	verteporfin
AMD	age-related macular degeneration
PTX	paclitaxel
mPAC	metastatic pancreatic adenocarcinoma

DOI: 10.1201/9781003463191-14

LV	leucovorin
QDs	quantum dots
Gd	gadolinium

11.1 INTRODUCTION

The name *cancer* originates from the Greek word "Karkinos (carcinos)," which also refers to crab or crayfish. Hippocrates coined this word to describe the crab-like form of the spreading cancerous projections, which resembled fingers. Cancers are a sizable family of diseases that can penetrate other portions of the body, owing to anomalous development of cells (M. A. Obeid et al. 2018). Depending on the origin, cancer is classified into five main categories, namely, carcinoma, which typically starts in epithelial cells; sarcoma (connective or supportive tissue of bone, cartilage, muscle, etc.); leukemia, which starts in the bone marrow; lymphoma; and multiple myeloma (Hanahan and Weinberg 2011). A collection of diseases known as cancer is distinguished by aberrant cell proliferation that has possibility to spread to other bodily tissues or organs. Over 100 different forms of cancer exist, making it the major causes of deaths globally (Underwood and Cross 2009).

About 90.5 million individuals had cancer diagnoses in 2015 (Vos et al. 2015). About 19.3 million novel cases were documented in 2020, and it was the cause of over 10 million fatalities that year (H. Wang et al. 2016; Sciacovelli et al. 2020; Deo, Sharma, and Kumar 2022). Most instances and deaths resulting from this ailment, encompassing 57% of cases and 65% of cancer-related fatalities, occur in low- and middle-income countries (Cancer Control: A Global Snapshot in 2015, Summary of Results from the 2015 Who NCD Country Capacity Survey Introduction). Lung, prostate, colorectal, stomach, and liver cancer are the utmost predominant malignancies in men, whereas in women, colorectal, breast, uterine/cervix, stomach, and lung cancer are further the most dominant cancers. The location, type, size, and degree of a cancer's impact on an organ or tissue all affect the signs and symptoms of the disease. Nevertheless, there are numerous general signs and indications of cancer, with the existence of an atypical protuberance, a tenacious cough or huskiness, an alteration in bowel patterns, weight loss, discomfort, sweating at night, etc. (Bruera et al. 1990).

Early detection has two main parts: education to inspire initial diagnosis and screening, which together increase the likelihood of a successful cancer therapy. Medical testing and a variety of indicators and markers can aid in the identification of cancer. Afterward, it would typically be further investigated with diagnostic imaging (such as nuclear scans, CT scans, magnetic resonance imaging [MRI], ultrasounds, X-rays, and PET scans) and validated with a biopsy (Connal et al. 2023).

11.2 CANCER THERAPY

By altering or eliminating its primary risk factors, about 30% of cancer deaths could be prevented. Early detection, accurate diagnosis, and efficient care, such as pain management and relaxing care, may increase cancer survival rates and decrease suffering. Cancer may be cured by means of a diversity of procedures, comprising surgery, chemotherapy, hormone treatment, stem cell therapies, immunotherapy, photodynamic therapy (PDT), radiotherapy, (CAR)-T cell therapies, and gene treatment (Singhal, Nie, and Wang 2010; M. Obeid et al. 2020; Q. Zhang et al. 2020).

Cancer remedy is fraught with difficulties due to violent tumor creation and spread in various organs, resistance to medicines, metastatic heterogeneity, and blood–brain hindrance for brain metastasis, among other factors (Valastyan and Weinberg 2011). Chemotherapy is the commonly used treatment, although it is linked with a variety of serious and long-term adverse effects that have a substantial impression on the condition of the patient. The two key revolutions that have revolutionized cancer therapy outlines are aiming actionable changes in oncogene-driven malignancies and immuno-oncology. Both approaches of cancer therapy have significant hurdles. Although sequencing technologies are increasingly being used in clinical research for molecular prescreening, clinical elucidations of vast genomic data limit their clinical use. Furthermore, tumor heterogeneousness and attained resistance are key barriers to precision oncology's success, while extended survival advantages with immunological checkpoint blockers are limited to a small subset of affected persons, and no prognostic markers have been robustly confirmed (Masucci, Elayoubi, and Sayrac 2016; Zugazagoitia et al. 2016).

Chemotherapies, radiation therapy, surgery, and gene therapy are among the treatment options (Singhal, Nie, and Wang 2010). Chemotherapies contain substances that disrupt cell propagation and division, leading to cell self-destruction and demise (Li and Huang 2010). Current chemotherapeutic medicines frequently confront unacceptable cytotoxicity, vague action, unpredictable drug amount within the tumor location, and increased resistance to drugs combined with extended usage. As these treatments target the inhibition of rapidly dividing cells, they affect both normal and malignant cells; this is what causes undesired side effects, like hair loss, nausea, exhaustion, and vomiting. As a result, new therapeutic choices are desperately needed. Drug delivery technology development is regarded as one strategy to improve current therapy choices, by boosting precision and specificity at the tumor location, lowering undesired acquaintance to regular cells (Misra, Acharya, and Sahoo 2010; Li and Huang 2010).

11.3 LIPID-BASED NANOMATERIALS IN DISEASES DIAGNOSIS

In many scientific domains, particularly the biological sciences, nanotechnology is an effective strategy that is rapidly expanding. It offers NPs in a variety of application forms, opening the door to more effective treatment, diagnosis, and sophisticated multifunctional nanomedicines. Advanced imaging technology has been devised for the identification of diverse cancer types. Various nanoparticle types, such as metallic, magnetic, polymeric, metal oxide, quantum dots, graphene, fullerene, liposomes, carbon nanotubes, and dendrimers, play a crucial role in diagnosing breast, colon, and cervical cancers. Moreover, they serve essential functions in certain imaging processes (Alrushaid et al. 2023). Research indicates that nanoparticles persist in the bloodstream for an extended duration before reaching target cells, navigating through various biological barriers like cell membranes, and interacting with biological systems. It has been reported that the detection of methylation patterns and mutations has been used as a marker for cancer diagnosis. It has been suggested that more studies are required before using extracellular vesicles, circulating tumor cells, and cell-free RNA in clinical diagnosis (Schiffman, Fisher, and Gibbs 2015). Various metallic nanoparticles have shown better sensitivity in detecting tumor cells, as they can be conjugated with cancer-specific antibodies and penetrate cancer cells more effectively. Studies have reported that nanocomposites containing more than one type of nanoparticle, such as gold, platinum, silver, copper, and cobalt, are better candidates for cancer detection and imaging. The nanocomposites help penetrate breast and colon cancer cells with great accuracy and produce better signals, which help diagnose cancer. The unique optical, magnetic, and chemical properties of materials at the nanoscale allow the creation of imaging probes with improved contrast enhancement, increased sensitivity, controlled biodistribution, better spatial and temporal information, multifunctionality, and multimodal imaging across MRI, PET, SPECT, and ultrasound. These features could ultimately translate to clinical advantages, such as earlier detection, real-time assessment of disease progression, and personalized medicine (Bobo et al. 2016; Ventola 2017). Lipid-based NPs are among the nanocarriers that are most appealing for use in biomedicine because of their beneficial qualities, including biocompatibility, simplicity in manufacturing, and encapsulation of various functional chemicals (Mirahadi et al. 2018). In SLNs, nanostructured lipid carriers, and liposomes, the use of lipid-based NPs in diagnostic and medical imaging has been extensively studied (Mussi and Torchilin 2013; Mirahadi et al. 2018; Aljabali and Obeid 2019).

Solid lipids with relatively low toxicity that are stabilized by surfactant make up the majority of SLNs. Extremely cleansed triglycerides, fatty acids, and complex glyceride mixes steadied by a combination of surfactants or polymers are the most typical lipids utilized to make SLNs (Pardeike,

Hommoss, and Müller 2008; Mehnert and Mäder 2012; Mirahadi et al. 2018). With beneficial characteristics like site-specific targeting, drug release control, physical stability, easy manufacturing, and industrial scaling-up, SLNs serve as an effective and versatile colloidal drug carrier. It is also capable of avoiding or minimizing medication breakdown when loaded. Technetium-99, 64Cu, and quantum dots (QDs) are only a few of the many kinds of diagnostic chemicals that have been transferred using SLNs as a pharmacological tool (Mehnert and Mäder 2012; Mussi and Torchilin 2013; Mirahadi et al. 2018). Quantum dots and paclitaxel combined with SLNs displayed anticancer action against human lung carcinoma cells, and the intense fluorescence from the quantum dots within the SLNs suggested the picturing of the intracellular translocation of SLNs in cancer cells (Bae et al. 2013). This indicates value of SLNs as a multifunctional nanocarrier for therapeutic and diagnostic instruments.

The use of liposomes in investigative medical imaging is a relatively novel and expanding subject. The purpose of liposomes in imaging is to enable adequate imaging and to provide distinguishable differences between diseased and normal tissues (Mirahadi et al. 2018). Lipid-based nanomaterials in detection, QDs, gadolinium, and manganese; radionuclides like Ga, ^{111}In, and ^{99m}Tc; iodine-based agents; and even gases can be used to label liposomes as diagnostic tools (Mukundan et al. 2006; Laurent et al. 2014; Aljabali and Obeid 2019). The flexibility of the liposome structure makes it possible to incorporate imaging agents into either the interior or the bilayer, making them efficient carriers for contrast intensification (Kao et al. 2003; Y. Chen, Bose, and Bothun 2010). For improved tumor diagnostics, liposomes-containing components like gadolinium (Gd) have proven to be useful. Pure Gd is rapidly decreased in the intravascular plasma and distributed extracellularly, whereas Gd that has been conjugated or encapsulated in a liposomal formulation has a lengthy retention duration in the circulation (X. Li et al. 2014). Furthermore, ^{64}Cu-encapsulated liposomes have distinctive imaging features. It can prevent ^{64}Cu from exchanging because the liposome's protective layer shields it from the biological surrounding's membrane, leading to a high concentration of ^{64}Cu inside the liposomes. Since they are suitable for PET/CT imaging, these liposomes offer a non-intrusive visualization and measurement approach (Petersen et al. 2011). By facilitating the distribution of therapeutic substances with precision to the target tissues, these applications highlight the growing usage of lipophilic nanoparticles in the field of disease, predominantly in the diagnosis, monitoring, and treatment of cancer.

11.4 NANOPARTICLE USE IN TRANSPORT OF DRUG

A promising cancer treatment has been developed using cancer nanotechnology for the transport of anticancer drugs (Bor, Azmi, and Yaghmur 2018). Nanoparticle sizes range between 1 and 1,000 nm. They serve as an effective device to enhance targeting of drug, increase drug bioavailability, and reduce many drugs' toxicities (Miele et al. 2012; García-Pinel et al. 2019). Different criteria are used to categorize nanoparticles, some of which depend on the particle's size, form, and source, whereas others rely on the chemical composition, identifying them as organic or inorganic. Nanoparticles have established a lot of consideration due to their diverse physicochemical characteristics, elevated ratio of volume to surface that is significantly higher in comparison to other particles. Due to this property, nanoscale particles have a very little volume for carrying load but a very broad area of coverage for interacting with biological membranes (De Jong and Borm 2008).

The main difficulty in medicine administration is getting the drug to the place of action while preventing collateral effects that are off-target and on healthy tissues. Nanoparticles are the best drug carriers because they have a variety of properties that make them ideal for drug targeting, including controllable size, which encourages the accumulation of tumor cells, allows penetration through various biological barricades and cell membranes, and reverses functionality to avoid devastation by lysosomes after endocytosis. The perfect nanoparticle must therefore be immune-free, biocompatible, biodegradable, non-toxic, and capable of avoiding early hepatic or renal clearance (M. A. Obeid et al. 2018).

Large molecules like nucleic acids, peptides, and medications that are not membrane-permeable but are just weakly water-soluble can all be delivered by means of nanoparticle drug transporters. The medicine might be bonded covalently to the nanoparticles' outer surface or encapsulated inside their core; when the delivery system reaches the intended location, the medication frequently detaches from the nanoparticles by degradation, swelling, or diffusion. In this chapter, we highlight lipid formulations among the many nanoparticle-based cancer preparations available, since their preparation and alternate compositions have advanced significantly in the last several years (Johoon Kim et al. 2017). Doxil (liposomal doxorubicin) and AmBisome (liposomal amphotericin B) were a couple of the first drugs made with lipid-based nanoparticles to hit the market (Allen and Cullis 2013; Díaz and Vivas-Mejia 2013; Ozpolat, Sood, and Lopez-Berestein 2014).

11.5 LIPID-BASED NANOPARTICLES IN CANCER TREATMENT

Lipids are materials that are not water-soluble but nevertheless dissolve in diethyl ether, chloroform, and alcohol (IUPAC 1997). Among the various types of lipids are fats, steroids, waxes, and fatty acids. Lipids are occasionally referred to as aquaphobic or amphipathic minorparticles. Due to the amphiphilic characteristics of different lipids, structures such as vesicles and large uniflagellar liposomes can be created in an aquatic environment. Figure 11.2 depicts the structural components of solid lipid nanoparticles, liposomes, and micelles (Sheoran et al. 2022).

As of the commencement of the pharmaceutical era, lipids have drawn significant attention for their biocompatibility in transportation. Because of their strong hydrophobic nature, they exhibit limited oral absorption (Tang, Sun, and He 2007). Consequently, efforts to broaden the spectrum of potential uses for these carriers were unsuccessful and were not utilized in propulsion systems until 1900, when incorporated into colloidal delivery systems (Humberstone and Charman 1997; Pouton and Porter 2008; Patel and Velikov 2011; Kuentz 2012). Lipid nanoparticles (LNPs) have been utilized extensively for drug administration since they were shown to be more advantageous than polymeric nanoparticles for development of nanoparticle-based distribution structures (R. H. Müller, Mäder, and Gohla 2000). These lipid-based structures are known as "nano safe" carriers, as LNPs are made from physiological or biodegradable lipids. Solid lipid nanoparticles (SLNs), established in the 1990s, are a very effective form of LNP production (Gasco 1993; Lucks and Muller 1996; Pardeike, Hommoss, and Müller 2009; Doktorovova, Souto, and Silva 2014).

The main lipid-based nanoparticles are liposomes, solid lipid nanoparticles, niosomes, micelles, and lipidoid nanoparticles (Figure 11.1).

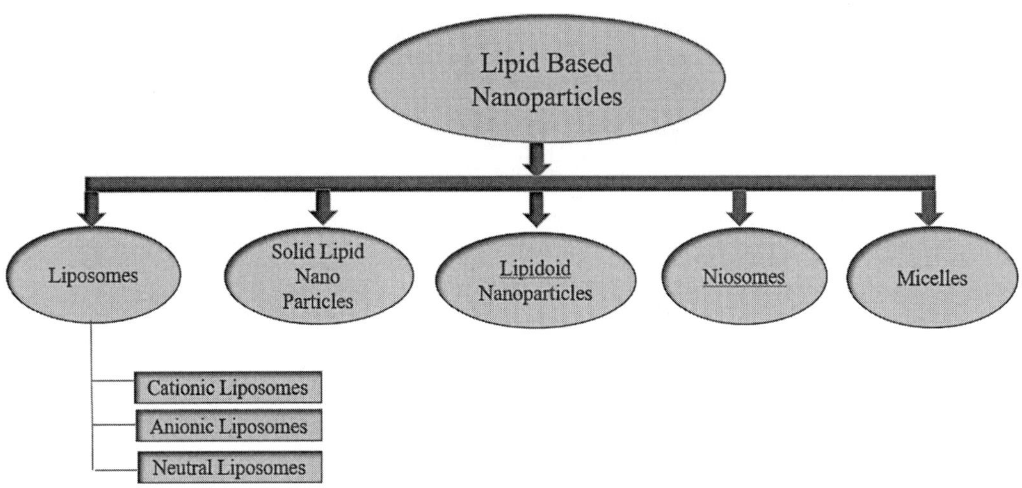

FIGURE 11.1 Types of lipid-based nanoparticles. A schematic diagram depicting the frequently employed lipid-based nanoparticles for the delivery of anticancer drugs.

11.5.1 Liposomes

Liposomes were reported originally in 1965 by Bangham; it was discovered that they exhibited a number of physical, structural, and functional characteristics that were comparable to those of biological membranes. Since then, liposomes have been completely inspected and are well-established as drug delivery systems. The first lipid-based system to receive clinical approval were liposomes, which have received the most research attention (A D Bangham, Standish, and Watkins 1965; Gregoriadis 1976; Qaraghuli et al. 2017; Beltran et al. 2019). Liposomes, formerly acknowledged as spherules, are amid the utmost sophisticated drug distribution mechanisms. They are sphere-shaped artificial vesicles (typically 50–500 nm in diameter) made up of phospholipid bilayers (Sun et al. 2014; Jha, Sharma, and Malviya 2016). Liposomes firstly emerged as one of the most comprehensive drug delivery arrangements (Sercombe et al. 2015). Liposomes offer significant potential as a drug dispersal scheme in cancer chemotherapy because of their passive, selective medication targeting, enhanced healing effectiveness, adaptability for linking with unique ligands for each location to attain dynamic aiming, improved drug firmness, and lower noxiousness of capturing agents with better pharmacokinetic effects (Mare et al. 2018).

Liposomes are mostly made up of phospholipids, although they also comprise cholesterol and lipids linked with polymers. Phospholipids consist of a water-attracting (hydrophilic) head and a water-repelling (hydrophobic) tail, which autonomously assemble, forming a double layer when exposed to water (Akbarzadeh et al. 2013; Nakhaei et al. 2021; Wu et al. 2021). Hydrophilic chemotherapy medications (for example, cytarabine) may be captured by encasing them in the liposomes' aqueous center, whereas hydrophobic anticancer drugs, anthracyclines, can be encapsulated by including them in entering the liposomes' lipid bilayer (Allen 1998).

Natural phospholipids utilized in liposome preparations include phosphatidyl choline (PC) and phosphatidylethanolamine (PE). PE is often employed in small doses in liposome formulations due to its capability to create nonbilayer structures and disrupt the liposome membrane under physiological conditions. PC is the primary lipid component of the liposome membrane. Other phospholipids, viz. phosphatidyl glycerol (PG), phosphatidyl serine (PS), and phosphatidylinositol (PI), could also be utilized (Ellens, Bentz, and Szoka 1986; Vemuri and Rhodes 1995). Cholesterol-enclosed phospholipid bilayers contribute to decreased lipid membrane bilayer fluidity, reduced hydrophilic molecule permeability, and enhanced firmness of these vesicles within the bloodstream (Yingchoncharoen, Kalinowski, and Richardson 2016).

11.5.2 Categories of Liposomes

There are several ways to classify liposomes, that is, how they were made, the quantity of bilayers encased inside the liposomal vesicle, or their dimensions (Vemuri and Rhodes 1995) (Figure 11.2).

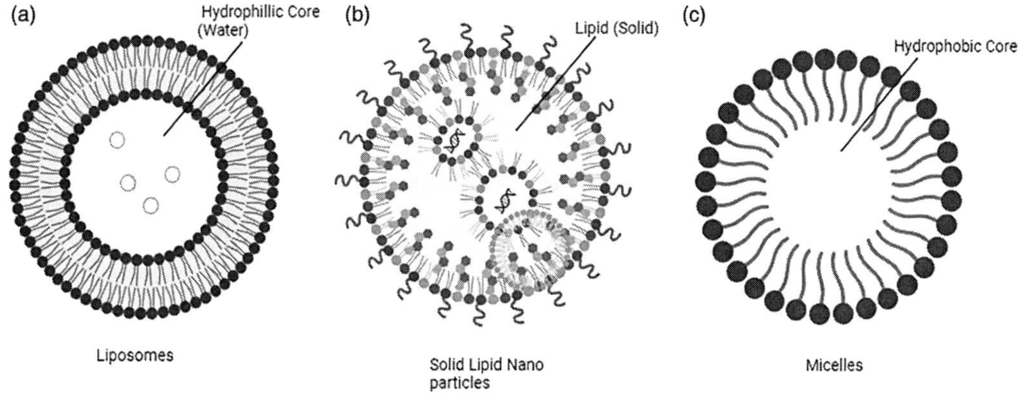

FIGURE 11.2 Types of lipid-based nanoparticles. A schematic representation of structure of different type of lipids: (a) liposomes, (b) solid lipid nanoparticles, and (c) micelles.

The most common categories of liposomes, however, are unilamellar vesicles (ULVs), which are further separated into small (SUVs, particle size 20–200 nm), large (LUVs, particle size 0.2–1 μm), and giant (GUVs particle size >1 μm), and multilamellar vesicles (MLVs, particle size 0.5–10 μm) (Yingchoncharoen, Kalinowski, and Richardson 2016).

The behavior of these nanoparticles in vivo is greatly influenced by their physiochemical qualities, which will have influence on their anticancer effects. Liposomes are conventionally divided into cationic, anionic, and neutral based on their surface charges (Sercombe et al. 2015). The amount of cellular absorption and dispersal of nanoparticles depends on their surface charges (Albanese, Tang, and Chan 2012; Hühn et al. 2013). Compared to cationic nanoparticles, which tend to attract serum proteins to their surfaces, promoting opsonization and recognition by the reticuloendothelial system, neutral and negatively charged nanoparticles exhibit prolonged in vivo circulation half-lives (Honeywell-Nguyen and Bouwstra 2005; Alexis et al. 2008; Hong-Xia Wang et al. 2016).

11.5.2.1 Positively Charged Liposomes

Liposomes with a positive charge are created by incorporating lipids like dioleoylphosphatidylethanolamine (DOPE), didioleoylphosphatidylethanolamine, 1, 2-dioleoyl-3-trimethylammoniumpropane (DOTAP), and dimethyldioctadecyl ammonium bromide. These liposomes have been widely utilized as a delivery mechanism inside of mammal cells because they can produce firm complexes through healing agents with a negative charge, siRNA to produce complexes of higher capability to facilitate siRNA transport (A. Laouini et al. 2012; J.-M. Lee, Yoon, and Cho 2013; Ozpolat, Sood, and Lopez-Berestein 2014). Modulating the apparent acid dissociation constant (pKa) of ionizable cationic liposomes has improved their design, and it has been shown that pKa values of 7 or below are critical for siRNA encapsulation and in vivo activity. In clinical trials right now, cationic liposomes with pKa values of 6.2 to 6.5 are the most active ones (Y. Tam, Chen, and Cullis 2013; M. Draz et al. 2014; Wan, Allen, and Cullis 2014). The usage of positively charged liposomes for delivering anticancer medications has been studied by numerous research teams. EndoTAG-1 is the primary clinically tested preparation of positively charged liposomes containing paclitaxel. Models of animal tumors like B16 and Sk-Mel 28 melanoma were used in preclinical programs to study how EndoTAG-1 affected tumor progression. Furthermore, it was discovered that the cationic liposomal method could successfully lower bcl-2 levels by capturing siRNA aiming human oncogene bcl-2 mRNA (Chang and Yeh 2012). Although cationic liposomes, particularly for siRNA, offer tremendous benefits as delivery vehicles, possible toxicities must be taken into account before further clinical deployment. When cationic liposomes are used excessively, they can cause pulmonary inflammation, hepatotoxicity, and dose-dependent toxicity by encouraging the production of reactive oxygen molecules and raising intracellular calcium levels (J.-M. Lee, Yoon, and Cho 2013; J. Zhang, Li, and Huang 2014; Ozpolat, Sood, and Lopez-Berestein 2014).

Numerous PEG-coated cationic liposome formulations regarding the orderly administration of nucleic acids to induce gene silencing have been produced. Among these preparations, the stabilized nucleic acid lipid particles (SNALPs) developed are particularly notable. Cationic lipids prone to ionization, for example, DL in DMA or DL in KC2-DMA, a lipid known for its elevated temperature of transition, namely, 1,2-distearoyl-sn-glycero-3-phosphocholine, cholesterol, and lipids improved with PEG, make up the structure. This lipid combination enables effective taking up by cells and successful seepage of nucleic acid cargo from endosomes. SNALPs have been effectively examined for the systemic siRNA administration and have a typical particle size of 100 nm. The PEG covering on SNALPs protects, stabilizes, and delays vesicle evacuation (Gomes-da-Silva et al. 2012; Ozpolat, Sood, and Lopez-Berestein 2014; J. Zhang, Li, and Huang 2014; Zhou, Zhang, and Liang 2014).

11.5.2.2 Anionic Liposomes

The main building blocks of cell membranes are phospholipids containing anionic head groups, which are crucial for both the integrity of the membrane and intracellular trafficking. Natural anionic lipid includes phosphatidylglycerol (PG), phosphatidylinositol (PI), phosphatidylserine (PS), and phosphatidic acids present in cell membranes and crucial for membrane trafficking, lipoprotein association, and cell signaling (Draz et al. 2014; Wan, Allen, and Cullis 2014). Kaur stated that anionic liposomes demonstrated enhanced lymphatic uptake in comparison to cationic liposomes (Kaur, Nahar, and Jain 2008). Doxorubicin's antileukemic action was significantly boosted by anionic liposomes, while its long-term cardiac toxicity was decreased. As a substitute to cationic liposomes for the transfer of siRNA, stable anionic lipid–siRNA complexes have been created by means of calcium, a divalent cationic bridging agent. Anionic nanocomplexes are gaining increased technical interest for the complete administration of siRNA in order get past the shortcomings of cationic liposomes, for example, poisonousness and quick removal from the bloodstream. Anionic liposomes were created by Tagalakis for the transport of siRNA, and this system's effectiveness was examined in vitro along with its physical characteristics, biocompatibilities, and cytotoxicity. However, more study is required to improve the composition, preparation, and characterization of the anionic nanocomplexes, even if they demonstrated encouraging results in vitro when an anionic formulation was used. Furthermore, researchers developed a liposome with a negative charge, composed of DOPG (sodium salt of 1,2-dioleoyl-sn-glycero-3-phospho-(1′-rac-glycerol) DOPE (dioleoylphosphatidylethanolamine) (in a 40:60 molar ratio). This liposome is designed to transport siRNA using calcium bridges, and they achieved a successful encapsulation of over 99% of the siRNA with this method (Kapoor and Burgess 2012; J. Zhang, Li, and Huang 2014; Tagalakis et al. 2014; Tseu and Kamaruzaman 2023).

11.5.2.3 Neutral Liposomes

The success in DNA formulation was initially attributed to the usage of charged lipids for siRNA transport; however, toxicity issues with the cationic constituent and lipids continue to be key obstacles for such formulations. The toxicity and additional issues linked to positively charged liposomes have been proven to be solved by neutral liposomes, which have great delivery efficiencies for goods like siRNA and are made of neutral lipids like 1,2-dioleoyl-sn-glycero-3-phosphatidylcholine (DOPC) (Buyens et al. 2012; J. Zhang, Li, and Huang 2014). Due to their lack of interaction with serum and blood's negatively charged proteins, neutral liposomes have a prolonged circulation period and less cytotoxicity than cationic liposomes (Buyens et al. 2012). Additionally, neutral liposomes were found to be more prevalent in tumors and inflammatory locations than cationic liposomes because neutral liposomes are more amenable to active targeting tactics than cationic liposomes due to the nonspecific electrostatic interactions that they exhibit (Bozzuto and Molinari 2015). Doxorubicin is encapsulated into tiny neutral unilamellar liposomes featuring surface-bound PEG to create liposomal doxorubicin (Doxil), an FDA-approved anticancer treatment. Additionally, DaunoXome is a liposome formulation made solely of neutral lipids, distearoylphosphatidylcholine, and cholesterol and, as a result, has a neutral charge on surface. Both preparations show prolonged circulation and significant accretion in tumor tissues. The transport of nucleic acids using neutral liposomes has also been investigated. Merritt demonstrated that their liposomal formulations were very active in an in vivo context, aiming to decrease the expression of genes in an ovarian cancer model in mice by targeting the proangiogenic cytokine interleukin 8 and the oncoprotein EphA2 (Mamot et al. 2003; Merritt et al. 2008).

When a neutral liposome is delivered to a mass, it will be rapidly cleared, in divergence to anionic and cationic liposomes. Anionic liposomes are recognized as external substances that eventually enter the reticuloendothelial system. As for positively charged liposomes, they have a propensity to bind with plasma proteins, ensuing in the creation of a protein halo on their surface, and subsequently being adorned with antibodies that are subsequently ingested by scavenger cells to be drawn to plasma proteins, producing a corona layer on their surface, and coated with antibodies, which are later consumed by scavenger cell. These results suggest that, given the constraints, it is not feasible to create a functional liposome using just one kind of lipid. However, the properties can be changed, and the carrier made more useful by combining different kinds of lipids (Xiong, Mi, and Gu 2011; Digiacomo et al. 2020).

11.5.3 Lipid Nanoparticles in Solid Form

New generations of lipid-based nanoparticles have been proposed as superior substitutes that combine the benefits and get around the main drawbacks of conventional colloidal systems like liposomes and polymeric NPs (R. Müller, Mäder, and Gohla 2000). These solid lipid-based nanomaterials comprise of lipid–drug conjugates (LDCs), solid lipid nanoparticles (SLNs), and nanostructured lipid carriers (NLCs) (Wissing, Kayser, and Müller 2004). They are lipid-based particles that range in size from 50 to 1,000 nm and continue to be solid at both standard body temperature and ambient conditions (Wong et al. 2007). The benefits of these particles include easy preparation, high stability, flexible chemistry, and regulated drug release. Solid lipids like phospholipids, glycerides, glyceride mixtures, lipid acids or waxes, and cholesterol are used to create SLNs. To increase the stability of SLNs, surfactants like lecithin, Tween 80, and sodium glycholate are added to the SLN engineering methodology (D.-B. Chen et al. 2001; Feng and Mumper 2013).

Several research has been undertaken on the administration of anticancer medications like paclitaxel using SLNs (D.-B. Chen et al. 2001; M.-K. Lee, Lim, and Kim 2007). These lipid nanoparticles have substantial advantages, viz., targeting particular sites, physical firmness over prolonged duration, the capability for precise release of mutually water-soluble and fat-soluble medications, safeguarding of sensitive substances, cost-effectiveness, ease of production, and safety (Shahgaldian et al. 2003; Wong et al. 2007; Mydin and Moshawih 2019). Drug ejection during storage and poor drug loading capacity are potential drawbacks of these formulations (Mehnert and Mäder 2001). The application of these lipid nanoparticles as a transport platform for an array of water-soluble and ionic compounds is being extended with the progress of newer versions of SLNs that overcome the drawbacks of older versions (M. A. Obeid et al. 2018).

According to the major contributions from the previous year, SLNs can be used to encapsulate anticancer medications. The formulation of niclosamide-loaded solid lipid nanoparticles boosted cellular acceptance and the effectiveness of antitumor activity against triple-negative breast cancer cells (TNBC). *Triple-negative cancer* means breast cancer devoid of the receptors typically present in common breast cancer types (Chintamaneni, Pindiprolu, and Krishnamurthy 2018). The Eskiler group developed talazoparib loaded onto SLNs in 2018, enhancing the drug's therapeutic index against TNBC cells (Guney Eskiler et al. 2018). In order to regulate temperature-dependent drug release, other magnetic SLN formulations of paclitaxel PTX were developed. These formulations used magnetic hyperthermia to cause regulated PTX discharge from the magnetic SLNs. Alternative illustration is the anti-inflammatory action of SLNs that were loaded with citral and geraniol in the RAW 264.7 cell line. These SLNs also had improved ability to block NO generation (Oliveira et al. 2018; Zielińska et al. 2018). SLNs can positively carry labile anticancer medications to the site of action while protecting them from degradation, such as camptothecin and doxorubicin (Yang and Zhu 2002; Wong et al. 2006).

11.5.4 Lipidoid Nanoparticles

Lipidoid nanoparticles use cholesterol and PEG-coated lipids and are a characteristic family of lipid-based compounds. The word *lipidoid* comes from the Greek and means "lipid-like"(Akinc et al. 2008). With the aid of the Michael addition reaction, huge degradable or nondegradable combinatorial libraries can be easily and quickly created by conjugating an amine to acrylates or acrylamides. Chemically, the library's components mimic lipids, protecting and improving the uptake of their siRNA payload (Akinc et al. 2009; Goldberg 2012). An examination of this unusual class of materials reveals that these special substances have the form of a structure that is a cross amid positively charged lipids and dendrimers of the initial generation. Members of this library differ from conventional positively charged lipids in that lipidoids are positive charged because of the presence of amine groups that can undergo reversible protonation, in contrast to conventional cationic lipids, which consist of a positively charged head group and two hydrophobic tails. Lipidoids can either be employed in place of cationic lipids in the creation of cationic liposomes or used straight as carriers for siRNA (Goldberg 2012; Tam, Chen, and Cullis 2013). Moreover, it was observed that these formulations achieved gene silencing with lower siRNA doses compared to traditional nanoparticles, thereby reducing the potential for toxicity. The widely adopted lipidoid-based nanocarriers designed for siRNA delivery, aiming at genes like FVII or apolipoprotein B (ApoB) factor, exhibited a substantial reduction in the manifestation of these targets in hepatocytes among nonhuman primates and mice afflicted with liver cancer. These findings hold promise for the distribution of siRNA targeting the HoxA1 gene for breast cancer treatment. Brock created a lipidoid delivery system. They discovered that the lipidoid system efficiently inhibited cell growth, lowered the frequency of mammary tumors in mice, and allowed contacts with cell membrane and endosomal outflow (Brock et al. 2014).

11.5.5 Niosomes

The non-ionic surfactant vesicles (NISV) acknowledged as niosomes are lipid-derived structures that resemble liposomes in relation to construction (Pandey and Kartikeyan 2008). They are made up of an aqueous component that is encased by lipid bilayers, making them capable of encasing pharmaceuticals and acting as drug carriers. Since then, there has been an increase in interest in niosomes as a medication delivery mechanism. Researchers in the cosmetic business were the first to describe and use them (Uchegbu and Vyas 1998). The surfactants derived from alkyl or di-alkyl polyglycerol ethers and cholesterol, which cannot be ionized and coupled with other substances, including charge-inducing compounds. Alkyl ethers, Tweens, Spans (sorbitan fatty acid esters), and alkyl glyceryl ethers are frequently employed to create niosomes (Marianecci et al. 2014; Paecharoenchai et al. 2014). These surfactants exhibit amphiphilic properties, featuring a hydrophilic head and a hydrophobic tail. Niosomes possess a bilayer structure resembling that of liposomes, permitting them to contain hydrophilic materials within both their hydrophobic particles and watery core. Because it can impact vesicle cohesion, mechanical strength, water permeability, and membrane rigidity, cholesterol is a noteworthy feature in the growth of NISVs (G. P. Kumar and Rajeshwarrao 2011; Moghassemi and Hadjizadeh 2014). Supplementary additives include charged compounds that improve the niosomes' overall stability during storage by reducing the agglomeration of vesicles due to electrostatic attraction. Niosomal formulations have garnered increased attention because of their ability to transport and encapsulate a varied array of medications, coupled with their advantages, including cost-effectiveness, excellent steadiness, and storing convenience. These attributes position them as promising liposomal substitutes (M. A. Obeid et al. 2022). Anticancer medications, gene transfer, inflammation and infection-fighting medicines, and numerous other pharmaceuticals have all been studied as potential drug delivery systems using niosomes (Vyas et al. 2005; Balakrishnan et al. 2009; Pardakhty et al. 2007; Zidan, Rahman, and Khan 2011; Tavano, Vivacqua, et al. 2013; Pawar and Vavia 2015).

A lot of interest has been focused on niosomes as a possible anticancer transport mechanism. In order to deliver doxorubicin to Michigan Cancer Foundation-7 (MCF-7) and M.D. Anderson Metastasis Breast Cancer (MDA-MB-231) human breast cancer cell lines, Tavano, in 2013, created transferrin (TF)conjugate niosomes (Tavano, Muzzalupo et al. 2013). Polyethylene glycol (PEG)niosomes were effectively created by Hong to deliver hydroxycamptothecin to solid tumors after intravenous treatment (Hong et al. 2009). This method exhibited significant cytotoxicity and demonstrated a high level of cellular uptake when tested in vitro against KB, K562, and S180 cancer cell lines. Furthermore, it displayed potent antitumor activity against S180 tumors in mice. Niosomes loaded with 5-fluorouracil have been created for topical treatment of various types of skin cancer (Paolino et al. 2008).

11.5.6 Micelles

These are tiny colloidal structures with sizes between 5 and 100 nm that are created when amphiphilic molecules self-assemble (Hanafy, El-Kemary, and Leporatti 2018). Three types of micelles are formed: lipid, polymeric, or lipid-polymeric hybrid micelles (Sawant and Torchilin 2010). Lipid micelles arrange themselves into a monolayer where the hydrophilic heads are oriented toward the aqueous surroundings, whereas lipophilic tails constitute the inner core. This is distinct from liposomes or niosomes, which possess a lipid bilayer assembly surrounding a watery core (Arleth et al. 2005; Feng and Mumper 2013). Depending on their constituent elements, micelles can assume various shapes, such as spherical, ellipsoidal, or rod-like structures. The critical micelle concentration (CMC) represents the lowest concentration of amphiphilic components required for the initiation of micelle formation of ellipsoidal or spherical rod-like assemblies. CMC is the lowermost concentration of amphiphilic fragments at which micelles begin to form. Assembly of the molecules is triggered by a decrease in free energy at this concentration. Drugs that are hydrophobic are usually supplied via nanocarrier micelles and retained within the micellar inner core. (Mu, Elbayoumi, and Torchilin 2005). Lipid micellar nanostructures have a comparatively limited hydrophobic capacity, which constrains the amount of medication they can accommodate. Additionally, when diluted to a concentration below CMC, whether in vivo or in vitro, lipid micelles are prone to dissolution. The micellar structure has been used in the administration of anticancer medications in numerous applications. Genexol-PM is the first class of polymeric micelles that encapsulate paclitaxel. When compared to the Taxol commercial formulation, the micellar delivery system for paclitaxel developed by Hamaguchi had a 25 times enhanced drug accretion in colon cancers in mice and a comparable improvement in anticancer action (Hamaguchi et al. 2005; Tawfik et al. 2020). Furthermore, Gill established a micelle-centric preparation containing paclitaxel and parthenolide within a modified vitamin E micellar system. Parthenolide is a medication known to inhibit nuclear factor kappa B, which contributes to paclitaxel resistance. This approach exhibited significantly superior efficacy when compared to the individual administration of paclitaxel or parthenolide in in vitro studies (Gill, Kaddoumi, and Nazzal 2012).

11.6 METHODS FOR PRODUCING LIPID-BOUND NANOPARTICLE

Regardless of technique used, the fundamental idea behind the creation of lipid-based nanoparticles is the hydrophilic/hydrophobic contact among lipid–water and lipid–lipid fragments, which is aided by the addition of energy to help the lipid components arrange themselves into double layer or micelles (M. Mozafari 2005). Top-down and bottom-up methodologies are frequently used in the preparation of nanoparticles. The Turkeyvich method, block copolymer synthesis, gas phase synthesis, and microbial synthesis are all used in the bottom-up strategy to nucleate atomic-sized materials into nanoparticles (Hadinoto, Sundaresan, and Cheow 2013; Shafique et al. 2023). Milling, spark ablation, and laser ablation are used in the top-down strategy to actually separate bulk materials into nanosized pieces (V. Kumar et al. 2012).

11.6.1 Traditional Preparation Methods

Lipid-based nanoparticles are prepared using four traditional techniques. The techniques differ in how the lipids are disseminated again in aqueous medium after being extracted from the organic solvent (M. Mozafari 2005). To avoid toxicity, residues of these organic solvents, which are used in high quantities in these processes, must be eliminated from the formulation's final product (Abdallah Laouini et al. 2012).

11.6.2 Hydration-Based Thin Lipid Film Formation

The easiest and most popular technique, referred to as the Bangham approach and initially reported in 1965, is widely used to create lipid-based nanoparticles at both laboratory and industrial scale

(Bangham, Standish, and Watkins 1965). An organic solvent is used to disperse a combination of lipids during this operation to achieve homogeneity, most frequently methanol, chloroform, ether, methylene chloride, ethanol, or a combination of solvents (Kohli et al. 2014). A slender lipid film is created on the flask's sidewalls as the solvent is separated at by means of rotary evaporator (Ganesan and Narayanasamy 2017). The lipid suspension is first hydrated, and then it is repeatedly pushed through a filter with uniform pore diameters to produce lipid nanoparticles of a consistent size. The size and polydispersity of created nanoparticles depend on a number of factors, including temperature, extrusion force, membrane pore size, and applied pressure (Tenchov et al. 2021). The required drug can either be dispersed with lipid components for hydrophobic drugs or added to the aqueous hydration media for water-loving drugs in order to create the generated vesicles (Ranade and Hollinger 2011). Large multilamellar vesicles with diverse diameters are prepared using this technique. Despite being simple and popular, this approach achieves a drug encapsulation efficacy of only 5–15% for water-soluble medicines (Yingchoncharoen, Kalinowski, and Richardson 2016).

11.6.3 Using Inversion-Phase Evaporation Method

The process includes dispersing lipids in an organic solvent, such as a 1:1 mixture of diethyl ether and chloroform, diethyl ether and isopropyl ether, or a 2:1 v/v combination of chloroform and methanol, which promotes the creation of upturned micelles (Szoka Jr and Papahadjopoulos 1978; Pidgeon et al. 1987; Shi and Qi 2021). When there is surplus of organic phase present, an emulsion of lipids and buffer, where water is dispersed in an oil phase, is first prepared mechanically or by sonication, and then the organic phase is eliminated under vacuum (Vemuri and Rhodes 1995). The elimination of organic phase from blend results in the creation of massive unilamellar and oligolamellar vesicles that enclose aqueous media. Large hydrophilic molecules can be encapsulated in the particles created by this approach thanks to their high aqueous-volume-to-lipid ratio. It is feasible to capture approximately 30–45% of the aqueous volume, and under ideal circumstances, this (Figure 11.3) can go up to 65% (Szoka and Papahadjopoulos 1978). Though this technique

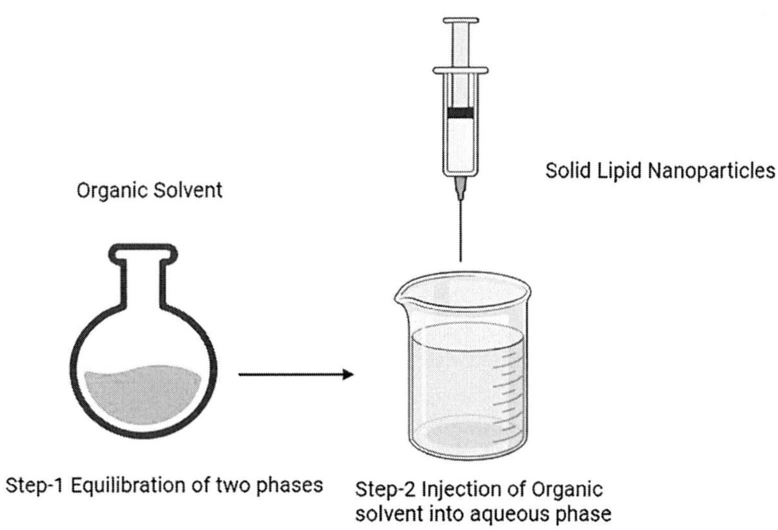

FIGURE 11.3 Solvent injection method. A schematic representation of preparation of lipid-based nanoparticles. Lipids are dispersed in ethanol or ether, and the resulting solution is then delivered through syringe-type infusion pumps into an excessive volume of aqueous medium.

Source: New (1990); Lasch, Weissig, and Brandl (2003); H. Zhang and D'Souza (2017).

could yield greater drug encapsulation, it exposes the drug to organic solvents and mechanical agitation. Since the drugs that are to be placed in the liposomes are in direct contact with an organic solvent, this approach is not suited for subtle particles (peptides). Finally, mechanical stirring and direct contact with the organic solvent could lead to alterations in the conformation of biomolecules, potentially resulting in effects like protein denaturation and DNA strand breaks for substances such as enzymes, proteins, or oligonucleotides (Szoka Jr and Papahadjopoulos 1978; Pidgeon et al. 1987; Shi and Qi 2021).

11.6.4 Solvent Injection Method

In order to create the nanoparticles via this approach, lipids are dispersed in ethanol or ether, and the resulting solution is then delivered through syringe-type infusion pumps into an excessive volume of aqueous medium (New 1990; Lasch, Weissig, and Brandl 2003; H. Zhang and D'Souza 2017). When ethanol is employed as a solvent, the lipids dissolved in the aqueous phase can autonomously form tiny particles, since ethanol is miscible with water and can be diluted to the necessary concentration (Lasic 1995). The ether injection technique comprises introducing a solution of ether and lipids into a heated aqueous phase. Following the injection, the ether evaporates, and the dispersed lipids primarily shape large unilamellar vesicles (LUVs), which effectively encapsulate water-soluble drugs (Deamer and Bangham 1976).

11.6.5 Detergent Depletion Method

Detergent hydrates and solubilizes lipids to form mixed micelles (Jiskoot et al. 1986), which are then eliminated via precise dialysis, column chromatography, or adsorption to produce consistent LUVs or MLVs, reliant on the category of detergent and the process of detergent elimination (Ollivon et al. 2000; Torchilin 2005). In this process, commonly used detergents with a high critical micelle concentration (CMC) include sodium cholate, Triton X-100, alkyl glycoside, and sodium deoxycholate (Vemuri and Rhodes 1995).

11.6.6 Modern Techniques of Preparation

11.6.6.1 Heating Method

The most recent techniques for creating lipid-based nanoparticles without using organic solvent has been published. In this process, lipid constituents are first dissolved in aqueous medium and heated with stirring, up to 120°C (M. R. Mozafari et al. 2004). A polyol such as glycerol, which increases the stability of the vesicles, is added in this procedure at a concentration of 3% (v/v). The method's key benefit is that it does not use hazardous or volatile organic solvents. The kind and charge of lipids and rate of stirring all can affect the particle size (M. Mozafari 2005; Durak et al. 2020).

11.6.6.2 Freeze-Drying of Double Emulsions

Lipid-based nanoformulations used in water-soluble drugs are typically prone to leakage during manufacturing and shelf storage. Additionally, active medicines may degrade prior to usage in drug delivery systems due to potential oxidation processes and other chemical interactions (Lombardo and Kiselev 2022). So to overcome these problems, freeze-drying method was developed. A transparent isotropic monophasic solution is created by dispersing lipid components uniformly in water and tert-butyl alcohol in proper ratios. After that, under carefully monitored circumstances and low pressure, the solution is sterilized and freeze-dried. When aqueous media is added to the freeze-dried product and shaken afterward, somewhat-homogenous MLV dispersions develop on their own (Patil and Jadhav 2014). The produce can be kept in its freeze-dried state when not in use and then rehydrated immediately as needed. The obstacles preventing the widespread adoption of this method include the instability of particle sizes during the freeze-drying process, the high cost associated with the procedure, and the variability in the encapsulation efficiency of the resulting particles (Ranade and Cannon 2011).

11.6.6.3 Reverse-Phase Supercritical Evaporation

This method was firstly described by Otake et al., who used supercritical CO_2 to dissolve phospholipids (Otake et al. 2001). In the procedure, lipid constituents are initially disseminated in compressed carbon dioxide with ethanol. Speedy depressurization and instantaneous mingling of the precipitated lipids into the aqueous phase result in the formation of the vesicles. This approach produces sizable unilamellar particles, eliminating the organic solvent through vacuum extraction. Subsequently, the particles can be size-controlled using either filtration or extrusion. With this single-step approach, it is possible to produce nanoparticles with a high level of encapsulation efficiency (Frederiksen et al. 1997). Imura et al.'s study demonstrated the potential to regulate both the dimensions and trapping efficiency of generated liposomes by manipulating pressure and the concentration of organic co-solvent (Imura et al. 2003; Ranade and Cannon 2011; Akbarzadeh et al. 2013). Because carbon dioxide possesses antibacterial qualities, this approach has attracted attention. It produces sterile formulations that may be useful for creating lipid-based nanoparticles for use in medicine (Kraft et al. 2014; Lombardo and Kiselev 2022).

11.6.7 Modified Ethanol Injection Technique

11.6.7.1 Cross-Flow Injection Approach

This process entails dissolving lipids in ethanol and then injecting the solution into an aqueous buffer using the cross-flow injection technique, which employs two tubes connected at one end to create a cross-configuration with an injection orifice in the center. Different factors, including diameter of injection hole, flow rate of buffer, pressure during injection, the features of lipid particles formed, can be influenced by factors such as lipid composition and concentration. With this technique, pharmaceutical application particle preparation may be scaled up (A. Wagneret al. 2002; Abdallah Laouini et al. 2012).

11.6.7.2 Microfluidic Mixing Method

The microfluidic process is known as a very active procedure for the commercial manufacturing of several lipid nanoparticles (Pradhan et al. 2008; Ding et al. 2016). Due to the carefully regulated mingling of lipid and drug in microchannels, this approach is basically dependent on nanoprecipitation (Liu et al. 2022). When compared to conventional bulk mixing techniques, microfluidic devices' quick mixing at the microscale permits more homogeneous and repeatable nanoparticle creation. Additionally, the benefits of heat and mass transport provided by the tiny dimensions of microfluidic channels lead to greater size control and uniformity of LNPs (Pourabed et al. 2021).

In a microfluidic device, the channels with cross sections between 5 and 50 μm were used, which permit quick mixing via diffusion or convection (Whitesides 2006). The two main kinds of microfluidic devices used to create LNPs are capillary-based platforms and chip-based platforms. In capillary-based systems, a central tube serves as the introduction point for the organic solvent bounded by a series of manifold tubes to facilitate speedy dilution with the outgoing aqueous solution (Kurakazu and Takeuchi 2010). Various types of micromixers have been developed to create lipid-based nanoparticles, depending on the specific channel configurations. These methods encompass a staggered herringbone micromixer, resulting in turbulent advection mixing, and enable the elongating and folding of fluid streams across the microchannel's cross-sectional area, as well as T- or Y-shaped mixers, droplet-based microfluidic systems, and a microfluidic hydrodynamic focusing platform (Jahn et al. 2004; Teh et al. 2008). Microfluidics has the capability to generate nanoparticles within a diameter range of 20 to 100 nm while maintaining high efficiency. The size of particles is prejudiced by factors such as flow rates of both fluids, choice of aqueous media, and ratio of water and lipid phases (Pradhan et al. 2008; M. Obeid et al. 2017; Maeki et al. 2018, 2022).

11.6.7.3 Membrane Contractor Method

A modified ethanol injection technique serves as the foundation for the membrane contactor approach. The setup comprises of two pressure containers:(1) for organic phase (lipids) and (2) for an aqueous phase, detached by a unique permeable glass membrane that permits the flow of the organic phase (Lasch 2003; Jaafar-Maalej, Charcosset, and Fessi 2011; A. Laouini et al. 2012). The (other) polypropylene hollow fibers are frequently used as membrane because they enable bigger regions and homogeneous flows. After being dissolved in ethanol, the lipid phase is transferred via membrane having a predetermined pore diameter into aqueous phase using this technique. To assist the lipid phase in moving through pores, nitrogen gas is employed at a pressure lower than 5 bar (A. Laouini et al. 2011). While the vesicles produced are extracted from the apparatus, the aqueous phase concurrently runs along the surface of a membrane. The particle size is prejudiced by variables such as the pressure in the organic phase, the flow velocity in the aqueous phase, and the lipid concentration (Jaafar-Maalej, Charcosset, and Fessi 2011; A. Laouini et al. 2012; Abdallah Laouini et al. 2013).

11.6.8 Additional Techniques for Preparing Nanoparticles

SLN preparation also uses high-speed homogenization, ultrasonication, high-pressure homogenization, and thinning of microemulsions (Mehnert and Mäder 2001). The most often used techniques for preparing micelles are direct dissolving, film casting, dialysis, and oil-in-water emulsion (Letchford and Burt 2007; Lombardo and Kiselev 2022).

11.6.8.1 High-Pressure Homogenization (HPH)

First, a liquid formulation is created by dispersing or dissolving the medication in the melted lipid. A suspension of homogenized lipid particles with a smaller final size is formed when the liquid formulation is forced through a micrometric cavity by the high operating pressure (R. Müller, Mäder, and Gohla 2000). Excellent product qualities can be achieved by either performing it at normal temperature (cold homogenization) or at a higher temperature (hot homogenization). This technique's main drawbacks have been its high energy consumption and the polydispersity of the final formulations (Nastruzzi 2005). In order to overcome its initial limitations, the HPH approach has demonstrated some modifications/improvements to lipid-based nanomaterials in cancer healing and diagnosis. In this way, alternative concepts like microfluidics can be used to produce the narrowest droplet distributions while maintaining stable pressure. High-pressure homogenizers come in the form of microfluidics (Figure 11.4).

11.6.8.2 High-Speed Homogenization

High-speed stirrers or rotor mixers provide the external mechanical energy needed to generate the emulsion. The speed range that is utilized is 6,000–24,000 rpm (X. Wang et al. 2008). At the same temperature and with continuous stirring, the melted lipid and the surfactants in the aqueous phase are combined. This would allow the temperature to be maintained in an oil bath until the particles form. When the process is ramped up, higher stirring rates do not significantly improve repeatability, but they do reduce the polydispersity (Choi et al. 2014).

11.6.8.3 Ultrasonication

The three most crucial ultrasonication process parameters are irradiation power, ultrasonication time, and frequency. These parameters are tabulated in accordance with the manufacturer's guidelines and are connected to the probe tip's diameter. Lipid NP dispersion is produced when the final emulsion's temperature is gradually lowered below the lipid's crystallization temperature (Shah

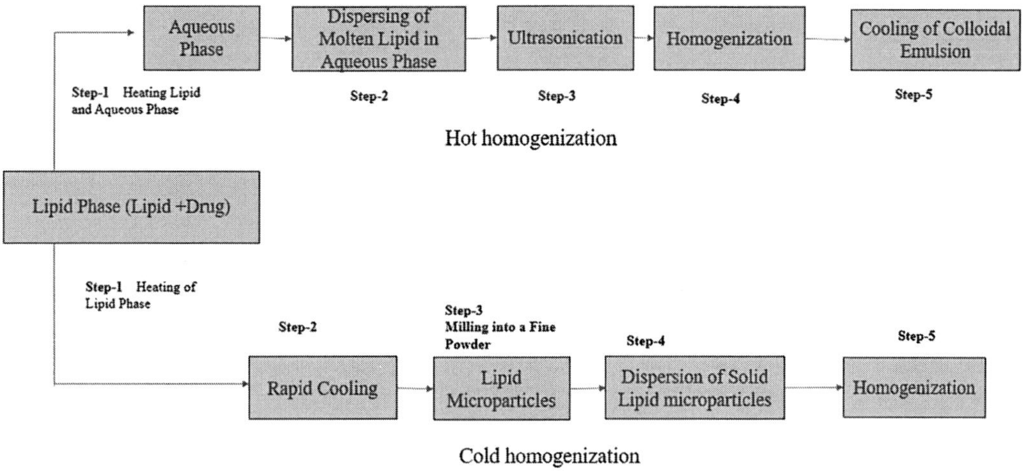

FIGURE 11.4 High-pressure homogenization. Schematic representation of homogenization technique for preparation of nanoparticle: (1) hot homogenization technique, (2) cold homogenization technique.

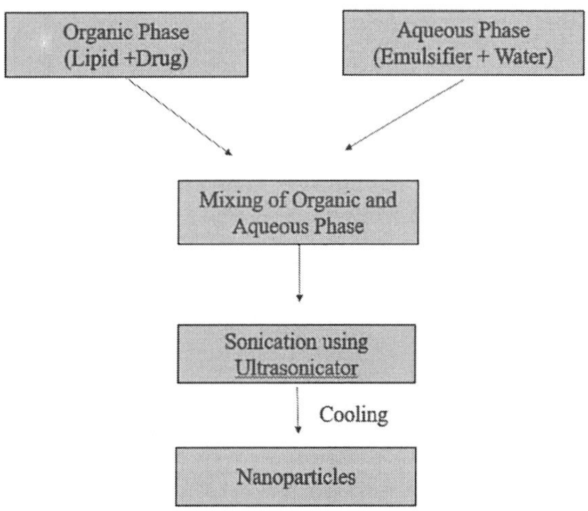

FIGURE 11.5 Sonication technique. A schematic representation of sonication technique for preparation of nanoparticle. Lipid NP dispersion is produced when the final emulsion's temperature is gradually lowered below the lipid's crystallization temperature.

Source: Shah et al. (2015).

et al. 2015). Ultrasonic irradiation preparations for emulsions are very reproducible; nevertheless, this technology is not easily scalable for the industry due to heat generation and probable metal contamination caused by ultrasonication (Abdullah, Malaki, and Baghizadeh 2012) (Figure 11.5).

11.7 LIPID-BASED NANOPARTICLE CHARACTERIZATION

Characterization of the manufactured nanoparticles is crucial for determining their effectiveness and quality. Following are the most popular approaches to characterize nanoparticles.

11.7.1 Morphology and Analysis of Particle Size

The performance of nanoparticles is greatly prejudiced by the shape, size, and morphology of particles. SLNs can have the following shapes: sphere, rod, pellet, or anisotropic. The desired characteristics of SLNs are obtained by determining particle size. SLNs range in diameter from 50 to 1m000 nm on average (Ferrari 2008; Lin et al. 2014). Dynamic light scattering (DLS), microscopy methods, size exclusion chromatography, and other methods are available for detecting particle size (Brar and Verma 2011). DLS has restricted usefulness for studying samples with heterogeneous dispersal (big PDI) and produces inaccurate results for non-spherical particles (Brar and Verma 2011; Uskoković 2012).

Microscopic methods such as scanning electron microscopy, atomic force microscopy, scanning tunneling microscopy, and transmission electron microscopy are useful in revealing shape, size and morphology, stability, and potential accumulation procedure of particles during stowage (Koçum, Çimen, and Pişkin 2004; Z. L. Wang 2004; Parot et al. 2007). In biological contexts, LNPs are greatly benefited by having a clearly defined and smooth surface shape because it increases steadiness and reduces the possibility of opsonization, in which serum proteins attach to surface and cause the removal of the immunological system. The seamless top reduces unfavorable interplays with biological elements, enabling positive LNP biodistribution, and confirming maximum healing effectiveness. However, in contrast, LNPs with uneven surface might interact with biological agents more frequently, which might affect biodistribution of LNP and complete healing effectiveness (Mehta et al. 2023).

11.7.2 Charge on the Outer Area

Charge on the outer part of a particle is defined as the total charge that particle absorbs in a given medium. It is a physical characteristic that may be found on the surface of any suspended particle and serves as a gauge for the likelihood of particle interactions (Abdallah Laouini et al. 2012). The strength of particles in the colloidal system is often predicted using surface charge measurement, normally assessed using zeta potential (ZP). ZP typically has a value of ±30 mV, used to deduce steadiness of particle; a value larger than 30 mV denotes stable state. ZP value of less than 30 mV implies an inclination for aggregation, coagulation, or instability flocculation (Andar et al. 2014; Lin et al. 2014). Zeta potential can be estimated with a variety of tools, such as a zeta sizer. Surface charge may have an impact on physiological barrier permeation and receptor binding. Positively charged nanoparticles have better cellular absorption than their negatively or neutrally charged counterparts, making cationic nanoparticles perfect for medication delivery to nucleic acids and tumors. However, compared to their negatively charged cousins, positively charged nanoparticles may be more harmful (Luyts et al. 2013).

11.7.3 Determination of Lamellarity

Lamellarity, or the number of bilayers in a liposome, has an impact on the liposomal product's implementation, encapsulation effectiveness, and drug release kinetics (A. Kumar, Gupta, and Braya 2021). The lamellarity of the particle can be ascertained using techniques based on how lipid markers' visual or fluorescence signals change when reagent is added (Fröhlich, Brecht, and Peschka-Süss 2001; Abdallah Laouini et al. 2012). Another technique for determining lamellarity is magnetic resonance, which has also been used to examine membrane structure and determine how lipids are distributed inside bilayers. Other methods for determining lamellarity include small-angle X-ray scattering (SAXS) and imaging techniques using electron microscopy. It can also be measured using 31P-NMR, freeze-fracture electron microscopy techniques (M. Müller, Mackeben, and Müller-Goymann 2004; Lin et al. 2014).

11.7.4 Stability of Particle

Nanomedicines' *stability* is defined as their capacity to maintain the similar properties after being produced for a set amount of time. Chemical, physical, and biological stability are all interlinked, are critical factors for ensuring the stability of vesicles. The assessment of these variables has a significant role in determining whether or not nanoparticles will be used in vitro or in vivo (Marianecci et al. 2014). The stability of nanoparticles might be impacted by elements like temperature, moisture, pH, surface charge, solvents, enzymatic degradation, or the inclusion of excipients in preparation (Briscoe and Hage 2009). In a broad sense, steadiness is evaluated by observing modifications in factors like zeta potential (ZP), drug release, or particle size over time and under different conditions, including variations in temperature and exposure to biological fluids (Celia et al. 2009).

11.7.5 Efficiency of Encapsulation

A portion of the medicine that is not encapsulated is present in the same blend as the encapsulated drug in lipid-based nanoparticle formulations. For assessing the preparation technique for drug encapsulation, drug EE is a crucial metric, and it may be written as follows:

$$EE = \left(\frac{amount\ entrapped}{total\ amount} \right) \times 100$$

The "total amount" refers to the extent of drug employed in the preparation (Marianecci et al. 2014).

High-performance liquid chromatography, UV-vis spectrometry, enzyme-based techniques, or gel electrophoresis are typically employed to measure the amount of drug contained in nanoparticles (Xu et al. 2021). Methanol or Triton X-100 is used to break up the lipidic structure and release the drug after it has been extracted from the lipid nanoparticles containing the drug. The direct approach and the indirect method are the two basic ways to measure EE. The indirect approach first analyzes the quantity of unencapsulated pharmaceuticals in the supernatant before calculating the EE, whereas the direct method directly determines the quantity of drug entrapped in nanoparticles (Charrois and Allen 2004; A. Laouini et al. 2011).

The percentage of pharmaceuticals that are successfully entrapped in carriers can only be understood with the usage of EE. A higher EE is ideal for applications involving drug delivery. The kinds, content, and crystallinity of the lipid components, as well as the drug's miscibility in the organic phase and water phase, all have influence on EE. Drugs in LNPs should typically have an EE of more than 70%. Because they include liquid lipids, NLCs often have higher EE than SLNs (Xu et al. 2021).

11.8 CLINICAL APPLICATIONS OF LIPID-BASED NANOMATERIALS

Numerous investigations have been conducted on the usage of NPs in the cure of different ailments, with a specific prominence on cancer. The first NP for the treatment of cancer, liposomal doxorubicin (Doxil), received clinical approval. Since then, numerous other formulations based on lipids have already been authorized, and a great deal more are in various stages of clinical research. Those in clinical trials are either newly created nanoformulations or ones that have already received approval (Anselmo and Mitragotri 2016). A few of them are featured here. Figure 11.6 shows the various steps of the clinical trial for the approval of newly created nanodrugs.

As an upgraded variant of the already-approved Doxil (Myocet and Caelyx/Doxil), Talidox (TLD-1) is a new PEGylated liposomal formulation of doxorubicin created by InnoMedica. Despite Caelyx's ability to prevent doxorubicin-related cardiotoxicity, TLD-1 was created as a remedy for

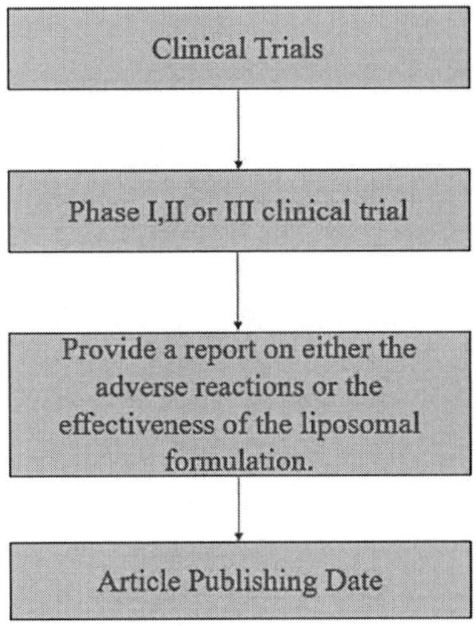

FIGURE 11.6 Steps of clinical trial.

the high incidence of palmar–plantar erythrodysesthesia (PPE) associated with its use. In terms of improved cytotoxicity and antitumor efficacy with lower toxicity, preclinical investigations showed that TLD-1 was superior to free doxorubicin and Caelyx (Broggini et al. 2017). In contrast to doxorubicin, annamycin is a better modern-era lipophilic anthracycline antibiotic which avoids multidrug confrontation and lacks cardiotoxicity. Individuals suffering from recalcitrant or recurrent acute myelic leukemia are being evaluated in two separate phase 1/2 trials using a liposomal formulation of annamycin created by Moleculin Biotech Inc. (Zou and Priebe 1995).

Mitomycin C's bioavailability was enhanced by delivering it as a lipid-based prodrug in liposomes that have been PEGylated, known as Promitil® (Gabizon et al. 2006). A stable liposomal formulation is created by encapsulating the prodrug within the bilayer; this prodrug is only released as the active drug by the thioredoxin–thioreductase system, which is overexpressed in tumors and improves tumor localization. In order to treat individuals with firm tumors, a preliminary study (phase 1) of Promitil, a drug created by Lipomedix Pharmaceuticals Inc., was conducted (Golan et al. 2015).

To upsurge drug bioavailability, stimuli-responsive liposomes have also been researched. One illustration is a doxorubicin liposomal formulation that responds to heat, called lyso-thermosensitive liposomal doxorubicin (LTLD), or ThermoDox, created by Celsion Corporation. When temperatures rise over 39.5°C, the PEGylated LTLDis designed to release its payload. Local heat is used after it has been administered intravenously because it helps maximize liposomal localization at tumor areas because of enhanced vasculature and because it causes the release of the chemotherapy drug doxorubicin. By using radiofrequency ablation (RAF), local heating can be achieved. ThermoDoxhas reached several phases of clinical study. Phase 1 of research, which also combined LTLD with RFA in patients of primary and metastatic liver tumors, is already complete. Phase 1 of the TARDOX trial, which combines targeted ultrasound with LTLD in patients with primary or secondary liver tumors, has shown encouraging results. Phase 1/2 of the DIGNITY trial has evaluated the usage of microwave-induced hyperthermia combined with LTD in order to treat breast cancer that has locally progressed or recurs (Poon and Borys 2011).

Polymeric micelles have been used efficaciously in clinical trials as chemotherapeutic drug delivery systems. A novel polymeric micellar formulation of paclitaxel is called Genexol PM, created by a biopharmaceutical corporation (John Kim et al. 2017). Genexol PM has been studied in a variety of clinical trials, including those for pancreatic cancer, either alone or in combination with gemcitabine; urothelial cancer (phase 2); lung cancer, combined with cisplatin (phase 2) and with gemcitabine; head and neck cancer, combined with cisplatin (phase 2); and ovarian cancer, combined with carboplatin (phase 1 and phase 2). To get around the toxicities associated with cisplatin, Nano Carrier Co. Ltd. created a unique sustained-release micellar formulation of cisplatin (Subbiah et al. 2017).

The first lipid-based nanomaterial, Onpattro, that was accepted for use in the healing of cancer marked a significant advancement in gene delivery, and many more are now being developed. SGT-94, which delivers plasmid DNA encoding the tumor suppressor gene RB94, and SGT-53, which delivers plasmid DNA encoding the typical human wild-type p53 suppressor gene, were created by SynerGene Therapeutics Inc. (Pirollo et al. 2008, 2016). A single-chain anti-transferrin (TfR) antibody fragment is attached to cationic liposomes, which target tumors by binding to TfR, in cancer cells. Furthermore, a phase 1b trial using SGT53 and docetaxel in individuals with solid tumors has been finished (Siefker-Radtke et al. 2016).

When united with cationic liposomes made of DOTAP and cholesterol, the tumor suppressor gene TUSC2 (FUS1) is deactivated in 82% of cases of non–small cell lung cancer and 100% of small cell lung cancer cases. An enduring trial of phase 1/2 examines the synergistic effect of this liposomal formulation in fusion with erlotinib in individuals with stage IV lung cancer cells (non–small cell) (Xiaobo et al. 2016). To transport EphA2-siRNA (EPHARNA) to the location of cancer cells overexpressing the EphA2 receptor, a neutral liposomal formulation including DOPE was created. To examine the formulation in cases of advanced or recurrent solid tumors, a phase 1 trial is now recruiting participants (M. Wagner et al. 2017).

The usage of lipid-derived nanoparticles for cancer immunotherapy, including vaccine administration, has also been investigated (Z. Gu et al. 2020). XEME Biopharma Inc. created Onco Quest-CLL, a liposomal product that delivers a vaccination made of whole-cell tumor lysates with IL-2 for the treatment of asymptomatic chronic lymphocytic leukemia (CLL). Multilamellar liposomes are used to deliver the patient's leukemia cell lysate and a recombinant human IL-2, creating customized cancer vaccinations. The safety and effectiveness of the vaccine in people with previously untreated CLL are being investigated in a phase 1b experiment. In phase 1 of the OLIVIA experiment, a liposomal mRNA vaccine against ovarian cancer is being tested in conjunction with carboplatin and paclitaxel (Ma and Platanias 2018; M. Obeid et al. 2020).

Radiotherapy delivery has also investigated the uses of lipid-based polymers in the healing of cancer. The treatment of glioblastoma with brachytherapy using convection-enhanced delivery of liposomes encapsulating the radionuclide rhenium-186 showed encouraging preclinical results (Phillips et al. 2012).

11.9 CLINICALLY APPROVED LIPID-BASED NP MEDICINES

Doxil®, licensed by FDA in 1995 to cure ovarian cancer and Kaposi's sarcoma allied with AIDS, was the first nanomedicine product to receive approval from the agency (Beltran et al. 2019; Yingchoncharoen, Kalinowski, and Richardson 2016; Almeida et al. 2020; M. Obeid et al. 2021). Liposomal formulation of doxorubicin, called Doxil®, was PEGylated, which means that PEG chains were bonded to the liposome surface. With reference to the standard non-PEGylated liposomes' short circulating half-life as a result of macrophage clearance occurring quickly, this formulation was developed to reduce those constraints. Additionally, Doxil® was found superior than free DOX in terms of improving drug levels in malignancies and reducing cardiotoxic adverse effects of doxorubicin (DOX) treatment. More effective and tolerant liposomal DOX formulations than free DOX, including Lipo-Dox®, were created. Furthermore, the European Medicines Agency (EMA) authorized the usage of Myocet®, a liposome-coated preparation of DOX and cyclophosphamide, to heal metastatic cancer of breast (Mussi and Torchilin 2013; Bobo et al. 2016; Bulbake et al. 2017).

Trials and approvals of liposomal delivery have increased in the 2000s. A photosensitizer-encapsulated liposome was first developed for photodynamic treatment (Ventola 2017). A verteporphin (VPF), a modified porphyrin that resembles chlorine, is delivered through the unilamellar phospholipid vesicle known as Visudyne®. It was the first light-activated medication to heal up age-related macular degeneration (AMD) persons with primarily choroidal neovascularization in the typical subfoveal region (Bobo et al. 2016; Bulbake et al. 2017; Beltran et al. 2019). The purpose of this formulation is to eliminate the aberrant blood vessels in the eye caused by diseases such as wet macular degeneration. The treatment of ovarian cancer uses the well-known medicinal medication paclitaxel (PTX). PTX has been developed in liposomal formulations, including Lipusu®, which was approved in China (Sike Pharmaceutical Co. Ltd.). A lot of approved liposomal formulation products for the healing of cancer are available. For instance, the bupivacaine liposomal injection form Exparel® is a multivesicular liposome based on DepofoamTM technology and is used to manage pain. Pacira Pharmaceutical, Inc. created Exparel®, which has FDA approval for local surgical site injection for postoperative discomfort following hemorrhoidectomy and bunionectomy (Mazloomdoost et al. 2017; Ventola 2017).

The FDA has authorized the use of three fresh liposomal formulations in clinical settings since 2015. The FDA and EMA authorized Merrimack Pharmaceuticals Inc.'s Onivyde® in 2015 to heal metastatic pancreatic adenocarcinoma (mPAC) patients who have previously had gemcitabine-based healing. Onivyde® is irinotecan formulation using PEGylated nanoliposomal hydrochloride. It is used in conjunction with 5-FU and leucovorin (LV) (Ventola 2017; Beltran et al. 2019; Almeida et al. 2020). These patients still have a very limited range of alternatives, and there is no accepted standard of care. Patients who received Onivyde® along with 5-FU/LV had a greater survival rate, it was discovered. Additionally, CPX-351 (VyxeosTM), which received FDA approval in 2017, is a liposomal drug that delivers daunorubicin and cytarabine for the cure of seriousmyeloid leukemia (Bulbake et al. 2017; Caster et al. 2016; Ventola 2017; Beltran et al. 2019).

Based on the evidence, liposomal drug delivery has been established to be a beneficial therapeutic tool, and as nanotechnology advances, this platform will carry on to develop into the upcoming generation of nanomedicines. Table 11.1 lists the products with liposomal formulations that have been authorized for clinical use.

TABLE 11.1
Clinically Approved Liposomal Formulation Items

Product Name	Nanosystem Type	Active Ingredient	Approving Organization	Indication	References
Doxil	Liposome	Doxorubicin hydrochloride	FDA (1995) EMA (1996)	Ovarian cancer	Yingchoncharoen, Kalinowski, and Richardson (2016); Beltran et al. (2019); Almeida et al. (2020)
Caelyx®	PEGylated liposome	Doxorubicin hydrochloride	EMA (1996)	Breast cancer, ovarian cancer	Beltran et al. (2019); Yingchoncharoen, Kalinowski, and Richardson (2016)
Myocet®	Liposome	Doxorubicin hydrochloride and an anthracycline cytotoxic agent	EMA (2000)	Breast cancer	Bulbake et al. (2017)
Lipodox®	Liposome	Doxorubicin hydrochloride	FDA (2013)	Ovarian cancer	Beltran et al. (2019)
Onivyde®	Liposome	Irinotecan	FDA (2015)	Pancreatic cancer	Ventola (2017); Bulbake et al. (2017)
Genexol-PM®	Micelle	Paclitaxel	FDA (2007)	Breast cancer	Ventola (2017)

TABLE 11.1 *(Continued)*
Clinically Approved Liposomal Formulation Items

Product Name	Nanosystem Type	Active Ingredient	Approving Organization	Indication	References
Apealea®	Micelle	Paclitaxel	FDA (2018)	Ovarian cancer, peritoneal cancer, fallopian tube cancer	Fetterly et al. (2008)
LEP-ETU	Liposome	Paclitaxel	-	Lung/ovarian/ breast cancer	J. A. Zhang et al. (2005); Fetterly et al. (2008)
Lipusu	Liposome	Paclitaxel	FDA (2005)	Gastric, ovarian, and lung cancer	W. Gu, Andrews, and Tian (2023); Beltrán-Gracia et al. (2019)

11.10 CONCLUSION AND FUTURE PROSPECTS

Diverse lipid-based nanomaterials offer effective avenues for enhancing the diagnosis and treatment of various cancer types. They achieve this by improving the detection of cancer-specific biomarkers, facilitating tumor and metastasis imaging, enabling specific drug delivery to target cells, and providing real-time monitoring of treatment progress. Among these nanomaterials, liposomes stand out as the most extensively researched and utilized lipid nanoparticles. Several lipid-based nanomedications have already entered the market, addressing these objectives, while others are in development or undergoing clinical trials. These advancements hold the promise of significantly improving the outcomes of anticancer therapeutics and diagnostics.

REFERENCES

Abdullah, Amir, Massoud Malaki, and E. Baghizadeh. 2012. "On the Impact of Ultrasonic Cavitation Bubbles." *Proceedings of the Institution of Mechanical Engineers, Part C: Journal of Mechanical Engineering Science* 226 (March): 681–94. https://doi.org/10.1177/0954406211414769.

Akbarzadeh, Abolfazl, Rogaie Rezaei-Sadabady, Soodabeh Davaran, Sang Woo Joo, Nosratollah Zarghami, Younes Hanifehpour, Mohammad Samiei, Mohammad Kouhi, and Kazem Nejati-Koshki. 2013. "Liposome: Classification, Preparation, and Applications." *Nanoscale Research Letters* 8 (1). Springer: 1–9. https://doi.org/10.1186/1556-276X-8-102.

Akinc, Akin, Michael Goldberg, June Qin, J. Robert Dorkin, Christina Gamba-Vitalo, Martin Maier, K. Narayanannair Jayaprakash, Muthusamy Jayaraman, Kallanthottathil G. Rajeev, and Muthiah Manoharan. 2009. "Development of Lipidoid-SiRNA Formulations for Systemic Delivery to the Liver." *Molecular Therapy* 17 (5). Elsevier: 872–9.

Akinc, Akin, Andreas Zumbuehl, Michael Goldberg, Elizaveta S. Leshchiner, Valentina Busini, Naushad Hossain, Sergio A. Bacallado, et al. 2008. "A Combinatorial Library of Lipid-Like Materials for Delivery of RNAi Therapeutics." *Nature Biotechnology* 26 (5): 561–9. https://doi.org/10.1038/nbt1402.

Albanese, Alexandre, Peter S. Tang, and Warren C. W. Chan. 2012. "The Effect of Nanoparticle Size, Shape, and Surface Chemistry on Biological Systems." *Annual Review of Biomedical Engineering* 14 (1). Annual Reviews: 1–16. https://doi.org/10.1146/annurev-bioeng-071811-150124.

Alexis, Frank, Eric Pridgen, Linda K. Molnar, and Omid C. Farokhzad. 2008. "Factors Affecting the Clearance and Biodistribution of Polymeric Nanoparticles." *Molecular Pharmaceutics* 5 (4). American Chemical Society: 505–15. https://doi.org/10.1021/mp800051m.

Aljabali, Alaa, and Mohammad Obeid. 2019. "Inorganic-Organic Nanomaterials for Therapeutics and Molecular Imaging Applications." *Nanoscience &Nanotechnology-Asia* 9 (August). https://doi.org/10.2174/2210681209666190807145229.

Allen, Theresa M. 1998. "Liposomal Drug Formulations." *Drugs* 56 (5): 747–56. https://doi.org/10.2165/00003495-199856050-00001.

Allen, Theresa M., and Pieter R. Cullis. 2013. "Liposomal Drug Delivery Systems: From Concept to Clinical Applications." *Advanced Drug Delivery Reviews* 65 (1): 36–48. https://doi.org/10.1016/j.addr.2012.09.037.

Almeida, Bethany, Okhil Nag, Katherine Rogers, and James Delehanty. 2020. "Recent Progress in Bioconjugation Strategies for Liposome-Mediated Drug Delivery." *Molecules* 25 (December): 5672. https://doi.org/10.3390/molecules25235672.

Alrushaid, Noor, Firdos Alam Khan, Ebtesam Abdullah Al-Suhaimi, and Abdelhamid Elaissari. 2023. "Nanotechnology in Cancer Diagnosis and Treatment." *Pharmaceutics* 15 (3): 1025. https://doi.org/10.3390/pharmaceutics15031025.

Andar, Abhay U., Renee R. Hood, Wyatt N. Vreeland, Don L. DeVoe, and Peter W. Swaan. 2014. "Microfluidic Preparation of Liposomes to Determine Particle Size Influence on Cellular Uptake Mechanisms." *Pharmaceutical Research* 31 (2): 401–13. https://doi.org/10.1007/s11095-013-1171-8.

Anselmo, Aaron, and Samir Mitragotri. 2016. "Nanoparticles in the Clinic." *Bioengineering & Translational Medicine* 1 (March). https://doi.org/10.1002/btm2.10003.

Arleth, Lise, Beena Ashok, Hayat Onyuksel, Pappannan Thiyagarajan, Jaby Jacob, and Rex P. Hjelm. 2005. "Detailed Structure of Hairy Mixed Micelles Formed by Phosphatidylcholine and PEGylated Phospholipids in Aqueous Media." *Langmuir* 21 (8). American Chemical Society: 3279–90. https://doi.org/10.1021/la047588y.

Bae, Ki, Jeong Yu Lee, Soo Lee, Tae Park, and Yoon Sung Nam. 2013. "Cancer Therapy: Optically Traceable Solid Lipid Nanoparticles Loaded with SiRNA and Paclitaxel for Synergistic Chemotherapy with In Situ Imaging (Adv. Healthcare Mater. 4/2013)." *Advanced Healthcare Materials* 2 (April). https://doi.org/10.1002/adhm.201200338.

Balakrishnan, Prabagar, Srinivasan Shanmugam, Won Seok Lee, Won Mo Lee, Jong Oh Kim, Dong Hoon Oh, Dae-Duk Kim, et al. 2009. "Formulation and in Vitro Assessment of Minoxidil Niosomes for Enhanced Skin Delivery." *International Journal of Pharmaceutics* 377 (1): 1–8. https://doi.org/10.1016/j.ijpharm.2009.04.020.

Bangham, Alec D., Malcolm M. Standish, and Jeff C. Watkins. 1965. "Diffusion of Univalent Ions Across the Lamellae of Swollen Phospholipids." *Journal of Molecular Biology* 13 (1): Elsevier: 238–58. https://doi.org/10.1016/S0022-2836(65)80093-6.

Beltran, Esteban, Adolfo López, I. Higuera-Ciapara, Jesus Velazquez, and Alba Adriana Vallejo. 2019. "Nanomedicine Review: Clinical Developments in Liposomal Applications." *Cancer Nanotechnology* 10 (December) BioMed Central Ltd. https://doi.org/10.1186/s12645-019-0055-y.

Bobo, Daniel, Kye Robinson, Jiaul Islam, Kristofer Thurecht, and Simon Corrie. 2016. "Nanoparticle-Based Medicines: A Review of FDA-Approved Materials and Clinical Trials to Date." *Pharmaceutical Research* 33 (October). https://doi.org/10.1007/s11095-016-1958-5.

Bor, Gizem, Intan Azmi, and Anan Yaghmur. 2018. "Nanomedicines for Cancer Therapy: Current Status, Challenges and Future Prospects." *Therapeutic Delivery* 10 (November). https://doi.org/10.4155/tde-2018-0062.

Bozzuto, Giuseppina, and Agnese Molinari. 2015. "Liposomes as Nanomedical Devices." *International Journal of Nanomedicine* 10 (February): 975. https://doi.org/10.2147/IJN.S68861.

Brar, Satinder K., and M. Verma. 2011. "Measurement of Nanoparticles by Light-Scattering Techniques." *TrAC Trends in Analytical Chemistry* 30 (1): 4–17. https://doi.org/10.1016/j.trac.2010.08.008.

Briscoe, Chad, and David Hage. 2009. "Factors Affecting the Stability of Drugs and Drug Metabolites in Biological Matrices." *Bioanalysis* 1 (April): 205–20. https://doi.org/10.4155/bio.09.20.

Brock, Amy, Silva Krause, Hu Li, Marek Kowalski, Michael S. Goldberg, James J. Collins, and Donald E. Ingber. 2014. "Silencing HoxA1 by Intraductal Injection of SiRNA Lipidoid Nanoparticles Prevents Mammary Tumor Progression in Mice." *Science Translational Medicine* 6 (217). American Association for the Advancement of Science: 217ra2.

Broggini, Massimo, Federica Guffanti, Roberta Affatato, Lavinia Morosi, Patrick Buschor, Christoph Matthieu, Florian Weiss, Andreas Konig, Peter Halbherr, and Stefan Halbherr. 2017. "Abstract 174: Preclinical Activity of New Liposomal Formulation of Doxorubicin (TLD-1)." *Cancer Research* 77 (July): 174. https://doi.org/10.1158/1538-7445.AM2017-174.

Bruera, Eduardo, Alfredo Navigante, Mario Barugel, Karen Macmillan, R. Neil MacDonald, and Reinaldo Chacon. 1990. "Treatment of Pain and Other Symptoms in Cancer Patients: Patterns in a North American and a South American Hospital." *Journal of Pain and Symptom Management* 5 (2): 78–82. https://doi.org/10.1016/S0885-3924(05)80020-X.

Bulbake, Upendra, Sindhu Doppalapudi, Nagavendra Kommineni, and Wahid Khan. 2017. "Liposomal Formulations in Clinical Use: An Updated Review." *Pharmaceutics* 9 (March): 12. https://doi.org/10.3390/pharmaceutics9020012.

Buyens, Kevin, Stefaan C. De Smedt, Kevin Braeckmans, Joseph Demeester, Liesbeth Peeters, Leo A. van Grunsven, Xavier de Mollerat du Jeu, et al. 2012. "Liposome Based Systems for Systemic SiRNA Delivery: Stability in Blood Sets the Requirements for Optimal Carrier Design." *Journal of Controlled Release* 158 (3): 362–70. https://doi.org/10.1016/j.jconrel.2011.10.009.

Cancer Control: A Global Snapshot in 2015 Summary of Results from the 2015 Who NCD Country Capacity Survey Introduction. https://www.who.int/publications-detail-redirect/cancer-control-a-global-snapshot-in-2015.

Caster, Joseph, Artish Patel, Tian Zhang, and Andrew Wang. 2016. "Investigational Nanomedicines in 2016: A Review of Nanotherapeutics Currently Undergoing Clinical Trials: Investigational Nanomedicines in 2016." *Wiley Interdisciplinary Reviews: Nanomedicine and Nanobiotechnology* 9 (June). https://doi.org/10.1002/wnan.1416.

Celia, Christian, Elena Trapasso, Donato Cosco, Donatella Paolino, and Massimo Fresta. 2009. "Turbiscan Lab® Expert Analysis of the Stability of Ethosomes® and Ultradeformable Liposomes Containing a Bilayer Fluidizing Agent." *Colloids and Surfaces B: Biointerfaces* 72 (1): 155–60. https://doi.org/10.1016/j.colsurfb.2009.03.007.

Chang, Hsin-I., and Ming-Kung Yeh. 2012. "Clinical Development of Liposome-Based Drugs: Formulation, Characterization, and Therapeutic Efficacy." *International Journal of Nanomedicine*. Taylor & Francis: 49–60.

Charrois, Gregory J. R., and Theresa M. Allen. 2004. "Drug Release Rate Influences the Pharmacokinetics, Biodistribution, Therapeutic Activity, and Toxicity of Pegylated Liposomal Doxorubicin Formulations in Murine Breast Cancer." *Biochimica et Biophysica Acta (BBA)—Biomembranes* 1663 (1): 167–77. https://doi.org/10.1016/j.bbamem.2004.03.006.

Chen, Da-Bing, Tian-Zhi Yang, Wang-Liang Lu, and Qiang Zhang. 2001. "In Vitro and in Vivo Study of Two Types of Long-Circulating Solid Lipid Nanoparticles Containing Paclitaxel." *Chemical and Pharmaceutical Bulletin*: 49.

Chen, Yanjing, Arijit Bose, and Geoffrey Bothun. 2010. "Controlled Release from Bilayer-Decorated Magnetoliposomes via Electromagnetic Heating." *ACS Nano* 4 (June): 3215–21. https://doi.org/10.1021/nn100274v.

Chintamaneni, Pavan, Sai Kiran Pindiprolu, and Praveen Krishnamurthy. 2018. "Formulation-Optimization of Solid Lipid Nanocarrier System of STAT3 Inhibitor to Improve Its Activity in Triple Negative Breast Cancer Cells." *Drug Development and Industrial Pharmacy* 45 (October). https://doi.org/10.1080/03639045.2018.1539496.

Choi, Jin-Seok, Jiafu Cao, Muhammad Naeem, Jinki Noh, Nurhasni Hasan, Hoo-Kyun Choi, and Jin-Wook Yoo. 2014. "Size-Controlled Biodegradable Nanoparticles: Preparation and Size-Dependent Cellular Uptake and Tumor Cell Growth Inhibition." *Colloids and Surfaces. B, Biointerfaces* 122 (July). https://doi.org/10.1016/j.colsurfb.2014.07.030.

Connal, Siobhan, James M. Cameron, Alexandra Sala, Paul M. Brennan, David S. Palmer, Joshua D. Palmer, Haley Perlow, and Matthew J. Baker. 2023. "Liquid Biopsies: The Future of Cancer Early Detection." *Journal of Translational Medicine* 21 (1): 118. https://doi.org/10.1186/s12967-023-03960-8.

Deamer, D., and A. D. Bangham. 1976. "Large Volume Liposomes by an Ether Vaporization Method." *Biochimica et Biophysica Acta (BBA)—Nucleic Acids and Protein Synthesis* 443 (3): 629–34. https://doi.org/10.1016/0005-2787(76)90527-X.

De Jong, Wim H., and Paul Ja Borm. 2008. "Drug Delivery and Nanoparticles: Applications and Hazards." *International Journal of Nanomedicine* 3.

Deo, S. V. S., Jyoti Sharma, and Sunil Kumar. 2022. "GLOBOCAN 2020 Report on Global Cancer Burden: Challenges and Opportunities for Surgical Oncologists." *Annals of Surgical Oncology* 29 (11): 6497–500. https://doi.org/10.1245/s10434-022-12151-6.

Díaz, Mónica Rivera, and Pablo E. Vivas-Mejia. 2013. "Nanoparticles as Drug Delivery Systems in Cancer Medicine: Emphasis on RNAi-Containing Nanoliposomes." *Pharmaceuticals* 6 (11): 1361–80. https://doi.org/10.3390/ph6111361.

Digiacomo, Luca, Daniela Pozzi, Sara Palchetti, Alessandra Zingoni, and Giulio Caracciolo. 2020. "Impact of the Protein Corona on Nanomaterial Immune Response and Targeting Ability." *WIREs Nanomedicine and Nanobiotechnology* 12 (January). https://doi.org/10.1002/wnan.1615.

Ding, Shukai, Nicolas Anton, Thierry F. Vandamme, and Christophe A. Serra. 2016. "Microfluidic Nanoprecipitation Systems for Preparing Pure Drug or Polymeric Drug Loaded Nanoparticles: An

Overview." *Expert Opinion on Drug Delivery* 13 (10). Taylor & Francis: 1447–60. https://doi.org/10.1080/17425247.2016.1193151.

Doktorovova, Slavomira, Eliana B. Souto, and Amélia M. Silva. 2014. "Nanotoxicology Applied to Solid Lipid Nanoparticles and Nanostructured Lipid Carriers–a Systematic Review of in Vitro Data." *European Journal of Pharmaceutics and Biopharmaceutics* 87 (1). Elsevier: 1–18.

Draz, Mohamed Shehata, Binbin Fang, Pengfei Zhang, Zhi Hu, Shenda Gu, Kevin Weng, Joe Gray, and Fanqing Chen. 2014. "Nanoparticle-Mediated Systemic Delivery of SiRNA for Treatment of Cancers and Viral Infections." *Theranostics* 4 (June): 872–92. Ivyspring International Publisher. https://doi.org/10.7150/thno.9404.

Durak, Saliha, Monireh Esmaeili Rad, Abuzer Alp Yetisgin, Hande Eda Sutova, Ozlem Kutlu, Sibel Cetinel, and Ali Zarrabi. 2020. "Niosomal Drug Delivery Systems for Ocular Disease—Recent Advances and Future Prospects." *Nanomaterials* 10 (6). MDPI: 1191.

Ellens, Harma, Joe Bentz, and Francis C Szoka. 1986. "Destabilization of Phosphatidylethanolamine Liposomes at the Hexagonal Phase Transition Temperature." *Biochemistry* 25 (2). American Chemical Society: 285–94. https://doi.org/10.1021/bi00350a001.

Feng, Lan, and Russell J. Mumper. 2013. "A Critical Review of Lipid-Based Nanoparticles for Taxane Delivery." *Cancer Letters* 334 (2): 157–75. https://doi.org/10.1016/j.canlet.2012.07.006.

Ferrari, Mauro. 2008. "Beyond Drug Delivery." *Nature Nanotechnology* 3 (3): 131–2. https://doi.org/10.1038/nnano.2008.46.

Fetterly, Gerald J., Thaddeus H. Grasela, Jeffrey W. Sherman, Jeanne L. Dul, Amy Grahn, Diane Lecomte, Jill Fiedler-Kelly, Nevena Damjanov, Mayer Fishman, and Michael P. Kane. 2008. "Pharmacokinetic/Pharmacodynamic Modeling and Simulation of Neutropenia During Phase I Development of Liposome-Entrapped Paclitaxel." *Clinical Cancer Research* 14 (18). AACR: 5856–63.

Frederiksen, Lene, Klaus Anton, Peter van Hoogevest, Hans Rudolf Keller, and Hans Leuenberger. 1997. "Preparation of Liposomes Encapsulating Water-Soluble Compounds Using Supercritical Carbon Dioxide." *Journal of Pharmaceutical Sciences* 86 (8): 921–8. https://doi.org/10.1021/js960403q.

Fröhlich, Margret, Volker Brecht, and Regine Peschka-Süss. 2001. "Parameters Influencing the Determination of Liposome Lamellarity by 31P-NMR." *Chemistry and Physics of Lipids* 109 (1): 103–12. https://doi.org/10.1016/S0009-3084(00)00220-6.

Gabizon, Alberto, Dinah Tzemach, Aviva Horowitz, Hilary Shmeeda, Jerry Yeh, and Samuel Zalipsky. 2006. "Reduced Toxicity and Superior Therapeutic Activity of a Mitomycin C Lipid-Based Prodrug Incorporated in Pegylated Liposomes." *Clinical Cancer Research: An Official Journal of the American Association for Cancer Research* 12 (April): 1913–20. https://doi.org/10.1158/1078-0432.CCR-05-1547.

Ganesan, Poovi, and Damodharan Narayanasamy. 2017. "Lipid Nanoparticles: Different Preparation Techniques, Characterization, Hurdles, and Strategies for the Production of Solid Lipid Nanoparticles and Nanostructured Lipid Carriers for Oral Drug Delivery." *Sustainable Chemistry and Pharmacy* 6: 37–56. https://doi.org/10.1016/j.scp.2017.07.002.

García-Pinel, Beatriz, Cristina Porras-Alcalá, Alicia Ortega-Rodríguez, Francisco Sarabia, Jose Prados, Consolación Melguizo, and Juan M. López-Romero. 2019. "Lipid-Based Nanoparticles: Application and Recent Advances in Cancer Treatment." *Nanomaterials* 9 (4). MDPI AG. https://doi.org/10.3390/nano9040638.

Gasco, Maria R. 1993. "Method for Producing Solid Lipid Microspheres Having a Narrow Size Distribution." Google Patents.

Gill, Kanwaldeep K., Amal Kaddoumi, and Sami Nazzal. 2012. "Mixed Micelles of PEG2000-DSPE and Vitamin-E TPGS for Concurrent Delivery of Paclitaxel and Parthenolide: Enhanced Chemosenstization and Antitumor Efficacy Against Non-Small Cell Lung Cancer (NSCLC) Cell Lines." *European Journal of Pharmaceutical Sciences* 46 (1): 64–71. https://doi.org/10.1016/j.ejps.2012.02.010.

Golan, Talia, Tal Grenader, Patricia Ohana, Yasmine Amitay, Hilary Shmeeda, Ninh (Irene) La-Beck, Esther Tahover, Raanan Berger, and Alberto Gabizon. 2015. "Pegylated Liposomal Mitomycin C Prodrug Enhances Tolerance of Mitomycin C: A Phase 1 Study in Advanced Solid Tumor Patients." *Cancer Medicine* 4 (July). https://doi.org/10.1002/cam4.491.

Goldberg, Michael. 2012. "Lipidoids: A Combinatorial Approach to SiRNA Delivery." In *RNA Interference from Biology to Therapeutics*, 143–60. Springer.

Gomes-da-Silva, Lígia C., Nuno A. Fonseca, Vera Moura, Maria C. Pedroso de Lima, Sérgio Simões, and João N Moreira. 2012. "Lipid-Based Nanoparticles for SiRNA Delivery in Cancer Therapy: Paradigms and Challenges." *Accounts of Chemical Research* 45 (7). American Chemical Society: 1163–71. https://doi.org/10.1021/ar300048p.

Gregoriadis, Gregory. 1976. "The Carrier Potential of Liposomes in Biology and Medicine." *The New England Journal of Medicine* 295 (October): 765–70. https://doi.org/10.1056/NEJM197609302951406.

Gu, Wenjie, Gavin P. Andrews, and Yiwei Tian. 2023. "Recent Clinical Successes in Liposomal Nanomedicines." *International Journal of Drug Discovery and Pharmacology* (February). Australia Academic Press Pty Ltd: 52–9. https://doi.org/10.53941/ijddp.0201009.

Gu, Zili, Candido da Silva, Koen van der Maaden, Ferry Ossendorp, and Luis Cruz. 2020. "Liposome-Based Drug Delivery Systems in Cancer Immunotherapy." *Pharmaceutics* 12 (November). https://doi.org/10.3390/pharmaceutics12111054.

Guney Eskiler, Gamze, Gulsah Cecener, Unal Egeli, and Berrin Tunca. 2018. "Synthetically Lethal BMN 673 (Talazoparib) Loaded Solid Lipid Nanoparticles for BRCA1 Mutant Triple Negative Breast Cancer." *Pharmaceutical Research* 35 (September). https://doi.org/10.1007/s11095-018-2502-6.

Hadinoto, Kunn, Ajitha Sundaresan, and Wean Sin Cheow. 2013. "Lipid-Polymer Hybrid Nanoparticles as a New Generation Therapeutic Delivery Platform: A Review." *European Journal of Pharmaceutics and Biopharmaceutics* 85 (3, Part A): 427–43. https://doi.org/10.1016/j.ejpb.2013.07.002.

Hamaguchi, T., Y. Matsumura, M. Suzuki, K. Shimizu, R. Goda, I. Nakamura, I. Nakatomi, M. Yokoyama, K. Kataoka, and T. Kakizoe. 2005. "NK105, a Paclitaxel-Incorporating Micellar Nanoparticle Formulation, Can Extend in Vivo Antitumour Activity and Reduce the Neurotoxicity of Paclitaxel." *British Journal of Cancer* 92 (7): 1240–6. https://doi.org/10.1038/sj.bjc.6602479.

Hanafy, Nemany, El-Kemary, and Stefano Leporatti. 2018. "Micelles Structure Development as a Strategy to Improve Smart Cancer Therapy." *Cancers* 10 (July): 238. https://doi.org/10.3390/cancers10070238.

Hanahan, Douglas, and Robert A. Weinberg. 2011. "Hallmarks of Cancer: The Next Generation." *Cell* 144 (5): 646–74. https://doi.org/10.1016/j.cell.2011.02.013.

Honeywell-Nguyen, P. Loan, and Joke A. Bouwstra. 2005. "Vesicles as a Tool for Transdermal and Dermal Delivery." *Drug Discovery Today: Technologies* 2 (1): 67–74. https://doi.org/10.1016/j.ddtec.2005.05.003.

Hong, Minghuang, Saijie Zhu, Yanyan Jiang, Guotao Tang, and Yuanying Pei. 2009. "Efficient Tumor Targeting of Hydroxycamptothecin Loaded PEGylated Niosomes Modified with Transferrin." *Journal of Controlled Release* 133 (2): 96–102. https://doi.org/10.1016/j.jconrel.2008.09.005.

Hühn, Dominik, Karsten Kantner, Christian Geidel, Stefan Brandholt, Ine De Cock, Stefaan J. H. Soenen, Pilar Rivera-Gil, et al. 2013. "Polymer-Coated Nanoparticles Interacting with Proteins and Cells: Focusing on the Sign of the Net Charge." *ACS Nano* 7 (4). American Chemical Society: 3253–63. https://doi.org/10.1021/nn3059295.

Humberstone, Andrew J., and William N Charman. 1997. "Lipid-Based Vehicles for the Oral Delivery of Poorly Water Soluble Drugs." *Advanced Drug Delivery Reviews* 25 (1). Elsevier: 103–28.

Imura, Tomohiro, Toshihiro Gotoh, Katsuto Otake, Satoshi Yoda, Yoshihiro Takebayashi, Shoko Yokoyama, Hitoshi Takebayashi, Hideki Sakai, Makoto Yuasa, and Masahiko Abe. 2003. "Control of Physicochemical Properties of Liposomes Using a Supercritical Reverse Phase Evaporation Method." *Langmuir* 19 (6): 2021–5. https://doi.org/10.1021/la020589a.

IUPAC. 1997. "Compendium of Chemical Terminology." In *The "Gold Book"*. Blackwell Scientific Publications.

Jaafar-Maalej, Chiraz, Catherine Charcosset, and Hatem Fessi. 2011. "A New Method for Liposome Preparation Using a Membrane Contactor." *Journal of Liposome Research* 21 (3). Taylor & Francis: 213–20.

Jahn, Andreas, Wyatt Vreeland, Michael Gaitan, and Laurie Locascio. 2004. "Controlled Vesicle Self-Assembly in Microfluidic Channels with Hydrodynamic Focusing." *Journal of the American Chemical Society* 126 (April): 2674–5. https://doi.org/10.1021/ja0318030.

Jha, Sheetal, Pramod K. Sharma, and Rishabha Malviya. 2016. "Liposomal Drug Delivery System for Cancer Therapy: Advancement and Patents." *Recent Patents on Drug Delivery & Formulation* 10 (3). Bentham Science Publishers: 177–83.

Jiskoot, Wim, Tom Teerlink, E. Coen Beuvery, and Daan J. A. Crommelin. 1986. "Preparation of Liposomes via Detergent Removal from Mixed Micelles by Dilution: The Effect of Bilayer Composition and Process Parameters on Liposome Characteristics." *Pharmaceutisch Weekblad* 8. Springer: 259–65.

Kao, Chen-Yu, Eric Hoffman, Kenneth Beck, Ravi Bellamkonda, and Ananth Annapragada. 2003. "Long-Residence-Time Nano-Scale Liposomal Iohexol for X-Ray-Based Blood Pool Imaging." *Academic Radiology* 10 (June): 475–83. https://doi.org/10.1016/S1076-6332(03)80055-7.

Kapoor, Mamta, and Diane J. Burgess. 2012. "Efficient and Safe Delivery of SiRNA Using Anionic Lipids: Formulation Optimization Studies." *International Journal of Pharmaceutics* 432 (1): 80–90. https://doi.org/10.1016/j.ijpharm.2012.04.058.

Kaur, Chanchal Deep, Manoj Nahar, and Narendra K Jain. 2008. "Lymphatic Targeting of Zidovudine Using Surface-Engineered Liposomes." *Journal of Drug Targeting* 16 (10). Taylor & Francis: 798–805. https://doi.org/10.1080/10611860802475688.

Kim, John, Young Do, Hong Song, Yoon Cho, Hun Ryoo, Sung Hwa Bae, Jong Kim, et al. 2017. "Multicenter Phase II Clinical Trial of Genexol-PM® with Gemcitabine in Advanced Biliary Tract Cancer." *Anticancer Research* 37 (March): 1467–73. https://doi.org/10.21873/anticanres.11471.

Kim, Johoon, Peter Chhour, Jessica Hsu, Harold I. Litt, Victor A Ferrari, Rachela Popovtzer, and David P. Cormode. 2017. "Use of Nanoparticle Contrast Agents for Cell Tracking with Computed Tomography." *Bioconjugate Chemistry* 28 (6). American Chemical Society: 1581–97. https://doi.org/10.1021/acs.bioconjchem.7b00194.

Koçum, Cengiz, Emel Kalaycioğlu Çimen, and Erhan Pişkin. 2004. "Imaging of Poly(NIPA-Co-MAH)-HIgG Conjugate with Scanning Tunneling Microscopy." *Journal of Biomaterials Science, Polymer Edition* 15 (12). Taylor & Francis: 1513–20. https://doi.org/10.1163/1568562042459706.

Kohli, Aditya G., Paul H. Kierstead, Vincent J. Venditto, Colin L. Walsh, and Francis C. Szoka. 2014. "Designer Lipids for Drug Delivery: From Heads to Tails." *Journal of Controlled Release* 190: 274–87. https://doi.org/10.1016/j.jconrel.2014.04.047.

Kraft, John C., Jennifer P. Freeling, Ziyao Wang, and Rodney J. Y. Ho. 2014. "Emerging Research and Clinical Development Trends of Liposome and Lipid Nanoparticle Drug Delivery Systems." *Journal of Pharmaceutical Sciences* 103 (1): 29–52. https://doi.org/10.1002/jps.23773.

Kuentz, Martin. 2012. "Lipid-Based Formulations for Oral Delivery of Lipophilic Drugs." *Drug Discovery Today: Technologies* 9 (2). Elsevier: e97–104.

Kumar, Amit, Madhu Gupta, and Simran Braya. 2021. "Liposome Characterization, Applications and Regulatory Landscape in US." *International Journal of Drug Regulatory Affairs* 9 (2). Society of Pharmaceutical Tecnocrats: 81–9. https://doi.org/10.22270/ijdra.v9i2.474.

Kumar, Gannu P., and Pogaku Rajeshwarrao. 2011. "Nonionic Surfactant Vesicular Systems for Effective Drug Delivery—an Overview." *Acta Pharmaceutica Sinica B* 1 (4): 208–19. https://doi.org/10.1016/j.apsb.2011.09.002.

Kumar, Vinay, Rojarani Komuravelli, Madhusudana Kuncha, Ramakrishna Sistla, and Prakash V. Diwan. 2012. "Increased Brain Uptake of Docetaxel and Ketoconazole Loaded Folate-Grafted Solid Lipid Nanoparticles." *Nanomedicine: Nanotechnology, Biology, and Medicine* 9 (March). https://doi.org/10.1016/j.nano.2012.03.003.

Kurakazu, T., and S. Takeuchi. 2010. "Generation of Lipid Vesicles Using Microfluidic T-Junctions with Pneumatic Valves." In *2010 IEEE 23rd International Conference on Micro Electro Mechanical Systems (MEMS)*, 1115–18. IEEE. https://doi.org/10.1109/MEMSYS.2010.5442406.

Laouini, A., C. Jaafar-Maalej, S. Gandoura-Sfar, C. Charcosset, and H. Fessi. 2012. "Spironolactone-Loaded Liposomes Produced Using a Membrane Contactor Method: An Improvement of the Ethanol Injection Technique." In *UK Colloids 2011: An International Colloid and Surface Science Symposium*, 23–8. Springer.

Laouini, A., C. Jaafar-Maalej, S. Sfar, C. Charcosset, and H. Fessi. 2011. "Liposome Preparation Using a Hollow Fiber Membrane Contactor—Application to Spironolactone Encapsulation." *International Journal of Pharmaceutics* 415 (1–2). Elsevier: 53–61. https://doi.org/10.1016/j.ijpharm.2011.05.034.

Laouini, Abdallah, Catherine Charcosset, Hatem Fessi, Richard G. Holdich, and G. T. Vladisavljević. 2013. "Preparation of Liposomes: A Novel Application of Microengineered Membranes-Investigation of the Process Parameters and Application to the Encapsulation of Vitamin E." *RSC Advances* 3 (15). Royal Society of Chemistry: 4985–94.

Laouini, Abdallah, Chiraz Jaafar-Maalej, Imen Blouza, Souad Sfar, Catherine Charcosset, and Hatem Fessi. 2012. "Preparation, Characterization and Applications of Liposomes: State of the Art." *Journal of Colloid Science and Biotechnology* 1 (December): 147–68. https://doi.org/10.1166/jcsb.2012.1020.

Lasch, J. 2003. *Preparation of Liposomes, in "Liposomes"*. Edited by V. P. Torchilin and V. Weissig. Oxford University Press.

Lasch, J., V. Weissig, and M. Brandl. 2003. *Liposomes: A Practical Approach*. Oxford University Press.

Lasic, D. D. 1995. "Mechanisms of Liposome Formation." *Journal of Liposome Research* 5 (3). Taylor & Francis: 431–41. https://doi.org/10.3109/08982109509010233.

Laurent, Sophie, Amirata Saei, Shahed Behzadi, Arash Panahifar, and Morteza Mahmoudi. 2014. "Superparamagnetic Iron Oxide Nanoparticles for Delivery of Therapeutic Agents: Opportunities and Challenges." *Expert Opinion on Drug Delivery* 29 (May): 1–22. https://doi.org/10.1517/17425247.2014.924501.

Lee, Jong-Min, Tae-Jong Yoon, and Young-Seok Cho. 2013. "Recent Developments in Nanoparticle-Based SiRNA Delivery for Cancer Therapy." Edited by John B. Vincent. *BioMed Research International.* Hindawi Publishing Corporation: 782041. https://doi.org/10.1155/2013/782041.

Lee, Mi-Kyung, Soo-Jeong Lim, and Chong-Kook Kim. 2007. "Preparation, Characterization and in Vitro Cytotoxicity of Paclitaxel-Loaded Sterically Stabilized Solid Lipid Nanoparticles." *Biomaterials* 28 (12): 2137–46. https://doi.org/10.1016/j.biomaterials.2007.01.014.

Letchford, Kevin, and Helen Burt. 2007. "A Review of the Formation and Classification of Amphiphilic Block Copolymer Nanoparticulate Structures: Micelles, Nanospheres, Nanocapsules and Polymersomes." *European Journal of Pharmaceutics and Biopharmaceutics* 65 (3): 259–69. https://doi.org/10.1016/j.ejpb.2006.11.009.

Li, Shyh-Dar, and Leaf Huang. 2010. "Stealth Nanoparticles: High Density but Sheddable PEG Is a Key for Tumor Targeting." *Journal of Controlled Release* 145 (3): 178–81. https://doi.org/10.1016/j.jconrel.2010.03.016.

Li, Xiang, Nicolas Anton, Guy Zuber, and Thierry Vandamme. 2014. "Contrast Agents for Preclinical Targeted X-Ray Imaging." *Advanced Drug Delivery Reviews* 76: 116–33. https://doi.org/10.1016/j.addr.2014.07.013.

Lin, Ping-Chang, Stephen Lin, Paul C. Wang, and Rajagopalan Sridhar. 2014. "Techniques for Physicochemical Characterization of Nanomaterials." *Biotechnology Advances* 32 (4): 711–26. https://doi.org/10.1016/j.biotechadv.2013.11.006.

Liu, Yun, Guangze Yang, Yue Hui, Supun Ranaweera, and Chun-Xia Zhao. 2022. "Microfluidic Nanoparticles for Drug Delivery." *Small* 18 (April). https://doi.org/10.1002/smll.202106580.

Lombardo, Domenico, and Mikhail A. Kiselev. 2022. "Methods of Liposomes Preparation: Formation and Control Factors of Versatile Nanocarriers for Biomedical and Nanomedicine Application." *Pharmaceutics* 14 (3): 543. https://doi.org/10.3390/pharmaceutics14030543.

Lucks, Stefan, and Rainer Muller. 1996. "Medication Vehicles Made of Solid Lipid Particles (Solid Lipid Nanospheres-SLN)." Google Patents.

Luyts, Katrien, Dorota Napierska, Ben Nemery, and Peter Hoet. 2013. "How Physico-Chemical Characteristics of Nanoparticles Cause Their Toxicity: Complex and Unresolved Interrelations." *Environmental Science-Processes & Impacts* 15 (January): 23–38. https://doi.org/10.1039/C2EM30237C.

Ma, Shuo, and Leonidas C. Platanias. 2018. "Can Early Intervention with Pharmacotherapy Reduce the Morbidity and Mortality of Chronic Lymphocytic Leukemia?" *Expert Opinion on Pharmacotherapy* 19 (11). Taylor & Francis: 1171–5. https://doi.org/10.1080/14656566.2018.1498844.

Maeki, Masatoshi, Niko Kimura, Yusuke Sato, Hideyoshi Harashima, and Manabu Tokeshi. 2018. "Advances in Microfluidics for Lipid Nanoparticles and Extracellular Vesicles and Applications in Drug Delivery Systems." *Advanced Drug Delivery Reviews* 128: 84–100. https://doi.org/10.1016/j.addr.2018.03.008.

Maeki, Masatoshi, Shuya Uno, Ayuka Niwa, Yuto Okada, and Manabu Tokeshi. 2022. "Microfluidic Technologies and Devices for Lipid Nanoparticle-Based RNA Delivery." *Journal of Controlled Release* 344: 80–96. https://doi.org/10.1016/j.jconrel.2022.02.017.

Mamot, Christoph, Daryl C. Drummond, Keelung Hong, Dmitri B. Kirpotin, and John W. Park. 2003. "Liposome-Based Approaches to Overcome Anticancer Drug Resistance." *Drug Resistance Updates* 6 (5): 271–9. https://doi.org/10.1016/S1368-7646(03)00082-7.

Mare, Rosario, Donatella Paolino, Christian Celia, Roberto Molinaro, Massimo Fresta, and Donato Cosco. 2018. "Post-Insertion Parameters of PEG-Derivatives in Phosphocholine-Liposomes." *International Journal of Pharmaceutics* 552 (1–2). Elsevier: 414–21.

Marianecci, Carlotta, Luisa Di Marzio, Federica Rinaldi, Christian Celia, Donatella Paolino, Franco Alhaique, Sara Esposito, and Maria Carafa. 2014. "Niosomes from 80s to Present: The State of the Art." *Advances in Colloid and Interface Science* 205: 187–206. https://doi.org/10.1016/j.cis.2013.11.018.

Masucci, A., S. E. Elayoubi, and B. Sayrac. 2016. "Flow Level Analysis of the Offloading Capacity of D2D Communications." In *2016 IEEE Wireless Communications and Networking Conference*, 1–6. IEEE. https://doi.org/10.1109/WCNC.2016.7565069.

Mazloomdoost, Donna, Rachel N. Pauls, Erin N. Hennen, Jennifer Y. Yeung, Benjamin C. Smith, Steven D. Kleeman, and Catrina C. Crisp. 2017. "Liposomal Bupivacaine Decreases Pain Following Retropubic Sling Placement: A Randomized Placebo-Controlled Trial." *American Journal of Obstetrics and Gynecology* 217: 598.e1–11. https://api.semanticscholar.org/CorpusID:13953400.

Mehnert, Wolfgang, and Karsten Mäder. 2001. "Solid Lipid Nanoparticles: Production, Characterization and Applications." *Advanced Drug Delivery Reviews* 47 (2): 165–96. https://doi.org/10.1016/S0169-409X(01)00105-3.

Mehnert, Wolfgang, and Karsten Mäder. 2012. "Solid Lipid Nanoparticles: Production, Characterization and Applications." *Advanced Drug Delivery Reviews* 47 (9): 165–96. https://doi.org/10.1016/S0169-409X(01)00105-3.

Mehta, Meenu, Thuy Anh Bui, Xinpu Yang, Yagiz Aksoy, Ewa M. Goldys, and Wei Deng. 2023. "Lipid-Based Nanoparticles for Drug/Gene Delivery: An Overview of the Production Techniques and Difficulties Encountered in Their Industrial Development." *ACS Materials Au* 3 (6): 600–19. American Chemical Society. https://doi.org/10.1021/acsmaterialsau.3c00032.

Merritt, William M., Yvonne G. Lin, Whitney A. Spannuth, Mavis S. Fletcher, Aparna A. Kamat, Liz Y. Han, Charles N. Landen, et al. 2008. "Effect of Interleukin-8 Gene Silencing With Liposome-Encapsulated Small Interfering RNA on Ovarian Cancer Cell Growth." *JNCI: Journal of the National Cancer Institute* 100 (5): 359–72. https://doi.org/10.1093/jnci/djn024.

Miele, Evelina, Gian Spinelli, Ermanno Miele, Enzo Di Fabrizio, Elisabetta Ferretti, Silverio Tomao, and Alberto Gulino. 2012. "Nanoparticle-Based Delivery of Small Interfering RNA: Challenges for Cancer Therapy." *International Journal of Nanomedicine* 7 (July): 3637–57. https://doi.org/10.2147/IJN.S23696.

Mirahadi, Mozhdeh, Saeed Ghanbarzadeh, Marjan Ghorbani, Amin Gholizadeh, and Hamed Hamishehkar. 2018. "A Review on the Role of Lipid-Based Nanoparticles in Medical Diagnosis and Imaging." *Therapeutic Delivery* 9 (August): 557–69. https://doi.org/10.4155/tde-2018-0020.

Misra, Ranjita, Sarbari Acharya, and Sanjeeb K Sahoo. 2010. "Cancer Nanotechnology: Application of Nanotechnology in Cancer Therapy." *Drug Discovery Today* 15 (19): 842–50. https://doi.org/10.1016/j.drudis.2010.08.006.

Moghassemi, Saeid, and Afra Hadjizadeh. 2014. "Nano-Niosomes as Nanoscale Drug Delivery Systems: An Illustrated Review." *Journal of Controlled Release* 185: 22–36. https://doi.org/10.1016/j.jconrel.2014.04.015.

Mozafari, M. 2005. "Liposomes: An Overview of Manufacturing Techniques." *Cellular & Molecular Biology Letters* 10 (February): 711–19.

Mozafari, Mohammad R., C. J. Reed, C. Rostron, and D. S. Martin. 2004. "Transfection of Human Airway Epithelial Cells Using a Lipid-Based Vector Prepared by the Heating Method." *Journal of Aerosol Medicine* 17: 100.

Mu, L., T. A. Elbayoumi, and V. P. Torchilin. 2005. "Mixed Micelles Made of Poly(Ethylene Glycol)-Phosphatidylethanolamine Conjugate and d-α-Tocopheryl Polyethylene Glycol 1000 Succinate as Pharmaceutical Nanocarriers for Camptothecin." *International Journal of Pharmaceutics* 306 (1): 142–9. https://doi.org/10.1016/j.ijpharm.2005.08.026.

Mukundan, Srini, Ketan Ghaghada, Cristian Badea, Chen-Yu Kao, Laurence Hedlund, James Provenzale, George Johnson, Emmanuel Chen, Ravi Bellamkonda, and Ananth Annapragada. 2006. "A Liposomal Nanoscale Contrast Agent for Preclinical CT in Mice." *AJR: American Journal of Roentgenology* 186 (March): 300–7. https://doi.org/10.2214/AJR.05.0523.

Müller, Markus, Stefan Mackeben, and Christel C Müller-Goymann. 2004. "Physicochemical Characterisation of Liposomes with Encapsulated Local Anaesthetics." *International Journal of Pharmaceutics* 274 (1): 139–48. https://doi.org/10.1016/j.ijpharm.2004.01.015.

Müller, Rainer H., Karsten Mäder, and Sven Gohla. 2000. "Solid Lipid Nanoparticles (SLN) for Controlled Drug Delivery—A Review of the State of the Art." *European Journal of Pharmaceutics and Biopharmaceutics : Official Journal of Arbeitsgemeinschaft Für PharmazeutischeVerfahrenstechnike V* 50 (August): 161–77. https://doi.org/10.1016/S0939-6411(00)00087-4.

Mussi, Samuel, and Vladimir Torchilin. 2013. "Recent Trends in the Use of Lipidic Nanoparticles as Pharmaceutical Carriers for Cancer Therapy and Diagnostics." *Journal of Materials Chemistry B* 1 (July): 5201–9. https://doi.org/10.1039/C3TB20990C.

Mydin, R. B. S. M. N., and S. Moshawih. 2019. "Nanoparticles in Nanomedicine Application: Lipid-Based Nanoparticles and Their Safety Concerns." In *Nanotechnology: Applications in Energy, Drug and Food*, eds. S. Siddiquee, G. Melvin, and M. Rahman. Springer. https://doi.org/10.1007/978-3-319-99602-8_10.

Nakhaei, Pooria, Ria Margiana, Dmitry O. Bokov, Walid Kamal Abdelbasset, Mohammad Amin Jadidi Kouhbanani, Rajender S. Varma, Faroogh Marofi, Mostafa Jarahian, and Nasrin Beheshtkhoo. 2021. "Liposomes: Structure, Biomedical Applications, and Stability Parameters with Emphasis on Cholesterol." *Frontiers in Bioengineering and Biotechnology* 9. Frontiers: 705886.

Nastruzzi, Claudio. 2005. *Lipospheres in Drug Targets and Delivery : Approaches, Methods, and Applications*. CRC Press.

New, Roger R. C. 1990. *Liposomes: A Practical Approach*. IRL Press.

Obeid, Mohammad A., Alaa Aljabali, Maryam Rezig, Haneen Amawi, Hanin Alyamani, Shatha Abdeljaber, and Valerie Ferro. 2021. "Use of Nanoparticles in Delivery of Nucleic Acids for Melanoma Treatment." *Methods in Molecular Biology (Clifton, N.J.)* 2265:591–620. https://doi.org/10.1007/978-1-0716-1205-7_41.

Obeid, Mohammad A., Mohammed Al Qaraghuli, Marta Ruano, Sirikwan Sangboonruang, Manal Alsaadi, Yingmanee Tragoolpua, and Valerie A. Ferro. 2022. "Lipid-Based Nanomaterials in Cancer Treatment and Diagnosis." In *Bionanotechnology: Next-Generation Therapeutic Tools*, 49–83. Bentham Science Publishers. https://doi.org/10.2174/9789815051278122010005.

Obeid, Mohammad, Ashref Elburi, Louise Young, Alexander Mullen, Rothwelle Tate, and Valerie Ferro. 2017. "Formulation of Nonionic Surfactant Vesicles (NISV) Prepared by Microfluidics for Therapeutic Delivery of SiRNA into Cancer Cells." *Molecular Pharmaceutics* 14 (June). https://doi.org/10.1021/acs.molpharmaceut.7b00352.

Obeid, Mohammad A., Rothwelle J. Tate, Alexander B. Mullen, and Valerie A. Ferro. 2018. "Lipid-Based Nanoparticles for Cancer Treatment." In *Lipid Nanocarriers for Drug Targeting*, 313–59. Elsevier. https://doi.org/10.1016/B978-0-12-813687-4.00008-6.

Obeid, Mohammad, Teeranun Teeravatcharoenchai, David Connell, Kanidta Niwasabutra, Muattaz Hussain, Katharine Carter, and Valerie Ferro. 2020. "Examination of the Effect of Niosome Preparation Methods in Encapsulating Model Antigens on the Vesicle Characteristics and Their Ability to Induce Immune Responses." *Journal of Liposome Research* 31 (May): 1–30. https://doi.org/10.1080/08982104.2020.1768110.

Oliveira, Relton, Marcus Carrião, Maiulle Pacheco, Luis Branquinho, Ana Ribeiro de Souza, A Bakuzis, and Eliana Lima. 2018. "Triggered Release of Paclitaxel from Magnetic Solid Lipid Nanoparticles by Magnetic Hyperthermia." *Materials Science and Engineering: C* 92 (July). https://doi.org/10.1016/j.msec.2018.07.011.

Ollivon, Michel, Sylviane Lesieur, Cécile Grabielle-Madelmont, and Maïté Paternostre. 2000. "Vesicle Reconstitution from Lipid-Detergent Mixed Micelles." *Biochimica et Biophysica Acta (BBA)-Biomembranes* 1508 (1–2). Elsevier: 34–50.

Otake, Katsuto, Tomohiro Imura, Hideki Sakai, and Masahiko Abe. 2001. "Development of a New Preparation Method of Liposomes Using Supercritical Carbon Dioxide." *Langmuir* 17 (13). ACS Publications: 3898–901.

Ozpolat, Bulent, Anil K. Sood, and Gabriel Lopez-Berestein. 2014. "Liposomal SiRNA Nanocarriers for Cancer Therapy." *Advanced Drug Delivery Reviews* 66: 110–16. https://doi.org/10.1016/j.addr.2013.12.008.

Paecharoenchai, Orapan, Nattisa Niyomtham, Lalita Leksantikul, Tanasait Ngawhirunpat, Theerasak Rojanarata, Boon-ek Yingyongnarongkul, and Praneet Opanasopit. 2014. "Nonionic Surfactant Vesicles Composed of Novel Spermine-Derivative Cationic Lipids as an Effective Gene Carrier In Vitro." *AAPS PharmSciTech* 15 (3): 722–30. https://doi.org/10.1208/s12249-014-0095-x.

Pandey, V. P., and D. Karthikeyan. 2008. "Non-Ionic Surfactant Based Vesicle 'Niosome' as a Potential Ocular Drug Delivery System - An Overview." *Pharmaceutical Reviews*.

Paolino, Donatella, Donato Cosco, Rita Muzzalupo, Elena Trapasso, Nevio Picci, and Massimo Fresta. 2008. "Innovative Bola-Surfactant Niosomes as Topical Delivery Systems of 5-Fluorouracil for the Treatment of Skin Cancer." *International Journal of Pharmaceutics* 353 (1): 233–42. https://doi.org/10.1016/j.ijpharm.2007.11.037.

Pardakhty, Abbas, Jaleh Varshosaz, and Abdolhossein Rouholamini. 2007. "In Vitro Study of Polyoxyethylene Alkyl Ether Niosomes for Delivery of Insulin." *International Journal of Pharmaceutics* 328 (2): 130–41. https://doi.org/10.1016/j.ijpharm.2006.08.002.

Pardeike, Jana, Aiman Hommoss, and Rainer Müller. 2008. "Lipid Nanoparticles (SLN, NLC) in Cosmetic and Pharmaceutical Dermal Products." *International Journal of Pharmaceutics* 366 (November): 170–84. https://doi.org/10.1016/j.ijpharm.2008.10.003.

Pardeike, Jana, Aiman Hommoss, and Rainer H. Müller. 2009. "Lipid Nanoparticles (SLN, NLC) in Cosmetic and Pharmaceutical Dermal Products." *International Journal of Pharmaceutics* 366 (1–2). Elsevier: 170–84.

Parot, Pierre, Yves Dufrêne, Peter Hinterdorfer, Christian Le Grimellec, Daniel Navajas, Jean-Luc Pellequer, and Simon Scheuring. 2007. "Past, Present and Future of Atomic Force Microscopy in Life Sciences and Medicine." *Journal of Molecular Recognition: JMR* 20 (November): 418–31. https://doi.org/10.1002/jmr.857.

Patel, A. R., and Krassimir P. Velikov. 2011. "Colloidal Delivery Systems in Foods: A General Comparison with Oral Drug Delivery." *LWT-Food Science and Technology* 44 (9). Elsevier: 1958–64.

Patil, Yogita P., and Sameer Jadhav. 2014. "Novel Methods for Liposome Preparation." *Chemistry and Physics of Lipids* 177: 8–18. https://doi.org/10.1016/j.chemphyslip.2013.10.011.

Pawar, Smita, and Pradeep Vavia. 2015. "Glucosamine Anchored Cancer Targeted Nano-Vesicular Drug Delivery System of Doxorubicin." *Journal of Drug Targeting* 24 (July): 1–12. https://doi.org/10.3109/1061186X.2015.1055572.

Petersen, Anncatrine, Tina Binderup, Palle Rasmussen, Jonas Henriksen, Dennis Elema, Andreas Kjaer, and Thomas Andresen. 2011. "64Cu Loaded Liposomes as Positron Emission Tomography Imaging Agents." *Biomaterials* 32 (March): 2334–41. https://doi.org/10.1016/j.biomaterials.2010.11.059.

Phillips, William, Beth Goins, Ande Bao, Daniel Vargas, Juan Guttierez, Abram Trevino, Jessica Miller, et al. 2012. "Rhenium-186 Liposomes as Convection-Enhanced Nanoparticle Brachytherapy for Treatment of Glioblastoma." *Neuro-Oncology* 14 (March): 416–25. https://doi.org/10.1093/neuonc/nos060.

Pidgeon, Charles, Susan McNeely, Tim Schmidt, and John E. Johnson. 1987. "Multilayered Vesicles Prepared by Reverse-Phase Evaporation: Liposome Structure and Optimum Solute Entrapment." *Biochemistry* 26 (1). ACS Publications: 17–29.

Pirollo, Kathleen, John Nemunaitis, Po Leung, Robert Nunan, Jana Adams, and Esther H. Chang. 2016. "Safety and Efficacy in Advanced Solid Tumors of Docetaxel in Combination with a Targeted Nanocomplex Carrying the P53 Gene: A Phase Ib Study." *Molecular Therapy* 24 (June). https://doi.org/10.1038/mt.2016.135.

Pirollo, Kathleen, Antonina Rait, Qi Zhou, Xin-Qiao Zhang, Jain Zhou, Chang-Soo Kim, William Benedict, and Esther H. Chang. 2008. "Tumor-Targeting Nanocomplex Delivery of Novel Tumor Suppressor RB94 Chemosensitizes Bladder Carcinoma Cells In Vitro and In Vivo." *Clinical Cancer Research: An Official Journal of the American Association for Cancer Research* 14 (April): 2190–8. https://doi.org/10.1158/1078-0432.CCR-07-1951.

Poon, Ronnie, and Nicholas Borys. 2011. "Lyso-Thermosensitive Liposomal Doxorubicin: An Adjuvant to Increase the Cure Rate of Radiofrequency Ablation in Liver Cancer." *Future Oncology (London, England)* 7 (August): 937–45. https://doi.org/10.2217/fon.11.73.

Pourabed, Amir, Tayyaba Younas, Chang Liu, Bhuvana K Shanbhag, Lizhong He, and Tuncay Alan. 2021. "High Throughput Acoustic Microfluidic Mixer Controls Self-Assembly of Protein Nanoparticles with Tuneable Sizes." *Journal of Colloid and Interface Science* 585: 229–36. https://doi.org/10.1016/j.jcis.2020.11.070.

Pouton, Colin W., and Christopher J. H. Porter. 2008. "Formulation of Lipid-Based Delivery Systems for Oral Administration: Materials, Methods and Strategies." *Advanced Drug Delivery Reviews* 60 (6). Elsevier: 625–37.

Pradhan, Prashant, Jingjiao Guan, Dongning Lu, Peng Wang, Ly Lee, and Robert Lee. 2008. "A Facile Microfluidic Method for Production of Liposomes." *Anticancer Research* 28 (March): 943–7.

Qaraghuli, Mohammed, Mohammad Obeid, O. Aldulaimi, and Valerie Ferro. 2017. "Control of Malaria by Bio-Therapeutics and Drug Delivery Systems." *Journal of Medical Microbiology & Diagnosis* 6 (October). https://doi.org/10.4172/2161-0703.1000260.

Ranade, Vasant V., and John B. Cannon. 2011. *Drug Delivery Systems*. CRC Press.

Ranade, Vasant V., and Mannfred A. Hollinger. 2011. *Drug Delivery Systems*, 2nd edition. CRC Press.

Sawant, Rupa R., and Vladimir P Torchilin. 2010. "Multifunctionality of Lipid-Core Micelles for Drug Delivery and Tumour Targeting." *Molecular Membrane Biology* 27 (7). Taylor & Francis: 232–46. https://doi.org/10.3109/09687688.2010.516276.

Schiffman, Joshua D., Paul G. Fisher, and Peter Gibbs. 2015. "Early Detection of Cancer: Past, Present, and Future." *American Society of Clinical Oncology Educational Book* 35 (1). American Society of Clinical Oncology Alexandria, VA: 57–65.

Sciacovelli, Marco, Christina Schmidt, Eamonn R. Maher, and Christian Frezza. 2020. "Metabolic Drivers in Hereditary Cancer Syndromes." *Annual Review of Cancer Biology* 4. Annual Reviews: 77–97.

Sercombe, Lisa, Tejaswi Veerati, Fatemeh Moheimani, Sherry Y. Wu, Anil K. Sood, and Susan Hua. 2015. "Advances and Challenges of Liposome Assisted Drug Delivery." *Frontiers in Pharmacology* 6. Frontiers Media SA: 286. www.frontiersin.org/articles/10.3389/fphar.2015.00286.

Shafique, Muhammad, Maqsood Rehman, Zul Kamal, Rami Alzhrani, Sameer Alshehri, Ali Alamri, Mohammed Bakkari, et al. 2023. "Formulation Development of Lipid Polymer Hybrid Nanoparticles of Doxorubicin and Its In-Vitro, in-Vivo and Computational Evaluation." *Frontiers in Pharmacology* 14 (February). https://doi.org/10.3389/fphar.2023.1025013.

Shah, Rohan, Daniel Eldridge, Enzo Palombo, and Ian Harding. 2015. *Lipid Nanoparticles: Production, Characterization and Stability*. Springer. https://doi.org/10.1007/978-3-319-10711-0.

Shahgaldian, Patrick, Eric Da Silva, Anthony W. Coleman, Beth Rather, and Michael J. Zaworotko. 2003. "Para-Acyl-Calix-Arene Based Solid Lipid Nanoparticles (SLNs): A Detailed Study of Preparation and Stability Parameters." *International Journal of Pharmaceutics* 253 (1): 23–38. https://doi.org/10.1016/S0378-5173(02)00639-7.

Sheoran, Sumit, Swati Arora, R. Samsonraj, Pilli Govindaiah, and Sugunakar Vuree. 2022. "Lipid-Based Nanoparticles for Treatment of Cancer." *Heliyon* 8 (5): e09403. https://doi.org/10.1016/j.heliyon.2022.e09403.

Shi, N. Q., and X. R. Qi. 2021. *Liposome-Based Drug Delivery Systems: Biomaterial Engineering*. Springer.

Siefker-Radtke, Arlene, Xin-Qiao Zhang, Charles Guo, Yu Shen, Kathleen Pirollo, Sharjeel Sabir, Chris Leung, et al. 2016. "A Phase 1 Study of a Tumor-Targeted Systemic Nanodelivery System, SGT-94, in Genitourinary Cancers." *Molecular Therapy* 24 (June). https://doi.org/10.1038/mt.2016.118.

Singhal, Sunil, Shuming Nie, and May D Wang. 2010. "Nanotechnology Applications in Surgical Oncology." *Annual Review of Medicine* 61 (1). Annual Reviews: 359–73. https://doi.org/10.1146/annurev.med.60.052907.094936.

Subbiah, Vivek, Juneko Grilley-Olson, Austin Combest, Neelesh Sharma, Richard Tran, Iulian Bobe, Atsushi Osada, et al. 2017. "Phase Ib/II Trial of NC-6004 (Nanoparticle Cisplatin) Plus Gemcitabine in Patients with Advanced Solid Tumors." *Clinical Cancer Research* 24 (October). https://doi.org/10.1158/1078-0432.CCR-17-1114.

Sun, Tianmeng, Yu Shrike Zhang, Bo Pang, Dong Choon Hyun, Miaoxin Yang, and Younan Xia. 2014. "Engineered Nanoparticles for Drug Delivery in Cancer Therapy." *Angewandte Chemie International Edition* 53 (46). Wiley Online Library: 12320–64.

Szoka Jr, Francis, and Demetrios Papahadjopoulos. 1978. "Procedure for Preparation of Liposomes with Large Internal Aqueous Space and High Capture by Reverse-Phase Evaporation." *Proceedings of the National Academy of Sciences* 75 (9): 4194–8. https://doi.org/10.1073/pnas.75.9.4194.

Tagalakis, Aristides D., Do Hyang D. Lee, Alison S. Bienemann, Haiyan Zhou, Mustafa M. Munye, Luisa Saraiva, David McCarthy, et al. 2014. "Multifunctional, Self-Assembling Anionic Peptide-Lipid Nanocomplexes for Targeted SiRNA Delivery." *Biomaterials* 35 (29): 8406–15. https://doi.org/10.1016/j.biomaterials.2014.06.003.

Tam, Yuen Yi C., Sam Chen, and Pieter R. Cullis. 2013. "Advances in Lipid Nanoparticles for SiRNA Delivery." *Pharmaceutics* 5 (September): 498–507. https://doi.org/10.3390/pharmaceutics5030498.

Tang, Jing-Ling, Jin Sun, and Zhong-Gui He. 2007. "Self-Emulsifying Drug Delivery Systems: Strategy for Improving Oral Delivery of Poorly Soluble Drugs." *Current Drug Therapy* 2 (1). Bentham Science Publishers: 85–93.

Tavano, Lorena, Rita Muzzalupo, Loredana Mauro, Michele Pellegrino, Sebastiano Andò, and Nevio Picci. 2013. "Transferrin-Conjugated Pluronic Niosomes as a New Drug Delivery System for Anticancer Therapy." *Langmuir* 29 (41). American Chemical Society: 12638–46. https://doi.org/10.1021/la4021383.

Tavano, Lorena, Marco Vivacqua, Valentina Carito, Rita Muzzalupo, Maria Cristina Caroleo, and Fiore Nicoletta. 2013. "Doxorubicin Loaded Magneto-Niosomes for Targeted Drug Delivery." *Colloids and Surfaces B: Biointerfaces* 102: 803–7. https://doi.org/10.1016/j.colsurfb.2012.09.019.

Tawfik, Salah, Shavkatjon Azizov, Mohamed Elmasry, Mirkomil Sharipov, and Yong-Ill Lee. 2020. "Recent Advances in Nanomicelles Delivery Systems." *Nanomaterials* 11 (December): 70. https://doi.org/10.3390/nano11010070.

Teh, Shia-Yen, Robert Lin, Lung-Hsin Hung, and Abraham Lee. 2008. "Droplet Microfluidics." *Lab on a Chip* 8 (March): 198–220. https://doi.org/10.1039/b715524g.

Tenchov, Rumiana, Robert Bird, Allison E. Curtze, and Qiongqiong Zhou. 2021. "Lipid Nanoparticles—From Liposomes to MRNA Vaccine Delivery, a Landscape of Research Diversity and Advancement." *ACS Nano* 15 (11). American Chemical Society: 16982–7015. https://doi.org/10.1021/acsnano.1c04996.

Torchilin, Vladimir P. 2005. "Recent Advances with Liposomes as Pharmaceutical Carriers." *Nature Reviews Drug Discovery* 4 (2). Nature Publishing Group UK London: 145–60.

Tseu, Gloria Yi Wei, and Khairul Azfar Kamaruzaman. 2023. "A Review of Different Types of Liposomes and Their Advancements as a Form of Gene Therapy Treatment for Breast Cancer." *Molecules* 28 (3): 1498. https://doi.org/10.3390/molecules28031498.

Uchegbu, Ijeoma F., and Suresh P. Vyas. 1998. "Non-Ionic Surfactant Based Vesicles (Niosomes) in Drug Delivery." *International Journal of Pharmaceutics* 172 (1): 33–70. https://doi.org/10.1016/S0378-5173(98)00169-0.

Underwood, James C. E., and Simon S. Cross. 2009. *General and Systematic Pathology E-Book*. Elsevier Health Sciences.

Uskoković, Vuk. 2012. "Dynamic Light Scattering Based Microelectrophoresis: Main Prospects and Limitations." *Journal of Dispersion Science and Technology* 33 (12). Taylor & Francis: 1762–86. https://doi.org/10.1080/01932691.2011.625523.

Valastyan, Scott, and Robert A. Weinberg. 2011. "Tumor Metastasis: Molecular Insights and Evolving Paradigms." *Cell* 147 (2): 275–92. https://doi.org/10.1016/j.cell.2011.09.024.

Vemuri, Sriram, and C. T. Rhodes. 1995. "Preparation and Characterization of Liposomes as Therapeutic Delivery Systems: A Review." *Pharmaceutica Acta Helvetiae* 70 (2): 95–111. https://doi.org/10.1016/0031-6865(95)00010-7.

Ventola, C. 2017. "Progress in Nanomedicine: Approved and Investigational Nanodrugs." *P &T: A Peer-Reviewed Journal for Formulary Management* 42 (December): 742–55.

Vos, Theo, Ryan M. Barber, Brad Bell, Amelia Bertozzi-Villa, Stan Biryukov, Ian Bolliger, Fiona Charlson, Adrian Davis, Louisa Degenhardt, and Daniel Dicker. 2015. "Global, Regional, and National Incidence, Prevalence, and Years Lived with Disability for 301 Acute and Chronic Diseases and Injuries in 188 Countries, 1990–2013: A Systematic Analysis for the Global Burden of Disease Study 2013." *The Lancet* 386 (9995). Elsevier: 743–800.

Vyas, S. P., R. P. Singh, Sanyog Jain, Vivek Mishra, Sunil Mahor, Paramjit Singh, P. N. Gupta, A. Rawat, and P. Dubey. 2005. "Non-Ionic Surfactant Based Vesicles (Niosomes) for Non-Invasive Topical Genetic Immunization Against Hepatitis B." *International Journal of Pharmaceutics* 296 (1): 80–6. https://doi.org/10.1016/j.ijpharm.2005.02.016.

Wagner, Andreas, Karola Vorauer-Uhl, Günther Kreismayr, and Hermann Katinger. 2002. "The Crossflow Injection Technique: An Improvement of the Ethanol Injection Method." *Journal of Liposome Research* 12 (February): 259–70. https://doi.org/10.1081/LPR-120014761.

Wagner, Michael, Rahul Mitra, Mark Mcarthur, Wallace Baze, Kirstin Barnhart, Sherry Wu, Cristian Rodriguez, et al. 2017. "Preclinical Mammalian Safety Studies of EPHARNA (DOPC Nanoliposomal EphA2-Targeted SiRNA)." *Molecular Cancer Therapeutics* 16 (March). https://doi.org/10.1158/1535-7163.MCT-16-0541.

Wan, C., T. M. Allen, and P. R. Cullis. 2014. "Lipid Nanoparticle Delivery Systems for SiRNA-Based Therapeutics." *Drug Delivery and Translational Research* 4 (1): 74–83. https://doi.org/10.1007/s13346-013-0161-z.

Wang, Haidong, Mohsen Naghavi, Christine Allen, Ryan M. Barber, Zulfiqar A Bhutta, Austin Carter, Daniel C. Casey, Fiona J. Charlson, Alan Zian Chen, and Matthew M. Coates. 2016. "Global, Regional, and National Life Expectancy, All-Cause Mortality, and Cause-Specific Mortality for 249 Causes of Death, 1980–2015: A Systematic Analysis for the Global Burden of Disease Study 2015." *The Lancet* 388 (10053). Elsevier: 1459–544.

Wang, Hong-Xia, Zu-Qi Zuo, Jin-Zhi Du, Yu-Cai Wang, Rong Sun, Zhi-Ting Cao, Xiao-Dong Ye, Ji-Long Wang, Kam W Leong, and Jun Wang. 2016. "Surface Charge Critically Affects Tumor Penetration and Therapeutic Efficacy of Cancer Nanomedicines." *Nano Today* 11 (2): 133–44. https://doi.org/10.1016/j.nantod.2016.04.008.

Wang, Xiaoyong, Yan Jiang, Yu-Wen Wang, Mou-Tuan Huang, Chi-Tang Ho, and Qingrong Huang. 2008. "Enhancing Anti-Inflammation Activity of Curcumin through O/W Nanoemulsion." *Food Chemistry* 108 (May): 419–24. https://doi.org/10.1016/j.foodchem.2007.10.086.

Wang, Zhong Lin. 2004. "Zinc Oxide Nanostructures: Growth, Properties and Applications." *Journal of Physics: Condensed Matter* 16 (25). IOP Publishing: R829.

Whitesides, George M. 2006. "The Origins and the Future of Microfluidics." *Nature* 442 (7101): 368–73. https://doi.org/10.1038/nature05058.

Wissing, S. A., O. Kayser, and R. H. Müller. 2004. "Solid Lipid Nanoparticles for Parenteral Drug Delivery." *Advanced Drug Delivery Reviews* 56 (9): 1257–72. https://doi.org/10.1016/j.addr.2003.12.002.

Wong, Ho Lun, Reina Bendayan, Andrew M Rauth, Yongqiang Li, and Xiao Yu Wu. 2007. "Chemotherapy with Anticancer Drugs Encapsulated in Solid Lipid Nanoparticles." *Advanced Drug Delivery Reviews* 59 (6): 491–504. https://doi.org/10.1016/j.addr.2007.04.008.

Wong, Ho Lun, Andrew M. Rauth, Reina Bendayan, Janet L. Manias, Manisha Ramaswamy, Zengshe Liu, Sevim Z Erhan, and Xiao Yu Wu. 2006. "A New Polymer-Lipid Hybrid Nanoparticle System Increases Cytotoxicity of Doxorubicin Against Multidrug-Resistant Human Breast Cancer Cells." *Pharmaceutical Research* 23 (7): 1574–85. https://doi.org/10.1007/s11095-006-0282-x.

Wu, Xiaowen, Xingxing Dai, Yuyao Liao, Mengke Sheng, and Xinyuan Shi. 2021. "Investigation on Drug Entrapment Location in Liposomes and Transfersomes Based on Molecular Dynamics Simulation." *Journal of Molecular Modeling* 27. Springer: 1–10.

Xiaobo, Cao, Mourad Majidi, Meng Feng, Ruping Shao, Jing Wang, Yang Zhao, Veerabhadran Baladandayuthapani, et al. 2016. "TUSC2 (FUS1)-Erlotinib Induced Vulnerabilities in Epidermal Growth Factor Receptor (EGFR) Wildtype Non-Small Cell Lung Cancer (NSCLC) Targeted by the Repurposed Drug Auranofin." *Scientific Reports* 6 (1): 35741. https://doi.org/10.1038/srep35741.

Xiong, F., Z. Mi, and Ning Gu. 2011. "Cationic Liposomes as Gene Delivery System: Transfection Efficiency and New Application." *Pharmazie* 66 (3): 158–64. https://doi.org/10.1691/ph.2011.0768.

Xu, Letao, Xing Wang, Yun Liu, Guangze Yang, Robert Falconer, and Chun-Xia Zhao. 2021. "Lipid Nanoparticles for Drug Delivery." *Advanced NanoBiomed Research* 2 (November): 2100109. https://doi.org/10.1002/anbr.202100109.

Yang, Shi, and Jia Zhu. 2002. "Preparation and Characterization of Camptothecin Solid Lipid Nanoparticles." *Drug Development and Industrial Pharmacy* 28 (April): 265–74. https://doi.org/10.1081/DDC-120002842.

Yingchoncharoen, Phatsapong, Danuta Kalinowski, and Des Richardson. 2016. "Lipid-Based Drug Delivery Systems in Cancer Therapy: What Is Available and What Is Yet to Come." *Pharmacological Reviews* 68 (June): 701–87. https://doi.org/10.1124/pr.115.012070.

Zhang, H., and G. D'Souza. 2017. *Liposomes: Methods in Molecular Biology*. Humana Press.

Zhang, J. Allen, Gopal Anyarambhatla, Lan Ma, Sydney Ugwu, Tong Xuan, Tommaso Sardone, and Imran Ahmad. 2005. "Development and Characterization of a Novel Cremophor® EL Free Liposome-Based Paclitaxel (LEP-ETU) Formulation." *European Journal of Pharmaceutics and Biopharmaceutics* 59 (1). Elsevier: 177–87.

Zhang, Jing, Xiang Li, and Leaf Huang. 2014. "Non-Viral Nanocarriers for SiRNA Delivery in Breast Cancer." *Journal of Controlled Release* 190: 440–50. https://doi.org/10.1016/j.jconrel.2014.05.037.

Zhang, Qingyang, Jieming Ping, Zirui Huang, Xiaoli Zhang, Jingyi Zhou, Gangyang Wang, Shaoyang Liu, and Jianjun Ma. 2020. "CAR-T Cell Therapy in Cancer: Tribulations and Road Ahead." *Journal of Immunology Research* 2020 (January): 1–11. https://doi.org/10.1155/2020/1924379.

Zhou, Yinjian, Chunling Zhang, and Wei Liang. 2014. "Development of RNAi Technology for Targeted Therapy—A Track of SiRNA Based Agents to RNAi Therapeutics." *Journal of Controlled Release* 193: 270–81. https://doi.org/10.1016/j.jconrel.2014.04.044.

Zidan, Ahmed S., Ziyaur Rahman, and Mansoor A. Khan. 2011. "Product and Process Understanding of a Novel Pediatric Anti-HIV Tenofovir Niosomes with a High-Pressure Homogenizer." *European Journal of Pharmaceutical Sciences* 44 (1): 93–102. https://doi.org/10.1016/j.ejps.2011.06.012.

Zielińska, Aleksandra, Carlos Martins-Gomes, N. R. Ferreira, Amélia Silva, Izabela Nowak, and Eliana B. Souto. 2018. "Anti-Inflammatory and Anti-Cancer Activity of Citral: Optimization of Citral-Loaded Solid Lipid Nanoparticles (SLN) Using Experimental Factorial Design and LUMiSizer®." *International Journal of Pharmaceutics* 553 (October). https://doi.org/10.1016/j.ijpharm.2018.10.065.

Zou, Yiyu, and Waldemar Priebe. 1995. "Article in Clinical Cancer Research." http://clincancerres.aacrjournals.org/content/1/11/1369.

Zugazagoitia, Jon, Cristiano Guedes, Santiago Ponce, Irene Ferrer, Sonia Molina-Pinelo, and Luis Paz-Ares. 2016. "Current Challenges in Cancer Treatment." *Clinical Therapeutics* 38 (7): 1551–66. https://doi.org/10.1016/j.clinthera.2016.03.026.

12 Multifunctional Nanomaterials for Advanced Cancer Therapy

Akriti Sharma, Arundhati, and Divya Dhawal Bhandari

ABBREVIATIONS

Acronym	Full Form
CNM	carbon nanomaterial
GSM	signaling molecule
NP	nanoparticle
MRI	magnetic resonance imaging
CT	computed tomography
RNA	ribonucleic acid
EPR	enhanced permeability and retention
EV	extracellular vesicles

12.1 INTRODUCTION

Nanotechnology has garnered significant interest in the past few years. The concept of nanotechnology primarily relates to the manufacturing of innovative materials that possess a minimum dimension falling within a size spectrum ranging from 1 to 100 nm, which is equal to one billionth of a meter. It is presently being utilized in a wide array of sectors, including chemicals, cosmetics, textiles, agriculture, recycling, energy, electronics, and healthcare (McNeil 2005).

Recent developments in the field of nanotechnology have sparked a burgeoning enthusiasm for utilizing nanomaterials in the realm of medicine, with the aim of resolving a multitude of challenges involving therapeutic agents. The investigation of fabricated nanomaterials possessing distinctive physical and chemical attributes has been undertaken for the purpose of diagnostic and therapeutic utilization. In order to mitigate systemic toxicity, enhance solubility, extend the duration of circulation, diminish immunogenicity, and optimize distribution, therapeutic agents and nanoparticles have been combined (Seleci et al. 2016). A wide range of nanoparticles, about 100 nm in size, is being deployed for boosting drug absorption, internalization, and therapeutic efficacy. Furthermore, by adjusting these nanoparticles' chemical characteristics, dimensions, configurations, structures, morphologies, and surface attributes, their physicochemical and biological properties can be precisely altered (Xia 2014).

In recent times, the utilization of nanoparticle-based delivery platforms has been harnessed across diverse medical domains. These mechanisms are enticing since they are composed of well-characterized, biocompatible components that are relatively easy to functionalize (Tiwari, Patra, and Choi 2015). There are numerous biomedical applications of liposomes, dendrimers, polymeric nanoparticles, quantum dots, and metal nanoparticles. They are utilized in various capacities, including diagnostic assays (Donolato et al. 2015), enhancing the efficacy of radiotherapy (K. Kim et al. 2016), and facilitating the delivery of drugs (Look et al. 2015).

The potential of carbon nanomaterials (CNMs), specifically carbon nanotubes, graphene, fullerene, and carbon quantum dots, for both the detection and management of multiple health conditions

 DOI: 10.1201/9781003463191-15

has been thoroughly studied (Masoudi Asil et al. 2023). Carbon nanomaterials (CNMs) have been employed in non-invasive diagnostic approaches, namely, fluorescence and magnetic resonance imaging, in addition to being utilized in targeted drug delivery systems (Waris et al. 2022).

Several nanomaterials, such as carbon nanotube, metallic nanoparticles, and quantum dots, have been applied to neurological illnesses for imaging and therapeutic purposes (Liu et al. 2021). Nanotechnology has also been investigated in enhancing treatment efficacy in prostatitis diagnosis and therapy, where functional nanoparticles have exhibited great potential in augmenting the efficacy of treatment (Lugoloobi et al. 2023).

Furthermore, there have been advancements in the creation of hybrid nanoplatforms that allow for the precise delivery of gaseous signaling molecules (GSMs) like carbon monoxide, hydrogen sulfide, and nitric oxide. These GSMs possess promising therapeutic potential and can be administered in a controlled manner (Sundar Singh, Tiwari, and Tyagi 2021). In general, nanomaterials present a vast array of opportunities for multifaceted therapeutic implementations across diverse domains. Nanomaterials have unlocked a realm of transformative therapeutic applications across medicine. These minuscule structures, like liposomes, polymeric nanoparticles, and dendrimers, have revolutionized drug delivery, enabling targeted treatment to specific cells or tissues while minimizing side effects. Table 12.1 presents an overview of the therapeutic implementations of different nanomaterials.

The expedient advancement of nanotechnology has enabled the emergence of multifunctional nanomaterials that hold tremendous promise in the field of therapeutic applications. These versatile

TABLE 12.1
Applications of Nanomaterials as Groundbreaking Tools in Various Therapeutic Realms Due to Their Unique Properties at the Nanoscale

Research Envisaged	Nanomaterials	Applications	References
The potential of using fullerene, carbon quantum dots, graphene, and carbon nanotubes in biomedical fields is highlighted by Masoudi et al. in the study titled "Theranostic applications of multifunctional carbon nanomaterials," which reviewed the biomedical application of carbon nanomaterials and their latest breakthroughs in treatment and diagnosis.	The types of multifunctional nanomaterials for therapeutic applications in the present work include carbon nanotubes, carbon quantum dots, graphene, and fullerene.	• CNMs have potential applications in disease diagnosis and therapy. • Various types of CNMs have been studied and found to be safe and efficient for non-invasive diagnostic techniques and drug delivery.	Masoudi Asil et al. (2023)
The study "Therapeutic Applications of Functional Nanomaterials for Prostatitis" by Liu et al. highlights the treatment approaches for and challenges associated with prostatitis and describes the advantages of functional nanoparticles in improving treatment effectiveness and overcoming side effects, which is projected to be used in prostate cancer evaluation and therapy.	The research describes several types of multifunctional nanomaterials for therapeutic applications, including CuFeO2 and Fe3O4 NPs, nanohydrogels, photosensitive H2-generated nanosystems, and polydopamine nanoparticles.	• Nanotechnology shows promise in the diagnosis and treatment of prostatitis. • Functional nanoparticles can improve treatment effectiveness and overcome side effects.	Liu et al. (2021)

(*Continued*)

TABLE 12.1 *(Continued)*
Applications of Nanomaterials as Groundbreaking Tools in Various Therapeutic Realms Due to Their Unique Properties at the Nanoscale

Research Envisaged	Nanomaterials	Applications	References
In the work "Gaseous Signaling Molecule-Releasing Hybrid Nanomaterials for Therapeutic Applications," the authors conducted an extensive examination of the mechanisms underlying gas therapy, latest research on the controlled release of gaseous signaling molecules from hybrid nanoplatforms, as well as the utilization of these nanoplatforms in the management of diverse diseases.	The use of hybrid nanomaterials for the controlled release of gaseous signaling molecules (GSMs) in therapeutic applications has been discussed in the research.	• Hybrid nanomaterials can enhance the delivery of gaseous signaling molecules (GSMs). • GSM releasers have potential for therapeutic applications.	Lugoloobi et al. (2023)
An overview of radiolabeling methods for preparing anticancer agents that have been investigated recently in preclinical studies are provided, and the therapeutic applications and efficacy of α- or β-emitter-incorporated nanomaterials in animal models are discussed by Jeon and Jonghoin the work "Review of Therapeutic Applications of Radiolabeled Functional Nanomaterial."	Various types of nanomaterials, including inorganic, polymeric, carbon-based materials, and liposomes, have been delineated for their utilization in the realm of therapeutic applications within the domain of cancer therapy.	• Radiolabeled nanomaterials have potential for cancer therapy. • α- or β-emitter-incorporated nanomaterials show effectiveness in animal models.	Jeon 2019
Tambe et al., in the study "Carbon nanomaterials for therapeutic applications," highlighted the cutting-edge properties, mechanism of action, and advancements of carbon nanomaterials as DDS in a range of ailments, including cancer and inflammatory disorders.	The types of multifunctional nanomaterials for therapeutic applications, including single- and multi-walled carbon nanotubes, graphene, reduced graphene oxides, carbon dots, and fullerenes, have been outlined in the research.	• Carbon nanomaterials have potential for drug delivery systems. • Carbon nanomaterials show promise in biomedical applications.	Tambe et al. 2022
Current research on the state-of-the-art and emerging photonic nanomaterials for diverse biomedical applications is reviewed, and the remaining challenges and future prospects are discussed, in the study "Multifunctional Photonic Nanomaterials for Diagnostic, Therapeutic, and Theranostic Applications" by Kim et al.	The types of multifunctional nanomaterials for therapeutic applications discussed in the research include semiconductor quantum dots, plasmonic metal nanoparticles, organic carbon, and polymeric nanomaterials.	• Progress in photonic nanomaterials for biomedical applications.	H. Kim et al. (2018)

materials exhibit the potential to revolutionize drug delivery, imaging, and diagnostics, offering innovative solutions for the management of disease. The integration of multiple functionalities within a single nanomaterial platform represents a significant breakthrough, allowing for targeted and personalized therapies, reduced side effects, and improved patient outcomes. This review provides a deeper understanding of the rich field of multifunctional nanomaterials. It will explore the different types of nanomaterials, the methods employed in their synthesis, the therapeutic uses of multifunctional nanomaterials, the challenges that require attention, and the future directions.

12.2 TYPES OF MULTIFUNCTIONAL NANOMATERIALS FOR THERAPEUTIC APPLICATIONS

The broad field of medicine and healthcare has shown the immense potential that multifunctional nanomaterials hold for therapeutic applications. These nanoparticles have special characteristics that make them appropriate for a range of biomedical applications (Masoudi Asil et al. 2023). Graphene, fullerene, carbon nanotubes, and carbon quantum dots are examples of CNMs that have been used in non-invasive diagnostic methods like magnetic resonance imaging and fluorescence imaging (Waris et al. 2022). Moreover, they have been applied to cancer photothermal and photodynamic therapy, as well as to enhance the cell targeting of anticancer medications. Furthermore, the potential applications of multifunctional nanomaterials, such as magnetic nanoparticles, in tissue engineering, regenerative medicine, drug delivery, and extracellular vesicles (EV)–based illness detection have been investigated (Srinath et al. 2023). The physical, chemical, and biological characteristics of these nanomaterials can be tuned to improve the delivery, detection, and isolation of EVs and the biomolecules they are linked with. Multifunctional nanomaterials show potential for expanding medicinal uses in the biological sciences (Srinath et al. 2023).

Multifunctional nanomaterials for therapeutic applications include dendrimers, iron oxide nanoparticles, micelles, gold nanostructures, carbon dots, quantum dots, polymeric conjugates, and stimuli-responsive systems (Sahu, Biswas, and Das 2020). Proteins, peptides, polysaccharides, and nucleic acids are examples of biomolecule-based nanostructures that are being investigated for use in cancer nanomedicine (Jing Wang, Li, and Nie 2021). Organic nanomaterials like liposomal, dendrimer, polymer, and protein-based nanoparticles, as well as inorganic nanoparticles like silica, gold, and silver, exhibit potential in the treatment of disorders associated with inflammation and immunotherapy (Lenders et al. 2020), as given in Figure 12.1.

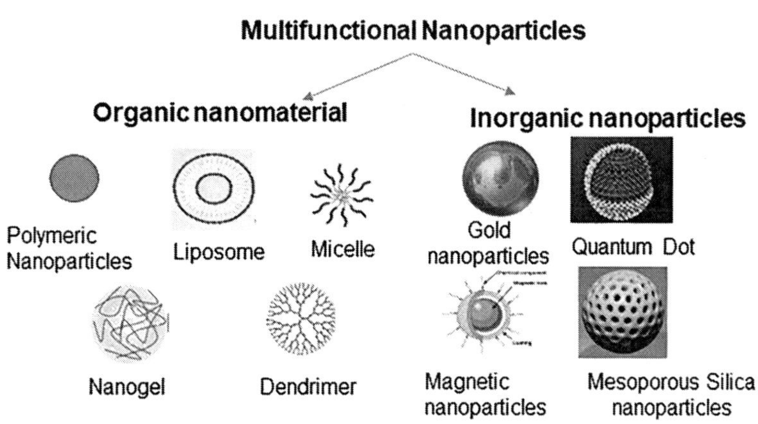

FIGURE 12.1 Structures representing various types of multifunctional nanoparticles used in drug delivery. The figure illustrates the two classes of multifunctional nanoparticles, which further include liposomes, micelles, nanogels, dendrimers, and polymeric nanoparticles under the class of organic nanoparticles, while quantum dot, gold, magnetic and mesoporous silica nanoparticles are under the class of inorganic nanoparticles.

TABLE 12.2
Multifunctional Nanomaterials as a Cutting-Edge Class of Compounds with Diverse Applications in Therapeutics, Offering a Fusion of Diagnostic, Therapeutic, and Targeting Functionalities within a Single Platform

Title of Paper	Types	Scope	References
"Stimuli-Responsive Nanomaterials for Drug Delivery"	The different types of nanomaterials, including metallic nanomaterials, sensors, mesoporous materials, biosensors, nanocomposites for potential therapeutic applications, are discussed in the present study.	• Stimuli-responsive nanomaterials have potential biomedical applications. • Different types of nanomaterials can be fabricated using various approaches.	López-Saucedo et al. (2019)
"Synthesis and Application of Nanomaterials for Biomedical Anticancer Therapy"	The study discusses various types of nanomaterials, such as gold, silver, titanium oxide, polymeric nanoparticles, iron oxide silica, platinum, and for therapeutic applications.	• Nanomaterials have significant potential in biomedical anticancer therapy. • Nanomaterials can be used to image cancer cells and as drug carriers.	Vallinayagam and Rajendran (2021)
"Multifunctional nanomedicines: potentials and prospects"	The current research mentions several types of pharmaceutical nanocarriers, such as nanoparticles, polymeric nanoparticles, micelles microspheres, and dendrimers that can be used for therapeutic applications.	• Multifunctional nanocarriers enhance therapeutic and diagnostic protocols. • Nanotechnology offers new tools for therapy, imaging, and diagnosis.	Agrawal et al. (2013)
"Multifunctional biomolecule nanostructures for cancer therapy"	This work presents biomolecule-based nanostructures, such as proteins, peptides, nucleic acids, and polysaccharides, and emphasizes how much design space they have for multipurpose nanomedicines.	• Biomolecule-based nanostructures have potential for cancer therapy. • Challenges in design, characterization, and clinical translation.	Jing Wang, Li, and Nie (2021)
"Biomedical nanomaterials for immunological applications: ongoing research and clinical trials"	The study discusses various types of nanomaterials, including inorganic nanoparticles, such as silver, gold, and silica, as well as organic nanomaterials, such as polymer, liposomal, dendrimer, and protein-based nanoparticles.	• Nanoparticles have the potential to enhance therapies for diseases. • Inorganic and organic nanomaterials have specific applications in drug delivery and immunotherapy.	Lenders et al. (2020)
"Functional Nanomaterials and Their Potential Applications in Antibacterial Therapy"	This work is focused on the antibacterial applications of four widely utilized nanomaterials—polymeric nanoparticles, graphene, nanogels, metal-based, and oxides or carbon-based nanomaterials.	• Nanomaterials have a promising future in biomedical application. • More research is needed in biocompatibility and biosafety.	Hong et al. (2019)

For antibacterial usage, nanomaterials such as graphene oxides, metal-based or carbon-based, polymeric nanoparticles, and nanogels have been formed (Hong et al. 2019). Furthermore, stimuli-responsive nanoparticles, such as mesoporous materials, nanomedicine, sensors, metallic nanomaterials, and biosensors, present a promising scope in biomedical applications (López-Saucedo et al. 2019). These multifunctional nanomaterials hold immense promise in medicine due to their ability to combine therapeutic, diagnostic, and targeting functionalities in a single platform. However, thorough evaluation of their biocompatibility, stability, and potential toxicity is crucial for their successful translation into clinical applications. Table 12.2 discusses the types of multifunctional nanomaterials for therapeutic applications.

12.3 METHODS USED FOR THE SYNTHESIS OF MULTIFUNCTIONAL NANOMATERIALS FOR THERAPEUTIC APPLICATIONS

Numerous methods have been explored for the production of nanoparticles. Utilizing magnetic nanoparticles as drug carriers is one such technique. These particles can be designed to exhibit a hyperthermia response when functionalized with biomolecules (Galarreta-Rodriguez et al. 2023). Also, high-performance nanomaterials have been designed and synthesized using bioinspired techniques for biomedical uses, such as cancer treatment (Tang et al. 2023). Green synthesis techniques, which use living organisms like fungi, bacteria, and plants, have become a biocompatible and environmentally friendly way to produce nanoparticles, with potential uses in the delivery of drugs for the treatment of cancer (Majithia and Barretto 2023). Since they are easily functionalized and have good biocompatibility, luminescent polymer nanomaterials have also been explored for therapeutic uses. These applications include drug delivery, biosensing, and bioimaging (Bu et al. 2023).

The synthesis of multifunctional nanomaterials for therapeutic purposes can be performed through hydrothermal synthesis, coprecipitation, seeding, microemulsion, chemical reduction, and so no electrode position (Habibi et al. 2020). Polymeric one-dimensional nanostructures can be synthesized using different techniques and functionalized for specific applications in biosensing and drug delivery (Nam and Luong 2019). Nanomaterials can be designed and characterized for drug delivery in cancer therapy, enhancing efficiency and reducing toxicity and side effects (Sayin et al. 2019). Additionally, a method involving the synthesis of Gd: CuS-coated Flu-coated TPE-coated alpha cd47-coated RGD nanoparticles has been developed for targeted tumor therapy (Rajabi, Srinivasan, and Mousa 2016). These methods and approaches provide prospects for the formation of multifunctional nanoparticles for therapeutic applications, addressing challenges in drug delivery and treatment of diseases. The synthesis of multifunctional nanomaterials for therapeutic applications involves several techniques tailored to produce nanoparticles with specific properties suitable for targeted drug delivery, imaging, and other therapeutic functions, as described in Table 12.3.

TABLE 12.3
Methods Used for the Synthesis of Multifunctional Nanomaterials for Therapeutic Applications Involving a Range of Sophisticated Methods Tailored to Create Nanoparticles with Specific Properties

Title of Paper	Description	Method Used	References
"Nanoparticles: synthesis and applications"	The research addresses several approaches to synthesizing and functionalizing metallic, semiconductor, magnetic, and multifunctional nanoparticles that can be applied to therapeutic usages.	• Chemical reduction, coprecipitation, seeding, microemulsion, sonoelectrodeposition. • Hydrothermal synthesis.	Nam and Luong (2019)

(Continued)

TABLE 12.3 *(Continued)*
Methods Used for the Synthesis of Multifunctional Nanomaterials for Therapeutic Applications Involving a Range of Sophisticated Methods Tailored to Create Nanoparticles with Specific Properties

Title of Paper	Description	Method Used	References
"Nanobiomaterials in drug delivery"	This study presents the introduction of the design and characterization of a diverse range of nanomaterials for drug delivery in order to effectively treat cancer.	• Synthesis and manipulation of nanomaterials. • Conjugation of small molecules to nanomaterials.	Rajabi, Srinivasan, and Mousa (2016)
"Multifunctional nanovesicle-bioactive conjugates prepared by a one-step scalable method using CO2-expanded solvents"	The present work aimed to introduce a one-step method using CO2-expanded solvents to prepare multifunctional nanovesicle–bioactive conjugates for therapeutic applications.	• One-step scalable method using CO2-expanded solvents. • DELOS-SUSP methodology for the preparation of nanovesicles.	Cabrera et al. (2013)
"Methods of synthesis of non-toxic multifunctional nanoparticles and applications"	The present invention involves methods for synthesizing multifunctional nanoparticles that can be utilized in biomedical approaches for therapeutic applications.	• Sol-gel chemistry, doping, and sonication.	Kuniyil et al. (2008)

12.4 MULTIFUNCTIONAL NANOMATERIALS FOR THERAPEUTIC APPLICATIONS

Due to their unique characteristics at the nanoscale, nanomaterials have a wide range of applications in multiple sectors. Here are some notable applications, like medicines and healthcare, electronics, energy, catalysis, material science, environmental remediation, textiles, food packaging, aerospace, cosmetics, construction, water purification, biotechnology, defense, transportation, etc. Their versatility and unique properties continue to drive innovation in science and technology across a wide range of industries. However, when it comes to exploring the therapeutic applications, the details are discussed in what follow.

12.4.1 Targeted Drug Delivery

Nanomaterial has unique properties which allow them to carry drugs to defined locations in the body. They have specialized size and surface properties that allow them to navigate through the bloodstream and reach the target tissues or cells much more effectively, as presented in Figure 12.2 and Figure 12.3. Various molecules, such as ligands, peptides, and antibodies, are functionalized to specifically bind with the receptors or biomarkers on the surface of target cells or tissues, which enhances the selectivity of drug delivery (Swarbrick 2013). The nanomaterials can be loaded with drugs. This encapsulation safeguards the medication from disintegration in the bloodstream and guarantees a gradual, controlled release of the medication. Nanomaterials can benefit from the increased permeability and retention (EPR) effect, because tumor tissues have weak lymphatic drainage and leaky blood vessels (Maeda 2001). Due to their size and leaky vasculature, tumor tissues can passively absorb nanomaterial. They can actively target

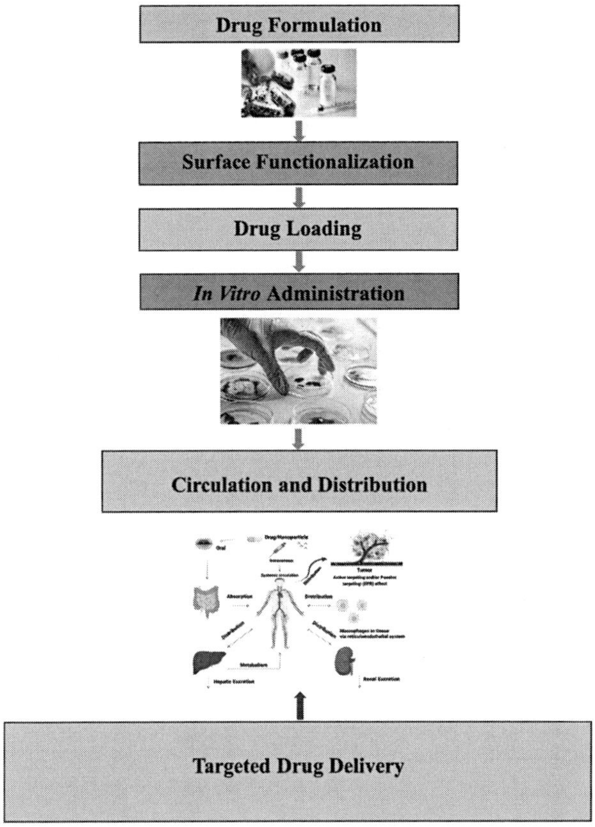

FIGURE 12.2 Various steps involved in the formulation of nanoparticles. The formulation of nanoparticles includes surface functionalization of available drug formulation, followed by the loading of drug onto the surface of nanoparticles. The so-formed formulation is administered *in vitro*, and a check is kept on its circulation and distribution in the body to achieve targeted drug delivery.

particular cells or tissues by adding particular ligands to the nanomaterials to functionalize them. For instance, in cancer therapy, nanoparticles can be created to specifically target cancer cells by identifying their distinctive surface markers (Lamprecht et al. 2001). In reaction to certain triggers, certain nanomaterials are programmed to release medications. Changes in pH, temperature, or the presence of enzymes that are common in particular infectious locations can all act as triggers. This guarantees that the medicine is released in the appropriate area. It is possible to build nanomaterials to degrade naturally. The danger of long-term side effects is decreased because, after drug administration, they can degrade into non-toxic metabolites and are removed from the body (Koo, Rubinstein, and Onyuksel 2006). Nanomaterials can provide controlled and sustained release of drugs for long term, reducing the need for repeated dosing and minimizing side effects. To reduce the toxicity, targeted drug delivery using nanomaterials can reduce healthy tissue exposure to the drug, minimizing systemic toxicity and side effects (Koo, Rubinstein, and Onyuksel 2006). Some nanomaterials can also be used for diagnostic purposes, helping to visualize disease sites and monitor the effectiveness of therapy. However, it is important to note that the development and clinical translation of nanomedicine involve various challenges, such as safety, scalability, and regulatory aspects that must be considered for successful clinical application (Koo, Rubinstein, and Onyuksel 2006).

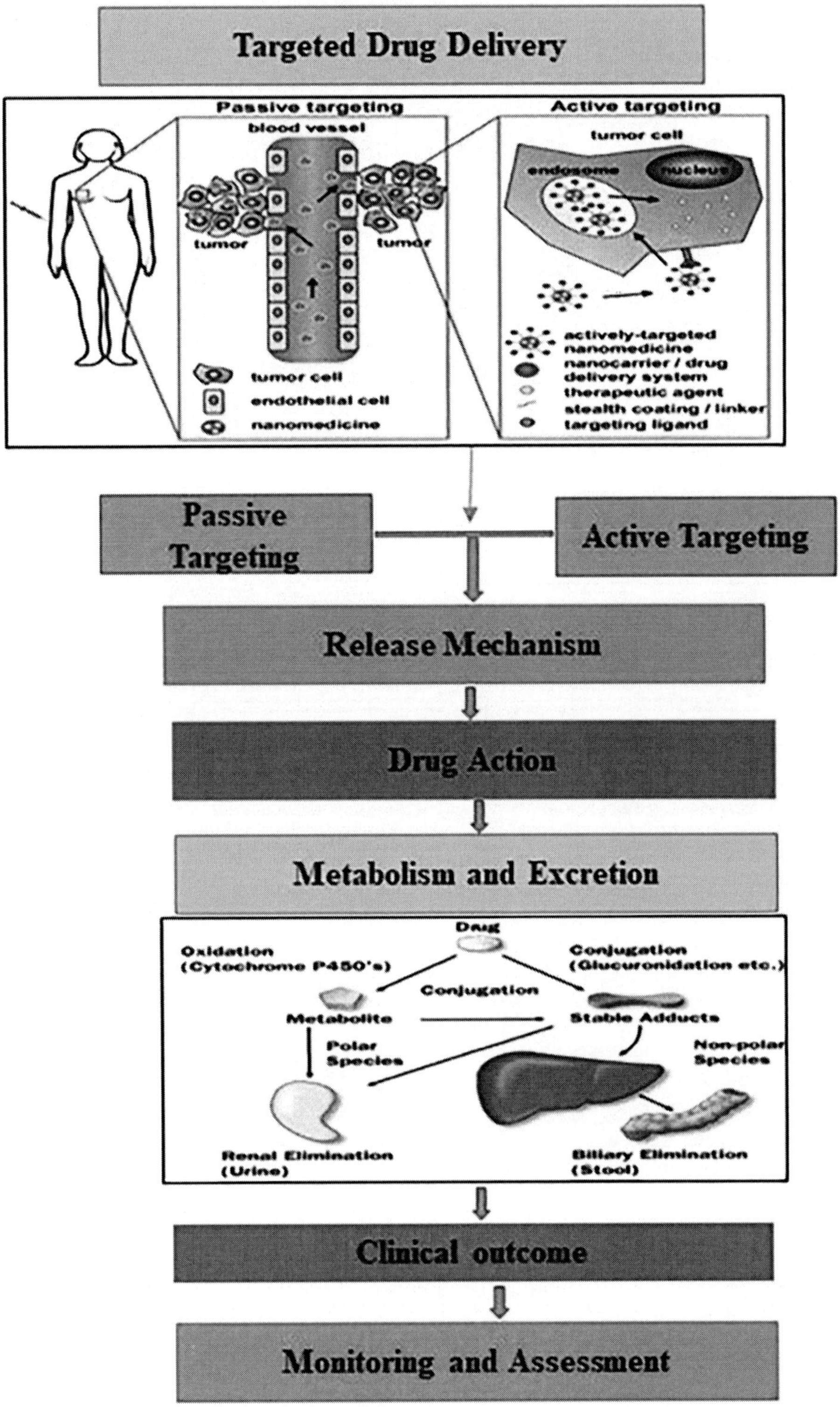

FIGURE 12.3 Various steps involved in the clinical delivery of nanoparticles. The flowchart illustrates the pharmacodynamics, that is, what the body does with the drug once it reaches its target. After the release, the drug will show its action, and then metabolized and excreted. The clinical delivery is being monitored afterward.

12.4.2 Image Enhancement

Imaging enhancement is, indeed, an important application of nanomaterials in medical diagnostics and imaging domain. In many different kinds of imaging processes, such as magnetic resonance imaging (MRI), ultrasound, and computed tomography (CT) scans, nanomaterials can serve as contrast agents. These nanoparticles are made to accumulate at particular bodily locations, like tumors or inflammatory wounds, making them easier to see on imaging tests (Jiang et al. 2023). MRI contrast agents often include superparamagnetic nanoparticles like iron oxide nanoparticles. They can greatly enhance the contrast between various biological tissues or structures, making it simple to identify abnormalities. For example, gold nanoparticles can be utilized as CT contrast materials. They offer superior contrast in CT scans by more effectively absorbing X-rays than the surrounding tissues. For example, gold nanoparticles can be utilized as CT contrast materials. They offer superior contrast in CT scans by effectively absorbing X-rays than the surrounding tissues. Nanomaterial-based microbubbles can improve ultrasound imaging. These microbubbles enable better imaging of blood arteries and other structures and can be directed to particular areas. Transition metal (TM)–based nanomaterials, gold (Au), bismuth (Bi), and lanthanide (Ln) are among the numerous contrast agents for CT imaging that have been reported to date (Lusic and Grinstaff 2013).

Nanotechnology has made significant advances in recent years. It has the potential to greatly benefit society and encourage scientific innovation. Many nanomaterials have been developed as potential tools for use in biology because of their distinct chemical and physical traits, such as regulated manufacturing and effortless surface modification (Riehemann et al. 2009; Guerrero-Martínez, Pérez-Juste, and Liz-Marzán 2010). Looking at the past records, different number of diseases have been considerably diagnosed using imaging techniques, like fluorescence imaging positron emission tomography and MRI (Kircher and Willmann 2012). For optical imaging methods, quantum dots and other fluorescent nanoparticles can be employed. When activated, they release particular wavelengths of light that make it possible to image biological structures with extreme sensitivity and clarity. Multimodal imaging, which integrates two or more imaging modalities, is a function of some nanomaterials (Basuki et al. 2013). For instance, a nanoparticle might be capable of both MRI and fluorescence, offering supplementary data for more precise diagnoses. Nanomaterials can be created with medicinal and diagnostic capabilities. They can act as imaging agents and deliver medications to particular locations. *Theranostics* is a concept that enables real-time monitoring of drug delivery and therapeutic efficacy (Zavaleta, Ho, and Chung 2018). Antibodies or ligands that precisely bind to disease indicators or receptors on target cells can be used to functionalize nanoparticles. The accuracy of imaging is increased, and the background signal is decreased, by this focused technique. Physiological characteristics in the body, such as pH levels, oxygen concentrations, or glucose levels, can be continuously monitored using nanosensors. These sensors can provide real-time data to healthcare providers for better patient management (Zavaleta, Ho, and Chung 2018).

12.4.3 Therapeutic Functions

Nanomaterials have successfully been used in treating cancer, diabetes management, and other ailments by enabling controlled drug delivery. As nanotechnology advances, it has the potential to fundamentally alter how we currently manage and treat diseases on an individual basis (Anjum et al. 2021). The controlled release of drugs from nanomaterials can be achieved through approaches such as encapsulation in nanocarriers, surface modification and functionalization, responsive nanomaterials, nanoparticle surface erosion or degradation, external stimuli-responsive systems (Anjum et al. 2021).

Drugs can be encapsulated within nanocarriers, such as micelles, dendrimers, liposomes, and polymeric nanoparticles. These nanocarriers shield the drug from getting degraded and clearance, allowing for regulated release over an extended period (Ahmad et al. 2021). The composition, size,

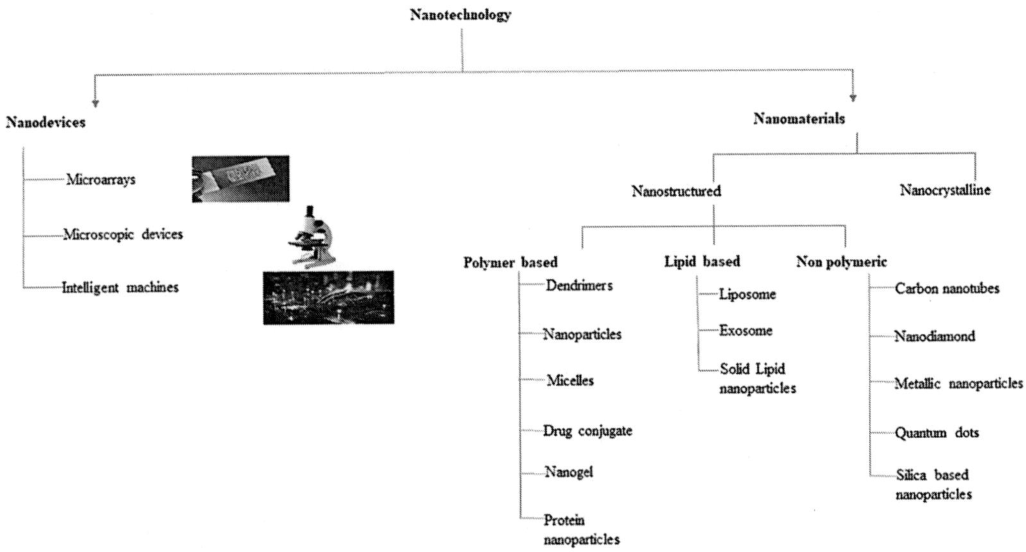

FIGURE 12.4 Various applications of nanoparticles in therapeutics. The flowchart depicts the applications of nanotechnology as nanomaterials and nanodevices. The available nanodevices include microscopic devices, microarrays, while nanomaterials include dendrimers, nanogels, carbon nanotubes, quantum dots, etc.

and surface characteristics of the nanocarriers can all be changed to control the rate of release. The surface of nanomaterials can be altered with particular functional groups or ligands that react to environmental factors like pH, temperature, light, or enzymes. By enabling triggered drug release at the target site, these modifications maximize therapeutic efficacy while reducing off-target effects, as given in (Osman et al. 2022) Figure 12.4.

Some nanomaterials are designed to respond to specific biological cues or environmental changes. As an example, stimuli-responsive hydrogels may experience volume-phase transitions in response to variations in pH or temperature, which will cause the drug to be released under control (Mohaghegh et al. 2022). In a similar manner, an external magnetic field can be used to direct magnetic nanoparticles to the desired location, facilitating site-specific drug delivery. Certain nanoparticles are engineered to degrade or erode gradually under physiological conditions. The encapsulated drugs are released in a steady and regulated manner as the nanomaterials break down, providing a prolonged therapeutic effect. This approach is particularly useful for the delivery of sensitive or potent drugs that require controlled dosing (Mohaghegh et al. 2022).

Nanomaterials can be developed to release drugs when exposed to external stimuli like light, magnetic fields, or ultrasound. For instance, light-responsive nanocarriers may be triggered by particular light wavelengths, causing the encapsulated drug to be released at the desired location (Sethuraman et al. 2021). This approach allows for spatiotemporal control over drug release, enhancing treatment precision. By leveraging these mechanisms, nanomaterials can be engineered to achieve controlled drug release, ensuring optimal therapeutic outcomes, reduced dosing frequency, and minimized adverse effects. The ability to precisely regulate drug release kinetics contributes to the advancement of personalized and targeted therapeutic strategies for numerous ailments and medical conditions. By harnessing the capabilities of multifunctional nanomaterials, personalized medicine can be advanced to a level where treatments can be customized to the unique clinical and biological profiles of individual patients. The integration of multifunctional nanomaterials in diagnostic, therapeutic, and monitoring platforms holds great promise for improving treatment efficacy, minimizing adverse effects, and ultimately enhancing patient outcomes and quality of life (Sethuraman et al. 2021).

12.4.4 Continuous Monitoring

Nanomaterials have demonstrated immense potential in revolutionizing the field of healthcare, particularly in enabling real-time health monitoring and diagnostics. They are impeccable for many different applications in biology and medicine, thanks to their distinctive qualities, which include a high surface-area-to-volume ratio, enhanced sensitivity, and customizable surface functionalities. Thereare some ways in which nanomaterials can be used to monitor a patient's health in real-time, like biosensors, implantable devices, nanoparticle-based imaging techniques, smart wearable devices (Pirzada and Altintas 2019).

Nanomaterial-based biosensors can detect specific biomarkers or molecules indicative of various health conditions. Functionalized nanoparticles, such as quantum dots or gold nanoparticles, can be engineered to bind to target molecules within the body (Contera, De La Serna, and Tetley 2020). Changes in the optical, electrical, or magnetic properties of these nanoparticles upon binding enable real-time detection and quantification of biomarkers, allowing for continuous monitoring of health parameters. Nanomaterials can be incorporated into implantable devices to monitor various physiological parameters, such as glucose levels, pH, temperature, or pressure. Nanosensors integrated into these devices can provide continuous data, enabling healthcare providers to track a patient's health status and intervene promptly in case of any abnormalities (Duan et al. 2020).

Fluorescence imaging, CT scan, and MRI are some of the cutting-edge imaging modalities made possible by quantum dots and superparamagnetic nanoparticles. These imaging techniques provide detailed insights into the internal biological processes and can aid in the real-time visualization of disease progression and treatment efficacy (Blasiak, Van Veggel, and Tomanek 2013). Nanomaterials integrated into wearable devices, such as smart clothing or patches, can continuously monitor vital signs, body movements, and biochemical parameters (Guk et al. 2019). These devices can transmit real-time data to a patient's smartphone or a healthcare provider's system, allowing for remote monitoring and timely intervention in case of any health concerns or emergencies (Huang et al. 2022). By leveraging the unique properties of nanomaterials, researchers and healthcare professionals can develop advanced monitoring systems that provide real-time insights into a patient's health status, facilitating early disease detection, personalized treatments, and improved overall healthcare management (Contera, De La Serna, and Tetley 2020).

Nanosensors, owing to their exceptional sensitivity, specificity, and capacity to detect and monitor various biological molecules, have found diverse applications in disease management and prevention. Some examples of nanosensors and their applications in the field of healthcare are glucose nanosensors, biomarker nanosensors, nanoparticle-based imaging agents, nanoparticle-based pathogen detection, nanobiosensors for drug monitoring (Javaid et al. 2021). The integration of nanosensors in disease management and prevention exemplifies the potential of nanotechnology in revolutionizing healthcare by enabling early detection, accurate diagnosis, personalized treatments, and improved patient outcomes (Javaid et al. 2021).

12.4.5 Combining Treatments

Combining multiple therapies using nanomaterials, often referred to as nanotheranostics, offers several significant advantages, revolutionizing the landscape of modern medicine and providing comprehensive and targeted treatments for various diseases. Combining different therapeutic modalities within a single nanosystem can lead to synergistic effects, enhancing the overall therapeutic efficacy compared to individual treatments (Jie Wang et al. 2021). The simultaneous delivery of multiple therapeutic agents can target various pathways involved in disease progression, leading to improved treatment outcomes and better patient responses. Nanomaterials can be made to carry multiple therapeutic agents to particular target sites in the body, thereby mitigating off-target effects and reducing systemic toxicity (Navya et al. 2019). By incorporating ligands or surface modifications, nanocarriers can selectively accumulate at the disease site, enabling precise and localized treatment delivery while minimizing damage to healthy tissues. Nanomaterials allow for the integration of diverse treatment modalities, including chemotherapy, immunotherapy, gene therapy, and photothermal therapy, within a single platform. This enables the development of multifaceted treatment regimens cutomized to the specific characteristics of the disease, thereby providing comprehensive and personalized therapeutic interventions for complex and multifactorial health conditions (Mosleh-Shirazi et al. 2022).

There aresome notable examples that demonstrate the synergistic effects of multifunctional nanomaterial-based treatments, showcasing the potential of combining various therapeutic modalities for enhanced treatment outcomes, like nanoparticle-based cancer therapy, combination nanomedicine for infectious diseases, theranostic nanoplatforms for cardiovascular disease (VanDyke et al. 2016). These underscore the ability of multifunctional nanomaterial-based treatments in achieving synergistic therapeutic effects, emphasizing the importance of integrated approaches for addressing complex and multifaceted diseases. To validate the effectiveness and safety of these nanotherapeutic strategies for translation into clinical practice, more research and clinical studies are required (Prasad et al. 2018).

Customized treatments, often referred to as personalized or precision medicine, hold significant promise for addressing complex medical conditions by leveraging advancements in technology and individualized patient data (Akhondzadeh 2014). Genomic profiling, biomarker analysis, theranostic nanomedicine, regenerative medicine and tissue engineering, and data-driven decision-makingare some key aspects that showcase the potential of customized treatments for complex medical conditions (Park and Na 2015). The integration of these personalized approaches in clinical practice highlights the transformative potential of customized treatments for addressing complex medical conditions. Healthcare professionals can optimize treatment plans, enhance patient outcomes, and advance the paradigm of precision medicine in the management of a variety of health conditions by focusing on unique patient characteristics and disease profiles (Bilkey et al. 2019).

The current innovations in multifunctional nanomaterials for therapeutic functions have shown great potential in the field of medicine. Nanomaterials, including biogenic nanoparticles, nanomedicines, and functional nanomaterials, offer personalized medicine with reduced toxicity and enhanced therapeutic performance (Bhagat et al. 2023). Multifunctional nanomaterials have proven to be effective in targeted therapy, tissue engineering, drug delivery, and imaging. Some of the developed uses of nanomedicine include scaffolds for tissue growth, nanoparticle-based medicinal formulations, nanozymes, and antimicrobials based on nanomaterials (Sanjay Singh 2021). Nanomaterials have been designed for antibacterial purposes, giving more effectiveness and fewer side effects than conventional antibiotics. Examples of nanomaterials include nanogels, polymeric nanoparticles, graphene oxides, or carbon-based and metal-based (Hong et al. 2019). Nanoparticles conjugated with therapeutic agents, such as liposomes, dendrimers, and gold nanoparticles, have been used in targeted therapy and investigation into cancer, including microRNA and RNA interference delivery (Jurj et al. 2017). The discovery of customized medicines and the improvement of therapeutic efficacy have been made possible by the development of multifunctional bionanomaterials composed of either synthetic or natural biopolymers, with potential uses in tissue engineering, treatment of cancer, and targeted delivery (Armentano et al. 2017). These advancements in nanotechnology have resulted in nanoparticle-based therapeutics for plenty of ailments, providing advantages such as improved solubility, bioavailability, and reduced toxicity (Saboktakin 2017).

12.5 CHALLENGES

Multifunctional nanomaterials for therapeutic applications face several challenges. The physicochemical and pharmacokinetic traits of nanoformulations can show difference from their parent drug molecules, affecting their absorption, distribution, elimination, and metabolism (Praveen, Kalarikkal, and Thomas 2021). As nanomaterials can cause cytotoxic and genotoxic responses, it is important to maintain the harmony between therapeutic efficiency and cytotoxicity (Ding and Ma

2017). The newly emerging nanomedicine is still in its budding stage, with limited success stories which are shown as clinical trials and medical practice (Wu, Wang, and Li 2020). Risk assessment and regulation of nanomaterials pose difficulties due to uncertainties regarding their potential adverse effects and exposure to humans and the environment (Rocks et al. 2014). Nanoparticle-based therapeutics require careful design, engineering, and analysis to achieve consistent product characteristics and pharmacological profiles (Desai 2012). The development and approval of multifunctional nanomaterials for therapeutic applications require addressing challenges related to their physicochemical properties, cytotoxicity, translation to clinical practice, risk assessment, and regulation.

12.6 FUTURE DIRECTIONS

Future directions for multifunctional nanomaterials for therapeutic applications include the creation of DNA nanostructures with novel preparation and design techniques, as well as the exploration of their ability in medical and biological applications (Ma et al. 2021). Nanotechnology has the power to boost the effectiveness of currently known therapeutics and facilitate the development of innovative therapeutic agents, by integrating both inorganic and organic nanostructures (Armentano et al. 2017). Advances in polymer science have contributed to the progress of polymeric nanomaterials for drug delivery usages, with a focus on self-assembly techniques and the engineering of different properties of the nanostructures (Sanjay Singh 2021). The use of biocompatible nanomaterials as platforms for multifunctional nanomedicine offers opportunities for synergistic anticancer effects, targeted therapy, smart drug delivery systems, and theranostics for real-time monitoring (Mishra 2017). These future directions aim to enhance the therapeutic performance of nanomedicines, reduce toxicity and side effects, and provide personalized therapies (Zhang 2012).

12.7 CONCLUSION

Multifunctional nanomaterials represent a remarkable frontier in the realm of therapeutic applications, offering versatile solutions to complex healthcare challenges. These nanomaterials have possessed the ability to transform targeted therapies, medication delivery, and diagnostics, enhancing the effectiveness and accuracy of medical interventions. Their multifaceted capabilities, such as simultaneous drug delivery and imaging, are reshaping the landscape of personalized medicine, promising more effective and patient-specific interventions. While there are obstacles to overcome, including safety concerns and regulatory issues, the ongoing collaboration between scientists, engineers, and healthcare professionals is steadily addressing these challenges. As we look ahead, the future of multifunctional nanomaterials is undeniably promising. With continual advancements in materials science and increasing insights into their biological interactions, these nanomaterials are poised to redefine healthcare, providing safer, more efficient, and customized therapeutic options that have the potential to enhance the well-being of patients worldwide.

REFERENCES

Agrawal, Udita, Madhu Gupta, Rajesh S. Jadon, Rajeev Sharma, and S. P. Vyas. 2013. "Multifunctional Nanomedicines: Potentials and Prospects." *Drug Delivery and Translational Research* 3 (5): 479–97. https://doi.org/10.1007/S13346-012-0123-X.

Ahmad, Razi, Sukriti Srivastava, Shubhrima Ghosh, and Sunil Kumar Khare. 2021. "Phytochemical Delivery Through Nanocarriers: A Review." *Colloids and Surfaces. B, Biointerfaces* 197 (January). https://doi.org/10.1016/J.COLSURFB.2020.111389.

Akhondzadeh, Shahin. 2014. "Personalized Medicine: A Tailor Made Medicine." *Avicenna Journal of Medical Biotechnology* 6 (4): 191. https://www.ncbi.nlm.nih.gov/pmc/articles/PMC4224657/.

Anjum, Sumaira, Sara Ishaque, Hijab Fatima, Wajiha Farooq, Christophe Hano, Bilal Haider Abbasi, and Iram Anjum. 2021. "Emerging Applications of Nanotechnology in Healthcare Systems: Grand Challenges and Perspectives." *Pharmaceuticals (Basel, Switzerland)* 14 (8). https://doi.org/10.3390/PH14080707.

Armentano, Ilaria, Nicoletta Rescignano, Eelna Fortunati, Samantha Mattioli, Francesco Morena, Sabata Martino, Luigi Torre, and Josè M. Kenny. 2017. "Multifunctional Nanostructured Biopolymeric Materials for Therapeutic Applications." *Nanostructures for Novel Therapy: Synthesis, Characterization and Applications* (January): 107–35. https://doi.org/10.1016/B978-0-323-46142-9.00005-0.

Basuki, Johan S., Hien T. T. Duong, Alexander Macmillan, Rafael B. Erlich, Lars Esser, Mia C. Akerfeldt, Renee Megan Whan, Maria Kavallaris, Cyrille Boyer, and Thomas P. Davis. 2013. "Using Fluorescence Lifetime Imaging Microscopy to Monitor Theranostic Nanoparticle Uptake and Intracellular Doxorubicin Release." *ACS Nano* 7 (11): 10175–89. https://doi.org/10.1021/NN404407G.

Bhagat, Devidas S., Wasudeo B. Gurnule, Gurvinder S. Bumbrah, Pankaj Koinkar, and Pooja A. Chawla. 2023. "Recent Advances in Biomedical Applications of Biogenic Nanomaterials." *Current Pharmaceutical Biotechnology* 24 (1): 86–100. https://doi.org/10.2174/1389201023666220513101628.

Bilkey, Gemma A., Belinda L. Burns, Emily P. Coles, Trinity Mahede, Gareth Baynam, and Kristen J. Nowak. 2019. "Optimizing Precision Medicine for Public Health." *Frontiers in Public Health* 7 (March). https://doi.org/10.3389/FPUBH.2019.00042.

Blasiak, Barbara, Frank C.J.M. Van Veggel, and Boguslaw Tomanek. 2013. "Applications of Nanoparticles for MRI Cancer Diagnosis and Therapy." *Journal of Nanomaterials* 12 (12) https://doi.org/10.1155/2013/148578.

Bu, Qingpan, Ping Li, Yunfei Xia, Die Hu, Wenjing Li, Dongfang Shi, and Kai Song. 2023. "Design, Synthesis, and Biomedical Application of Multifunctional Fluorescent Polymer Nanomaterials." *Molecules* 28 (9): 3819. https://doi.org/10.3390/MOLECULES28093819.

Cabrera, Ingrid, Elisa Elizondo, Olga Esteban, José Luis Corchero, Marta Melgarejo, Daniel Pulido, Alba Córdoba, et al. 2013. "Multifunctional Nanovesicle-Bioactive Conjugates Prepared by a One-Step Scalable Method Using CO2-Expanded Solvents." *Nano Letters* 13 (8): 3766–74. https://doi.org/10.1021/NL4017072/SUPPL_FILE/NL4017072_SI_001.PDF.

Contera, Sonia, Jorge Bernardino De La Serna, and Teresa D. Tetley. 2020. "Biotechnology, Nanotechnology and Medicine." *Emerging Topics in Life Sciences* 4 (6): 551. https://doi.org/10.1042/ETLS20200350.

Desai, Neil. 2012. "Challenges in Development of Nanoparticle-Based Therapeutics." *The AAPS Journal* 14 (2): 282. https://doi.org/10.1208/S12248-012-9339-4.

Ding, Hong Ming, and Yu Qiang Ma. 2017. "Computational Approaches to Cell-Nanomaterial Interactions: Keeping Balance Between Therapeutic Efficiency and Cytotoxicity." *Nanoscale Horizons* 3 (1): 6–27. https://doi.org/10.1039/C7NH00138J.

Donolato, Marco, Paula Antunes, Rebecca S. Bejhed, Teresa Zardán Gómez De La Torre, Frederik W. Østerberg, Mattias Strömberg, Mats Nilsson, et al. 2015. "Novel Readout Method for Molecular Diagnostic Assays Based on Optical Measurements of Magnetic Nanobead Dynamics." *Analytical Chemistry* 87 (3): 1622–9. https://doi.org/10.1021/AC503191V/SUPPL_FILE/AC503191V_SI_001.PDF.

Duan, Yixiang, Yongxin Li, Chuyan Zhang, Jing Chen, Rui Sun, Zhijun Huang, Zewei Luo, Chen Zhou, and Mengfan Wu. 2020. "The Recent Development of Hybridization Chain Reaction Strategies in Biosensors." *ACS Sensors* 5 (10): 2977–3000. https://doi.org/10.1021/ACSSENSORS.0C01453/SUPPL_FILE/SE0C01453_SI_001.PDF.

Galarreta-Rodriguez, Itziar, Mikel Etxebeste-Mitxeltorena, Esther Moreno, Daniel Plano, Carmen Sanmartín, Saad Megahed, Neus Feliu, et al. 2023. "Preparation of Selenium-Based Drug-Modified Polymeric Ligand-Functionalised Fe3O4 Nanoparticles as Multimodal Drug Carrier and Magnetic Hyperthermia Inductor." *Pharmaceuticals* 16 (7): 949. https://doi.org/10.3390/PH16070949/S1.

Guerrero-Martínez, Andrés, Jorge Pérez-Juste, and Luis M. Liz-Marzán. 2010. "Recent Progress on Silica Coating of Nanoparticles and Related Nanomaterials." *Advanced Materials (Deerfield Beach, Fla.)* 22 (11): 1182–95. https://doi.org/10.1002/ADMA.200901263.

Guk, Kyeonghye, Gaon Han, Jaewoo Lim, Keunwon Jeong, Taejoon Kang, Eun Kyung Lim, and Juyeon Jung. 2019. "Evolution of Wearable Devices with Real-Time Disease Monitoring for Personalized Healthcare." *Nanomaterials (Basel, Switzerland)* 9 (6). https://doi.org/10.3390/NANO9060813.

Habibi, Nahal, Daniel F. Quevedo, Jason V. Gregory, and Joerg Lahann. 2020. "Emerging Methods in Therapeutics Using Multifunctional Nanoparticles." *Wiley Interdisciplinary Reviews: Nanomedicine and Nanobiotechnology* 12 (4): e1625. https://doi.org/10.1002/WNAN.1625.

Hong, Le, Shu-Han Luo, Chen-Hao Yu, Yu Xie, Meng-Ying Xia, Ge-Yun Chen, and Qiang Peng. 2019. "Functional Nanomaterials and Their Potential Applications in Antibacterial Therapy." *Pharmaceutical Nanotechnology* 7 (2): 129–46. https://doi.org/10.2174/2211738507666190320160802.

Huang, Yu, Cihui Luo, Fan Xia, Yanlin Song, Lei Jiang, and Fengyu Li. 2022. "Multi-Analyte Sensing Strategies Towards Wearable and Intelligent Devices." *Chemical Science* 13 (42): 12309–25. https://doi.org/10.1039/D2SC03750E.

Javaid, Mohd, Abid Haleem, Ravi Pratap Singh, Shanay Rab, and Rajiv Suman. 2021. "Exploring the Potential of Nanosensors: A Brief Overview." *Sensors International* 2 (January). https://doi.org/10.1016/J.SINTL.2021.100130.

Jeon, Jongho. 2019. "Review of Therapeutic Applications of Radiolabeled Functional Nanomaterials." *International Journal of Molecular Sciences* 20 (9). https://doi.org/10.3390/IJMS20092323.

Jiang, Zeyu, Meihua Zhang, Peifeng Li, Yin Wang, and Qinrui Fu. 2023. "Nanomaterial-Based CT Contrast Agents and Their Applications in Image-Guided Therapy." *Theranostics* 13 (2): 483. https://doi.org/10.7150/THNO.79625.

Jurj, Ancuta, Cornelia Braicu, Laura Ancuta Pop, Ciprian Tomuleasa, Claudia Diana Gherman, and Ioana Berindan-Neagoe. 2017. "The New Era of Nanotechnology, an Alternative to Change Cancer Treatment." *Drug Design, Development and Therapy* 11 (September): 2871–90. https://doi.org/10.2147/DDDT.S142337.

Kim, Hyemin, Songeun Beack, Seulgi Han, Myeonghwan Shin, Taehyung Lee, Yoonsang Park, Ki Su Kim, et al. 2018. "Multifunctional Photonic Nanomaterials for Diagnostic, Therapeutic, and Theranostic Applications." *Advanced Materials* 30 (10): 1701460. https://doi.org/10.1002/ADMA.201701460.

Kim, Kyungim, Keun Sang Oh, Dal Yong Park, Jae Young Lee, Beom Suk Lee, In San Kim, Kwangmeyung Kim, Ick Chan Kwon, Yoon Kim Sang, and Soon Hong Yuk. 2016. "Doxorubicin/Gold-Loaded Core/Shell Nanoparticles for Combination Therapy to Treat Cancer Through the Enhanced Tumor Targeting." *Journal of Controlled Release: Official Journal of the Controlled Release Society* 228 (April): 141–9. https://doi.org/10.1016/J.JCONREL.2016.03.009.

Kircher, Moritz F., and Jürgen K. Willmann. 2012. "Molecular Body Imaging: MR Imaging, CT, and US. Part I. Principles." *Radiology* 263 (3): 633–43. https://doi.org/10.1148/RADIOL.12102394.

Koo, Otilia M.Y., Israel Rubinstein, and Hayat Onyuksel. 2006. "Camptothecin in Sterically Stabilized Phospholipid Nano-Micelles: A Novel Solvent PH Change Solubilization Method." *Journal of Nanoscience and Nanotechnology* 6 (9–10): 2996–3000. https://doi.org/10.1166/JNN.2006.460.

Kuniyil, Prabhakaran, and Geetha Prabhakaran. 2008. "Methods of Synthesis of Non-Toxic Multifunctional Nanoparticles and Applications." U.S. Patent Application 12/135,206, filed December 11.

Lamprecht, Alf, Nathalie Ubrich, Hiromitsu Yamamoto, Ulrich Schäfer, Hirofumi Takeuchi, Philippe Maincent, Yoshiaki Kawashima, and Claus-Michael Lehr. 2001. "Biodegradable Nanoparticles for Targeted Drug Delivery in Treatment of Inflammatory Bowel Disease." *Journal of Pharmacology and Experimental Therapeutics* 299 (2).

Lenders, Vincent, Xanthippi Koutsoumpou, Ara Sargsian, and Bella B. Manshian. 2020. "Biomedical Nanomaterials for Immunological Applications: Ongoing Research and Clinical Trials." *Nanoscale Advances* 2 (11): 5046–89. https://doi.org/10.1039/D0NA00478B.

Liu, Chun Ping, Zi De Chen, Zi Yan Ye, Dong Yue He, Yue Dang, Zhe Wei Li, Lei Wang, Miao Ren, Zhi Jin Fan, and Hong Xing Liu. 2021. "Therapeutic Applications of Functional Nanomaterials for Prostatitis." *Frontiers in Pharmacology* 12 (May). https://doi.org/10.3389/FPHAR.2021.685465.

Look, Jennifer, Nadine Wilhelm, Hagen Von Briesen, Nadja Noske, Christine Günther, Klaus Langer, and Erwin Gorjup. 2015. "Ligand-Modified Human Serum Albumin Nanoparticles for Enhanced Gene Delivery." *Molecular Pharmaceutics* 12 (9): 3202–13. https://doi.org/10.1021/ACS.MOLPHARMACEUT.5B00153/ASSET/IMAGES/MEDIUM/MP-2015-00153C_0011.GIF.

López-Saucedo, Felipe, Guadalupe G. Flores-Rojas, H. Iván Meléndez-Ortiz, Adriana Morfín-Gutierrez, Marco A. Luna-Straffon, and Emilio Bucio. 2019. "Stimuli-Responsive Nanomaterials for Drug Delivery." *Characterization and Biology of Nanomaterials for Drug Delivery: Nanoscience and Nanotechnology in Drug Delivery* (January): 375–424. https://doi.org/10.1016/B978-0-12-814031-4.00014-3.

Lugoloobi, Ishaq, Yuanmeng Fang, Faxing Jiang, Guoying Zhang, and Jinming Hu. 2023. "Gaseous Signaling Molecule-Releasing Hybrid Nanomaterials for Therapeutic Applications." *Giant* 14 (June): 100153. https://doi.org/10.1016/J.GIANT.2023.100153.

Lusic, Hrvoje, and Mark W. Grinstaff. 2013. "X-Ray Computed Tomography Contrast Agents." *Chemical Reviews* 113 (3): 1641–66. https://doi.org/10.1021/CR200358S.

Ma, Wenjuan, Yuxi Zhan, Yuxin Zhang, Chenchen Mao, Xueping Xie, and Yunfeng Lin. 2021. "The Biological Applications of DNA Nanomaterials: Current Challenges and Future Directions." *Signal Transduction and Targeted Therapy* 6 (1). https://doi.org/10.1038/S41392-021-00727-9.

Maeda, Hiroshi. 2001. "The Enhanced Permeability and Retention (EPR) Effect in Tumor Vasculature: The Key Role of Tumor-Selective Macromolecular Drug Targeting." *Advances in Enzyme Regulation* 41 (1): 189–207. https://doi.org/10.1016/S0065-2571(00)00013-3.

Majithia, Maithili, and Delicia A. Barretto. 2023. "Biocompatible Green-Synthesized Nanomaterials for Therapeutic Applications." *Advances in Nano and Biochemistry: Environmental and Biomedical Applications* (January): 285–367. https://doi.org/10.1016/B978-0-323-95253-8.00012-7.

Masoudi Asil, Shima, Erick Damian Guerrero, Georgina Bugarini, Joshua Cayme, Nydia De Avila, Jaime Garcia, Adrian Hernandez, et al. 2023. "Theranostic Applications of Multifunctional Carbon Nanomaterials." *View* 4 (2): 20220056. https://doi.org/10.1002/VIW.20220056.

McNeil, Scott E. 2005. "Nanotechnology for the Biologist." *Journal of Leukocyte Biology* 78 (3): 585–94. https://doi.org/10.1189/JLB.0205074.

Mishra, Munmaya K. 2017. *Concise Encyclopedia of Biomedical Polymers and Polymeric Biomaterials*. CRC Press . https://doi.org/10.1081/E-EBPPC.

Mohaghegh, Seraj, Ali Tarighatnia, Yadollah Omidi, Jaleh Barar, Ayuob Aghanejad, and Khosro Adibkia. 2022. "Multifunctional Magnetic Nanoparticles for MRI-Guided Co-Delivery of Erlotinib and L-Asparaginase to Ovarian Cancer." *Journal of Microencapsulation* 39 (4): 394–408. https://doi.org/10.1080/02652048.2022.2094487.

Mosleh-Shirazi, Sareh, Milad Abbasi, Mohammad Reza Moaddeli, Ahmad Vaez, Mostafa Shafiee, Seyed Reza Kasaee, Ali Mohammad Amani, and Saeid Hatam. 2022. "Nanotechnology Advances in the Detection and Treatment of Cancer: An Overview." *Nanotheranostics* 6 (4): 400. https://doi.org/10.7150/NTNO.74613.

Nam, Nguyen Hoang, and Nguyen Hoang Luong. 2019. "Nanoparticles: Synthesis and Applications." *Materials for Biomedical Engineering* (January): 211. https://doi.org/10.1016/B978-0-08-102814-8.00008-1.

Navya, P. N., Anubhav Kaphle, S. P. Srinivas, Suresh Kumar Bhargava, Vincent M. Rotello, and Hemant Kumar Daima. 2019. "Current Trends and Challenges in Cancer Management and Therapy Using Designer Nanomaterials." *Nano Convergence* 6 (1): 1–30. https://doi.org/10.1186/S40580-019-0193-2.

Osman, Nawras, Nikita Devnarain, Calvin A. Omolo, Victoria Fasiku, Yajna Jaglal, and Thirumala Govender. 2022. "Surface Modification of Nano-Drug Delivery Systems for Enhancing Antibiotic Delivery and Activity." *Wiley Interdisciplinary Reviews: Nanomedicine and Nanobiotechnology* 14 (1). https://doi.org/10.1002/WNAN.1758.

Park, Wooram, and Kun Na. 2015. "Advances in the Synthesis and Application of Nanoparticles for Drug Delivery." *Wiley Interdisciplinary Reviews: Nanomedicine and Nanobiotechnology* 7 (4): 494–508. https://doi.org/10.1002/WNAN.1325.

Pirzada, Muqsit, and Zeynep Altintas. 2019. "Nanomaterials for Healthcare Biosensing Applications." *Sensors (Basel, Switzerland)* 19 (23). https://doi.org/10.3390/S19235311.

Prasad, Minakshi, Upendra P. Lambe, Basanti Brar, Ikbal Shah, Manimegalai J, Koushlesh Ranjan, Rekha Rao, et al. 2018. "Nanotherapeutics: An Insight into Healthcare and Multi-Dimensional Applications in Medical Sector of the Modern World." *Biomedicine & Pharmacotherapy = Biomedecine & Pharmacotherapie* 97 (January): 1521–37. https://doi.org/10.1016/J.BIOPHA.2017.11.026.

Praveen, G., Nandakumar Kalarikkal, and Sabu Thomas. 2021. "Challenges in Nonparenteral Nanomedicine Therapy." *Theory and Applications of Nonparenteral Nanomedicines* (January): 27–54. https://doi.org/10.1016/B978-0-12-820466-5.00002-8.

Rajabi, Mehdi, Mathangi Srinivasan, and Shaker A. Mousa. 2016. "Nanobiomaterials in Drug Delivery." *Nanobiomaterials in Drug Delivery: Applications of Nanobiomaterials* (May): 1–37. https://doi.org/10.1016/B978-0-323-42866-8.00001-0.

Riehemann, Kristina, Stefan W. Schneider, Thomas A. Luger, Biana Godin, Mauro Ferrari, and Harald Fuchs. 2009. "Nanomedicine-Challenge and Perspectives." *Angewandte Chemie (International Ed. in English)* 48 (5): 872–97. https://doi.org/10.1002/ANIE.200802585.

Rocks, Sophie A., Huijun Zhu, Robert Dorey, and Philip Holmes. 2014. "Harmful or Helpful, the Toxicity and Safety of Nano-Sized Medicine." *Nanomedicine: Principles and Perspectives* 237–250. https://doi.org/10.1007/978-1-4614-2140-5_11.

Saboktakin, Mohammadrez. 2017. "The Biological and Biomedical Nanoparticles—Synthesis and Applications." *Advanced Material Science* 2 (3). https://doi.org/10.15761/AMS.1000127.

Sahu, Bhanu P., Nikhil Biswas, and Malay K. Das. 2020. "Multifunctional Nanoscale Particles for Theranostic Application in Healthcare." *Nano Medicine and Nano Safety*: 347–75. https://doi.org/10.1007/978-981-15-6255-6_14.

Sayin, Sezin, Ece Ozdemir, Egemen Acar, and Gozde Ozaydin Ince. 2019. "Multifunctional One-Dimensional Polymeric Nanostructures for Drug Delivery and Biosensor Applications." *Nanotechnology* 30 (41): 412001. https://doi.org/10.1088/1361-6528/AB2E2C.

Seleci, Muharrem, Didem Ag Seleci, Rebecca Joncyzk, Frank Stahl, Cornelia Blume, and Thomas Scheper. 2016. "Smart Multifunctional Nanoparticles in Nanomedicine." *BioNanoMaterials* 17 (1–2): 33–41. https://doi.org/10.1515/BNM-2015-0030/ASSET/GRAPHIC/J_BNM-2015-0030_FIG_003.JPG.

Sethuraman, Vaidevi, Kumar Janakiraman, Venkateshwaran Krishnaswami, and Ruckmani Kandasamy. 2021. "Recent Progress in Stimuli-Responsive Intelligent Nano Scale Drug Delivery Systems: A Special Focus Towards PH-Sensitive Systems." *Current Drug Targets* 22 (8): 947–66. https://doi.org/10.2174/1389450122999210128180058.

Singh, Sanjay. 2021. "Concluding Remarks and Future of Nanomedicines." *Emerging Trends in Nanomedicine* (January): 235–40. https://doi.org/10.1007/978-981-15-9920-0_8/COVER.

Singh, Sundar, S. B. Tiwari, and Sanjeev Tyagi. 2021. "Nanomaterials for Pharmaceutical Applications." *Emerging Trends in Nanotechnology* (January): 221–65. https://doi.org/10.1007/978-981-15-9904-0_8/COVER.

Srinath, M. K., R. Anusha, Shashi Prakash Dwivedi, Chitra Gupta, Hanaa Addai Ali, and Sorabh Lakhanpal. 2023. "Development of Multifunctional Nanomaterials and Devices for Biomedical Applications." *E3S Web of Conferences* 430 (October). https://doi.org/10.1051/E3SCONF/202343001123.

Swarbrick, James. 2013. *Encyclopedia of Pharmaceutical Technology*, volume 6. CRC Press. https://doi.org/10.1201/b19309.

Tambe, Prajakta, Shamala Mane, Bhushan P. Chaudhari, and Prabir Kumar Kulabhusan. 2022. "Carbon Nanomaterials for Therapeutic Applications." *Fundamentals of Bionanomaterials* (January): 293–325. https://doi.org/10.1016/B978-0-12-824147-9.00011-X.

Tang, Kai, Jianmin Xue, Yufang Zhu, and Chengtie Wu. 2023. "Design and Synthesis of Bioinspired Nanomaterials for Biomedical Application." *Wiley Interdisciplinary Reviews: Nanomedicine and Nanobiotechnology*: e1914. https://doi.org/10.1002/WNAN.1914.

Tiwari, Ashutosh, Hirak Kumar Patra, and Jeong Woo Choi. 2015. "Advanced Theranostics Materials." *Advanced Theranostics Materials* (July): 1–343. https://doi.org/10.1002/9781118998922.

Vallinayagam, Sugumari, and Karthikeyan Rajendran. 2021. "Synthesis and Application of Nanomaterials for Biomedical Anticancer Therapy." *Bio-Manufactured Nanomaterials: Perspectives and Promotion* (June): 339–73. https://doi.org/10.1007/978-3-030-67223-2_16/COVER.

VanDyke, D., P. Kyriacopulos, B. Yassini, A. Wright, E. Burkhart, S. Jacek, M. Pratt, C. R. Peterson, and P. Rai. 2016. "Nanoparticle Based Combination Treatments for Targeting Multiple Hallmarks of Cancer." *International Journal of Nano Studies & Technology* 4 (July): 1. https://doi.org/10.19070/2167-8685-SI04001.

Wang, Jie, Peng Chen, Yue Dong, Han Xie, Yachao Wang, Fernando Soto, Peng Ma, Xiaojun Feng, Wei Du, and Bi Feng Liu. 2021. "Designer Exosomes Enabling Tumor Targeted Efficient Chemo/Gene/Photothermal Therapy." *Biomaterials* 276 (September). https://doi.org/10.1016/J.BIOMATERIALS.2021.121056.

Wang, Jing, Yiye Li, and Guangjun Nie. 2021. "Multifunctional Biomolecule Nanostructures for Cancer Therapy." *Nature Reviews Materials* 6 (9): 766–83. https://doi.org/10.1038/s41578-021-00315-x.

Waris, Abdul, Asmat Ali, Atta Ullah Khan, Muhammad Asim, Doaa Zamel, Kinza Fatima, Abdur Raziq, et al. 2022. "Applications of Various Types of Nanomaterials for the Treatment of Neurological Disorders." *Nanomaterials (Basel, Switzerland)* 12 (13). https://doi.org/10.3390/NANO12132140.

Wu, Lin Ping, Danyang Wang, and Zibiao Li. 2020. "Grand Challenges in Nanomedicine." *Materials Science and Engineering: C* 106 (January): 110302. https://doi.org/10.1016/J.MSEC.2019.110302.

Xia, Younan. 2014. "Editorial: Are We Entering the Nano Era?" *Angewandte Chemie International Edition* 53 (46): 12268–71. https://doi.org/10.1002/ANIE.201406740.

Zavaleta, Cristina, Dean Ho, and Eun Ji Chung. 2018. "Theranostic Nanoparticles for Tracking and Monitoring Disease State." *SLAS Technology* 23 (3): 281–93. https://doi.org/10.1177/2472630317738699.

Zhang, Haijun. 2012. "Multifunctional Nanomedicine Platforms for Cancer Therapy." *Journal of Nanoscience and Nanotechnology* 12 (5): 4012–18. https://doi.org/10.1166/JNN.2012.6160.

13 Monoclonal Antibodies for Targeted Drug Delivery

Sujata Adhana, Jyoti Chaudhary, and Anil Kumar Mavi

ABBREVIATIONS

Acronym	Full Form
FDA	Food and Drug Administration
Abs	antibodies
mAbs	monoclonal antibodies
Ab	antibody
NPs	nanoparticles
ADCs	antibody–drug conjugates
B cells	B lymphocyte cells
Ig	immunoglobin
Fc	fragment crystallizable
Fab	antigen-binding fragment
HGPRT	hypoxanthine-guanine phosphoribosyltransferase
HAT	hypoxanthine-aminopterin-thymidine
CD	cell differentiation
IL-1ra	interleukin-1 receptor antagonist
IL-1	interleukin-1
PEG	polyethylene glycol
EPRPEG	enhanced permeability and retention effect
EGFR	epidermal growth factor receptor
HER	human epidermal growth factor receptor
MCF	Michigan Cancer Foundation
PE38KDEL	pseudomonas exotoxin A fragment 38 with a C-terminal lysine–aspartic acid–glutamic acid–leucine (KDEL)
PLGA	poly(lactide-co-glycolide)

13.1 INTRODUCTION

Modern medicine is characterized by a relentless pursuit of enhanced therapeutic precision and efficacy, which has led to groundbreaking innovations (Mahara et al. 2023). Conventional drug delivery methods, predominantly oral and injection routes, have constrained drug development progress (Adepu and Ramakrishna 2021). Many drugs are tailored for these routes, often lacking efficiency for specific therapies. The advent of biologic drugs like nucleic acids and protein necessitates innovative technologies of delivery to increase efficacy, reduce side effects, and recover patient compliance (Ezike et al. 2023). Meeting these challenges is crucial for advancing therapeutic interventions beyond the limitations of traditional delivery systems (Ezike et al. 2023).

Nanoparticle systems have had a great deal of interest in biomedical research and applications over the previous few decades (Rizvi and Saleh 2018). With the ability to customize biodistribution

 DOI: 10.1201/9781003463191-16

in vivo, nanoparticles fall within the nanometer size range and are typically made for better drug delivery and biocompatibility. Because tumors have leaky vasculatures that allow nanoparticles to escape and remain in the tumor tissues, a variety of nanoparticles has been studied to target and improve the accumulation of their payload in tumorous tissues (Lin, O'Reilly Beringhs, and Lu 2021). This phenomenon based on tumor physiology is known as the enhanced permeation and retention, or EPR, effect. Xenograft tumor model preclinical data have been surveyed recently, and the results show that the mean amount of dose based on injected nanoparticles that builds up in solid tumor tissues is less than 2 points (25 percent) (Wilhelm et al. 2016; Cheng et al. 2020). Moreover, higher-than-expected failure rates have been observed in phase 2/3 clinical trials utilizing nanomedicines for cancer therapy (Hua et al. 2018; D. Sun, Zhou, and Gao 2020; Rosenblum et al. 2018), which is partly due to the EPR effect's known variability and inconsistency between and within individuals (Rosenblum et al. 2018). Therefore, by utilizing active targeting techniques, particularly the use of antibodies or antibody fragments, scientists have attempted to use passive targeting to address these issues (Attia et al. 2019). Recently, platforms for imaging and diagnosis have been developed using nanoparticle–antibody conjugates for both in vivo and in vitro applications (Lin, O'Reilly Beringhs, and Lu 2021).

13.2 THE USE OF NANOTECHNOLOGY IN DRUG DELIVERY

The science of nanotechnology, which operates at the nanoscale, has been a catalyst for the transformation of many industries (Malik, Muhammad, and Waheed 2023). It is particularly relevant to drug delivery in medicine. Nanoscale materials exhibit unique and often unexpected properties, allowing them to be used to transport drugs precisely (De Jong and Borm 2008). In the human body, these tiny carriers are called nanoparticles and are capable of carrying therapeutic agents to specific locations with astonishing accuracy, minimizing off-target effects and reducing collateral damage often associated with systemic drug administration (Patra et al. 2018).

When combined with more established fields like engineering, molecular chemistry, applied health, pharmaceutical science, and optics, nanoscience can be a game changer (Sahu et al. 2021). Over the previous few decades, science and technology have been carefully combined to address issues in the medical and health sciences. The term "nanotechnology," originally used by Prof. N. Taniguchi in 1974 and later theorized by Drexler in 1986, has become an important figure in the development of therapeutic approaches and health science (Bayda et al. 2020). Nanotechnology, with its interdisciplinary focus on creating biological entities at the nanoscale (1–100 nm), offers special instruments and materials to investigate, comprehend, and solve biological problems, opening up new and exciting possibilities for illness treatment and diagnosis (Sheeparamatti, Sheeparamatti, and Kadadevaramath 2007). Since living cells function at the nanoscale and are crucial to many biological processes, nanotechnology is a prime contender for the development of therapeutic technologies (Kumar Dash et al. 2020). The primary usage of nanotechnology in the nanomedical field is the advancement of tools at the nanoscale for efficient medical treatment. It is essential for tissue engineering, imaging, disease diagnosis, and creating accurate drug delivery systems (Sim and Wong 2021). Deeper knowledge of human physiology is made possible by nanomedicine, which is especially helpful in the fight against diseases like cancer. The significance comes from its ability to develop drug delivery systems that are safer and effective (Mahesh and Viveka 2023).

In the health sciences, nanomedicine is starting to become the gold standard (Figure 13.1) (Mahesh and Viveka 2023). Consequently, there may be a variety of approaches available to tissue-specific drug targeting techniques to improve disease prognosis (Z. Zhao et al. 2020). Present years have observed an increase in interest in the wide arena of medical science in nanomaterials, particularly metal nanoparticles (Murthy 2007). Nowadays, a lot of research is being done on how to best synthesize nanomaterials, including liposomes, micelles, nanocapsules, dendrimers, polymers, emulsions, and nanoparticles (Patra et al. 2018). The FDA (Food and Drug Administration) has

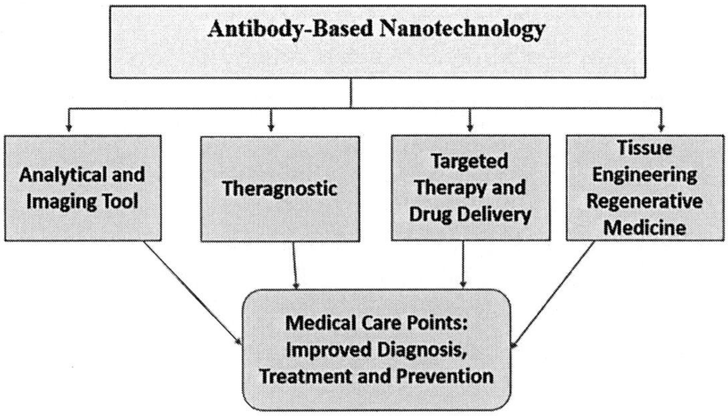

FIGURE 13.1 Applications of antibody-based nanotechnology in various fields of biomedical science. This image visually depicts the four applications (analytical and imaging tool, theragnostic, targeted therapy and drug delivery, tissue engineering and regenerative medicine) which are important and help in the medical care points, improved diagnosis, treatment and prevention.

approved around 51 nanomedicines; the remaining approximately 40% of the 77 products that are in the preclinical stage are undergoing clinical trials. Nanocrystal and polymeric liposomal formulations make up the bulk of these approved nanomaterials. Still, scientists think that more potent substances, like micelles, protein-based nanoparticles (NPs), and different inorganic and metallic particles, ought to be created for clinical trials.

13.3 EXPLORING ALTERNATIVES IN DRUG DELIVERY SYSTEMS

The following nanomaterials are commonly used in mechanisms to achieve alternative drug delivery: metals, silicon-based materials, polymers, biologics, and carbon- or silicon-based materials (Table 13.1). These materials have nanoscale and, more recently, microscale structures (Berillo et al. 2021). Table 13.1 summarizes nanoscale materials and structures under investigation for drug delivery applications (Quinteros et al. 2017).

13.4 OPPORTUNITIES AND CHALLENGES FOR NANOPARTICLES IN MEDICINE

Nanoparticles, which are between 10 and 100 nm in size, are a crucial part of nanotechnology and are categorized according to their dimensionality, morphology, state, and chemical structure. Nanoparticles, such as platinum (Pt), gold (Au), and silver (Ag), are classified into different dimensions, such as 0D and 1D, and they have distinct physiochemical properties (M. Sun and Sen Gupta 2020). Because nanotechnology is compatible with the natural systems of living cells, which function at the nanoscale, its use in medicine is becoming more and more common. This review examines the rapidly expanding field of nanotechnology in medicine, with particular attention to surgical advancements, cancer treatment, and related risks.

13.4.1 Cancer Treatment

By tackling the problems caused by multistage carcinogenesis, the treatment of cancer may be totally changed by nanotechnology (Rasool et al. 2022). Chemoresistance and serious side effects are two drawbacks of traditional methods like chemotherapy. Nanoparticles provide targeted drug delivery that minimizes side effects and develops the effectiveness of treatment.

TABLE 13.1
Nanoscale Drug Delivery Technologies

Drug delivery technology	Materials	Nanostructure forms
Biologic	Peptides	Nanoparticles
	Lipids	Vesicles, nanotubes, rings
	Polysaccharides	
	Nucleic acids	
	Viruses	
Polymeric	Poly(glycolic acid)	Micelles, dendrimers
	Poly(lactic acid)	Vesicles, spheres, nanoparticles
	Poly(3-hydroxybutanoicacid)	
	Poly(alkylcyanoacrylate)	
	Poly(organophosphazene)	
	Poly(ethylene glycol)	
	Poly(ethylene oxide)	
	Poly(caprolactone)	
	Poly(propylene imine)	
	Poly(L-glutamic acid)	
	Poly(amidoamine)	
	Poly(ethyleneimine)	
Silicon-based	Silicon dioxide	Nanoneedles
	Silicon	Porous nanoparticles
Carbon-based	Carbon	Nanotubes, fullerenes
Metallic	Silver	
	Gold	Nanoparticles, nanoshells
	Palladium	
	Platinum	

Source: Hughes (2005).

13.4.2 Improvements in Surgery

By altering traditional surgical blades, nanotechnology advances the field of surgical instruments. By improving qualities like low physical adhesion to tissues, coating blades with materials like diamond and gold or with metal-coated diamond nanolayers presents advances in surgical practices (Protti et al. 2017).

13.4.3 Risk Assessment

Despite the possible advantages, a great deal of research has been done because of worries about the toxicity of nanoparticles. Pulmonary inflammations can result from inhaling nanoparticles, such as titanium dioxide (TiO2) nanoparticles (Lu et al. 2014). Comprehending these hazards is imperative for the secure and conscientious utilization of nanotechnology in the medical field.

13.5 ANTIBODIES AS A TARGETING AGENT

B cells have antibodies on their surface that can recognize, bind, and neutralize target antigens by secreting them or acting as BCR (B cell antigen receptors) (Lkhagvasuren 2017). Nowadays, antibodies are frequently utilized in clinical settings, particularly for cancer treatment. They can function as a targeting ligand in addition to being used in direct antibody treatment (Adler and Dimitrov 2012). Antibodies are categorized as immunoglobulin D (IgD), immunoglobulin M (IgM), immunoglobulin A (IgA), immunoglobulin G (IgG), and immunoglobulin E (IgE) based on the structures and characteristics of the C regions (Lkhagvasuren 2017). The IgG antibody is the most prevalent isotype amongst the five in human plasma. It is divided into four subclasses based on the variations in the Fc region's amino acid composition: IgG2, IgG3, IgG1, and IgG4 (Shaw et al. 2019). Each of the four polypeptide chains that make up an IgG antibody contains a variable (V) and constant (C) region that binds antigen. Based on their respective functions, they can be separated into two fragments: the fragment crystallizable (Fc) region and the antigen-binding fragment (Fab) (Nelson 2010). It is possible to split IgG antibodies into smaller pieces using various enzymes. It is possible to produce single-chain variable fragments (scFv), which include the variable light and variable heavy domains, by using recombinant antibody technologies. Despite having a smaller molecular size, scFv can exhibit good affinity and alter specificity toward specific targets due to its antigen-binding (two) domains being connected by a flexible peptide (Ahmad et al. 2012).

13.6 IMMUNE RESPONSE AND THERAPEUTIC USES OF ANTIBODIES (ABS)

Antibodies (Abs) are a highly diverse class of proteins that the body needs to produce in order to defend itself against a variety of pathogens. The production of Abs is the primary function of the adaptive immune system. In order to identify and neutralize foreign antigens, B cells secrete glycoproteins known as antibodies (Abs), which belong to the immunoglobulin (Ig) superfamily. Three types of heavy chains make up the two heavy and two light chains that comprise an Abs structure. Comprising the hypervariable regions of the heavy and light chains, the antigen binding site forms the fragment antigen binding domain (Fab). The fragment crystallizable suppressor.functions.

(Fc) domain consists of two constant domains. As a result of this configuration, the IgG (bivalent) molecule has an extended serum half-life, which is made possible by Ab recycling via the nascent Fc receptor that is pH-dependent. Antibodies production plays an important role in both therapeutic applications and immune response due to their complex structure and wide range of functions. Because of these structural characteristics, antibodies are crucial for a number of medical uses, such as the treatment of cancer (Janeway et al. 2001)

13.7 PRODUCTION OF MONOCLONAL ANTIBODIES

Monoclonal antibody (mAbs) production techniques have advanced significantly since the 1970s, moving from hybridoma technology (Köhler and Milstein 1975) (Figure 13.2) to advanced recombinant engineering technologies (Brüggemann et al. 1989a, 1989b; Steinitz et al. 1977). These developments allow for the creation of customized mAbs, resulting in the creation of fully human, chimeric, and humanized mAbs (Riechmann et al. 1988; Lonberg 2005; Brüggemann et al. 1989a, 1989b). The process of producing monoclonal antibodies involves a clever fusion technique in which tumor cells derived from B cells—which can grow long-term but may not secrete antibodies—are fused with lymphocytes B, which are responsible for production of desired antibodies but are incapable of sustained growth in culture. The resulting fusion, which is aided by substances such as polyethylene glycol, produces tetraploid hybrid cells. Mutant tumor cells, hypoxanthine guanine phosphoribosyltransferase (HGPRT)–deficient, are utilized for fusion in order to prevent the tumor cells from consuming the fusion product. Cells can use guanine and hypoxanthine for purine monophosphate synthesis. The growth of unfused tumor cells is stopped by adding aminopterin, which inhibits de novo purine biosynthesis; on the other hand, the hybrids grow further because the B

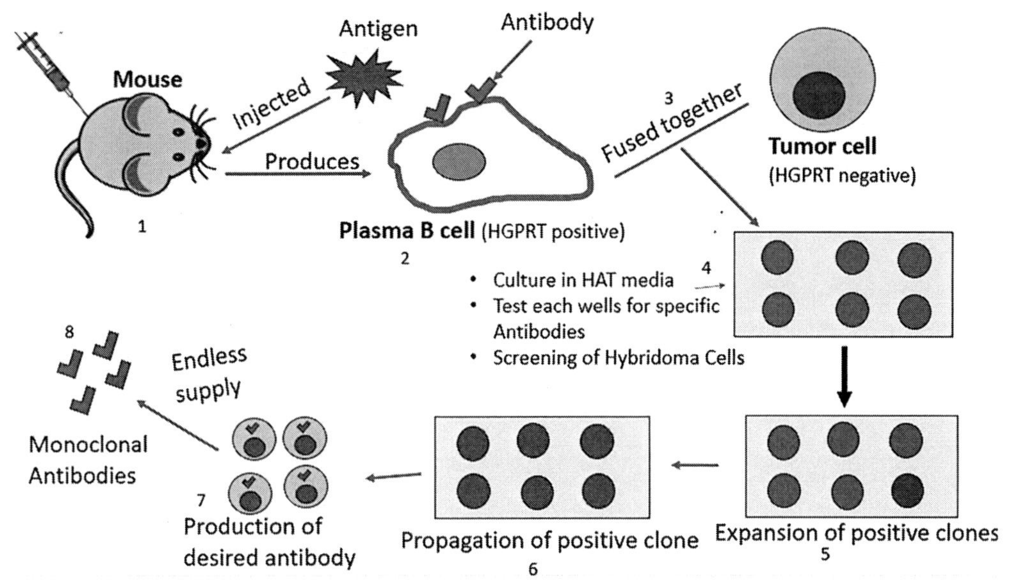

FIGURE 13.2 Representation of the production of monoclonal antibodies. (1) The first step involves injecting the laboratory mice with a selected antigen. (2) Stimulation and production of plasma B cells. (3) Plasma B cells then fuse with tumor cells. (4) Incubating the cell mixture in HAT-containing medium. (5) Selection of hybrid cells (which contain HGPRT gene). (6) Expansion of hybrid cell. (7) Propagation of hybrid cell. (8) Gene of the B cell lineage present in the hybrid cell (hybridoma cells) produces a specific antibody with a specific epitope; this antibody is known as "monoclonal antibody." (8) Number of monoclonal antibodies produced.

cell parent provides them with the required HGPRT gene product. Through this process, which is carried out in HAT (hypoxanthine-aminopterin-thymidine) selective medium supplemented with thymidine and hypoxanthine, hybrid B cell myeloma cells that produce antibodies are created. The clone secreting the desired antibody is then chosen through a rigorous screening process (Quinteros et al. 2017; Mitra and Tomar 2021; Berger, Shankar, and Vafai 2002).

Numerous difficulties arose in scaling up mAbs production for therapeutic uses. Attaining large drug quantities at a reasonable cost was the principal concern. Production became costly and time-consuming in the 1980s. Developing a culture medium that promotes the best possible growth for hybridomas involved the formation of a hybrid cell, clone selection that secretes Mabs in high amount, and other steps. There were 50 or more ingredients in this type of media, so it was difficult to scale up quality control, because the amounts of each nutrient had to be precisely determined. When given too much glucose, for example, hybridomas would stop secreting mAbs (Quinteros et al. 2017).

13.8 ANTIBODY–DRUG CONJUGATES (ADCS)

Targeted therapies are being revolutionized by a novel class of therapeutic agents called ADCs, or antibody–drug conjugates, which combine the precision of monoclonal antibodies (mAbs) with cytotoxic drug potency. This novel strategy uses chemical linkers to covalently link cytotoxic drugs to antibodies, using antibody–drug conjugates as prodrugs. Prodrugs are derivatives that are less active but that, through enzymatic or chemical transformations, become potent and active once they have reached their intended target (Quinteros et al. 2017; Bander 2013; Pettinato 2021).

13.8.1 Methods of Conjugation

Covalent binding and adsorption are the two main techniques of conjugation used in antibody functionalization (El-Sayed and Kamel 2020; Juan et al. 2020). The capability of the antibodies to be immobilized is indicated by conjugation efficiency, which represents the proportion of conjugated antibodies to total antibodies (Chen et al. 2019). Antibody immobilization on nanoparticle surfaces can be non-site-specific or site-specific, depending on the conjugation technique used. Antibody orientation is largely determined by the binding sites (Parracino, Martín, and Grazú 2019). When the antibody's Fc region binds to the nanoparticle, the Fab regions can interrelate with the antigen in the right way, resulting in optimal orientation (Ju, Lai, and Yan 2017). On the other hand, standard procedures could lead to random antibody orientation (Arruebo, Valladares, and González-Fernández 2009), which might result in a decrease in binding ability even though it is common.

13.8.2 Absorption

One of the most basic conjugation techniques involves both ionic and physical interactions: adsorption. During this process, intrinsic surface forces, such as van der Waals forces, hydrogen bonds, hydrophobic interactions, and electrostatic forces, help antibodies stick to material surfaces. Interestingly, this technique is mild, allowing for the immobilization of fragile antibodies on surfaces with low damage (Tallawi et al. 2015). But this method's ease of use has a cost: compared to covalent binding, it frequently results in less physical stability. As a result, conjugation retention and efficiency may be compromised (A. C. Marques et al. 2020). Furthermore, random antibody orientations are a consequence of the ionic and physical interactions' inherent lack of specificity.

13.8.3 Covalent Binding

Covalent bonds are resistant to disassembly, which makes covalent binding an excellent technique with high stability and remarkable reproducibility (Ou et al. 2013). Stronger conjugation with an ordered antibody orientation is the result of this feature, which is a significant benefit over adsorption. Two of the most popular covalent binding techniques for conjugating nanoparticles with antibodies are maleimide and carbodiimide chemistry.

13.8.3.1 Maleimide Chemistry

This type of conjugation comprises binding through the sulfhydryl (-SH) or thiol groups in the antibody. It is a site-selective method. Proteins containing cysteine amino acid side chains contain sulfhydryls, which oxidatively form disulfide bonds (Borges and Sherma 2014). These bonds are generally seen on the of IgG antibodies hinge region. Antibodies are broken into monovalent halves by disulfide bond reduction, which does not change the antigen-binding effectiveness and 3D structure (Robotham and Kelly 2019; Fra, Yoboue, and Sitia 2017). However, the chemistry of maleimides requires free sulfhydryl groups, which necessitates the reduction of disulfide bonds through the addition of sulfhydryl groups.

13.8.3.2 Carbodiimide Chemistry

Carbodiimide chemistry is a cross-linking technique that links carboxylic acids to primary amines by using substances such as 1-ethyl-3-(3-dimethylaminopropyl) carbodiimide (EDC) and N, N′-dicyclohexylcarbodiimide (DCC) (Cammarata, Hughes, and Ofner 2015; Iwasawa et al. 2007). Antibodies are rich in amine groups, which are highly reactive on their own without further chemical processing (Polo et al. 2013). When combined with EDC, N-hydroxysulfosuccinimide (NHS) or N-hydroxysuccinimide (sulfo-NHS) improves coupling efficiency, creates a more stable intermediate, and inhibits intra- and intermolecular cross-linking of antibodies (Conde et al.

2014; Yao et al. 2016; Jang and Keng 2008). However, because of amine groups' reactivity in the Fab region, carbodiimide chemistry can cause antibodies to randomly immobilize on nanoparticles, which can affect the antibodies' biological ability and activity to targets (Polo et al. 2013; Fuentes et al. 2005)

13.8.3.3 Click Chemistry

It refers to a class of general chemical reactions that are highly efficient and stereospecific. It is a great platform for biomedical applications because of its minimal by-product generation, selective nature, and orthogonal properties to the majority of known reactions. Four categories comprise click chemistry: cycloadditions, additions to carbon–carbon multiple bonds, non-aldol carbonyl, and nucleophilic ring-openings chemistry. The cycloaddition reaction is the most generally used technique for creating antibody nanoparticle conjugates among them. In particular, popular click chemistry techniques used in nanoparticle–antibody conjugates include copper-catalyzed azide-alkyne cycloaddition (CuAAC) reaction, inverse electron-demand Diels–Alder reactions, and strain-promoted alkyne-azide cycloadditions. Their use demonstrates how important they are for obtaining precise and effective conjugation, which advances biomedical research (Lin, O'Reilly Beringhs, and Lu 2021; Hein, Liu, and Wang 2008; Gole and Murphy 2008; Yi et al. 2018; Hainfeld et al. 2011).

13.9 THERAPEUTICS APPLICATIONS OF MONOCLONAL ANTIBODIES

Monoclonal antibodies (mAbs) are essential for both therapeutics and diagnostics because of their exceptional ability to selectively recognize a wide range of molecules, including disease-associated proteins. mAbs are essential in clinical settings because they aid in the detection of numerous markers, hormones, and molecules linked to tumors in diagnostics. Because mAbs target antigens on tumor cells and serve as carriers for payloads like toxins and medications, they have revolutionized the field of therapeutics, particularly in the treatment of cancer. When it comes to managing infections like cancer, monoclonal antibodies (mAbs) are crucial. Their therapeutic potential is demonstrated by their versatility in treating a wide range of disorders, such as skeletal disorders and neurological conditions. Moreover, mAbs are at the forefront of personalized medicine, providing a way to track a patient's response to therapy in addition to novel medications. The combination of mAbs and therapeutic agents to form immunoconjugates is a potent approach to targeted and precision therapy, demonstrating the diverse effects of mAbs in the advancement of medical interventions (Mahmuda et al. 2017; Degu, Endashaw, and Fesseha 2020; Berger, Shankar, and Vafai 2002; Castelli, McGonigle, and Hornby 2019).

13.10 ANTIBODY-BASED NANOTECHNOLOGY

A revolutionary era in antibody-based applications began in the 1970s with the development of Milstein and Köhler's groundbreaking mouse hybridoma technology. This novel approach changed the course of antibody research and application by opening the door to important breakthroughs (Köhler and Milstein 1975). Muromonab CD3 (OKT3), the first therapeutic mAb, was authorized over 30 years ago. This was a turning point that led to the rapid expansion of the therapeutic mAb market. Currently, more than 50 mAbs are approved for a variety of disease phenotypes, and there are about 540 mAbs in clinical development (Shukla et al. 2017; Nelson, Dhimolea, and Reichert 2010). mAbs are among the most popular biopharmaceutical therapeutic modalities (Ecker, Jones, and Levine 2015). Over the past 20 years, the use of mAbs has increased into diagnostics and research in addition to therapeutic applications. Sturdy production systems make it easier for antibody-based technologies to transition from drug discovery to clinical and commercial success. Antibody-based nanoparticles and antibody-based ordered nanostructures for targeted drug delivery, antibody-based nanomachines, and nanobiosensors for diagnostics are just a few of the novel developmental paths made possible by the unique structural and recognition qualities of antibodies. Because of their wide range of specificities, antibodies can now be integrated into generic nanotechnology platforms, which makes it easier to identify different biomolecules with high sensitivity and specificity.

13.10.1 Functionalization of Nanoparticles with Monoclonal Antibodies

When monoclonal antibodies and nanoparticles are combined, the true potential of nanotechnology is revealed. The term "functionalization" describes the process of binding of particular antibodies to nanoparticles surface. It is possible to precisely design monoclonal antibodies to identify and bind to antigens (specific) on target cells (Abuhelwa, Alloghbi, and Nagasaka 2022; Ana Camila Marques et al. 2023). These antibodies are homing devices that provide remarkable specificity in directing therapeutic payloads to their desired locations when coupled to nanoparticles (Abuhelwa, Alloghbi, and Nagasaka 2022; Quinteros et al. 2017). Functionalized nanoparticles have two benefits: they specifically target monoclonal antibodies while also improving the stability, controlled release, and targeting precision of the nanoparticles (Ana Camila Marques et al. 2023). The significance of monoclonal antibodies in precision therapy and the complexities of fusing nanotechnology and monoclonal antibodies to create novel drug delivery systems are discussed (Ezike et al. 2023; Rosenblum et al. 2018).

13.10.2 Non-Invasive Tumor Surface Antigen Detection with Nanoparticle–Antibody Conjugates

Accurate treatment strategies depend on the validation of antibody nanoparticle conjugates through imaging due to the variability and heterogeneity in tumor surface antigen expression levels. Targeted nanoparticles with imaging agents integrated show robust affinities to particular tumor surface antigens, offering comprehensive details on antigen density and localization in the tissue. For this, various types of imaging modalities have been used, like MRI (magnetic resonance imaging), optical imaging, and photoacoustic imaging. Fluorochrome-labeled nanoparticles have been used in optical imaging, a non-invasive method that uses fluorescent or luminescent probes. These nanoparticles, especially the ones conjugated with antibodies, improve signal contrast and enhance targeting features, allowing for detailed tumor morphology information. Compared to optical imaging, photoacoustic imaging provides superior tissue penetration. It is a hybrid modality that causes thermoelastic tissue expansion. In this modality, metal nanoparticles such as silver, gold, and iron oxide, as well as polymeric nanoparticles like PLGA (poly(lactide-co-glycolide)), have been studied as imaging probes. When these nanoparticles are coupled with antibodies, they allow for the visualization of tumor surface antigens that are overexpressed. MRI (magnetic resonance imaging): using sup, MRI is a commonly used clinical imaging technique (Zhan et al. 2017; Xiao et al. 2013; X. Li et al. 2018; Xiong et al. 2019).

13.10.3 Improved Antibody–Nanoparticle Conjugates Accumulation, Tumor Retention, and Cell Internalization

Antibody–nanoparticle conjugates are essential for enhancing the interactions between nanoparticles and cells, which may lead to better tumor retention and enhanced imaging capabilities. These conjugates increase residence time in tumor tissues by promoting internalization and interactions, which makes them easier to visualize using multimodal imaging techniques. Longer tumor retention than small-molecule contrast agents provides improved signal enhancement, less dose-required multiple contrast agent administration, and streamlined logistics between contrast administration and imaging (Johnston and Scott 2018).

13.10.4 Nanoparticles

Nanoparticles display distinct physical and chemical properties. These include metals, polymers, lipids, and carbon-based compounds. Because of the large surface-area-to-volume ratios that their small size imparts, which affect reactivity and conductivity, they are incredibly versatile in a variety of fields, such as materials science, electronics, and medicine. Monoclonal antibody-based nanoparticles are a prime example of how nanotechnology and medicine are coming together in the context of cancer treatment. Nanoparticles and precisely engineered monoclonal antibodies (mAbs) that are intended to target particular molecules on cancer cells are intricately combined to provide powerful vehicles for targeted drug delivery. By skillfully delivering the mAbs to the tumor site, these nanoparticles serve as carriers, reducing the likelihood of side effects and maximizing the effectiveness of treatment. This novel combination of monoclonal antibodies and nanoparticles offers individualized and effective treatments, especially for cancer-related illnesses. It is a game changer in personalized medicine (Khan, Saeed, and Khan 2019).

13.10.5 Gold Nanoparticles

When gold nanoparticles are combined with antibodies, like cetuximab, which targets the EGFR (epidermal growth factor receptor), the intake of the particles by cells is boosted, which prolongs their stay in tumor tissues. PEG surface modification reduces nonspecific uptake by extending the duration of blood circulation. The ideal particle size is between 15 and 30 nm. This helps improve intratumoral distribution and doubles the amount of tumor contrast in X-ray CT (computed tomography) when compared to iodinated small-molecule contrast agents. A number of factors can affect the effectiveness of antibody targeting, including the density and configuration of the antibodies, the size of the nanoparticles, and the levels of antigen expression on the targeted cells (Reuveni et al. 2011; Aydogan et al. 2010; Lijowski et al. 2009; I. C. Sun et al. 2009).

13.10.6 Albumin Nanoparticle

Proteins found in human plasma are mostly made up of hepatocytes, which also produce albumin, which makes up about half of all the proteins in plasma. Stabilizing osmotic pressure of plasma and promoting communication between extracellular, intracellular, and tissue fluids are two of its vital functions in preserving physiological balance. The body uses albumin to bind to heavy metal ions and use it as a natural detoxifier in addition to its role in fluid dynamics. Fused HSA (human serum albumin) to the IL-1ra (interleukin-1 receptor antagonist) of carboxyl terminus creates a recombinant protein, which was then successfully expressed using *Pichia pastoris*. IL-1ra, a naturally occurring protein that is essential for controlling the immune system, is interleukin-1 receptor antagonist. The pro-inflammatory cytokine interleukin-1 (IL-1), which is involved in a variety of immune responses and inflammatory processes, is countered by IL-1ra, as its name implies. By attaching itself to the same receptors that IL-1 uses, IL-1ra blocks IL-1's ability to cause inflammation. Albumin and IL-1Ra direct fusion was beneficial because the resultant fusion protein had an extended serum half-life and maintained the IL-1Ra biological activity. Interestingly, the fusion protein showed longer accumulation during joint inflammation in comparison to the administration of IL-1Ra alone, and lower distribution rates were seen in the kidney, liver, lung, and other organs. This result established the protein fusion superior targeting capabilities and emphasized its therapeutic efficacy.

13.10.7 Polymeric Nanoparticle

Predominantly in the arena of cancer treatment, polymeric nanoparticles—which use polymers to encapsulate drugs—have become adaptable platforms for both active and passive targeted drug delivery. Notably, monoclonal antibodies have been included as ligands in advances in active targeted delivery methods for lung cancer therapy. Combining RNA aptamer with PLGA-b-PEG nanopolymersomes allows for the selective targeting of the extracellular domain of epithelial cell adhesion molecules (EpCAM). The study demonstrated how these nanoparticles could be used to treat lung cancer using the SK-MES-1 and A549 cell lines (Jeevanandam et al. 2018; Malhotra et al. 2021; Alibolandi et al. 2015).

13.10.8 Spion Nanoparticle

A particular kind of nanoparticle known as superparamagnetic iron oxide nanoparticles (SPION) is made up of crystals of magnetite (Fe_3O_4) with a cubic lattice face centered and a solid foundation based on oxygen. While Fe_3+ occupies a tetrahedral area opposing the field in the tetrahedral region, ferrous (Fe_2+) and iron (Fe_3+) ions have octahedral sites that run parallel to the magnetic field outside. These nanoparticles have favorable physicochemical characteristics, such as surface modifiability, low toxicity, and high sensitivity. SPION is widely used in therapeutics and diagnostics, having a hydrodynamic diameter that falls between 5 and 300 nm. Interestingly, delivery and treatment of lung cancer using SPION, whether by passive or active delivery using ligand monoclonal antibodies, show promise (Yan et al. 2018; Lammers, Mertens, and Kiessling 2015; Kowalik et al. 2020).

13.10.9 Lipid–Based Nanoparticle

Liposomes and other lipid-based nanoparticles as well as lipid carriers with nanostructure have attracted a lot of attention in the fields of cancer treatment and medication development. The multifunctional nanoparticles demonstrate the ability to transfer hydrophilic and hydrophobic substances with very less toxicity. Lipid nanoparticles have a longer half-life, which prolongs therapeutic efficacy. Lipid nanoparticles are useful therapeutic carriers in the field of cancer treatment. Interestingly, by conjugated ligand monoclonal antibodies, they have been engineered for active targeted delivery, offering selectivity for particular receptors (Haron et al. 2018; Pindiprolu et al. 2019; Ninomiya et al. 2014).

13.10.10 Silica Nanoparticle and Mesoporous Silica

A class of nanomaterials which is chemically and thermally stable with regulated porosity and morphology is represented by mesoporous silica nanoparticles. These nanoparticles have been extensively used in the field of drug delivery for the therapy of lung cancer. Silica nanoparticles conjugated with monoclonal antibodies is the process of synthesis. Mesoporous silica self-assembly on reduced graphene oxide nanosheets containing gold nanoparticles (AuNPs) aligned with their nanogaps is specifically one novel approach. Then, this structure was encased and dispersed throughout the mesoporous silica layer's nanopores. According to Chen et al., these new nanoparticles present an exceptional nanotheragnostic system with notable cell tracking and targeting properties and a large photothermal therapy potential (Haron et al. 2018; Pindiprolu et al. 2019; Ninomiya et al. 2014).

13.11 CASE STUDY: NANOPARTICLE–BASED TARGETED THERAPY IN ONCOLOGY

13.11.1 Background

Nanoparticle-based drug delivery systems have shown potential in refining the effectiveness and reduce the side effects of cancer treatments.

13.11.2 Case Study

One notable example is the use of doxorubicin (Doxil) liposomal in the treatment of ovarian cancer. Doxorubicin is a potent chemotherapeutic drug, but its use is limited by its side effects. Liposomal Doxil is encapsulated within lipid nanoparticles, which allows for targeted delivery to tumor cells while minimizing exposure to healthy tissues (Norouzi et al. 2020).

13.11.3 Outcome

Liposomal Doxil demonstrated improved drug target to tumor sites, reduced side effects, and improved overall survival in patients with recurrent ovarian cancer. This case highlights the potential of nanotechnology to enhance the therapeutic index of cancer treatments.

These case studies highlight the practical applications of nanotechnology and monoclonal antibodies in the development of targeted therapies in various medical fields, including oncology. These innovative approaches have the potential to develop the effectiveness and safety of treatments for a wide range of conditions.

13.12 MONOCLONAL ANTIBODY-BASED TARGETING

To form immuno-nanoparticles, monoclonal antibodies (mAbs) can be attached to nanoparticle surfaces, which can be selectively targeted by antigens or receptors overexpressed in tumors (Figure 13.3). One of the mAb targets with a higher clinical relevance is EGFR, which is overexpressed in breast, ovarian, prostate, bladder, non–small cell lung, head, and neck cancers and glioblastoma. We conjugated an EGFR antibody with polymeric poly(lactide-coglycolide) nanoparticles loaded with rapamycin to target the extracellular ligand binding domain of EGFR specifically. It was found that this method was superior to free rapamycin and nanoparticles without a targeting

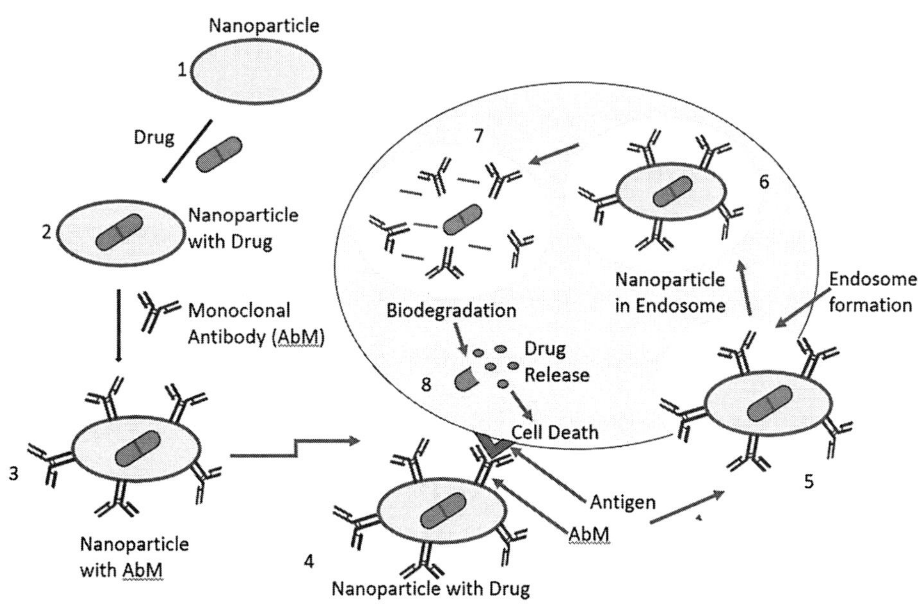

FIGURE 13.3 A monoclonal antibody and nanoparticle-based targeted medication delivery system: (1) nanoparticle, (2) drug with nanoparticle, (3) nanoparticle–antibody conjugation, (4) adhesion of monoclonal antibody on tumor cell, (5) endocytosis of nanoparticle, (6) endosome formation, (7) biodegradation of nanoparticle by endosomal enzymes, (7) drug release and cell death.

moiety in terms of antiproliferative activity and uptake by malignant MCF-7 breast cancer cells. Another member of the EGFR family, HER2, which is overexpressed in both ovarian and breast cancers, has also been shown to cause apoptosis and cell cycle arrest when injected with the active targeted particles. When anti-HER2 antibodies are conjugated to polymeric nanoparticles, their intracellular accumulation is encouraged due to receptor-mediated endocytosis.

In order to effectively target ovarian tumor cells that overexpress HER2 receptors, Cirstoiu-Hapca and colleagues (Cirstoiu-Hapca et al. 2009) created paclitaxel-loaded poly(DL-lactic acid) immuno-nanoparticles with anti-HER2 mAbs (trastuzumab, Herceptin) covalently conjugated to their surface. Comparing these immuno-nanoparticles to other paclitaxel formulations (either the same nanoparticles without the targeting moiety, with irrelevant mAbs, or the free drug), in vitro studies revealed the enhanced cytotoxic effects of these nanoparticles at low drug concentrations (Cirstoiu-Hapca et al. 2009). Bioluminescence imaging in a disseminated xenograft ovarian cancer mouse model proved the formulation's superior therapeutic efficacy by demonstrating the polymeric immuno-nanoparticles' higher antitumor activity compared to free paclitaxel. The longer survival rate of mice treated with immuno-nanoparticles as compared to mice treated with trastuzumab alone, paclitaxel-loaded nanoparticles with an insignificant amount of rituximab, or free paclitaxel (Cirstoiu-Hapca et al. 2009) supported these findings. Non-toxic human serum albumin (HSA) nanoparticles have also been associated with HER2 antibodies (trastuzumab) for the targeted delivery of methotrexate to tumors (Taheri et al. 2012). The cytotoxicity of these trotaguzumab-conjugated methotrexate-loaded human serum albumin nanoparticles was higher than that of non-functionalized particles or free methotrexate. Additionally, HER2 positive cells absorbed the nanoparticles more readily than non-targeted ones (Taheri et al. 2012), in addition to being employed as instruments for small-mole delivery.

Polymeric immune nanoparticles serve two purposes: in addition to carrying small molecules, they also help move larger molecules, like proteins or genes, along with small drug molecules. In a specific application, fragments of antigen-binding Fab' derived from a humanized anti-HER2 monoclonal antibody (mAb) were linked to the nanoparticles using carbodiimide chemistry. Poly(lactic-co-glycolic acid) (PLGA) immuno-nanoparticles containing PE38KDEL were produced as a result of this method. The addition of the anti-HER2 Fab increased the in vitro cytotoxicity of the PE38KDEL-loaded nanoparticles against breast cancer cell lines that overexpress HER2 receptors. In tumor-bearing mice, the immuno-nanoparticles showed increased antitumor efficacy in comparison to the control immunotoxin (anti-HER2Fab coupled to PE38KDEL). Additionally, the immuno-nanoparticles showed a greater suppression of tumor growth in a tumor xenograft model overexpressing the HER2 receptor. The toxicity of PE38KDEL on normal tissues was greatly decreased by the toxin's inclusion to the PLGA nanoparticles. Kos and colleagues (112) employed poly(D, L-lactide-co-glycolide) (PLGA) nanoparticles with a cytokeratin-specific Mabs (anti-cytokeratin mAb) linked to their surface in order to specifically target MCF-10A neoT invasive breast epithelial cells. The particles contained cystatin, a potent protease inhibitor. It was feasible to distinguish between malignant cells that overexpress cytokeratin and those that release the inhibitor into lysosomes or endosomes using polymeric nanocarrier technology.

13.13 METHODS FOR ANTIBODY CONJUGATION TO NANOCARRIERS

Therapeutic agents can be delivered at disease site by nanocarriers, which are the size of nanometers (Schroeder et al. 2012; Arias 2011). Their distinct physicochemical characteristics are intended to enhance a drug molecule's pharmacokinetics and biodistribution (S. D. Li and Huang 2008), as well as to deliver a substantial quantity of drug molecules. Al-Jamal and Kostarelos (Al-Jamal and Kostarelos 2011) identified lipid-based particles as an example of therapeutic nanocarriers, while Kedar (Kedar et al. 2010) identified as well nanoparticles (Shi et al. 2010), polymersomes (Levine et al. 2008), and dendrimers (Svenson 2009). Certain ones have been suggested as potential treatments for a range of illnesses, such as cancer (Dhar et al. 2011), blood vessel disorders (Chan et al. 2011), and rheumatoid arthritis (Thomas et al. 2011). The distinct architecture of cancer, namely, the permeability of the tumoral vasculatures, allows for nanocarriers' passive transport through the EPR effect (Maeda et al. 2003). Yet depending on the kind of tumor, the porosity of the blood vessels within it may change (Bae 2009). The ability of the nanocarriers to internalize inside the cancer cells is necessary even in the event that the EPR effect is successful in delivering them (Gradishar et al. 2005).

Active and passive targeting are entwined in a novel drug delivery paradigm. Ligands that are targeted, like antibodies (Mamot et al. 2005), proteins (Srinivasan, Marchant, and Gupta 2010), tiny molecules (Kukowska-Latallo et al. 2005), or aptamers, according to Farokhzad et al. (2006), can be affixed to a nanocarrier's surface. The therapeutic payloads are released by the cells via receptor-mediated endocytosis once the carriers have recognized and attached to the cell-surface receptors. Additionally, the multivalent impact can significantly raise the targeted nanocarriers' binding affinity.

Antibodies are among the most well-known targeting ligands due to their high specificity, binding affinity, and availability for various biomarkers disease (Manjappa et al. 2011). A nanocarrier's surface can easily absorb an antibody through hydrophobic and/or electrostatic interactions (Sokolov et al. 2003). This method could, however, induce a random orientation of the absorbed antibody on the surface and lose its binding affinity. Additionally, in vivo, the antibody may trade places with other endogenous proteins (Nobs et al. 2004). As a result, antibodies are typically chosen for their covalent attachment to the nanocarriers (Arruebo, Valladares, and González-Fernández 2009). A variety of functional groups makes up an antibody, offering a wide range of bioconjugation possibilities (Manjappa et al. 2011). For the compound to form, streptavidin and biotin are typically used as adapter molecules. The separation and selective quantification of *Escherichia coli* O157:H7 in ground beef in the presence of other bacteria is accomplished by attaching biotin-labeled polyclonal goat anti–*Escherichia coli* antibodies to streptavidin-coated magnetic nanoparticles.

13.14 ADVANCEMENTS IN NANOPARTICLE-MEDIATED THERAPIES: REVOLUTIONIZING CANCER

13.14.1 Interventions

The use of antibody-conjugated nanoparticles in cancer therapy and diagnosis has fundamentally changed the field of medical interventions. Even though they are sensitive, traditional diagnostic techniques for microbial infections frequently require time-consuming steps and lengthy readout times. The introduction of nanoparticles has become a sensitive and quick substitute because of their distinct electrical, magnetic, luminescent, and catalytic properties. Superparamagnetic iron oxide nanoparticles (SPION), an example of an antibody-conjugated nanoparticle, are essential for a variety of in vivo uses, such as medicine delivery, immunoassays, and magnetic resonance imaging. As demonstrated by their effectiveness against *E. coli*, these nanoparticles improve bioanalysis by permitting quick and accurate identification of pathogenic bacteria (*E. coli* O157:H7). Furthermore, ultrasensitive methods for microbial detection and bioassays are provided by antibody-conjugated silica nanoparticles and fluorescent bioconjugated nanoparticles.

The combination of antibodies and nanoparticles is a key strategy for improving specificity and efficacy in cancer treatment. Particularly, targeted drug delivery appears promising for iron oxide and gold nanoparticles, where antibodies are essential for improving specificity. By precisely targeting tumors with potent anticancer agents, advanced antibody–drug conjugates (ADCs) have overcome previous limitations and are now able to provide improved monitoring, early detection, and surgical guidance. Through targeted drug delivery, this deliberate conjugation of nanoparticles with antibodies not only minimizes side effects but also increases therapeutic efficacy. Nanotechnology's ongoing paradigm-shifting advances have the potential to significantly improve cancer therapy outcomes. The combination of nanotechnology and antibodies offers a revolutionary method to cancer therapy and medical diagnostics, even with associated challenges. This opens the door to targeted and individualized interventions (Das and Chandra 2022) (Table 13.2).

TABLE 13.2
Integration of Antibodies with Chemotherapeutic Agents in Nanoparticulate Systems

System	Antibody	Loaded Drug	Pathology/ Target	References
Fe_3O_4/Au magnetic/gold nanoparticles	Bevacizumab anti-VEGF antibody	Doxorubicin	–	Ramos-Tejada et al. (2015)
PEG liposomes	Anti-MT1-MP (Fab')	Doxorubicin	–	Hatakeyama et al. (2007)
Chitosan nanoparticle	Anti-HER2 monoclonal antibodies	Doxorubicin	Cancer therapy (breast, ovary)	Yousefpour et al. (2011)
Liposomes	Anti-HER2 monoclonal antibodies (trastuzumab)	Doxorubicin	Tumor xenograft nude mouse models	Banerjee, Harfouche, and Sengupta (2011); Praetorius and Mandal (2008)
Chitosan scaffold-PLGA nanoparticles	Bevacizumab anti-VEGF antibody	5-Fluorouracil	Brain cancer	Kutlu, Çakmak, and Gumusderelioglu (2014)
Human albumin serum (HAS) protein-based nanoparticle	Trastuzumab	Doxorubicin	Breast cancer therapy	Anhorn et al. (2008)
Poly(propylene imine) dendrimer	Primary antibody (mAbK1)	Paclitaxel	Ovarian cancer therapy	Jain et al. (2015)
PLGA nanoparticles	Cetuximab	Paclitaxel Palmitate	Lung cancer therapy	Karra et al. (2013)
Micellar nanoparticles	AntiHER2 antibody	Docetaxel	Breast cancer therapy	Mi, Zhao, and Feng (2013); J. Zhao et al. (2012)
Poly(lactide-*co*-glycolide) (PLGA) nanoparticles	IgG isotype control	Camptothecin	Prostate cancer therapy	McCarron et al. (2008)
Polylactide (PLA)–based nanoparticles	AntiHER2 antibody	Docetaxel	Colorectal cancer therapy	J. Zhao et al. (2012)
Poly(D,L-lactide-co-glycolide)/montmorillonite (PLGA/MMT) nanoparticle	Trastuzumab	Paclitaxel	Breast cancer therapy	B. Sun, Ranganathan, and Feng (2008)
Liposomes	Antibody fragments scFv antibodies	Topotecan	Prostate cancer therapy	Roth et al. (2007)

Source: Quinteros et al. (2017).

13.15 REGULATORY CONSIDERATIONS IN DEVELOPING TARGETED THERAPIES

Regulatory factors are essential to the creation and acceptance of targeted treatments. The effectiveness, safety, and caliber of these treatments are guaranteed by the regulatory framework (Schuck et al. 2018). Essential factors consist of the following.

13.15.1 Clinical Trials

Validating the safety and efficacy of targeted medicines requires extensive clinical trials. When planning these trials, the target and specific patient population should be taken into account.

13.15.2 Biomarker Validation

To identify patients, benefit from targeted therapies, and stratify patients, biomarkers must be developed and validated.

13.15.3 Regulatory Agencies

Various nations have their own regulatory bodies (e.g., FDA within the United States and EMA [European Medicines Agency] in Europe) that have their own procedures for approval. For market approval, adherence to these agencies' requirements is necessary.

13.15.4 Pharmacovigilance

After approval, it is critical to continuously monitor the safety and effectiveness of targeted therapies, and regulatory bodies may call for post-marketing surveillance.

13.15.5 Intellectual Property

Targeted therapy development and commercialization are heavily reliant on intellectual property rights, particularly patents. This may affect these treatments' inventiveness and cost-effectiveness.

13.15.6 Global Harmonization

Harmonizing regulatory norms and collaborating internationally can expedite the clearance process and make targeted therapies more widely accessible.

13.16 CONCLUSION

The integration of monoclonal antibodies and nanotechnology represents a powerful and innovative approach to drug delivery and cancer treatment. This synergy capitalizes on the precision of monoclonal antibodies to selectively recognize specific biomarkers on diseased cells and the versatility of nanotechnology to engineer drug delivery methods with enhanced properties. The combination of these two technologies offers several advantages, which follow.

13.16.1 Improved Targeting

Monoclonal antibodies can guide drug delivery to specific cells or tissues with high precision, minimizing off-target effects.

13.16.2 Enhanced Drug Efficacy

Nanotechnology allows for controlled drug release, ensuring that the therapeutic payload reaches the intended site in the desired concentration.

13.16.3 Reduced Side Effects

By minimizing exposure to healthy tissues, the synergy of these technologies can reduce the often-debilitating side effects associated with traditional therapies.

13.16.4 Personalized Medicine

The ability to tailor treatments to individual patient characteristics through the use of nanotechnology and monoclonal antibodies offers the promise of personalized medicine.

13.16.5 Innovative Therapeutic Strategies

Treatment for a number of diseases, including infectious diseases and cancer, could be completely changed by the development of combination medicines and smart drug delivery systems.

REFERENCES

Abuhelwa, Ziad, Abdurahman Alloghbi, and Misako Nagasaka. 2022. "A Comprehensive Review on Antibody-Drug Conjugates (ADCs) in the Treatment Landscape of Non-Small Cell Lung Cancer (NSCLC)." *Cancer Treatment Reviews* 106: 102393. https://doi.org/10.1016/j.ctrv.2022.102393.

Adepu, Shivakalyani, and Seeram Ramakrishna. 2021. "Controlled Drug Delivery Systems: Current Status and Future Directions." *Molecules* 26 (19): 5905. https://doi.org/10.3390/molecules26195905.

Adler, Mark J., and Dimiter S. Dimitrov. 2012. "Therapeutic Antibodies Against Cancer." *Hematology/Oncology Clinics of North America* 26 (3): 447–81, vii. https://doi.org/10.1016/j.hoc.2012.02.013.

Ahmad, Zuhaida Asra, Swee Keong Yeap, Abdul Manaf Ali, Wan Yong Ho, Noorjahan Banu Mohamed Alitheen, and Muhajir Hamid. 2012. "ScFv Antibody: Principles and Clinical Application." *Clinical and Developmental Immunology* 2012: 980250. https://doi.org/10.1155/2012/980250.

Alibolandi, Mona, Mohammad Ramezani, Khalil Abnous, Fatemeh Sadeghi, Fatemeh Atyabi, Mohsen Asouri, Ali Asghar Ahmadi, and Farzin Hadizadeh. 2015. "In Vitro and in Vivo Evaluation of Therapy Targeting Epithelial-Cell Adhesion-Molecule Aptamers for Non-Small Cell Lung Cancer." *Journal of Controlled Release* 209: 88–100. https://doi.org/10.1016/j.jconrel.2015.04.026.

Al-Jamal, Wafa T., and Kostas Kostarelos. 2011. "Liposomes: From a Clinically Established Drug Delivery System to a Nanoparticle Platform for Theranostic Nanomedicine" *Accounts of Chemical Research* 44 (10): 1094–104. https://doi.org/10.1021/ar200105p.

Anhorn, Marion G., Sylvia Wagner, Jörg Kreuter, Klaus Langer, and Hagen Von Briesen. 2008. "Specific Targeting of HER2 Overexpressing Breast Cancer Cells with Doxorubicin-Loaded Trastuzumab-Modified Human Serum Albumin Nanoparticles." *Bioconjugate Chemistry* 19 (12): 2321–31. https://doi.org/10.1021/bc8002452.

Arias, José L. 2011. "Advanced Methodologies to Formulate Nanotheragnostic Agents for Combined Drug Delivery and Imaging." *Expert Opinion on Drug Delivery* 8 (12): 1589–608. https://doi.org/10.1517/17425247.2012.634794.

Arruebo, Manuel, Mónica Valladares, and África González-Fernández. 2009. "Antibody-Conjugated Nanoparticles for Biomedical Applications." *Journal of Nanomaterials* 37: 1–24. https://doi.org/10.1155/2009/439389.

Attia, Mohamed F., Nicolas Anton, Justine Wallyn, Ziad Omran, and Thierry F. Vandamme. 2019. "An Overview of Active and Passive Targeting Strategies to Improve the Nanocarriers Efficiency to Tumour Sites." *Journal of Pharmacy and Pharmacology* 71 (8): 1185–98. https://doi.org/10.1111/jphp.13098.

Aydogan, Bulent, Ji Li, Tijana Rajh, Ahmed Chaudhary, Steven J. Chmura, Charles Pelizzari, Christian Wietholt, Metin Kurtoglu, and Peter Redmond. 2010. "AuNP-DG: Deoxyglucose-Labeled Gold Nanoparticles as X-Ray Computed Tomography Contrast Agents for Cancer Imaging." *Molecular Imaging and Biology* 12 (5): 463–67. https://doi.org/10.1007/s11307-010-0299-8.

Bae, You Han. 2009. "Drug Targeting and Tumor Heterogeneity." *Journal of Controlled Release* 133 (1): 2–3. https://doi.org/10.1016/j.jconrel.2008.09.074.

Bander, Neil H. 2013. "Antibody-Drug Conjugate Target Selection: Critical Factors." *Methods in Molecular Biology* 1045: 29–40. https://doi.org/10.1007/978-1-62703-541-5_2.

Banerjee, Deboshri, Rania Harfouche, and Shiladitya Sengupta. 2011. "Nanotechnology-Mediated Targeting of Tumor Angiogenesis." *Vascular Cell* 3 (1): 3. https://doi.org/10.1186/2045-824X-3-3.

Bayda, Samer, Muhammad Adeel, Tiziano Tuccinardi, Marco Cordani, and Flavio Rizzolio. 2020. "The History of Nanoscience and Nanotechnology: From Chemical-Physical Applications to Nanomedicine." *Molecules* 25 (1): 112. https://doi.org/10.3390/molecules25010112.

Berger, Mitchell, Vidya Shankar, and Abbas Vafai. 2002. "Therapeutic Applications of Monoclonal Antibodies." *American Journal of the Medical Sciences* 324 (1): 14–30. https://doi.org/10.1097/00000441-200207000-00004.

Berillo, Dmitriy, Zharylkasyn Zharkinbekov, Yevgeniy Kim, Kamila Raziyeva, Kamila Temirkhanova, and Arman Saparov. 2021. "Stimuli-Responsive Polymers for Transdermal, Transmucosal and Ocular Drug Delivery." *Pharmaceutics* 13 (12): 2050. https://doi.org/10.3390/pharmaceutics13122050.

Borges, Chad R., and Nisha D. Sherma. 2014. "Techniques for the Analysis of Cysteine Sulfhydryls and Oxidative Protein Folding." *Antioxidants and Redox Signaling* 21 (3): 511–31. https://doi.org/10.1089/ars.2013.5559.

Brüggemann, Marianne, H. M. Caskey, C. Teale, H. Waldmann, G. T. Williams, M. A. Surani, and M. S. Neuberger. 1989a. "A Repertoire of Monoclonal Antibodies with Human Heavy Chains from Transgenic Mice." *Proceedings of the National Academy of Sciences of the United States of America* 86 (17): 6709–13. https://doi.org/10.1073/pnas.86.17.6709.

Brüggemann, Marianne, Greg Winter, Herman Waldmann, and Michael S. Neuberger. 1989b. "The Immunogenicity of Chimeric Antibodies." *Journal of Experimental Medicine* 170 (6): 2153–57. https://doi.org/10.1084/jem.170.6.2153.

Cammarata, Christopher R., Mitchell E. Hughes, and Clyde M. Ofner. 2015. "Carbodiimide Induced Cross-Linking, Ligand Addition, and Degradation in Gelatin." *Molecular Pharmaceutics* 12 (3): 783–93. https://doi.org/10.1021/mp5006118.

Castelli, María Sofía, Paul McGonigle, and Pamela J. Hornby. 2019. "The Pharmacology and Therapeutic Applications of Monoclonal Antibodies." *Pharmacology Research & Perspectives* 7 (6): e00535. https://doi.org/10.1002/prp2.535.

Chan, Juliana M., June Wha Rhee, Chester L. Drum, Roderick T. Bronson, Gershon Golomb, Robert Langer, and Omid C. Farokhzad. 2011. "In Vivo Prevention of Arterial Restenosis with Paclitaxel-Encapsulated Targeted Lipid-Polymeric Nanoparticles." *Proceedings of the National Academy of Sciences of the United States of America* 108 (48): 19347–52. https://doi.org/10.1073/pnas.1115945108.

Chen, Han, Jiajia Lin, Yongqi Shan, and Lu Zhengmao. 2019. "The Promotion of Nanoparticle Delivery to Two Populations of Gastric Cancer Stem Cells by CD133 and CD44 Antibodies." *Biomedicine and Pharmacotherapy* 115: 108857. https://doi.org/10.1016/j.biopha.2019.108857.

Cheng, Yi Hsien, Chunla He, Jim E. Riviere, Nancy A. Monteiro-Riviere, and Zhoumeng Lin. 2020. "Meta-Analysis of Nanoparticle Delivery to Tumors Using a Physiologically Based Pharmacokinetic Modeling and Simulation Approach." *ACS Nano* 14 (3): 3075–95. https://doi.org/10.1021/acsnano.9b08142.

Cirstoiu-Hapca, A., F. Buchegger, L. Bossy, M. Kosinski, R. Gurny, and F. Delie. 2009. "Nanomedicines for Active Targeting: Physico-Chemical Characterization of Paclitaxel-Loaded Anti-HER2 Immunonanoparticles and in Vitro Functional Studies on Target Cells." *European Journal of Pharmaceutical Sciences* 38 (3): 230–37. https://doi.org/10.1016/j.ejps.2009.07.006.

Conde, João, Jorge T. Dias, Valeria Grazú, Maria Moros, Pedro V. Baptista, and Jesus M. de la Fuente. 2014. "Revisiting 30 Years of Biofunctionalization and Surface Chemistry of Inorganic Nanoparticles for Nanomedicine." *Frontiers in Chemistry* 2: 48. https://doi.org/10.3389/fchem.2014.00048.

Das, Kaushik Pratim, and J. Chandra. 2022. "Nanoparticles and Convergence of Artificial Intelligence for Targeted Drug Delivery for Cancer Therapy: Current Progress and Challenges." *Frontiers in Medical Technology* 4: 1067144. https://doi.org/10.3389/fmedt.2022.1067144.

Degu, Tadesse, Dereje Endashaw, and Haben Fesseha. 2020. "Therapeutic Application of Monoclonal Antibodies: A Review." *Journal of Life Science and Biomedicine* 10 (5): 59–69. https://doi.org/10.51145/jlsb.2020.8.

Dhar, Shanta, Nagesh Kolishetti, Stephen J. Lippard, and Omid C. Farokhzad. 2011. "Targeted Delivery of a Cisplatin Prodrug for Safer and More Effective Prostate Cancer Therapy in Vivo." *Proceedings of the National Academy of Sciences of the United States of America* 108 (5): 1850–55. https://doi.org/10.1073/pnas.1011379108.

Ecker, Dawn M., Susan Dana Jones, and Howard L. Levine. 2015. "The Therapeutic Monoclonal Antibody Market." *Mabs* 7 (1): 9–14. https://doi.org/10.4161/19420862.2015.989042.

El-Sayed, Amr, and Mohamed Kamel. 2020. "Advances in Nanomedical Applications: Diagnostic, Therapeutic, Immunization, and Vaccine Production." *Environmental Science and Pollution Research* 27 (16): 19200–213. https://doi.org/10.1007/s11356-019-06459-2.

Ezike, Tobechukwu Christian, Ugochukwu Solomon Okpala, Ufedo Lovet Onoja, Chinenye Princess Nwike, Emmanuel Chimeh Ezeako, Osinachi Juliet Okpara, Charles Chinkwere Okoroafor, et al. 2023. "Advances in Drug Delivery Systems, Challenges and Future Directions." *Heliyon* 9 (6): e17488. https://doi.org/10.1016/j.heliyon.2023.e17488.

Farokhzad, Omid C., Jianjun Cheng, Benjamin A. Teply, Ines Sherifi, Sangyong Jon, Philip W. Kantoff, Jerome P. Richie, and Robert Langer. 2006. "Targeted Nanoparticle-Aptamer Bioconjugates for Cancer Chemotherapy in Vivo." *Proceedings of the National Academy of Sciences of the United States of America* 103 (16): 6315–20. https://doi.org/10.1073/pnas.0601755103.

Fra, Annamaria, Edgar D. Yoboue, and Roberto Sitia. 2017. "Cysteines as Redox Molecular Switches and Targets of Disease." *Frontiers in Molecular Neuroscience* 10: 167. https://doi.org/10.3389/fnmol.2017.00167.

Fuentes, Manuel, Cesar Mateo, J. M. Guisán, and Roberto Fernández-Lafuente. 2005. "Preparation of Inert Magnetic Nano-Particles for the Directed Immobilization of Antibodies." *Biosensors and Bioelectronics* 20 (7): 1380–87. https://doi.org/10.1016/j.bios.2004.06.004.

Gole, Anand, and Catherine J. Murphy. 2008. "Azide-Derivatized Gold Nanorods: Functional Materials for 'Click' Chemistry." *Langmuir* 24 (1): 266–72. https://doi.org/10.1021/la7026303.

Gradishar, William J., Sergei Tjulandin, Neville Davidson, Heather Shaw, Neil Desai, Paul Bhar, Michael Hawkins, and Joyce O'Shaughnessy. 2005. "Phase III Trial of Nanoparticle Albumin-Bound Paclitaxel Compared with Polyethylated Castor Oil-Based Paclitaxel in Women with Breast Cancer." *Journal of Clinical Oncology* 23 (31): 7794–803. https://doi.org/10.1200/JCO.2005.04.937.

Hainfeld, James F., M. J. O'Connor, F. A. Dilmanian, D. N. Slatkin, D. J. Adams, and H. M. Smilowitz. 2011. "Micro-CT Enables Microlocalisation and Quantification of Her2-Targeted Gold Nanoparticles within Tumour Regions." *British Journal of Radiology* 84 (1002): 526–33. https://doi.org/10.1259/bjr/42612922.

Haron, Aminah Suhaila, Sharifah Sakinah Syed Alwi, Latifah Saiful Yazan, Rohaina Abd Razak, Yong Sze Ong, Fatin Hannani Zakarial Ansar, and Henna Roshini Alexander. 2018. "Cytotoxic Effect of Thymoquinone-Loaded Nanostructured Lipid Carrier (TQ-NLC) on Liver Cancer Cell Integrated with Hepatitis B Genome, Hep3B." *Evidence-Based Complementary and Alternative Medicine* 2018: 1549805. https://doi.org/10.1155/2018/1549805.

Hatakeyama, Hiroto, Hidetaka Akita, Emi Ishida, Koichi Hashimoto, Hideo Kobayashi, Takanori Aoki, Junko Yasuda, et al. 2007. "Tumor Targeting of Doxorubicin by Anti-MT1-MMP Antibody-Modified PEG Liposomes." *International Journal of Pharmaceutics* 342 (1–2): 194–200. https://doi.org/10.1016/j.ijpharm.2007.04.037.

Hein, Christopher D., Xin Ming Liu, and Dong Wang. 2008. "Click Chemistry, a Powerful Tool for Pharmaceutical Sciences." *Pharmaceutical Research* 25 (10): 2216–30. https://doi.org/10.1007/s11095-008-9616-1.

Hua, Susan, Maria B. C. de Matos, Josbert M. Metselaar, and Gert Storm. 2018. "Current Trends and Challenges in the Clinical Translation of Nanoparticulate Nanomedicines: Pathways for Translational Development and Commercialization." *Frontiers in Pharmacology* 9: 790. https://doi.org/10.3389/fphar.2018.00790.

Hughes, Gareth A. 2005. "Nanostructure-Mediated Drug Delivery." *Nanomedicine: Nanotechnology, Biology, and Medicine* 1 (1): 22–30. https://doi.org/10.1016/j.nano.2004.11.009.

Iwasawa, Tetsuo, Paul Wash, Christoph Gibson, and Julius Rebek. 2007. "Reaction of an Introverted Carboxylic Acid with Carbodiimide." *Tetrahedron* 63 (28): 6506–11. https://doi.org/10.1016/j.tet.2007.03.075.

Jain, Narendra K., Manoj S. Tare, Vijay Mishra, and Pushpendra K. Tripathi. 2015. "The Development, Characterization and in Vivo Anti-Ovarian Cancer Activity of Poly (Propylene Imine) (PPI)-Antibody Conjugates Containing Encapsulated Paclitaxel." *Nanomedicine: Nanotechnology, Biology, and Medicine* 11 (1): 207–18. https://doi.org/10.1016/j.nano.2014.09.006.

Janeway Jr, Charles A., Paul Travers, Mark Walport, and Mark J. Shlomchik. 2001. "The Structure of a Typical Antibody Molecule." *Immunobiology* 14102. Garland Science.

Jang, Ling Sheng, and Hao Kai Keng. 2008. "Modified Fabrication Process of Protein Chips Using a Short-Chain Self-Assembled Monolayer." *Biomedical Microdevices* 10 (2): 203–11 https://doi.org/10.1007/s10544-007-9126-7.

Jeevanandam, Jaison, Ahmed Barhoum, Yen S. Chan, Alain Dufresne, and Michael K. Danquah. 2018. "Review on Nanoparticles and Nanostructured Materials: History, Sources, Toxicity and Regulations." *Beilstein Journal of Nanotechnology* 9: 1050–74. https://doi.org/10.3762/bjnano.9.98.

Johnston, Michael C., and Christopher J. Scott. 2018. "Antibody Conjugated Nanoparticles as a Novel Form of Antibody Drug Conjugate Chemotherapy." *Drug Discovery Today: Technologies* 30: 63–69. https://doi.org/10.1016/j.ddtec.2018.10.003.

Jong, Wim H. De, and Paul J. A. Borm. 2008. "Drug Delivery and Nanoparticles: Applications and Hazards." *International Journal of Nanomedicine* 3 (2): 133–49. https://doi.org/10.2147/ijn.s596.

Ju, Huangxian, Guosong Lai, and Feng Yan. 2017. *Immunosensing for Detection of Protein Biomarkers*. ISBN 978-0-08-101999-3. https://doi.org/10.1016/C2016-0-01168-3.

Juan, Alberto, Francisco J. Cimas, Iván Bravo, Atanasio Pandiella, Alberto Ocaña, and Carlos Alonso-Moreno. 2020. "An Overview of Antibody Conjugated Polymeric Nanoparticles for Breast Cancer Therapy." *Pharmaceutics* 12 (9): 802. https://doi.org/10.3390/pharmaceutics12090802.

Karra, Nour, Taher Nassar, Alina Nemirovski Ripin, Ouri Schwob, Jürgen Borlak, and Simon Benita. 2013. "Antibody Conjugated PLGA Nanoparticles for Targeted Delivery of Paclitaxel Palmitate: Efficacy and Biofate in a Lung Cancer Mouse Model." *Small* 9 (24): 4221–36. https://doi.org/10.1002/smll.201301417.

Kedar, Uttam, Prasanna Phutane, Supriya Shidhaye, and Vilasrao Kadam. 2010. "Advances in Polymeric Micelles for Drug Delivery and Tumor Targeting." *Nanomedicine: Nanotechnology, Biology, and Medicine* 6 (6): 714–29. https://doi.org/10.1016/j.nano.2010.05.005.

Khan, Ibrahim, Khalid Saeed, and Idrees Khan. 2019. "Nanoparticles: Properties, Applications and Toxicities." *Arabian Journal of Chemistry* 12(7): 908–31. https://doi.org/10.1016/j.arabjc.2017.05.011.

Köhler, G., and C. Milstein. 1975. "Continuous Cultures of Fused Cells Secreting Antibody of Predefined Specificity." *Nature* 256 (5517): 495–97. https://doi.org/10.1038/256495a0.

Kowalik, Przemyslaw, Jakub Mikulski, Anna Borodziuk, Magdalena Duda, Izabela Kamińska, Karolina Zajdel, Jaroslaw Rybusinski, et al. 2020. "Yttrium-Doped Iron Oxide Nanoparticles for Magnetic Hyperthermia Applications." *Journal of Physical Chemistry C* 124 (12): 6871–83. https://doi.org/10.1021/acs.jpcc.9b11043.

Kukowska-Latallo, Jolanta F., Kimberly A. Candido, Zhengyi Cao, Shraddha S. Nigavekar, Istvan J. Majoros, Thommey P. Thomas, Lajos P. Balogh, Mohamed K. Khan, and James R. Baker. 2005. "Nanoparticle Targeting of Anticancer Drug Improves Therapeutic Response in Animal Model of Human Epithelial Cancer." *Cancer Research* 65 (12): 5317–24. https://doi.org/10.1158/0008-5472.CAN-04-3921.

Kumar Dash, Deepak, Rajni Kant Panik, Anil Kumar Sahu, and Vaibhav Tripathi. 2020. "Role of Nanobiotechnology in Drug Discovery, Development and Molecular Diagnostic." In *Applications of Nanobiotechnology*. https://doi.org/10.5772/intechopen.92796.

Kutlu, Ceren, Anil S. Çakmak, and Menemşe Gumusderelioglu. 2014. "Double-Effective Chitosan Scaffold-PLGA Nanoparticle System for Brain Tumour Therapy: In Vitro Study." *Journal of Microencapsulation* 31 (7): 700–07. https://doi.org/10.3109/02652048.2014.913727.

Lammers, T., M. E. Mertens, and F. Kiessling. 2015. "Theranostic Tissue Engineering: MR Imaging of Uspio-Labeled Collagen Scaffolds and Vascular Grafts." *Molecular Imaging and Biology* 8 (1054): 20150207. https://pubmed.ncbi.nlm.nih.gov/25969868.

Levine, Dalia Hope, P. Peter Ghoroghchian, Jaclyn Freudenberg, Geng Zhang, Michael J. Therien, Mark I. Greene, Daniel A. Hammer, and Ramachandran Murali. 2008. "Polymersomes: A New Multi-Functional Tool for Cancer Diagnosis and Therapy." *Methods* 46 (1): 25–32. https://doi.org/10.1016/j.ymeth.2008.05.006.

Li, Shyh Dar, and Leaf Huang. 2008. "Pharmacokinetics and Biodistribution of Nanoparticles." *Molecular Pharmaceutics* 5: 496–504. https://doi.org/10.1021/mp800049w.

Li, Xuelin, Dong Wang, Haitao Ran, Lan Hao, Yang Cao, Meng Ao, Nan Zhang, et al. 2018. "A Preliminary Study of Photoacoustic/Ultrasound Dual-Mode Imaging in Melanoma Using MAGE-Targeted Gold Nanoparticles." *Biochemical and Biophysical Research Communications* 502 (2): 255–61. https://doi.org/10.1016/j.bbrc.2018.05.155.

Lijowski, Michal, Shelton Caruthers, Grace Hu, Huiying Zhang, Michael J. Scott, Todd Williams, Todd Erpelding, et al. 2009. "High Sensitivity: High-Resolution SPECT-CT/MR Molecular Imaging of Angiogenesis in the Vx2 Model." *Investigative Radiology* 44 (1): 15–22. https://doi.org/10.1097/RLI.0b013e31818935eb.

Lin, Xinhao, André O'Reilly Beringhs, and Xiuling Lu. 2021. "Applications of Nanoparticle-Antibody Conjugates in Immunoassays and Tumor Imaging." *AAPS Journal* 23 (2): 43. https://doi.org/10.1208/s12248-021-00561-5.

Lkhagvasuren, Enkhhsaikhan. 2017. "Janeway's Immunobiology, 9th Edition." *Central Asian Journal of Medical Sciences* 3 (1): 100—01. https://doi.org/10.24079/cajms.2017.01.015.

Lonberg, Nils. 2005. "Human Antibodies from Transgenic Animals." *Nature Biotechnology* 23 (9): 1117–25. https://doi.org/10.1038/nbt1135.

Lu, Xuefei, Tao Zhu, Chunying Chen, and Ying Liu. 2014. "Right or Left: The Role of Nanoparticles in Pulmonary Diseases." *International Journal of Molecular Sciences* 15 (10): 17577–600. https://doi.org/10.3390/ijms151017577.

Maeda, Hiroshi, Jun Fang, Takao Inutsuka, and Yasunori Kitamoto. 2003. "Vascular Permeability Enhancement in Solid Tumor: Various Factors, Mechanisms Involved and Its Implications." *International Immunopharmacology* 3: 319–28. https://doi.org/10.1016/S1567-5769(02)00271-0.

Mahara, Gehendra, Cuihong Tian, Xiaojia Xu, and Wei Wang. 2023. "Revolutionising Health Care: Exploring the Latest Advances in Medical Sciences." *Journal of Global Health* 13: 03042. https://doi.org/10.7189/JOGH.13.03042.

Mahesh, K. P., and S. Viveka. 2023. "Understanding Drug Delivery System for Safe Dispensing and Good Therapeutic Efficacy: A Review." *Acta Scientific Dental Sciences* 7 (4): 32–39. https://doi.org/10.31080/asds.2023.07.1601.

Mahmuda, Aliyu, Faruku Bande, Khalid Jameel Kadhim Al-Zihiry, Noor Abdulhaleem, Roslaini Abd Majid, Rukman Awang Hamat, Wan Omar Abdullah, and Zasmy Unyah. 2017. "Monoclonal Antibodies: A Review of Therapeutic Applications and Future Prospects." *Tropical Journal of Pharmaceutical Research.* 16 (3): 713. https://doi.org/10.4314/tjpr.v16i3.29.

Malhotra, Sahil, Shweta Dumoga, Akshay Joshi, Sujata Mohanty, and Neetu Singh. 2021. "Polymeric Micelles Coated with Hybrid Nanovesicles Enhance the Therapeutic Potential of the Reversible Topoisomerase Inhibitor Camptothecin in a Mouse Model." *Acta Biomaterialia* 121: 579–91. https://doi.org/10.1016/j.actbio.2020.11.049.

Malik, Shiza, Khalid Muhammad, and Yasir Waheed. 2023. "Nanotechnology: A Revolution in Modern Industry." *Molecules* 28 (2): 661. https://doi.org/10.3390/molecules28020661.

Mamot, Christoph, Daryl C. Drummond, Charles O. Noble, Verena Kallab, Zexiong Guo, Keelung Hong, Dmitri B. Kirpotin, and John W. Park. 2005. "Epidermal Growth Factor Receptor-Targeted Immunoliposomes Significantly Enhance the Efficacy of Multiple Anticancer Drugs in Vivo." *Cancer Research* 65 (24). https://doi.org/10.1158/0008-5472.CAN-05-1093.

Manjappa, Arehalli S., Kiran R. Chaudhari, Makam P. Venkataraju, Prudhviraju Dantuluri, Biswarup Nanda, Chennakesavulu Sidda, Krutika K. Sawant, and Rayasa S. Ramachandra Murthy. 2011. "Antibody Derivatization and Conjugation Strategies: Application in Preparation of Stealth Immunoliposome to Target Chemotherapeutics to Tumor." *Journal of Controlled Release* 150 (1): 2–22. https://doi.org/10.1016/j.jconrel.2010. 11.002.

Marques, Ana Camila, Paulo C. Costa, Sérgia Velho, and Maria Helena Amaral. 2020. "Functionalizing Nanoparticles with Cancer-Targeting Antibodies: A Comparison of Strategies." *Journal of Controlled Release* 320: 180–200. https://doi.org/10.1016/j.jconrel.2020.01.035.

Marques, Ana Camila, Paulo C. Costa, Sérgia Velho, and Maria Helena Amaral. 2023. "Lipid Nanoparticles Functionalized with Antibodies for Anticancer Drug Therapy." *Pharmaceutics* 15 (1): 216. https://doi.org/10.3390/pharmaceutics15010216.

McCarron, Paul A., Waleed M. Marouf, Derek J. Quinn, Francois Fay, Roberta E. Burden, Shane A. Olwill, and Christopher J. Scott. 2008. "Antibody Targeting of Camptothecin-Loaded PLGA Nanoparticles to Tumor Cells." *Bioconjugate Chemistry* 19 (8): 1561–69. https://doi.org/10.1021/bc800057g.

Mi, Yu, Jing Zhao, and Si Shen Feng. 2013. "Targeted Co-Delivery of Docetaxel, Cisplatin and Herceptin by Vitamin E TPGS-Cisplatin Prodrug Nanoparticles for Multimodality Treatment of Cancer." *Journal of Controlled Release* 169 (3): 185–92. https://doi.org/10.1016/j.jconrel.2013.01.035.

Mitra, Sanchita, and Pushpa Chaudhary Tomar. 2021. "Hybridoma Technology; Advancements, Clinical Significance, and Future Aspects." *Journal of Genetic Engineering and Biotechnology* 19 (1): 159. https://doi.org/10.1186/s43141-021-00264-6.

Murthy, Shashi K. 2007. "Nanoparticles in Modern Medicine: State of the Art and Future Challenges." *International Journal of Nanomedicine* 2 (2): 129–41. https://pubmed.ncbi.nlm.nih.gov/17722542/.

Nelson, Aaron L. 2010. "Antibody Fragments: Hope and Hype." *Mabs* 2 (1): 77–83. https://doi.org/10.4161/mabs.2.1.10786.

Nelson, Aaron L., Eugen Dhimolea, and Janice M. Reichert. 2010. "Development Trends for Human Monoclonal Antibody Therapeutics." *Nature Reviews Drug Discovery* 9 (10): 767–74. https://doi.org/10.1038/nrd3229.

Ninomiya, Kazuaki, Shinya Kawabata, Hiroyuki Tashita, and Nobuaki Shimizu. 2014. "Ultrasound-Mediated Drug Delivery Using Liposomes Modified with a Thermosensitive Polymer." *Ultrasonics Sonochemistry* 21 (1): 310–16. https://doi.org/10.1016/j.ultsonch.2013.07.014.

Nobs, Leila, Franz Buchegger, Robert Gurny, and Eric Allémann. 2004. "Current Methods for Attaching Targeting Ligands to Liposomes and Nanoparticles." *Journal of Pharmaceutical Sciences* 93 (8): 1980–92. https://doi.org/10.1002/jps.20098.

Norouzi, Mohammad, Vinith Yathindranath, James A. Thliveris, Brian M. Kopec, Teruna J. Siahaan, and Donald W. Miller. 2020. "Doxorubicin-Loaded Iron Oxide Nanoparticles for Glioblastoma Therapy: A Combinational Approach for Enhanced Delivery of Nanoparticles." *Scientific Reports* 10 (1): 11292. https://doi.org/10.1038/s41598-020-68017-y.

Ou, Xiaowei, Lang Jiang, Penglei Chen, Mingshan Zhu, Wenping Hu, Minghua Liu, Junfa Zhu, and Huanxin Ju. 2013. "Highly Stable Graphene-Based Multilayer Films Immobilized via Covalent Bonds and Their Applications in Organic Field-Effect Transistors." *Advanced Functional Materials* 23 (19): 2422–35. https://doi.org/10.1002/adfm.201202586.

Parracino, María Antonietta, Beatriz Martín, and Valeria Grazú. 2019. "State-of-the-Art Strategies for the Biofunctionalization of Photoactive Inorganic Nanoparticles for Nanomedicine." In *Photoactive Inorganic Nanoparticles: Surface Composition and Nanosystem Functionality*, 211–57, ISBN 9780128145319. Elsevier is the publisher. https://doi.org/10.1016/B978-0-12-814531-9.00009-9.

Patra, Jayanta Kumar, Gitishree Das, Leonardo Fernandes Fraceto, Estefania Vangelie Ramos Campos, Maria Del Pilar Rodriguez-Torres, Laura Susana Acosta-Torres, Luis Armando Diaz-Torres, et al. 2018. "Nano Based Drug Delivery Systems: Recent Developments and Future Prospects." *Journal of Nanobiotechnology* 16 (1): 71. https://doi.org/10.1186/s12951-018-0392-8.

Pettinato, Mark C. 2021. "Introduction to Antibody-Drug Conjugates." *Antibodies* 10 (4): 42. https://doi.org/10.3390/antib10040042.

Pindiprolu, Sai Kiran S. S., Pavan Kumar Chintamaneni, Praveen T. Krishnamurthy, and Kinnera Ratna Sree Ganapathineedi. 2019. "Formulation-Optimization of Solid Lipid Nanocarrier System of STAT3 Inhibitor to Improve Its Activity in Triple Negative Breast Cancer Cells." *Drug Development and Industrial Pharmacy* 45 (2): 304–13. https://doi.org/10.1080/03639045.2018.1539496.

Polo, Ester, Sara Puertas, María Moros, Pilar Batalla, José M. Guisán, Jesús M. De La Fuente, and Valeria Grazú. 2013. "Tips for the Functionalization of Nanoparticles with Antibodies." *Methods in Molecular Biology* 1051: 149–63. https://doi.org/10.1007/978-1-62703-550-7_11.

Praetorius, Natalie, and Tarun Mandal. 2008. "Engineered Nanoparticles in Cancer Therapy." *Recent Patents on Drug Delivery & Formulation* 1 (1): 37–51. https://doi.org/10.2174/187221107779814104.

Protti, Stefano, Angelo Albini, Radhika Viswanathan, and Alexander Greer. 2017. "Targeting Photochemical Scalpels or Lancets in the Photodynamic Therapy Field—The Photochemist's Role." *Photochemistry and Photobiology* 93 (5): 1139–53. https://doi.org/10.1111/php.12766.

Quinteros, Daniela A., José M. Bermúdez, Soledad Ravetti, Alicia Cid, Daniel A. Allemandi, and Santiago D. Palma. 2017. "Therapeutic Use of Monoclonal Antibodies: General Aspects and Challenges for Drug Delivery." In *Nanostructures for Drug Delivery*, 807–33. https://doi.org/10.1016/b978-0-323-46143-6.00025-7.

Ramos-Tejada, María del Mar, Julian L. Viota, Katarzyna Rudzka, and Angel V. Delgado. 2015. "Preparation of Multi-Functionalized Fe3O4/Au Nanoparticles for Medical Purposes." *Colloids and Surfaces B: Biointerfaces*: 128: 1-7. https://doi.org/10.1016/j.colsurfb.2015.02.002.

Rasool, Mahmood, Arif Malik, Sulayman Waquar, Mahwish Arooj, Sara Zahid, Muhammad Asif, Sumaira Shaheen, Abrar Hussain, Hamid Ullah, and Siew Hua Gan. 2022. "New Challenges in the Use of Nanomedicine in Cancer Therapy." *Bioengineered* 13 (1): 759–73. https://doi.org/10.1080/21655979.2021.2012907.

Reuveni, Tobi, Menachem Motiei, ZimamRomman, Aron Popovtzer, and Rachela Popovtzer. 2011. "Targeted Gold Nanoparticles Enable Molecular CT Imaging of Cancer: An in Vivo Study." *International Journal of Nanomedicine* 6: 2859–64. https://doi.org/10.2147/ijn.s25446.

Riechmann, Lutz, Michael Clark, Herman Waldmann, and Greg Winter. 1988. "Reshaping Human Antibodies for Therapy." *Nature* 332 (6162): 323–27. https://doi.org/10.1038/332323a0.

Rizvi, Syed A. A., and Ayman M. Saleh. 2018. "Applications of Nanoparticle Systems in Drug Delivery Technology." *Saudi Pharmaceutical Journal* 26 (1): 64–70. https://doi.org/10.1016/j.jsps.2017.10.012.

Robotham, Anna C., and John F. Kelly. 2019. "Detection and Quantification of Free Sulfhydryls in Monoclonal Antibodies Using Maleimide Labeling and Mass Spectrometry." *Mabs* 11 (4): 757–66. https://doi.org/10.1080/19420862.2019.1595307.

Rosenblum, Daniel, Nitin Joshi, Wei Tao, Jeffrey M. Karp, and Dan Peer. 2018. "Progress and Challenges Towards Targeted Delivery of Cancer Therapeutics." *Nature Communications* 9 (1): 1410. https://doi.org/10.1038/s41467-018-03705-y.

Roth, Audrey, Daryl C. Drummond, Fraser Conrad, Mark E. Hayes, Dmitri B. Kirpotin, Christopher C. Benz, James D. Marks, and Bin Liu. 2007. "Anti-CD166 Single Chain Antibody-Mediated Intracellular Delivery of Liposomal Drugs to Prostate Cancer Cells." *Molecular Cancer Therapeutics* 6 (10): 2737–46. https://doi.org/10.1158/1535-7163.MCT-07-0140.

Sahu, Tarun, Yashwant Kumar Ratre, Sushma Chauhan, L. V. K. S. Bhaskar, Maya P. Nair, and Henu Kumar Verma. 2021. "Nanotechnology Based Drug Delivery System: Current Strategies and Emerging Therapeutic Potential for Medical Science." *Journal of Drug Delivery Science and Technology*. 63: 102487. https://doi.org/10.1016/j.jddst.2021.102487.

Schroeder, Avi, Daniel A. Heller, Monte M. Winslow, James E. Dahlman, George W. Pratt, Robert Langer, Tyler Jacks, and Daniel G. Anderson. 2012. "Treating Metastatic Cancer with Nanotechnology." *Nature Reviews Cancer* 12 (1): 39–50. https://doi.org/10.1038/nrc3180.

Schuck, R., M. Pacanowski, J. Woodcock, *et al.* 2018. "Regulatory Policy for the Development of Targeted Therapies for Low-Frequency Molecular Subtypes of Disease." *Nature Review Drug Discovery* 17: 79–80. https://doi.org/10.1038/nrd.2017.231.

Shaw, Alan, Ian T. Hoffecker, Ioanna Smyrlaki, Joao Rosa, Algirdas Grevys, Diane Bratlie, Inger Sandlie, Terje Einar Michaelsen, Jan Terje Andersen, and Björn Högberg. 2019. "Binding to Nanopatterned Antigens Is Dominated by the Spatial Tolerance of Antibodies." *Nature Nanotechnology* 14 (2): 184–90. https://doi.org/10.1038/s41565-018-0336-3.

Sheeparamatti, B. G., R. B. Sheeparamatti, and J. S. Kadadevaramath. 2007. "Nanotechnology: Inspiration from Nature." *IETE Technical Review (Institution of Electronics and Telecommunication Engineers, India)* 24 (1): 5–8.

Shi, Jinjun, Alexander R. Votruba, Omid C. Farokhzad, and Robert Langer. 2010. "Nanotechnology in Drug Delivery and Tissue Engineering: From Discovery to Applications." *Nano Letters* 10 (9): 3223–30. https://doi.org/10.1021/nl102184c.

Shukla, Abhinav A., Leslie S. Wolfe, Sigma S. Mostafa, and Carnley Norman. 2017. "Evolving Trends in MAb Production Processes." *Bioengineering & Translational Medicine* 2 (1): 58–69. https://doi.org/10.1002/btm2.10061.

Sim, Serjay, and Nyet Kui Wong. 2021. "Nanotechnology and Its Use in Imaging and Drug Delivery (Review)." *Biomedical Reports* 14 (5): 42. https://doi.org/10.3892/br.2021.1418.

Sokolov, Konstantin, Michele Follen, Jesse Aaron, Ina Pavlova, Anais Malpica, Reuben Lotan, and Rebecca Richards-Kortum. 2003. "Real-Time Vital Optical Imaging of Precancer Using Anti-Epidermal Growth Factor Receptor Antibodies Conjugated to Gold Nanoparticles." *Cancer Research* 63 (9): 1999–2004. https://pubmed.ncbi.nlm.nih.gov/12727808/.

Srinivasan, Rekha, Roger E. Marchant, and Anirban Sen Gupta. 2010. "In Vitro and in Vivo Platelet Targeting by Cyclic RGD-Modified Liposomes." *Journal of Biomedical Materials Research—Part A* 93 (3): 1004–15. https://doi.org/10.1002/jbm.a.32549.

Steinitz, Michael, George Klein, Saiji Koskimies, and Olli Makel. 1977. "EB Virus-Induced B Lymphocyte Cell Lines Producing Specific Antibody." *Nature* 269 (5627): 420–22. https://doi.org/10.1038/269420a0.

Sun, Bingfeng, Balu Ranganathan, and Si Shen Feng. 2008. "Multifunctional Poly (d,l-Lactide-Co-Glycolide)/Montmorillonite (PLGA/MMT) Nanoparticles Decorated by Trastuzumab for Targeted Chemotherapy of Breast Cancer." *Biomaterials* 29 (4): 475–86. https://doi.org/10.1016/j.biomaterials.2007.09.038.

Sun, Duxin, Simon Zhou, and Wei Gao. 2020. "What Went Wrong with Anticancer Nanomedicine Design and How to Make It Right." *ACS Nano* 14 (10): 12281–90. https://doi.org/10.1021/acsnano.9b09713.

Sun, In Cheol, Dae Kyung Eun, Jin Hee Na, Seulki Lee, I. I. Jin Kim, In Chan Youn, Chang Yong Ko, et al. 2009. "Heparin-Coated Gold Nanopartieles for Liver-Specific CT Imaging." *Chemistry—A European Journal* 15 (48): 13341–47. https://doi.org/10.1002/chem.200902344.

Sun, Michael, and Anirban Sen Gupta. 2020. "Vascular Nanomedicine: Current Status, Opportunities, and Challenges." *Seminars in Thrombosis and Hemostasis* 46 (5): 524–44. https://doi.org/10.1055/s-0039-1692395.

Svenson, Sonke. 2009. "Dendrimers as Versatile Platform in Drug Delivery Applications." *European Journal of Pharmaceutics and Biopharmaceutics* 71 (3): 445–62. https://doi.org/10.1016/j.ejpb.2008.09.023.

Taheri, Azade, Rassoul Dinarvand, Fatemeh Atyabi, Mohammad Hossein Ghahremani, and Seyed Nasser Ostad. 2012. "Trastuzumab Decorated Methotrexate-Human Serum Albumin Conjugated Nanoparticles for Targeted Delivery to HER2 Positive Tumor Cells." *European Journal of Pharmaceutical Sciences* 47 (2): 331–40. https://doi.org/10.1016/j.ejps.2012.06.016.

Tallawi, Marwa, Elisabetta Rosellini, NiccolettaBarbani, Maria Grazia Cascone, Ranjana Rai, Guillaume Saint-Pierre, and Aldo R. Boccaccini. 2015. "Strategies for the Chemical and Biological Functionalization of Scaffolds for Cardiac Tissue Engineering: A Review." *Journal of the Royal Society Interface* 12 (108): 20150254. https://doi.org/10.1098/rsif.2015.0254.

Thomas, Thommey P., Sascha N. Goonewardena, Istvan J. Majoros, Alina Kotlyar, Zhengyi Cao, Pascale R. Leroueil, and James R. Baker. 2011. "Folate-Targeted Nanoparticles Show Efficacy in the Treatment of Inflammatory Arthritis." *Arthritis and Rheumatism* 63 (9): 2671–80. https://doi.org/10.1002/art.30459.

Wilhelm, Stefan, Anthony J. Tavares, Qin Dai, Seiichi Ohta, Julie Audet, Harold F. Dvorak, and Warren C.W. Chan. 2016. "Analysis of Nanoparticle Delivery to Tumours." *Nature Reviews Materials* 1: 16014. https://doi.org/10.1038/natrevmats.2016.14.

Xiao, J., X. M. Tian, C. Yang, P. Liu, N. Q. Luo, Y. Liang, H. B. Li, et al. 2013. "Ultrahigh Relaxivity and Safe Probes of Manganese Oxide Nanoparticles for in Vivo Imaging." *Scientific Reports* 3: 3424. https://doi.org/10.1038/srep03424.

Xiong, Jun, Jia Li Feng, Lihua Qiu, Zhi Gao, Pan Li, Liang Pang, and Zewei Zhang. 2019. "SDF-1-Loaded PLGA Nanoparticles for the Targeted Photoacoustic Imaging and Photothermal Therapy of Metastatic Lymph Nodes in Tongue Squamous Cell Carcinoma." *International Journal of Pharmaceutics* 554: 93–104. https://doi.org/10.1016/j.ijpharm.2018.10.064.

Yan, Lesan, Ahmad Amirshaghaghi, Dennis Huang, Joann Miller, Joel M. Stein, Theresa M. Busch, Zhiliang Cheng, and Andrew Tsourkas. 2018. "Protoporphyrin IX (PpIX)-Coated Superparamagnetic Iron Oxide Nanoparticle (SPION) Nanoclusters for Magnetic Resonance Imaging and Photodynamic Therapy." *Advanced Functional Materials* 28 (16): 1707030. https://doi.org/10.1002/adfm.201707030.

Yao, Virginia J., Sara D'Angelo, Kimberly S. Butler, Christophe Theron, Tracey L. Smith, Serena Marchiò, Juri G. Gelovani, et al. 2016. "Ligand-Targeted Theranostic Nanomedicines against Cancer." *Journal of Controlled Release* 240: 267–86. https://doi.org/10.1016/j.jconrel.2016.01.002.

Yi, Gawon, Jihwan Son, Jihye Yoo, Changhee Park, and Heebeom Koo. 2018. "Application of Click Chemistry in Nanoparticle Modification and Its Targeted Delivery." *Biomaterials Research* 22: 13. https://doi.org/10.1186/s40824-018-0123-0.

Yousefpour, Parisa, Fatemeh Atyabi, Ebrahim Vasheghani-Farahani, Ali Akbar Mousavi Movahedi, and Rassoul Dinarvand. 2011. "Targeted Delivery of Doxorubicin-Utilizing Chitosan Nanoparticles Surface-Functionalized with Anti-Her2 Trastuzumab." *International Journal of Nanomedicine* 6: 1977–90. https://doi.org/10.2147/ijn.s21523.

Zhan, Yonghua, Sixiang Shi, Emily B. Ehlerding, Stephen A. Graves, Shreya Goel, Jonathan W. Engle, Jimin Liang, Jie Tian, and Weibo Cai. 2017. "Radiolabeled, Antibody-Conjugated Manganese Oxide Nanoparticles for Tumor Vasculature Targeted Positron Emission Tomography and Magnetic Resonance Imaging." *ACS Applied Materials and Interfaces* 9 (44): 38304–12. https://doi.org/10.1021/acsami.7b12216.

Zhao, Jing, Yu Mi, Yutao Liu, and Si Shen Feng. 2012. "Quantitative Control of Targeting Effect of Anticancer Drugs Formulated by Ligand-Conjugated Nanoparticles of Biodegradable Copolymer Blend." *Biomaterials* 33 (6): 1948–58. https://doi.org/10.1016/j.biomaterials.2011.11.051.

Zhao, Zongmin, Anvay Ukidve, Jayoung Kim, and Samir Mitragotri. 2020. "Targeting Strategies for Tissue-Specific Drug Delivery." *Cell* 181 (1): 151–67. https://doi.org/10.1016/j.cell.2020.02.001.

14 Nanoparticles in Immunotherapy for Viral-Related Cancers

Akash Tripathi Satsangi, Soumya Upadhyay, Jyoti, and Anil Kumar Mavi

ABBREVIATIONS

Acronym	Full Form
WHO	World Health Organization
DNA	deoxyribonucleic acid
RNA	ribonucleic acid
HPV	human papillomavirus
BCG	Bacillus Calmette–Guérin
NPs	Nanoparticles
EBV	Epstein–Barr virus
BL	Burkitt's lymphoma
NPC	nasopharyngeal carcinoma
HD	Hodgkin's disease
PBNPs	Prussian blue nanoparticles
CTL	cytotoxic T lymphocytes
PTT	photothermal therapy
CC	cervical cancer
PAMAM	Polyamidoamine
AuNPs	gold nanoparticles
HBV	hepatitis B virus
HCC	hepatocellular carcinoma
DAAs	direct-acting antivirals
ETV	entecavir and tenofovir
HBsAg	hepatitis B surface antigen
VLPs	virus-like particles
HBcAg	hepatitis B core antigen
HCV	hepatitis C virus
mRNA	messenger ribonucleic acid
PEG	polyethylene glycol
DEAEMA	diethylaminoethyl methacrylate
DMAEMA	dimethylaminoethyl methacrylate
p53	tumor suppressor protein
pRB	tumor suppressor protein
HCVcAg	hepatitis C virus core antigen
HTLV-1	human T cell lymphotropic virus type 1
ATL	adult T cell leukemia

DOI: 10.1201/9781003463191-17

HBZ	HTLV-1 basic leucine zipper factor gene
TMC	Trimethylchitosan
CS	chitosan nanoparticles
TPP	Tripolyphosphate
pDNA	plasmid DNA
HHV-8	human herpesvirus-8
KSHV	Kaposi's sarcoma–associated herpesvirus
CHOP	(c)yclophosphamide, (h)ydroxydaunorubicin, (o)ncovin, (p)rednisone
MCPyV or MCV	Merkel cell polyomavirus
CMS5VP1	viral protein1

14.1 INTRODUCTION

Cancer has become one of the most important public health issues in the world, and the cases are predicted to rise. Microbes are estimated to underlie between 10% and 20% of all cancers worldwide (Tashiro and Brenner 2017; Sharma 2021). However, viruses alone are linked to around 63.4% of total 2.2 million cancer cases caused by microbes globally as per recent report of WHO-2022 based on GLOBOCAN-2018 data (de Martel et al. 2020). There are mainly seven types of viruses which can induce cancer worldwide. The first incidence of cancer caused by a virus was noticed in 1911 in chickens by pathologist Frances Peyton (Newman and Zloza 2017). However, in 2002, HPV (human papillomavirus) accounted for the largest global cancer burden, which was 5.2% of infection associated with cancers (Colón-López, Ortiz, and Palefsky 2010).

Viruses enter the host by introducing their own DNA or RNA into the cell. A cell may be pushed toward cancer when DNA or RNA modifies the genes of the host cell. Cancer cells are able to avoid immune identification and escape destruction (Kallingal et al. 2023). The knowledge gained and methods developed over time through tumor virology were found instrumental in the development of the first cancer vaccines. Initially, tumor vaccine was developed utilizing tuberculosis vaccine BCG combining with an appropriate adjuvant which worked against bladder cancer, and it was established as first immunotherapy against human cancer (Jiang and Redelman-Sidi 2022). Currently, the strategies of immunotherapy are being used, and it has become a clinically proven therapeutic option for many malignancies (Farkona, Diamandis, and Blasutig 2016). In contrast to conventional cancer treatments that are unable to differentiate between infected and healthy cells, immunotherapies are specifically designed to target malignancies linked to viruses (Liao 2006; Tashiro and Brenner 2017).

However, immunotherapy has demonstrated several drawbacks, such as immune system resistance or minimal bioavailability of drug, and some patients do not get relief. Consequently, novel approaches involving the use of nanoparticles (NPs) are arising in an effort to augment the effectiveness of immunotherapies (Mikelez-Alonso, Aires, and Cortajarena 2020).

14.2 NANOPARTICLES UTILIZED IN IMMUNOTHERAPY FOR VIRAL CANCERS

Cancer immunotherapy has become a viable therapeutic option through boosting the body's own immune system to cure a variety of cancer types caused by viruses (Tashiro and Brenner 2017; Tan, Li, and Zhu 2020). The potent antitumor immune response does not only eliminate tumor cells but, nonetheless, also stop them from happening again. A number of intractable obstacles confront therapeutic cancer immunotherapy, such as toxicity linked with excess of immunity, poor and unintended transport of cancer antigens to immune cells that impose adverse effects on the host. However, there are ways to overcome such restrictions with nanotechnology exploiting the nanoparticles, which can increase the effectiveness of immunotherapy. This review is concentrating

TABLE 14.1
Types and Advantages of Nanoparticles for the Treatment of Cervical Cancer

Nanoparticles	Types	Advantages	References
Lipid-based	PEGylated liposomes	Improved bioavailability, biocompatibility	Mishra, Webster, and Davis (2004); Singh et al. (2020)
	Tween 80–modified liposomes	High physical stability	Thumrongsiri et al. (2022)
	Lipid nanoparticles	High encapsulation property	Sheoran et al. (2022); X.-Y. Yang et al. (2013)
Polymeric	PLGA nanoparticles	Increases prolonged drug release and more stability	Pandita, Kumar, and Lather (2015)
	PAMAM nanoparticles	High transfection ability	Xiao et al. (2015); Li et al. (2021)
Inorganic	AuNPs (gold nanoparticles)	High physical stability, provide large surface-area-to-volume ratio	Artiga et al. (2019); Goddard et al. (2020)
	Mesoporous silica nanoparticles	Increased biocompatibility, provide large surface-area-to-volume ratio	Dajun Xu, Song, et al. (2021); Shahabi et al. (2015)
Exosomes	Genetically engineered exosomes	Biocompatibility, high targeting	Stremersch et al. (2016)
	Chemically modified exosomes	Facilitate controllable process	Haney et al. (2015)

on the use of nanoparticles in immunotherapy for viral-related cancers (Shao et al. 2015; Dang et al. 2024) (Tables 14.1, 14.2, 14.3).

14.2.1 Nanoparticles in Immunotherapy of EBV (Epstein–Barr Virus) Causing Stomach Cancer

In the 1960s, for the first time, EBV (Epstein–Barr virus) was coincidentally discovered during a study on Burkitt's lymphoma (BL), also known as non-Hodgkin's lymphoma, and successfully cultivated in vitro (Epstein 2012). More than 90% of people on earth are infected latently by it. EBV is a member of the herpesvirus family, and it harbors inactively the only host human (Thompson and Kurzrock 2004). Cancers are the most terrifying long-term effects of EBV. Once the virus gets activated, it may result into Hodgkin's lymphoma and nasopharyngeal carcinoma (NPC) (Kang and Kieff 2015). Oral secretions are the primary mode of viral transmission. The oropharynx is the route by which primary infection is caused and transforms the B-lymphocytes present in the circulation and coming in the contact to deactivate T lymphocyte (Rickinson 1996). Immunotherapeutic strategies for EBV are based on the latency-associated EBV proteins that are produced in tumor cells and offer strong antigenic targets. EBV-specific CTL is used to treat patients of Hodgkin's disease (HD) (Herbst et al. 1992; Gulley et al. 1994; Rooney et al. 1998). The predominant location for non-Hodgkin's lymphomas, which is related to stomach cancer caused by EBV, has a low incidence rate in general, making up fewer than 5% of all gastric cancers (Hosseini and Dehghan 2014). A novel approach towards the development of immunotherapy utilizing nanoparticles against EBV exploited a bioconjugation method that attaches nanoparticles to the cell surface in a stable manner. This involves the use of Prussian blue nanoparticles (PBNPs) in conjugation with antigen-specific cytotoxic T lymphocytes (CTL) (Burga et al. 2016). This combination of particles takes the advantage of both the photothermal therapy (PTT) properties of PBNPs and the ability of Epstein–Barr virus (EBV) antigen-specific CTL to travel to and kill target cells that express EBV antigen (Burga et al. 2016). A cell–nanoparticle hybrid has the ability to use the inherent qualities, such as antitumor responses, as well as treatment linked to the CTL and the nanoparticles (Zhang et al. 2015). The functioning of the nanoparticle has been shown through a diagram represented in Figure 14.1.

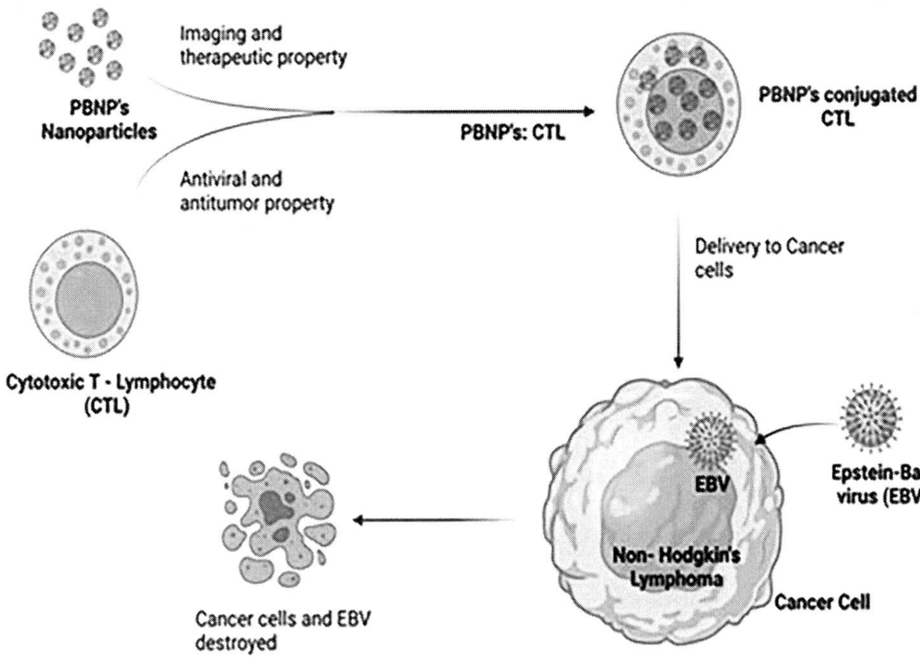

FIGURE 14.1 Nanoparticles in immunotherapy of EBV (Epstein–Barr virus).

Schematic representation of nanoparticle-mediated immunomodulation in EBV-associated non-Hodgkin's lymphoma. PBNP's nanoparticles (blue) enhance the activation and function of immune cells, such as Cytotoxic T cells (CTL; green), by boosting the body's ability to recognize and eliminate EBV-infected cancer cells. Immunotherapy involves (1) the introduction of PBNPs conjugated with antigen-specific CTL against EBV protein expressed by cancer cells infected with Epstein–Barr virus (yellow) into the host body, and (2) the nanoparticles enhancing the immune system's ability to detect and eliminate cancer cells infected with Epstein–Barr virus by killing target cells by inducing its antitumor responses against cancer cell.

14.2.2 Nanoparticles in Immunotherapy for Human Papilloma Virus (HPV) Causing Cervical Cancer

Most HPV infections are very common to everyone in their daily life and affect mucous membrane and produce warts only that are generally cured easily or go on their own. However, some variety of HPV infection which persists for a longer time can be a serious health issue when it is carcinogenic. HPV suppresses p53 and pRB antitumor proteins (Ferrall et al. 2021). HPV infection is responsible for approximately 5% of the total cancer cases in the world (Sharma 2021). HPV mostly infects sexually active people, irrespective of gender, and infection is generally localized to sex organs. The high-risk HPV can cause many types of cancer, including rare penile, vaginal, anal, and vulvar cancer, to oropharyngeal and cervical cancer. According to WHO (World Health Organization), cervical cancer (CC) is the fourth most frequently occurring malignancy in women around the world (World Health Organization 2020). HPV produces many regulatory proteins to carry throughout the life cycle, and among those, E6 and E7 are essential viral oncoproteins, produced during infection, and are the preferred antigens for preparing cervical cancer therapeutic vaccines (Miles, Safran, and Monk 2017). Immunotherapy of cervical cancer involves many strategies, which include live vector vaccine (ADXS11–001; prepared from live bacterium *Listeria monocytogenes*), peptide-based vaccine (SGN-00101; conjugation of E7 protein of HPV and heat shock protein of Mycobacterium), nucleic acid–based (hybrid of HPV E6/E7 and DNA/RNA), and adoptive cell therapy (personalized vaccine) (Zhou et al. 2022). Immunotherapy for cervical cancer is

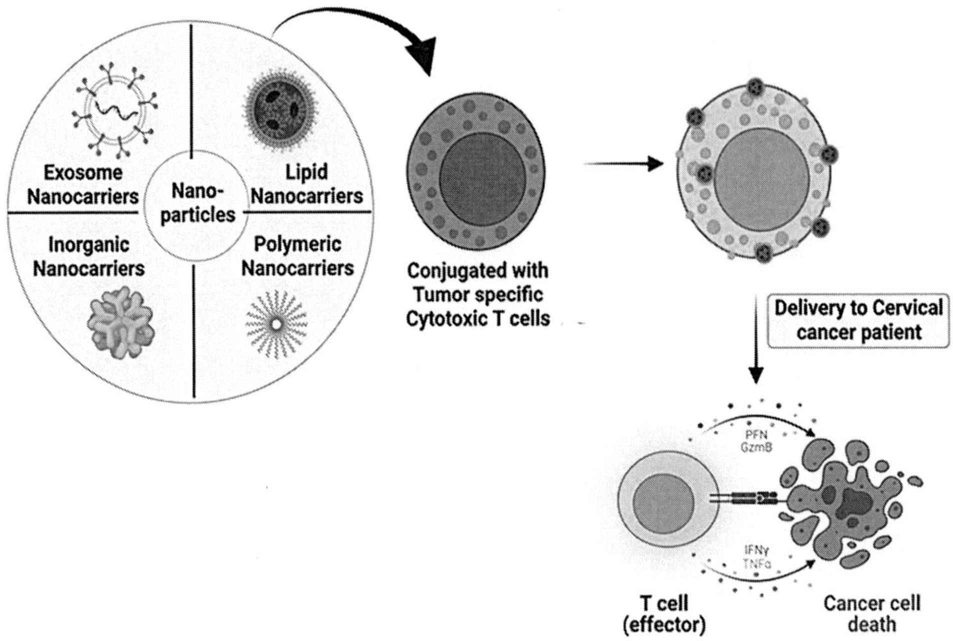

FIGURE 14.2 Nanoparticles in immunotherapy of HPV (human papilloma virus).

The figure depicts that currently there are many nanoparticle carriers developed, which include polymeric, inorganic, exosomes, and lipid-based nanocarriers conjugated with antigen-specific CTL (green) then destruction of cancer cells caused by HPV occurs.

still facing difficulties, including poor immunogenicity, ineffective targeting, and immunotoxicity (Song et al. 2015). Currently, there are many nanoparticle carriers that have been developed, which include polymeric, inorganic, exosomes, and lipid-based nanocarriers. These nanoparticles can be utilized either through chemotherapeutic or through immunotherapeutic ways (J. Yang et al. 2022; Bolhassani 2023). These nanoparticles-mediated immunotherapies have enhanced efficiency of the existing vaccine properties, especially by activating tumor-specific cytotoxic T cells for the treatment of cancer caused by HPV. These nanoparticles, with their types and advantages, are given in Table 14.1. The treatment of HPV causing a number of malignancies, including cervical cancer, in sexually active people by utilizing many different types of nanoparticles as a carrier for existing immunotherapeutics has been shown, through a diagram represented in Figure 14.2 and Table 14.1.

Nanoparticles conjugated with antigen-specific CTL against HPV can be used to deliver therapeutic agents, such as antigens or adjuvants, to enhance the T effector immune response against HPV by inducing its antitumor effect against HPV.

14.2.3 Nanoparticles in Immunotherapy for Hepatitis B Virus (HBV) Causing Liver Cancer

The hepatitis B virus (HBV) causes hepatitis B, which is an illness of the liver and characterized by liver cirrhosis and/or HCC (hepatocellular carcinoma) or liver cancer (Lampertico et al. 2017). HBV is a DNA virus and different from hepatitis C virus, which is an RNA virus (Bertoletti and Le Bert 2018). Furthermore, the available immunoregulatory medications for treating hepatitis B are IFN-α, and a few direct-acting antivirals (DAAs), like entecavir and tenofovir (ETV), do not provide adequate cure (D. Wang et al. 2021; Lee, Lee, and Ahn 2020). Preventive vaccines have a significant control on HBV, but it cannot help in case a patient has chronic infection, because of the challenges faced to achieve an improved and HBV-specific immune response, although efforts have been made to get success in developing a vaccine with specific immune response (D. Wang, Fu, and Wei 2022). On the other hand, parallelly, nanovaccines developed and licensed first in 1986 have provided unmatched benefits over traditional immunizations. A few nanoparticles-based delivery systems for anti-HBV vaccines have been proposed and reported for an effective viral clearance.

Among those is a SpyTag–ferritin nanoparticle vaccine, which was developed by Wang (W. Wang et al. 2020)and can deliver anti–hepatitis B preS1 antibody to certain myeloid cells, such as lymphatic sinus-associated SIGNR1+ macrophages and dendritic cells, which can activate B cells and T follicular helper cells. Another one, developed by Zhu and co-workers (Zhu et al. 2020), was found to elicit high-level monoprophylaxis, reported using mannose-modified poly-(D,L-lactide-co-glycolic acid) nanoparticles to load HBsAg (hepatitis B surface antigen) as a model antigen for targeted and sustained administration of the hepatitis B vaccine by subcutaneous injection. As a targeted alteration, mannose may boost humoral and cellular immune responses as well as immune cell absorption of nanoparticles. Another type of nanoparticle is based on VLPs (virus-like particles), which utilize HBcAg (hepatitis B core antigen) and improve VPL-based vaccine for the treatment of hepatitis B (Mobini et al. 2020). The nanoparticles with their types are given in Table 14.2. The diagrammatic representation for the treatment of liver infected with hepatitis B by currently used immunotherapeutic methods in combination with nanoparticles is shown in Figure 14.3.

14.2.4 Nanoparticles in Immunotherapy for Hepatitis C Virus (HCV) Causing Liver Cancer

Hepatitis C viral infections in the liver are caused by the hepatitis C virus, which contains RNA as a genetic material. Its infection affects 70 million people worldwide and has left many people with liver cirrhosis and liver cancer (Chung, Lee, and Zhang 2023). Although immune cells provide defense to liver cells and create memory against the antigens, but infections can be lethal if the body's immunological response is inadequate (Esper et al. 2010). Conventional methods of treatments, including vaccinations made of modified viruses or antigens, could be economically feasible, but it takes a lot of time. In addition, gene therapy can make alterations in non-targeted healthy cells produce genotoxicity in them (Lin, Revia, and Zhang 2021), whereas in an immunotherapeutic method, the immune system can be primed to identify tumor or virus-infected cells via messenger RNA (mRNA) coding for particular tumor antigens. These cells thus become susceptible to apoptosis brought on by the body's innate, cytotoxic immune cells. Although the benefits are achieved, poor stability and high immunogenicity are the disadvantages.

Use of nanoparticles can help the mRNA for its targeted and stable delivery to the specific cells and tissue in the treatment of liver cancer (Chung, Lee, and Zhang 2023). Most commonly used nanoparticle vectors for the mRNA are lipid nanoparticles, polymeric nanoparticles, and protein-based nanoparticles. There are a variety of lipid molecules which are being used, and one with

TABLE 14.2
Types of Nanoparticles Used for the Treatment of Hepatitis B

Nanoparticles	Type	Vaccine Component	Reference
Polymeric	SpyTag–ferritin based	PreS1 antibody	W. Wang et al. (2020)
	Mannose-modified poly(D,L-lactide-co-glycolic acid) based	HBsAg	Zhu et al. (2020)
Virus-like particles (VPLs)	HBcAg-based	HBsAg	Mobini et al. (2020)

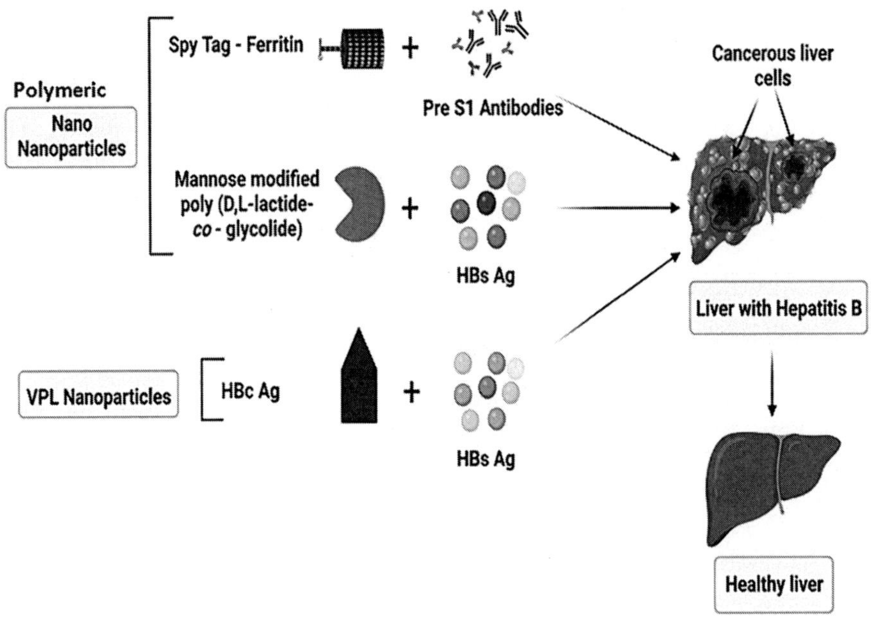

FIGURE 14.3 Nanoparticles in immunotherapy of HBV (hepatitis-B virus).

In the figure, SpyTag–ferritin nanoparticle vaccine can deliver anti–hepatitis B preS1 antibody (purple) to myeloid cells, such as lymphatic sinus-associated SIGNR1+ macrophages and dendritic cells, which can activate B cells and T follicular helper cells. SpyTag–ferritin (black and gray) nanoparticles vaccines are surface-modified with targeting ligands, such as anti–hepatitis B preS1 antibody (purple), to achieve selective binding to specific immune cells, such as lymphatic sinus-associated SIGNR1+ macrophages and dendritic cells, which can activate B cells and T follicular helper cells. The figure shows how to elicit high-level monoprophylaxis, reported using mannose-modified poly(D, L-lactide-co-glycolic acid) nanoparticles (sky blue) and VPL nanoparticle HBcAg (Brown) to load a model antigen HBsAg (hepatitis B surface antigen) for targeted and sustained administration of the hepatitis B vaccine by subcutaneous injection. As a targeted alteration, mannose may boost humoral (B cell response), cellular immune responses (T cell response), as well as immune cell absorption of nanoparticles.

cationic nature, which forms a bond with negatively charged nucleic acid, while some others work with phospholipids, cholesterol, and polyethylene glycol (PEG) (Ulkoski et al. 2021). Polymeric nanoparticles such as diethylaminoethyl methacrylate (DEAEMA) and dimethylaminoethyl methacrylate (DMAEMA) have been found as a suitable vector for the delivery of mRNA and/or other nucleic acids. In actuality, there are a number of mRNA-based cancer vaccines in clinical testing that are based on the lipid nanoparticles that were utilized to improve the mRNA vaccines' therapeutic advantages. The transfected cells by the mRNA cancer vaccines are immune cells rather than tumor cells. The idea behind this method involves expressing tumor antigens in order to activate cytotoxic immunity, which works against tumor cells. There are many mRNA-based vaccines under trial, and one which uses lipid nanoparticles as carrier to deliver mRNA coding for the tumor-associated genes that suppress tumor (p53) and produce apoptotic proteins against cancer cells, mRNA coding for the production of cytokines (IL-12) to polarize macrophages, and mRNA coding for the tumor antigens HCVcAg (hepatitis C virus core antigen) for the activation of T cells for the killing of cancer cells of the liver (Chung, Lee, and Zhang 2023). The diagrammatic representation for the treatment of liver infected with hepatitis C virus utilizing the most advocated immunotherapeutic method, that is, the use of mRNA vaccine exploiting the benefits of nanoparticles, is shown in Figure 14.4.

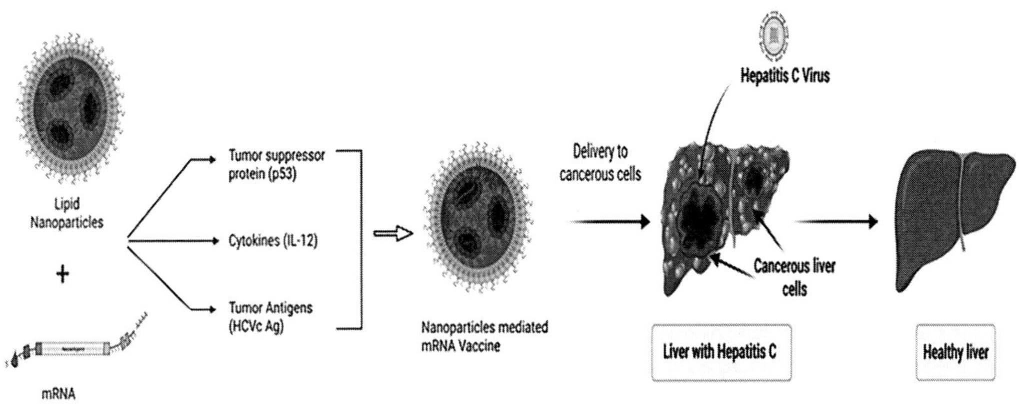

FIGURE 14.4 Nanoparticles in immunotherapy of HCV (hepatitis-C virus).

Schematic representation of the application of nanoparticles in the immunotherapy of HCV. (a) Nanoparticles loaded with mRNA (light blue) coding for the tumor-associated genes that suppress tumor and produce apoptotic proteins against cancer cells, mRNA coding the production cytokines (IL-12) to polarize macrophages, and mRNA coding for the tumor antigens HCVcAg (hepatitis C virus core antigen) for the activation of T cells for the killing of cancer cells of liver. (b) Representation of nanoparticles engineered with mRNA (yellow and blue spheres) inducing immune modulations, that is, suppresses tumor, and producing apoptotic proteins against cancer cells, mRNA coding the production cytokines (IL-12) to polarize macrophages, and mRNA coding for the tumor antigens HCVcAg (hepatitis C virus core antigen) for the activation of T cells killing the cancer cells of liver promoting anti-HCV immune responses. (c) View displaying the interaction between nanoparticles and HCV-infected cells (light-blue sphere) within the host.

14.2.5 Nanoparticles in Immunotherapy for Human T Cell Lymphotropic Virus-1 (HTLV-1) Causing ATL (Adult T Cell Leukemia/Lymphoma)

Adult T cell leukemia (ATL) is a fast-growing cancer associated with malignancy of $CD4^+$ T cells. It is caused by the human T cell lymphotropic virus type 1 (HTLV-1) (Mozhgani et al. 2020). A number of HTLV-1 proteins are essential for alteration in a cell and immortalization of T cells that are infected. As of right now, HTLV-1 infection is incurable. The HTLV-1 viral protein HBZ-based peptide vaccine has the lowest immunogenicity (Sugata et al. 2015). Nanoparticles such as trimethyl chitosan (TMC) and chitosan (CS) can be used to potentiate peptide antigens in order to boost immune responses against ATL (Amirnasr et al. 2016). In addition, nucleic acid–based vaccine constituted of nanoparticle chitosan (CS)–tripolyphosphate (TPP) in combination with plasmid DNA (pDNA) encoding HPV-E7 protein-based vaccine was formulated that can work well against ATL (Nunes et al. 2022) Table 14.3. The diagrammatic representation of the treatment of HTLV-1 taking advantages of CS-TPP-pDNA and other nanoparticles facilitating effective killing of cancerous $CD4^+$ T cells is shown in Figure 14.5.

14.2.6 Nanoparticles in Immunotherapy for Human Herpesvirus-8 (HHV-8) or Kaposi's Sarcoma-Associated Herpesvirus (KSHV) Causing Skin Cancer

Human herpesvirus-8 (HHV-8), referred to as Kaposi's sarcoma–associated herpesvirus (KSHV), is known as the eighth herpesvirus. It causes skin cancer (Kaposi 1982). Presently, there is no KSHV vaccine available. According to a study, the idea of generating a vaccine depends on the identification of the three virus proteins—gpK8.1, gB, and gH/gL—into KSHV-like particles similar to EBV virion, which develops a strong antibody response and could be an strong candidate for vaccine

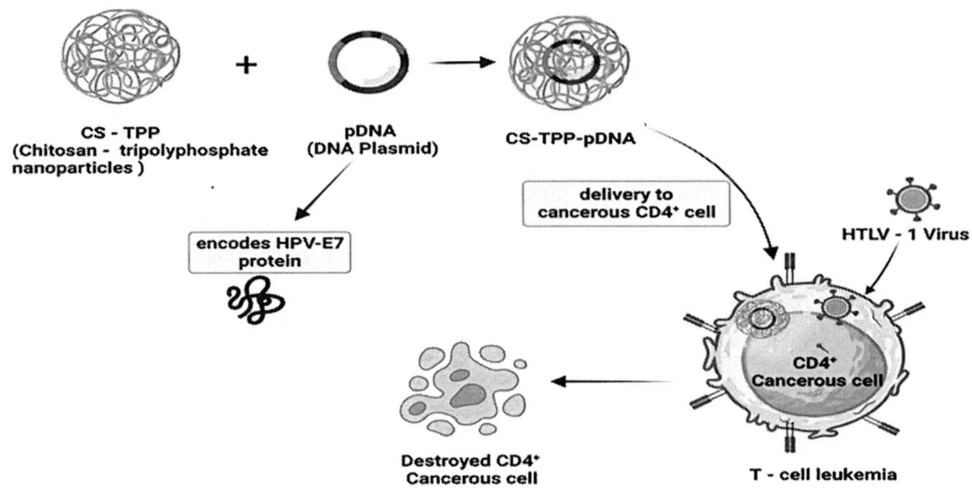

FIGURE 14.5 Nanoparticles in immunotherapy of HTLV-1 (human T cell lymphotropic virus). Schematic representation of the application of nanoparticles trimethylchitosan (TMC) and chitosan (CS) used to increase the potential of peptide antigens in order to boost immune responses against ATL in the immunotherapy of HTLV-1. Nanoparticles such as nucleic acid–based vaccine constituted of nanoparticle chitosan (CS)–tripolyphosphate (TPP) (light-yellow 3D sphere) in combination with plasmid DNA (pDNA, multicolor circular ring) encoding HPV-E7 protein was designed that works well against ATL (green sphere). The diagrammatic representation of the treatment of HTLV-1 taking advantages of CS-TPP-pDNA facilitating effective killing of cancerous $CD4^+$ T cells and generating immune response.

development (Granato 2021). Patients with γ-herpesvirus infections devoid of immunotherapy are treated with a variety of drugs, including bortezomib, the CHOP cocktail, and natural substances like curcumin or quercetin (Yoo et al. 2016; Granato 2021). These medications cause autophagy and apoptosis, which prevent these cancers from proliferating and from progressing through the cell cycle. However, nanoparticles (NPs) entrapped on the polyethylene glycol (PEG) surface contain some medications therein to move into particular tissues, and then the actions performed by drugs are more effective (Nunes et al. 2022) Table 14.3.

14.2.7 Nanoparticles in Immunotherapy for Merkel Cell Polyomavirus (MCPyV or MCV) Causing Skin Cancer

Merkel cell polyomavirus (MCPyV or MCV) is a rare cancer type in human and causes skin cancer with high mortality rate (Spurgeon and Lambert 2013; Dan Xu, Jiang, et al. 2021). A vaccine was developed with viral protein1 (VP1) target inducing both CD4+ and CD8+ T cells against CMS5-VP1 tumors in mice. Immunotherapy with this vaccine offers a unique therapeutic strategy for the management of MCV-related cancer in humans (Arora, Chang, and Moore 2012). Immunogenicity can be raised by dosage escalation or using lipid- and/or nucleic acid–based nanoparticles delivery methods, but currently, there is no such nanoparticles-based immunotherapy licensed so far for humans (Dan Xu, Jiang, et al. 2021) Table 14.3.

14.3 CONCLUSION

The advancement of nanotechnology has been crucial to the development of immunotherapeutics potential and to overcome the barriers in the treatment of various infectious diseases and cancers induced by viruses. Nanoparticles have been demonstrated in enhancing the effectiveness

TABLE 14.3
Nanoparticles Used in Immunotherapeutics of Virus Related to Cancer

Types of Oncoviruses	Cancer Type	Immunotherapeutic Agents	Nanoparticles Used	References
Epstein–Barr virus (EBV)	Stomach cancer Hodgkin's lymphoma, non-Hodgkin's lymphoma	Latency-associated EBV proteins	Prussian blue nanoparticles (PBNPs)	Burga et al. (2016)
Human papillomavirus (HPV)	Cervical cancer	E6 and E7 viral oncoproteins	Lipid-based nanoparticles, polymeric nanoparticles, inorganic nanoparticles, and exosomes-based nanoparticles	Zhou et al. (2022)
Hepatitis B viruses (HBV)	Liver cancer	PreS1, HBsAg, VPL	SpyTag–ferritin nanoparticle, mannose-modified poly(D,L-lactide-co-glycolic acid), and HBcAg	W. Wang et al. (2020); Zhu et al. (2020)
Hepatitis C viruses (HCV)	Liver cancer	mRNA coding antigen	Diethylaminoethyl methacrylate (DEAEMA), dimethylaminoethyl methacrylate (DMAEMA), lipid-based	Chung, Lee, and Zhang (2023)
Human Tcell lymphotropic virus-1 (HTLV-1)	Adult Tcell leukemia/ lymphoma	Peptide-coding antigen	Trimethyl-chitosan (TMC) and chitosan (CHT)	Amirnasr et al. (2016)
Human herpesvirus-8 (HHV-8) or KSHV	Skin cancer	Virus proteins—gpK8.1, gB, and gH/gL	N/A	Granato (2021)
Merkel cell polyomavirus (MCPyV)	Skin cancer	Viral protein1 (VP1)	N/A	Dan Xu, Jiang, et al. (2021)

N/A: currently, there are no nanoparticles available.

of currently available immunomodulators and vaccines. Nanoparticles stabilize and improve the cellular uptake and expression of mediums generating immune cells. Despite the advancement in nanoparticles-based immunotherapy, challenges still remain. Nano-immunotherapeutics needs more human clinical trials to ease the applications in treatment of viral-related cancers.

REFERENCES

Amirnasr, Maryam, Mojtaba Sankian, Abdorrahim Rezaei, and Mohsen Tafaghodi. 2016. "Immunization Against HTLV-I with Chitosan and Tri-Methylchitosan Nanoparticles Loaded with Recombinant env23 and env13 Antigens of Envelope Protein Gp46." *Microbial Pathogenesis* 97: 38–44.

Arora, Reety, Yuan Chang, and Patrick S Moore. 2012. "MCV and Merkel Cell Carcinoma: A Molecular Success Story." *Current Opinion in Virology* 2 (4): 489–98.

Artiga, Álvaro, Inés Serrano-Sevilla, Laura De Matteis, Scott G Mitchell, and Jesús M de la Fuente. 2019. "Current Status and Future Perspectives of Gold Nanoparticle Vectors for siRNA Delivery." *Journal of Materials Chemistry B* 7 (6): 876–96.

Bertoletti, Antonio, and Nina Le Bert. 2018. "Immunotherapy for Chronic Hepatitis B Virus Infection." *Gut and Liver* 12 (5): 497.
Bolhassani, Azam. 2023. "Lipid-Based Delivery Systems in Development of Genetic and Subunit Vaccines." *Molecular Biotechnology* 65 (5): 669–98.
Burga, Rachel A., Shabnum Patel, Catherine M. Bollard, Conrad Russell Y. Cruz, and Rohan Fernandes. 2016. "Conjugating Prussian Blue Nanoparticles onto Antigen-Specific T Cells as a Combined Nanoimmunotherapy." *Nanomedicine* 11 (14): 1759–67.
Chung, Seokhwan, Chan Mi Lee, and Miqin Zhang. 2023. "Advances in Nanoparticle-Based mRNA Delivery for Liver Cancer and Liver-Associated Infectious Diseases." *Nanoscale Horizons* 8 (1): 10–28.
Colón-López, Vivian, Ana P Ortiz, and Joel Palefsky. 2010. "Burden of Human Papillomavirus Infection and Related Comorbidities in Men: Implications for Research, Disease Prevention and Health Promotion Among Hispanic Men." *Puerto Rico Health Sciences Journal* 29 (3): 232.
Dang, Bao-Toan Nguyen, Taeg Kyu Kwon, Sooyeun Lee, Jee-Heon Jeong, and Simmyung Yook. 2024. "Nanoparticle-Based Immunoengineering Strategies for Enhancing Cancer Immunotherapy." *Journal of Controlled Release* 365: 773–800.
de Martel, Catherine, Damien Georges, Freddie Bray, Jacques Ferlay, and Gary M Clifford. 2020. "Global Burden of Cancer Attributable to Infections in 2018: A Worldwide Incidence Analysis." *The Lancet Global Health* 8 (2): e180–90.
Epstein, A. 2012. "Burkitt Lymphoma and the Discovery of Epstein–Barr Virus." *British Journal of Haematology* 156 (6): 777–79.
Esper, Raúl Carrillo, Estela Pérez Bustos, Sofía Ornelas Arroyo, Jorge Albores Saavedra, and Misael Uribe. 2010. "Liver Involvement in Severe Human Influenza a H1N1." *Annals of Hepatology* 9 (1): 107–11.
Farkona, Sofia, Eleftherios P. Diamandis, and Ivan M. Blasutig. 2016. "Cancer Immunotherapy: The Beginning of the End of Cancer?" *BMC medicine* 14 (1): 1–18.
Ferrall, Louise, Ken Y. Lin, Richard B. S. Roden, Chien-Fu Hung, and T.-C. Wu. 2021. "Cervical Cancer Immunotherapy: Facts and Hopes." *Clinical Cancer Research* 27 (18): 4953–73.
Goddard, Zoë Rachael, María J. Marín, David A. Russell, and Mark Searcey. 2020. "Active Targeting of Gold Nanoparticles as Cancer Therapeutics." *Chemical Society Reviews* 49 (23): 8774–89.
Granato, Marisa. 2021. "Nanotechnology Frontiers in γ-Herpesviruses Treatments." *International Journal of Molecular Sciences* 22 (21): 11407.
Gulley, Margaret L., Phyllis A. Eagan, Leticia Quintanilla-Martinez, Anabelle L. Picado, Bassam N. Smir, Craig Childs, Cory D. Dunn, Fiona E. Craig, J. W. Williams Jr, and Peter M. Banks. 1994. "Epstein-Barr Virus DNA Is Abundant and Monoclonal in the Reed-Sternberg Cells of Hodgkin's Disease: Association with Mixed Cellularity Subtype and Hispanic American Ethnicity." *Blood* 83: 1595–602.
Haney, Matthew J., Natalia L. Klyachko, Yuling Zhao, Richa Gupta, Evgeniya G. Plotnikova, Zhijian He, Tejash Patel, Aleksandr Piroyan, Marina Sokolsky, and Alexander V. Kabanov. 2015. "Exosomes as Drug Delivery Vehicles for Parkinson's Disease Therapy." *Journal of Controlled Release* 207: 18–30.
Herbst, Hermann, Erik Steinbrecher, Gerald Niedobitek, Lawrence S. Young, Louise Brooks, Nikolaus Muller-Lantzsch, and Harald Stein. 1992. "Distribution and Phenotype of Epstein-Barr Virus-Harboring Cells in Hodgkin's Disease." *Blood* 80: 1595–602.
Hosseini, Sare, and Parvaneh Dehghan. 2014. "Primary Non-Hodgkin Lymphoma of the Stomach: Clinicopathological Characteristics and Prognostic Factors in Iranian Patients." *Iranian Journal of Cancer Prevention* 7 (4): 219.
Jiang, Song, and Gil Redelman-Sidi. 2022. "BCG in Bladder Cancer Immunotherapy." *Cancers* 14 (13): 3073.
Kallingal, Anoop, Mateusz Olszewski, Natalia Maciejewska, Wioletta Brankiewicz, and Maciej Baginski. 2023. "Cancer Immune Escape: The Role of Antigen Presentation Machinery." *Journal of Cancer Research and Clinical Oncology*: 1–11.
Kang, Myung-Soo, and Elliott Kieff. 2015. "Epstein-Barr Virus Latent Genes." *Experimental & Molecular Medicine* 47 (1): e131.
Kaposi, Moriz. 1982. "Idiopathic Multiple Pigmented Sarcoma of the Skin." *CA: A Cancer Journal for Clinicians* 32 (6): 342–7.
Lampertico, Pietro, Kosh Agarwal, Thomas Berg, Maria Buti, Harry L. A. Janssen, George Papatheodoridis, Fabien Zoulim, and Frank Tacke. 2017. "EASL 2017 Clinical Practice Guidelines on the Management of Hepatitis B Virus Infection." *Journal of Hepatology* 67 (2): 370–98.
Lee, Hye Won, Jae Seung Lee, and Sang Hoon Ahn. 2020. "Hepatitis B Virus Cure: Targets and Future Therapies." *International Journal of Molecular Sciences* 22 (1): 213.
Li, Lin, Peng Zhang, Congcong Li, Yan Guo, and Kaoxiang Sun. 2021. "In Vitro/Vivo Antitumor Study of Modified-Chitosan/Carboxymethyl Chitosan 'Boosted' Charge-Reversal Nanoformulation." *Carbohydrate Polymers* 269: 118268.

Liao, John B. 2006. "Cancer Issue: Viruses and Human Cancer." *The Yale Journal of Biology and Medicine* 79 (3–4): 115.

Lin, Guanyou, Richard A. Revia, and Miqin Zhang. 2021. "Inorganic Nanomaterial-Mediated Gene Therapy in Combination with Other Antitumor Treatment Modalities." *Advanced Functional Materials* 31 (5): 2007096.

Mikelez-Alonso, Idoia, Antonio Aires, and Aitziber L. Cortajarena. 2020. "Cancer Nano-Immunotherapy from the Injection to the Target: The Role of Protein Corona." *International Journal of Molecular Sciences* 21 (2): 519.

Miles, Brett, Howard P. Safran, and Bradley J. Monk. 2017. "Therapeutic Options for Treatment of Human Papillomavirus-Associated Cancers-Novel Immunologic Vaccines: ADXS11-001." *Gynecologic Oncology Research and Practice* 4: 1–13.

Mishra, Swaroop, Paul Webster, and Mark E. Davis. 2004. "PEGylation Significantly Affects Cellular Uptake and Intracellular Trafficking of Non-Viral Gene Delivery Particles." *European Journal of Cell Biology* 83 (3): 97–111.

Mobini, Saeed, Milad Chizari, Ladan Mafakher, Elmira Rismani, and Elham Rismani. 2020. "Computational Design of a Novel VLP-Based Vaccine for Hepatitis B Virus." *Frontiers in Immunology* 11: 2074.

Mozhgani, Sayed-Hamidreza, Hanie Ahmadzade Kermani, Mehdi Norouzi, Mohsen Arabi, and Saber Soltani. 2020. "Nanotechnology Based Strategies for HIV-1 and HTLV-1 Retroviruses Gene Detection." *Heliyon* 6 (5).

Newman, Jenna H., and Andrew Zloza. 2017. "Infection: A Cause of and Cure for Cancer." *Current Pharmacology Reports* 3: 315–20.

Nunes, Renato, Ana Sofia Serra, Aiva Simaite, and Ângela Sousa. 2022. "Modulation of Chitosan-TPP Nanoparticle Properties for Plasmid DNA Vaccines Delivery." *Polymers* 14 (7): 1443.

Pandita, Deepti, Sandeep Kumar, and Viney Lather. 2015. "Hybrid Poly (Lactic-Co-Glycolic Acid) Nanoparticles: Design and Delivery Prospectives." *Drug Discovery Today* 20 (1): 95–104.

Rickinson, A. B. 1996. "Epstein-Barr Virus." *Fields Virology*: 2397–466.

Rooney, Cliona M., Marie A. Roskrow, Colton A. Smith, Malcolm K. Brenner, and Helen E. Heslop. 1998. "Immunotherapy for Epstein-Barr Virus-Associated Cancers." *JNCI Monographs* 1998 (23): 89–93.

Shahabi, Shakiba, Svea Döscher, Tobias Bollhorst, Laura Treccani, Michael Maas, Ralf Dringen, and Kurosch Rezwan. 2015. "Enhancing Cellular Uptake and Doxorubicin Delivery of Mesoporous Silica Nanoparticles Via Surface Functionalization: Effects of Serum." *ACS Applied Materials & Interfaces* 7 (48): 26880–91.

Shao, Kun, Santiswarup Singha, Xavier Clemente-Casares, Sue Tsai, Yang Yang, and Pere Santamaria. 2015. "Nanoparticle-Based Immunotherapy for Cancer." *ACS Nano* 9 (1): 16–30.

Sharma, Rajesh. 2021. "Global, Regional, National Burden of Breast Cancer in 185 Countries: Evidence from GLOBOCAN 2018." *Breast Cancer Research and Treatment* 187: 557–67.

Sheoran, Sumit, Swati Arora, R. Samsonraj, and Pilli Govindaiah. 2022. "Lipid-Based Nanoparticles for Treatment of Cancer." *Heliyon* 8 (5): e09403.

Singh, Archu, Yub Raj Neupane, Sadat Shafi, Bharti Mangla, and Kanchan Kohli. 2020. "PEGylated Liposomes as an Emerging Therapeutic Platform for Oral Nanomedicine in Cancer Therapy: In Vitro and in Vivo Assessment." *Journal of Molecular Liquids* 303: 112649.

Song, Hao, Xiao Su, Kaixuan Yang, Fangfang Niu, Jun Li, Jinjing Song, Huaiwen Chen, Bohua Li, Wei Li, and Weizhu Qian. 2015. "CD20 Antibody-Conjugated Immunoliposomes for Targeted Chemotherapy of Melanoma Cancer Initiating Cells." *Journal of Biomedical Nanotechnology* 11 (11): 1927–46.

Spurgeon, Megan E., and Paul F. Lambert. 2013. "Merkel Cell Polyomavirus: A Newly Discovered Human Virus with Oncogenic Potential." *Virology* 435 (1): 118–30.

Stremersch, Stephan, Roosmarijn E. Vandenbroucke, Elien Van Wonterghem, An Hendrix, Stefaan C. De Smedt, and Koen Raemdonck. 2016. "Comparing Exosome-Like Vesicles with Liposomes for the Functional Cellular Delivery of Small RNAs." *Journal of Controlled Release* 232: 51–61.

Sugata, Kenji, Jun-Ichirou Yasunaga, Yuichi Mitobe, Michi Miura, Paola Miyazato, Michinori Kohara, and Masao Matsuoka. 2015. "Protective Effect of Cytotoxic T lymphocytes Targeting HTLV-1 bZIP Factor." *Blood, the Journal of the American Society of Hematology* 126 (9): 1095–105.

Tan, Shuzhen, Dongpei Li, and Xiao Zhu. 2020. "Cancer Immunotherapy: Pros, Cons and Beyond." *Biomedicine & Pharmacotherapy* 124: 109821.

Tashiro, Haruko, and Malcolm K. Brenner. 2017. "Immunotherapy Against Cancer-Related Viruses." *Cell Research* 27 (1): 59–73.

Thompson, Matthew P., and Razelle Kurzrock. 2004. "Epstein-Barr Virus and Cancer." *Clinical Cancer Research* 10 (3): 803–21.

Thumrongsiri, Nutthanit, Paweena Dana, Rand Bawab, Prattana Tanyapanyachon, Chaichana Treetidnipa, Nattika Saengkrit, and Sith Sathornsumetee. 2022. "Assessment of Therapeutic Effect of CD20-Targeted

Immunoliposome in Primary Central Nervous System Lymphoma." *Biomedicine & Pharmacotherapy* 150: 112979.

Ulkoski, David, Michael J. Munson, Max E. Jacobson, Christian R. Palmer, Carcia S. Carson, Alan Sabirsh, John T. Wilson, and Venkata R. Krishnamurthy. 2021. "High-Throughput Automation of Endosomolytic Polymers for MRNA Delivery." *ACS Applied Bio Materials* 4 (2): 1640–54.

Wang, Dongyao, Binqing Fu, Xiaokun Shen, Chuang Guo, Yanyan Liu, Junfei Zhang, Rui Sun, Ying Ye, Jiabin Li, and Zhigang Tian. 2021. "Restoration of HBV-Specific CD8+ T-Cell Responses by Sequential Low-Dose IL-2 Treatment in Non-Responder Patients After IFN-α Therapy." *Signal Transduction and Targeted Therapy* 6 (1): 376.

Wang, Dongyao, Binqing Fu, and Haiming Wei. 2022. "Advances in Immunotherapy for Hepatitis b." *Pathogens* 11 (10): 1116.

Wang, Wenjun, Xiaoxiao Zhou, Yingjie Bian, Shan Wang, Qian Chai, Zhenqian Guo, Zhenni Wang, Ping Zhu, Hua Peng, and Xiyun Yan. 2020. "Dual-Targeting Nanoparticle Vaccine Elicits a Therapeutic Antibody Response Against Chronic Hepatitis B." *Nature Nanotechnology* 15 (5): 406–16.

World Health Organization. 2020. "World Health Organization 2021." In *COVID-19: Operational Guidance for Maintaining Essential Health Services During an Outbreak-Interim Guidance*, 25. World Health Organization.

Xiao, Shili, Rita Castro, João Rodrigues, Xiangyang Shi, and Helena Tomás. 2015. "PAMAM Dendrimer/pDNA Functionalized-Magnetic Iron Oxide Nanoparticles for Gene Delivery." *Journal of Biomedical Nanotechnology* 11 (8): 1370–84.

Xu, Dajun, Xiaoxiao Song, Jiahong Zhou, Xueliang Ouyang, Jinping Li, and Dawei Deng. 2021. "Virus-Like Hollow Mesoporous Silica Nanoparticles for Cancer Combination Therapy." *Colloids and Surfaces B: Biointerfaces* 197: 111452.

Xu, Dan, Sheng Jiang, Yue He, Xiang Jin, Gan Zhao, and Bin Wang. 2021. "Development of a Therapeutic Vaccine Targeting Merkel Cell Polyomavirus Capsid Protein VP1 Against Merkel Cell Carcinoma." *NPJ Vaccines* 6 (1): 119.

Yang, Jieru, Armira Azuar, Istvan Toth, and Mariusz Skwarczynski. 2022. "Liposomes for the Delivery of Lipopeptide Vaccines." *Vaccine Design: Methods and Protocols, Volume 3. Resources for Vaccine Development*: 295–307.

Yang, Xiao-Yan, Yun-Xia Li, Min Li, Li Zhang, Li-xia Feng, and Na Zhang. 2013. "Hyaluronic Acid-Coated Nanostructured Lipid Carriers for Targeting Paclitaxel to Cancer." *Cancer Letters* 334 (2): 338–45.

Yoo, Ji Young, Alena Cristina Jaime-Ramirez, Chelsea Bolyard, Hongsheng Dai, Tejaswini Nallanagulagari, Jeffrey Wojton, Brian S. Hurwitz, Theresa Relation, Tae Jin Lee, and Michael T. Lotze. 2016. "Bortezomib Treatment Sensitizes Oncolytic HSV-1-Treated Tumors to NK Cell Immunotherapy." *Clinical Cancer Research* 22 (21): 5265–76.

Zhang, Peipei, Yu-Chieh Chiu, Lisa H. Tostanoski, and Christopher M. Jewell. 2015. "Polyelectrolyte Multilayers Assembled Entirely from Immune Signals on Gold Nanoparticle Templates Promote Antigen-Specific T Cell Response." *ACS Nano* 9 (6): 6465–77.

Zhou, Xuyan, Haiying Lian, Hongpeng Li, Meiling Fan, Wei Xu, and Ye Jin. 2022. "Nanotechnology in Cervical Cancer Immunotherapy: Therapeutic Vaccines and Adoptive Cell Therapy." *Frontiers in Pharmacology* 13: 1065793.

Zhu, Jiahuan, Fuhua Qin, Zhonghua Ji, Weidong Fei, Zeng Tan, Ying Hu, and Caihong Zheng. 2020. "Mannose-Modified PLGA Nanoparticles for Sustained and Targeted Delivery in Hepatitis B Virus Immunoprophylaxis." *AAPS PharmSciTech* 21: 1–9.

15 Sequential Catalytic Nanomedicine-Enabled, Chemotherapy-Based Synergetic Cancer Treatments

Priyanka Chambial, Rhea Vas, and Neelam Thakur

ABBREVIATIONS

Acronym	Full Form
CDT	chemodynamic therapy
HER-2	human epidermal growth factor receptor 2
CPX-351	cytarabine and daunorubicin
TNF	tumor necrosis factor
PEG-THIOL	thiol-containing polyethylene glycol
CRLX101	colorectal cancer radiosensitizer
CaO2/MnO2	calcium peroxide, manganese dioxide
HIF-1/P-gp	hypoxia-inducible factor-1/P-glycoprotein
MCF-7	Michigan Cancer Foundation 7 (breast cancer cell line)
PDA	pancreatic ductal adenocarcinoma
AuNPs	silver nanoparticles
CPT	camptothecin
LTDC	light-triggered drug delivery system
PtNPs	platinum nanoparticles
Ce6	chlorine e6
TPZ	tirapazamine
CUR	curcumin
TACE	transarterial chemoembolization
VDA	vascular disruption agents
GOx	glucose oxidase
MDSCs	myeloid-derived suppressor cells
Tregs	regulatory T cells
NKT cells	natural killer T cells
DCs	dendritic cells
LPS	lipopolysaccharides
CpG-ODN	CpG oligodeoxynucleotides
PAMAM	poly(amidoamine)
TAAs	tumor-associated antigens
NO	nitric oxide
Inos	inducible nitric oxide synthase
PIC	polyriboinosinic: polyribocytidylic acid

DOI: 10.1201/9781003463191-18

HMPB	hollow mesoporous Prussian blue
DSF	drug disulfiram
PVP	polyvinylpyrrolidone
CuS	copper sulfide
RNP	ribonucleoprotein
Mpeg	methoxypolyethylene glycol
SPN	semiconducting polymer nanoparticle
MAPK	mitogen-activated protein kinase
CuL-2	Cullin
MMP-2	matrix metalloproteinase-2

15.1 INTRODUCTION

Cancer's pathological process is intricate. Lack of selectivity, cytotoxicity, generation of multidrug resistance, and stem-like cell proliferation are just some of the issues with current chemotherapy (Shi et al. 2016). Although treatment choices have improved over the years, serious side effects from hostile chemotherapies still exist, despite decades of research revealing the ever-changing nature of the disease (Zhu et al. 2022). Treatment centers have long relied on chemotherapy as the gold standard for both primary and secondary malignant tumors. There are a variety of ways to treat cancer, including chemotherapy, starvation therapy, targeted therapy, and immunotherapy (Tilsed et al. 2022). The main distinction between them is depicted in Table 15.1. Chemotherapy and targeted therapy both are effective cancer treatment options, but chemotherapy also damages healthy cells in addition to malignant cells. Targeted therapy, on the other hand, favorably picks out and destroys cancer cells while allowing healthy cells to survive. Since the end of the Second Great War, there has been a critical expansion in the number of imaginative chemotherapy prescriptions that have been found or fabricated. Be that as it may, chemotherapy might cause various disagreeable incidental effects, and it can likewise prompt different medication obstructions (Hassan et al. 2022).

TABLE 15.1
Distinction between Various Cancer Treatment Approaches

	Chemotherapy	Targeted Therapy	Starvation Therapy	Immunotherapy	References
Working	Rapidly target dividing cancerous cells	Usually target the proteins required for cancer growth	Targeted inhibition of angiogenic factors	Uses immune systems against cancer growth	Chen et al. (2018); Sandesh et al. (2021)
Limitations	Not specific Cancer cells develop resistance to chemotherapy	Cancer cells develop resistance	Low targeted efficacy Elevated tumor hypoxia Metastasis risk	Tailored Expensive	Chen et al. (2018); Mishra et al. (2022)
Side effects	Nausea Hair loss Intestinal damage	Skin problems Liver problems Vomiting Nausea Blood test abnormalities	Fatigue Lowered immunity	Autoimmune effect	Chen et al. (2018); Mishra et al. (2022)

Both of these variables improve the probability that malignant growth treatment will not find lasting success. Inadmissible clinical outcomes might be ascribed to the antagonistic microenvironment of growths, which makes it challenging for synthetic drugs to infiltrate the cancer (Rezvantalab et al. 2018). Patients with malignant growths that undergo oncogenic transformations will have persistent carcinogenic replications, followed by metastases to normal organs. This is notwithstanding the chemotherapy's unavoidable damage to ordinary tissues and organs. Subsequently, there is little inquiry that the quest for and advancement of malignant growth treatment regimens that are both more compelling and more secure are of colossal importance to both exploration and clinical practice (Zhang et al. 2022).

Researchers have shown that cancer metastasis treatments are substantially more effective when they use nanomedicine, which is based on a targeted medication delivery mechanism. Therefore, nanotechnology-based techniques represent a potentially beneficial research topic for both the detection of cancer at an early stage and the development of novel, highly effective treatments for the disease. On average, chemotherapy relies on cytotoxic antineoplastic drugs to eradicate cancer cells (Hou et al. 2022). Drugs or other substances used in targeted cancer therapy interfere with specific molecules essential to the growth and spread of tumors, hence halting their development and spreading. As a result of the quick development of nanotechnology, it is presently conceivable to successfully fabricate an assortment of multifunctional specialists at the nanoscale. These specialists show a lot of commitment as nanomedicines in the determination, counteraction, and treatment of diseases. Nanodotedimers (NDDSs) have drawn a great deal of interest as of late, especially in the field of malignant growth treatment (Entzian and Aigner 2021). As of late, the FDA has given its approval to various nano-definitions for use in clinical malignant growth treatment (for instance, paclitaxel egg whites–bound nanoparticles [Abraxane], liposomal irinotecan [Onivyde], etc.), and a lot more nanomedicines are, at present, going through clinical testing. Since designed nanomedicine can specifically, or even on request, discharge their freight in light of explicit excitements at the growth tissues, it is feasible to amplify the restorative impact while limiting the poisonous secondary effects (Jani and Gohil 2018). In contrast, subatomic synthetic drugs exhibit limited efficacy in targeting a specific disease (Man et al. 2018). Even though nanomedicine-enabled chemotherapy has demonstrated promising efficacy in treating cancer, a singular chemotherapy approach frequently proves insufficient in eradicating cancer cells, hence increasing the risk of cancer recurrence and jeopardizing the patient's life and well-being (Niza et al. 2021). Recent breakthroughs in nanomedicine-based chemotherapy have demonstrated a shift from monotherapy to multimodal synergistic treatment for cancer (Norouzi and Hardy 2021). The multimodal synergistic therapy of tumors is made possible by multifunctional nanoplatforms that incorporate the benefits of diverse therapeutic approaches. Smart nano-stages can also reliably coordinate various therapeutic modalities, such as photothermal therapy, photodynamic therapy, chemodynamic therapy, etc. In this context, we have discussed recent advances in multimodal treatments for malignant growth that make use of nanomedicine and a synergistic approach between chemotherapy and other disciplines (Xie et al. 2020). Nanomedicine-based chemotherapy may have synergistic benefits when combined with other treatments, such as phototothermotherapy, photodynamic therapy, chemotherapy-actuated photodynamic therapy (CDT), immunotherapy, and calorie deprivation (Figure 15.1). This comprehensive review includes the specifics of the multimodal synergistic treatment based on nanomedicine-enhanced chemotherapy, as well as its current challenges, prospects, and everything in between. In many cases, the synergistic effects of a combination of therapy modalities will improve clinical outcomes. Cancers as varied as non–small cell lung cancer and gastric cancer benefit from a multimodal approach to treatment (Pham et al. 2020).

Nanomedicines have the potential to enhance the effectiveness of traditional chemotherapy by efficiently transporting drugs into cells. NDDSs can be reproduced and modified to become multifunctional nanoplatforms for energy storage in vivo or in vitro conditions. However, blocking

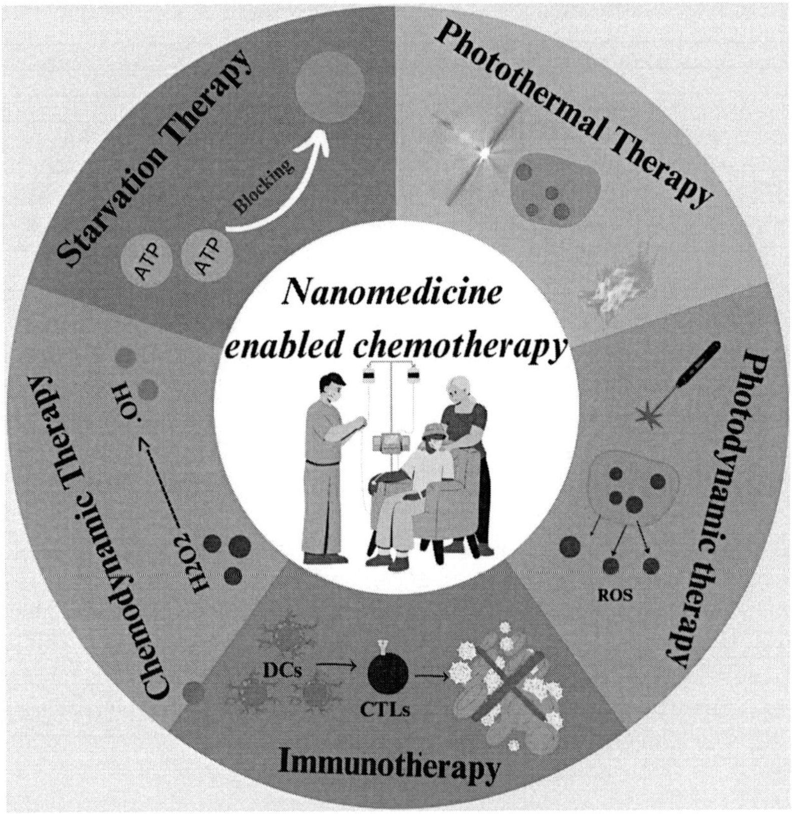

FIGURE 15.1 Detailed summary of synergistic chemotherapy-based strategies and their related modalities. These modalities include immunotherapy, chemodynamic therapy, starvation therapy, photothermal therapy, and photodynamic therapy.

natural growth impediments and designing malignant growth microenvironments can lead to unappealing clinical results. Nano-experts, such as size/surface charge-inconsistent nanomedicines and particle shape–variable nanoparticles, can address these issues. P-glycoprotein (P-gp) can also be used to siphon cytotoxic molecules from cells. Nanomedicine-enabled chemotherapy combined with Pgp inhibitors can overcome multidrug barriers in threatening development by converting non-toxic substances into cytotoxic ones, reducing adverse effects on various organs due to its exceptional biocatalytic performance (Liu et al. 2016).

15.2 NANOMEDICINE-BASED CHEMOTHERAPY

Traditionally, nanotechnology has been employed in cancer drugs to improve the pharmacokinetics of chemotherapy and reduce its systemic toxicities through the targeted delivery of anticancer agents to tumor tissues. By enclosing chemotherapeutics in nanoformulations or attaching them to the surfaces of nanoparticles, nanosized carriers improve the therapeutic index of the administered drug (Wu et al. 2022). Chemotherapy is one of the most popular clinical therapies nowadays because of how easily it can be administered. Multiple in vivo screens performed on tumors transplanted in laboratory mice demonstrated that paclitaxel possessed a broad spectrum of antitumor effects. With the approval of the polymer–protein conjugate Zinostatin stimalamer

100 in Japan for the treatment of hepatocellular carcinoma and the introduction of the PEGylated liposome Doxil® in the United States for the treatment of ovarian cancer, nanoformulations have been marketed for medical use against cancer since the early 1990s. The FDA has approved some chemotherapeutic drugs for use in treating cancer. Examples include Taxol, carboplatin, and Herceptin for HER2/neu-positive tumors and Platinol (cisplatin) and Navelbine for the treatment of non–small cell lung cancer. However, because of differences in pharmacokinetics and biodistribution of drugs, merely delivering two or more treatments at once is inefficient (Wei et al. 2021). The emergence of nanotechnology offers the potential to address the problem. Maintaining the physicochemical properties of the chemotherapeutic drugs used in chemotherapy combination therapy improves their efficacy in shrinking tumors. Several nanomedicines with two active ingredients have been the subject of preclinical and clinical studies or clinical trials in recent years; these include irinotecan, paclitaxel, cytarabine/daunorubicin, etc. Finding the optimal dosage ratio of two medications at which their combined effects can produce the best results is one of the important components of chemotherapy combination therapy. Cytarabine and daunorubicin in CPX-351 have an optimized molar ratio of 5:1, which can produce the most therapeutic benefit for acute myeloid leukemia.

One treatment modality under investigation at the moment is targeted chemotherapy, which administers a tumor necrosis factor (TNF) agent to malignant tumors. Thiol-derivatized polyethylene glycol (PEG-THIOL) and a gold nanoparticle are used to conceal the TNF-carrying nanoparticle from the immune system. Therefore, the nanoparticle is safe to transport through the circulatory system. Another experimental targeted chemotherapy treatment that employs CRLX101 is in the works (Spadavecchia et al. 2016). This innovative form of chemotherapy is being developed by Cerulean Pharma. The usage of manganese dioxide nanoparticles, which are designed to concentrate in a tumor and create oxygen, has been proven to increase the efficacy of doxorubicin as a drug used for chemotherapeutics. Mesoporous silica nanoparticles have been used successfully by researchers to deliver the chemotherapeutic medication irinotecan to pancreatic cancer tumors. According to studies done on mice, this technique lessens the toxicity of the treatment. University of Georgia researchers are developing a strategy to combat prostate cancer. In this case, nanoparticles are used to transport a chemical called IPA-3 to the cancer cells. Preliminary studies in mice suggest that IPA-3 can inhibit the development of prostate cancer cells (Filadi et al. 2023). There are some options for treating cancer, but many of them are impractical against multidrug-resistant (MDR) forms of the disease. The development of resistance to many anticancer drugs is an alarming threat, and this issue of MDR cannot be overlooked. The number of biomedical research efforts aimed at developing chemotherapeutics that can avoid or reverse MDR is rising rapidly (Zhang et al. 2021). In this context, researchers devised and built a calcium peroxide–covered lipid monostearin (MS) vehicle to drastically enhance DOX transport and overcome MDR. Using this vehicle, we were able to finally combat MDR. Once cancer cells have taken up the nanomedicine and it has been latently improved in cancer areas via EPR influence, the disease cells will undergo the following improvements: At first, the dynamic prescription's core was hidden by the MS layers of the NPs, but this was unraveled when the NPs were exposed to the extremely transmitted lipase in malignant growth cells (Lee et al. 2018). As soon as ten minutes have passed, the exposed DOX-CaO centers will react with the water, ushering in the potentially lethal arrival of DOX and oxygen. Later, the drug that was draining P-gp's activity was overcome by the oxygen-activated HIF-1/P-gp hindrance. This resulted in a longer duration, during which DOX was maintained intracellularly, which was crucial for achieving increased anticancer viability. Another multifunctional nanomedicine successfully developed by the researchers delivers siRNA to inhibit P-gp protein expression, hence increasing DOX chemotherapy's efficacy. Hence, in recent times, there has been a growing interest in investigating combination strategies to augment the effectiveness of cancer treatment, as indicated in Table 15.2.

TABLE 15.2
Combination with Chemotherapy Treatment Approaches

Combination	Nanoplatform	Agent	Cancer (In Vitro)	References
Combination with PTT	ZrC@prodrug Au/Fe3O4/ PVA-10%DXL DOX/MNP-PMs F@PDA-TPP/SS/ DOX	SN38-Nif + ZrC NSs DXL + AuNPs DOX + iron oxide nanoparticles DOX + PDA	A549 and SMMC- 7721 MCF-7 A549 B16F10	Kemp et al. (2016) Wang et al. (2017); Liu et al. (2020); Taheri-Ledari et al. (2020)
Combination with PDT	CPT-TK-HPPH/Pt NP PCT@HCCT DOX-loaded; H-LTDC TPZ/AI-NVs	CPT + PtNP Cisplatin + Ce6 DOX + Ps TPZ + Ce6	CT26 4T1 HCT-116 HepG2	Hao et al. (2020); Lei et al. (2020)
Combination with CDT	iRPPA@TMZ/MnO DOX@Cu2O-PEG NCs AMSNs/DOX Vk3@MOF-199 NPs 4T1	TMZ + MnO DOX + Cu (II) DOX + MnO2 Vitamin K3 + Cu²+	C6 MCF-7 Huh-7 4T1	Tian et al. (2021) Gu et al. (2020)
Combination with immunotherapy	PEG-CDM-PEI-P(CURDT) CM@MON@DOX LMWH/PPD/CpG TA-OBL	CUR + NLG919 DOX + anti-PD-L1 DOX + CpG Oxaliplatin + ApoA1 mimic peptide	B16F10 4T1 B16F10 4T1	Yu et al. (2021)

15.3 STARVATION THERAPY AND SYNERGISTIC CHEMOTHERAPY USING NANOMEDICINES

Signaling pathways and cell metabolism dysfunction are the two main hallmarks of cancer. Reactive oxygen species (ROS) play an important role in the growth of cancer, yet paradoxically, they also offer a promising approach to cancer treatment. They cause DNA damage, which is the main mechanism underlying cancer formation, and act as signaling molecules that promote the most challenging aspects of tumor progression, such as metastasis and drug resistance. While chemodynamic therapy and certain chemotherapies have shown success in the laboratory, their clinical application is complex due to the challenge of effectively increasing ROS levels within cancer cells without inducing excessive apoptosis (Liu et al. 2019). Many types of cancer cells are killed by silver (Ag) ions by increasing intracellular oxidative stress, destroying mitochondria, and initiating cell autophagy. Researchers created a glucose oxidase (GOx)–conjugated silver nanocube (AgNC-GOx) for Ag ion administration to take advantage of the synergy between starvation and metal ion therapy. In the presence of AgNC-GOx, glucose was broken down into gluconic acid and hydrogen peroxide after being taken up by tumor cells. Increased acidity of TME due to accumulated gluconic acid sped up the breakdown of silver nanocomposite and the production of Ag ions at the tumor site (Liu et al. 2017). Transarterial chemoembolization (TACE), vascular disruption agents (VDAs), and angiogenesis inhibitory agents (AIAs) can all cut off a tumor's blood supply and stop the delivery of nutrients. Poor targeting efficiency, increased tumor hypoxia-induced resistance to medicines, and increased risk of tumor dissemination are just some of the problems these treatments can cause

(Wang et al. 2021). When used in conjunction with other cancer treatment modalities, combination therapy of cancer-starving drugs is a successful technique for addressing these obstacles and increasing therapeutic efficiency. There are two primary approaches to the development of starving nanotherapeutics. The blood supply to a tumor can be cut off or reduced in two ways: by directly constricting blood vessels or by blocking or disrupting angiogenesis. The other strategy involves limiting the tumor's access to food and oxygen by limiting the tumor's intake of food and oxygen. Mesoporous silica nanoparticles (MSNs) can improve the targeting efficacy of tanshinone IIA, an angiogenesis inhibitor, to hypoxia-inducible factor (HIF-1) overexpression in a mouse model (HT-29), leading to enhanced antiangiogenesis action (Yu et al. 2019).

Combinations of chemotherapeutics and angiogenesis inhibitors have been widely employed to address the limitations of chemotherapeutics and improve the efficacy of cancer treatment. Antiangiogenic nanotherapeutics tailored for combination therapy have recently emerged. For instance, angiogenesis inhibitors have been employed in conjunction with chemotherapeutics to improve anticancer activity, according to a 2019 research published in the journal *Theranostics* (Prasad et al. 2013). Combination cancer therapy now includes the use of engineered antiangiogenic nanotherapeutics. For instance, doxorubicin and mitomycin C (MMC) co-loaded polymer–lipid hybrid nanoparticles showed better animal survival and tumor cure rate compared to liposomal DOX in multidrug-resistant human mammary tumor xenografts. Camptothecin (CPT) and sorafenib were co-delivered using a nanocarrier responsive to matrix metalloproteinase-2 (MMP-2) in another trial, and their synergistic effect against colorectal cancer seemed promising. Starving cancer cells by inhibiting their abnormal metabolism is a promising new direction in cancer treatment. It is possible to limit the metabolism of cancer cells by blocking both glycolysis and oxidative phosphorylation at the same time, resulting in cell death. Several methods have been developed to "starve" cancer cells, including interfering with tumor angiogenesis by inhibiting angiogenic factors or their receptors and integrins, cutting off the blood supply to tumors through embolization or compression, and interfering with the metabolic process of tumors by blocking the signal pathways of mitochondria. Various sequential multimodal therapies were developed for the cancer microenvironment and achieved high therapeutic efficacy and amplification, in part by combining starvation therapy and activated chemotherapy (H. Li et al.).

A well-planned nanosystem utilizing starvation therapy and PtNP-based chemotherapy should be used to eradicate tumors. By coating GOx and PtNPs in poly(lactic-co-glycolic acid) (PLGA), we were able to build a functional nanosystem (GOx-Pt-NS) that enhanced the cellular uptake of PtNPs, as shown in Figure 15.2. Nanoparticles' increased permeability and retention (EPR) effect caused GOx-Pt-NS to concentrate more strongly in tumors. The protective qualities of the GOx-Pt-NS allowed it to overcome several of the shortcomings of GOx: weaknesses of GOx include its short half-life in vivo, high immunogenicity, and systemic toxicity (Meng et al. 2022).

15.4 SYNERGISTIC CHEMOTHERAPY AND IMMUNOTHERAPY–BASED NANOMEDICINE

Immunotherapy is currently receiving a lot of attention as a potential treatment for cancer, from "cold tumors" like pancreatic and cervical cancer to "hot tumors" like lung cancer and melanoma. The credibility of combining cancer immunotherapy with traditional therapeutic methods has been bolstered in recent years by many clinical trials demonstrating the therapeutic efficacy of such combination medicines (Galluzzi et al. 2020). The synergistic anticancer impact of polymer NP medication delivery is achieved by encapsulating treatments such as immunotherapy and chemotherapy. Combining immunotherapy and chemotherapeutics can improve cancer treatment by conveying a cell death signal and increasing antitumor immunogenicity, which is further potentiated by immune stimulation (Vanneman and Dranoff 2012). The immunogenicity of tumors can be improved, and antitumor immune responses can be sparked by chemotherapeutic drugs that promote immunogenic cell death (ICD). Damage-associated molecular patterns (DAMPs) are released, which aid in this

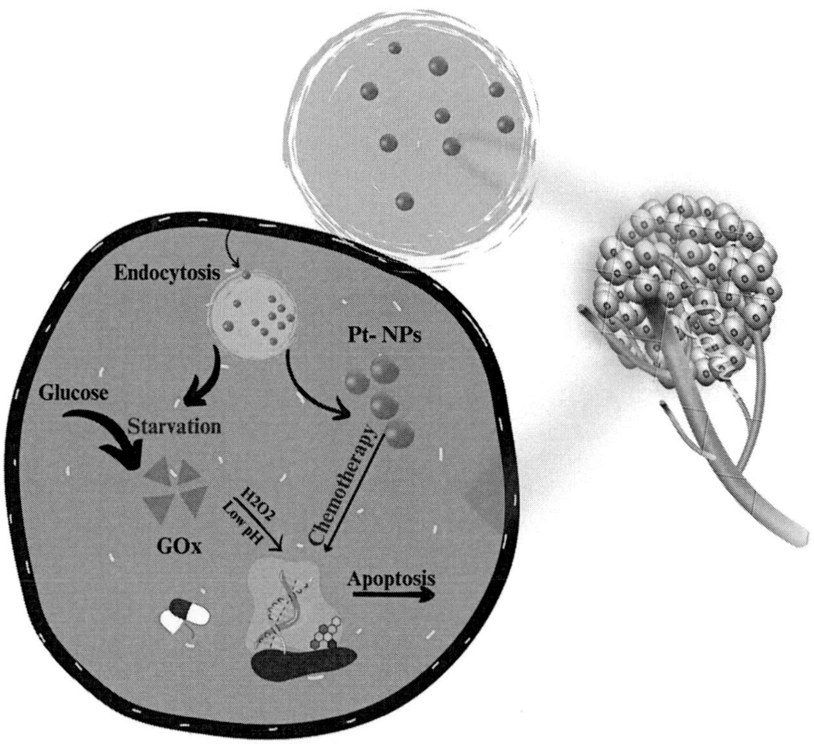

FIGURE 15.2 Diagrammatic representation of GOx and PtNPs coated with PLGA to create a functional nanosystem (GOx-Pt-NS). This will improve PtNPs' cellular absorption. Through the nanoparticles' EPR action, the accumulation of GOx-Pt-NS in tumors considerably increased.

process. Some examples of DAMPs are CRT, ATP, and high-mobility group protein B1 (HMGB). These DAMPs are essential for the development of mature dendritic cells (DCs) and the presentation of antigens to T cells. To boost the cellular immune response against tumors, activated T cells draw in cytotoxic T cells (CTLs). The anticancer effects of chemotherapy are boosted by the immune system's activation in this way (X. Li et al. 2022).

Immunotherapy is hampered by the tumor microenvironment, which frequently displays immunosuppressive features, such as the adenosine pathway. To combat this problem, scientists have created thermally sensitive, E-selectin-modified micelles that may simultaneously transport a chemotherapeutic drug (DOX) and an A2A adenosine receptor antagonist. These micelles, when exposed to microwaves, can have a dual chemo- and immunotherapeutic impact. This strategy tries to improve therapy outcomes by increasing the immune response and inhibiting the immunosuppressive adenosine pathway, both of which the tumor cells are targeted with DOX (Ahmed and Tait 2020).

By increasing the immunogenicity of tumors, as in ICD, certain chemotherapeutic drugs are used. High-mobility group protein B1, adenosine triphosphate (ATP), and calreticulin (CRT) are all examples of DAMPs that are released during ICD. These DAMPs are essential for the development of mature dendritic cells (DCs) and the presentation of antigens to T cells. A stronger cellular immune reaction against the tumor results. Immunosuppressive cells in the TME can also be removed with chemotherapy. Cells like Tregs and MDSCs dampen the body's natural defenses against cancer and allow the malignancy to flourish. To restore the immune system and kill tumor cells, chemotherapy can slow down and eliminate these immunosuppressive cells. Tumor cells can be made more vulnerable to immunological attack by chemotherapy. Chemotherapy helps the immune system identify and kill any leftover cancer cells by damaging tumor cells and producing inflammation. The immune system and chemotherapy working together have been shown to increase treatment results and overall survival (Qi et al. 2021).

In the surveyed studies, various immunotherapy agents have been employed in NP-mediated cancer immunotherapy to elicit specific outcomes. The synthesis of chemotherapeutic medicines and cytokines by carrier-mediated mechanisms was succinctly presented in Table 15.3. It has been demonstrated to be highly effective to combine chemotherapy with immune cell–based therapies, such as T cells and NKT cells, in the treatment of cancer. These immune cells recognize tumor cells and kill them by several different mechanisms, because of their powerful antitumor cytotoxicity. By stimulating particular pathways, chemotherapy may increase their cytotoxicity. Alendronate activates T cells, and doxorubicin co-encapsulated in a PEGylated liposome resulted in a synergistic antitumor impact. Similarly, the maximum level of apoptosis was observed in breast cancer cell

TABLE 15.3
Integration of Immunostimulants and Chemotherapeutics via Carrier

Carrier	Immunotherapy Agent	Chemotherapy Agent	Synergistic Effect	Cancer	Reference
Lipophilic prodrugs nanoassemblies/IV	TLR7 agonist		Effective apoptosis induction, tumor growth and angiogenesis suppression, and absence of tumor recurrence, TAAs and R837 working together to stimulate DCs result in a powerful tumor-specific immune response.	Breast	Lee et al. (2011) Roy et al. (2013)
Polymeric NPs (PEG-PEI/Tail vein)	TLR2 agonist	DOX	Higher activation of apoptosis and prevention of tumor growth.	Breast	Seth et al. (2014)
G4-Arga/PLGA-PEG-PLGA hydrogel/IV	L- arg	DOX	Synergistic immune therapy through the production of NO by providing a substrate.	Breast	Han et al. (2018)
PLGA/peritumoral	LPS		Greater antitumor immune response than with PTX and P-LPS alone at the TME.	Melanoma	Li et al. (2019)
Aptamer-G4 PAMAM bioconjugate/IV)	CpG, ODN		When compared to mice treated with free DOX, combined treatment had excellent antitumor activity.	Prostate	Kang et al. (2019)
γ-PGA/intratumoral	TLR-7 agonist	PTX	Extreme repression of tumor development. Enhanced DC activation and proliferation, as well as increased PIC and Th1 cytokine production.	Lung, Cervical	Ha and Kim (2021)
HDL nanodiscs/ intratumoral	TLR-9 agonist, ODN	DTX	Optimal tumor-killing power with the fewest possible unintended consequences. Mice given both treatments outlived mice given DTX alone by a significant margin.	Colon	Ha and Kim (2021)

lines when PTX was used first, followed by zoledronic acid. Sensitizing tumor cells to immunotherapy by administering chemotherapeutic drugs before immune cell treatment avoids the potential of immune cell suppression that can occur with simultaneous administration (Luo et al. 2019).

To improve the efficacy of DOX in chemo-immunotherapy, the team created Cu-Wear, a self-assembled nanosized oxidative stress amplifier. To induce immunogenic chemotherapy, Cu-Wear uses the coupling of Cu^{2+}, DOX, and NLG919. After accumulating in tumor tissue, the Cu-Wear nanoparticles' GSH-responsive drug release property enables them to release DOX via the EPR effect. Increased immunogenic cell death (ICD) results from induced oxidative stress, which is amplified by Cu^{2+}-mediated GSH depletion. NLG919 has been shown to reactivate the immune response and modify the immunosuppressive tumor microenvironment by simultaneously inhibiting indoleamine 2,3-dioxygenase 1 (IDO-1). The patient's immune system will be better able to spot and kill tumors, both locally and systemically, as a result of this approach (Prendergast et al. 2018).

15.5 NANOMEDICINE-BASED SYNERGISTIC CHEMOTHERAPY AND PTT

In numerous preclinical animal investigations, synergistic phototherapy and chemotherapy have shown their capacity to increase therapeutic efficacies, minimize adverse effects, and exhibit many distinct advantages over conventional chemotherapy. The term "photothermal therapy" describes the use of light-induced heat to treat cancer. This therapeutic approach has been viewed as a promising anticancer treatment since it can be spatially and temporally controlled, preventing harm to unintended areas. Photothermal therapy (PTT) is a relatively novel physical mechanism that utilizes the absorption of electromagnetic energy by an agent, such as nanoparticles, to generate heat upon irradiation with a laser (He et al. 2023). This heat can induce cell damage, similar to hyperthermia. However, photothermal therapy has an additional advantage in that it can trigger drug release from nanoassemblies. Since tissues are only partially transparent to light in the near-infrared (NIR) range (650–900 nm), photothermal therapy can obtain great light responsiveness even at modest laser strengths by utilizing nanoparticles with strong absorption in this range. This allows for precise and controlled treatment. Furthermore, the ability of NIR light to penetrate deeply into tissues enables the use of low concentrations of the photothermal agent, minimizing potential side effects. Overall, photothermal therapy holds promise as a targeted and efficient approach for both hyperthermia-based cell damage and controlled drug release, making it a valuable tool in the field of cancer treatment. To treat cancer, researchers have recently investigated the use of BMNPs (biomimetic magnetic nanoparticles) as photothermal agents, specifically in the context of combining guided chemotherapy and photothermal therapy. To explore this possibility, researchers produced DOXO-BMNP nanoassemblies by functionalizing bimetallic nanoparticles (BMNPs) with doxorubicin (DOXO) (Zou et al. 2016).

The aim was to analyze the response of these nanoassemblies to near-infrared (NIR) laser irradiation, which is commonly used in photothermal therapy. The NIR laser can generate localized hyperthermia, which releases the chemotherapy agent from the nanoassemblies and enhances its therapeutic efficacy. Additionally, the anticancer activity of these nanoassemblies was investigated (H. Li et al. 2022). To test the efficacy of this combined therapy, the HepG2 human hepatoma cell lines were used as a model. By combining directed chemotherapy with photothermal therapy using BMNPs, researchers aimed to achieve a synergistic effect, where the hyperthermia induced by the NIR laser enhances the cytotoxicity of the chemotherapy agent. By more precisely focusing on tumor cells and reducing adverse effects on healthy tissue, this strategy may boost the effectiveness of cancer treatments (Jabalera et al. 2021).

Another research focuses on the development of a nanomedicine called Cu-HMPB, which is based on Prussian blue and contains empty mesopores. In this study, a Cu-HMPB nanomedicine was created and loaded with a chemotherapy drug called disulfiram (DSF). The goal was to enhance the effectiveness of DSF chemotherapy through a photothermal mechanism using a chelating reaction between DSF and Cu2+ (Peer et al. 2007; Jabalera et al. 2021).

PTT and chemotherapy are a promising combination for treating cancer. PTT uses nanoparticles, such as Cu-Wear nanoparticles, to absorb electromagnetic energy and produce heat, which, in turn, triggers medication release. This can improve drug sensitivity, lessen the likelihood of adverse effects, and lessen the likelihood of drug resistance, by encouraging the formation and penetration of drug carriers in tumors. However, chemotherapy can eliminate tumors that were not reached by laser irradiation and help with the removal of primary tumors by PTT. CuS-RNP/DOX@PEI is a NIR-activated smart switch that exemplifies this combo. By using near-infrared (NIR) light to activate this thermo-responsive mechanism twice, a synergistic photo-chemotherapy strategy is made possible. This strategy can enhance the results of cancer treatment by overcoming the limitations of PTT and chemotherapy individually. Using an improved double-emulsion approach, researchers created a novel porphyrin-based micelle that could be used to load DOX and paclitaxel concurrently. The micelle was synthesized when the amphiphilic polymer mPEG-PLGA-porphyrin was self-assembled (Feng et al. 2017). The dual-drug-loaded micelles could produce a lot of heat and release two medications simultaneously to destroy the cancer cells when exposed to NIR radiation. More significantly, the combination of PTT and chemotherapy increased cancer cells' chemosensitivity and led to tumor shrinkage with just a tenth of the usual medication dosage (Su et al. 2016).

15.6 NANOMEDICINE-BASED SYNERGISTIC CHEMOTHERAPY AND PDT

Using targeted multifunctional nanoparticles allows enhanced drug delivery and accumulation in tumor tissues. The zein/hyaluronate acid/tannin/Cu^{2}+ loaded with IR780 nanoparticles (ZHTC@IR780) specifically target cancer cells due to the overexpression of hyaluronate acid receptors. This targeted delivery system improves drug efficacy and reduces off-target effects, minimizing damage to healthy tissues. The combination of CDT and PDT provides a synergistic effect in cancer treatment. CDT utilizes the catalytic decomposition of endogenous hydrogen peroxide by ZHTC@IR780 nanoparticles, generating oxygen that can further react with oxygen to produce toxic singlet oxygen upon exposure to 808 nm laser irradiation. This process relieves the tumor's hypoxic microenvironment and induces cytotoxic effects (Cui et al. 2019). Moreover, the glutathione oxidase-like effects of ZHTC@IR780 nanoparticles generate Fenton-like cuprous ions and deplete glutathione (GSH), leading to the efficient production of hydroxyl radicals (•OH). The combination of CDT and PDT enhances the antitumor effect by inducing immunogenic cell death, increasing calreticulin eversion, releasing histones, and promoting apoptosis of tumor cells. Overall, the use of targeted multifunctional nanoparticles like ZHTC@IR780 provides a promising approach for synergetic cancer therapy. The combination of CDT and PDT, along with targeted drug delivery, improves treatment outcomes by enhancing the antitumor effect and stimulating the immune system's response. This approach holds great potential for effective and targeted cancer treatment with reduced side effects (Z . Li et al. 2022).

A semiconducting polymer with grafted polyethylene glycol was demonstrated by researchers. In addition to having photodynamic action, this polymer proved a good vehicle for the conjugation of other chemotherapeutic medicines, including bromoisophosphoramide. The hypoxia-activatable phototherapeutic polymeric prodrug systems were initially developed. This semiconducting polymer nano-prodrug (SPNpd) activates its chemotherapeutic activity in a hypoxic microenvironment by effectively producing singlet oxygen when exposed to near-infrared (NIR) photo-irradiation (Cui et al. 2019).

Researchers have found that self-assembly of the prodrug linoleic acid (LNA)-thioketal-cabazitaxel (LTK-CTX) and the photosensitizer chlorine e6 (L-Ce6) resulted in the formation of a nanoassembly. When exposed to near-infrared (NIR) light, the tumor cells that had taken up the co-assembled L-Ce6 component of the PSPC nanoassembly produced a large amount of ROS. The cytotoxicity of cabazitaxel was boosted thanks to this ROS production, which sped up the breakdown of the drug's thioketal (TK) bonds. Cabazitaxel also worked in tandem with photodynamic treatment (PDT) to kill tumor cells more effectively. It indicates the possibility of enhancing tumor

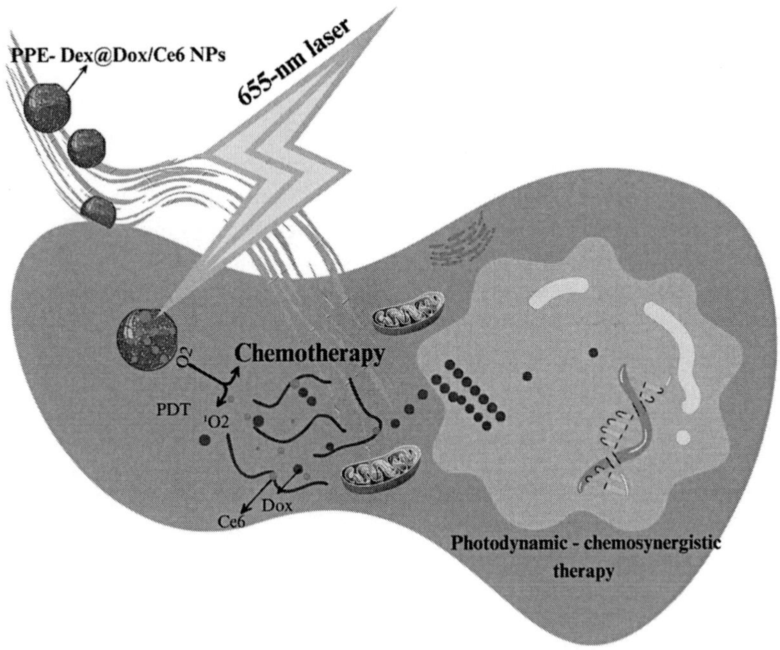

FIGURE 15.3 Diagrammatically shown PPE-Dex NPs, or poly(phenyleneethynylene)-dextrans nanoparticles, have shown remarkable potential in improving cancer treatment efficacy. Recent studies have demonstrated that PPE-Dex NPs can be used to co-deliver the chemotherapy drug doxorubicin (DOX) and the photosensitizer Ce6, resulting in synergistic therapeutic effects against cancer cells under irradiation.

therapy by combining self-assembling prodrugs with photosensitizers to generate a synergistic impact. Targeted ROS generation and increased antitumor effects are made possible by photoactivating the PSPC nanoassembly, making this a promising strategy for future cancer therapy methods (Huang et al. 2021).

Anticancer drugs like doxorubicin (Dox) and photosensitizers like chlorin e6 (Ce6) can be delivered to cancer cells together using a membrane-extrusion emulsification approach to create ROS-degradable nanoparticles based on phenylboronic pinacol ester-conjugated dextran. The medications contained within these nanoparticles can be released in response to ROS produced by Ce6 when exposed to laser irradiation. This double action causes not only considerable photodynamic treatment (PDT) effects in cancer cells but also PPE-Dex to be rapidly oxidized and degraded. Therefore, this results in rapid Dox release and increased Dox accumulation within nuclei, which improves the treatment's therapeutic efficacy, as shown in Figure 15.3 (Chen et al. 2019).

15.7 NANOMEDICINE–BASED SYNERGISTIC CHEMOTHERAPY AND CDT

CDT has gained attention in recent years due to its benefits of tumor specificity, low toxicity, and minimal side effects. The idea of CDT was put forth as a therapeutic approach that uses Fenton or Fenton-like reaction to generate hydroxyl radicals in the tumor site in light of the acidic and hydrogen peroxide overexpressed circumstances in TME. In the initial CDT study, iron-based nanomaterials produced ferrous ion, which might catalyze endogenous hydrogen peroxide breakdown into •OH under acidic TME conditions. CDT, in contrast to photothermal therapy (PTT), does not call for any external stimulation to be effective (Z. Li et al. 2022). When chemotherapy is combined with CDT, not only are the latter's negative effects mitigated, but the former's are also increased. For instance, scientists created a metal-organic framework termed MIL-100@DOX-HA (DMH) that is loaded with DOX and has been modified. DMH's superior DOX-loading efficiency enhanced the efficacy of chemotherapy (X. Li et al . 2022). DMH also produced copious quantities of poisonous •OH via Fenton reactions, which boosted CDT's efficacy. DMH nanoparticles may improve the therapeutic efficacy of DOX in breast cancer while decreasing its systemic toxicity. Since ferroptosis, an iron-based cell death process, is highly effective in killing cancer cells, its activation has received a lot of attention in cancer research. One mechanism to induce ferroptosis is through the upregulation of ROS via the Fenton reaction. Cisplatin, an activated chemotherapy drug, can elevate intracellular hydrogen peroxide levels through cascade reactions, making it an ideal partner for ferroptosis-assisted chemotherapy (CDT). For instance, researchers have developed a core-shell platform called PtH@FeP, combining cisplatin prodrug-based chemotherapy and chemodynamic treatment (CDT). The platform not only supplies hydrogen peroxide for the Fenton reaction, inducing ferroptosis, but also directly eliminates tumors (Zhang et al. 2023). This combination strategy amplifies intratumoral oxidative stress, resulting in a synergistic effect and promising applications in multidrug chemotherapy.

Exogenous $Cu^{2}+$ administration and the biodistribution of $Cu^{2}+$ in the body present substantial obstacles to the development of DSF chemotherapy. For the synergistic treatment of DSF by CDT, however, new research has concentrated on generating innovative nanocatalytic formulations for the accurate delivery of DSF and $Cu^{2}+$ in cancer. Such a formulation, such as the DSF@ PEG/Cu-HMSNs, uses uncoated mesoporous silica nanoparticles to transport the active ingredient. These nanoparticles collapse in the TME, rapidly releasing $Cu^{2}+$ and their cargo of DSF (Wu et al. 2019). Toxic CuET products are then formed when the co-released $Cu^{2}+$ ions react with DSF in situ via a chelation process. Furthermore, reactive oxygen species (ROS) are produced by a Fenton-like process involving Cu^{+} ions and overexpressed hydrogen peroxide. The TME is acidic enough to facilitate both of these reactions.

A pH-responsive nanoparticle (DSF/DOX@ZIF-8@Cu-TA) was produced in a recent study to improve chemotherapy using CDT. By enclosing DSF and DOX in zeolitic imidazole framework-8 (ZIF-8) and coating it with $Cu^{2}+$ and tannic acid (TA), a nanoparticle was produced. From 86.5 to 99.2 nm, the nanoparticle grew in size and underwent a shift from a hexagonal shape to a spherical shell. ZIF-8 nanoparticles assisted in the effective transport of the encapsulated medicines to the tumor site, where they were then released in the slightly acidic tumor microenvironment, where they generated large amounts of the very lethal CuL2 and ROS, as shown in Figure 15.4 (Meng et al. 2021). Improved therapeutic efficacy of CDT-coordinated chemotherapy was seen due to the nanoparticle's ability to block reactive oxygen species mitogen-activated protein kinases (ROS-MAPK) signaling pathways, which, in turn, amplified the anticancer action of DOX.

15.8 CHALLENGES TO OVERCOME

Although first misconstrued as a panacea, nanomedicines cannot fully address the problems associated with cancer chemotherapy. Research in this area is still in its infancy. Several significant challenges must be addressed before nanomedicine-enabled chemotherapy can speedily move from the laboratory to the clinic or hospital. The improved metabolic kinetics that emerge from the chemical interactions between nanoparticle carriers and therapeutic medicines make targeted drug delivery more difficult (Rasool et al. 2022). Finding more efficient methods of synthesis and construction is crucial for the continued clinical translation of therapeutic nanomedicines for two reasons: (1) although nanomedicine has the potential to improve chemotherapy, the EPR effect requires a developed tumor microenvironment, which is not always present, and (2) the EPR effect is dependent on a tumor's genetic makeup, which can be altered by a variety of factors. The term "nanomaterial-induced endothelial leakage" (NanoEL) describes a second mechanism by which nanoparticles actively target tumors; nonetheless, more study is needed to considerably boost the tumoral accumulation efficacy of nanomedicines for enhanced therapeutic efficacy. Particularly in the tumor microenvironment, nanomedicines can catalyze processes that produce ROS or other

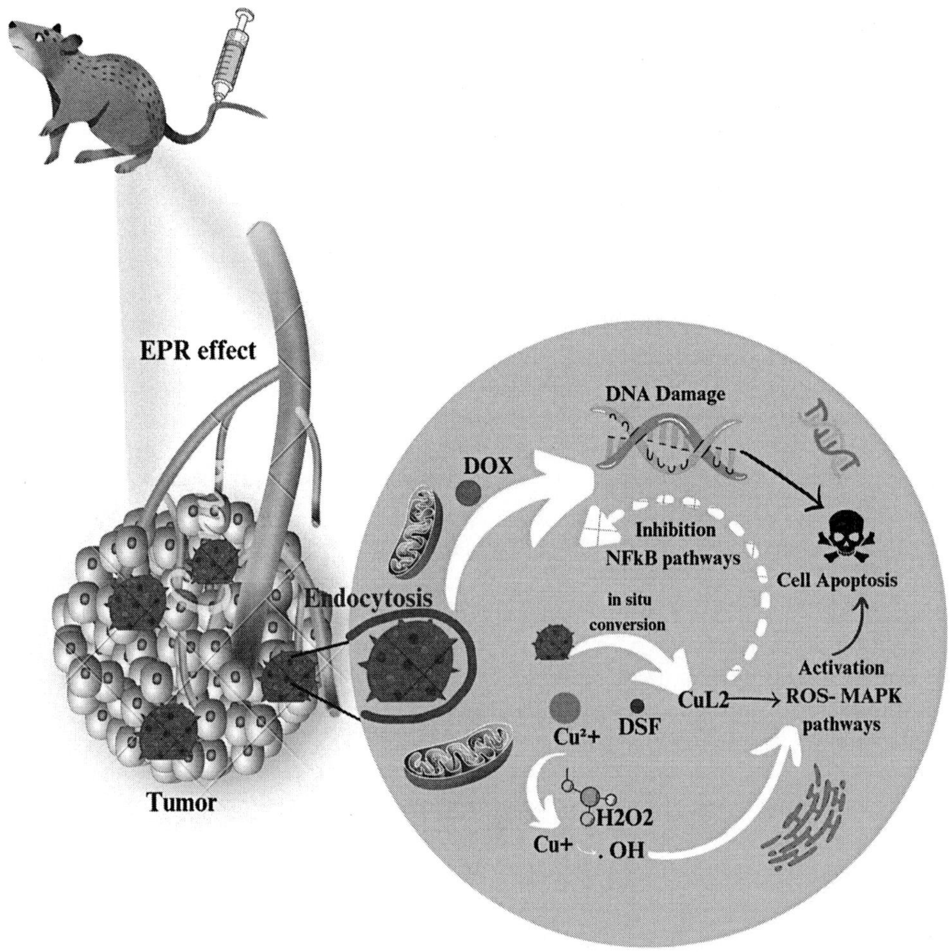

FIGURE15.4 This schematic diagram depicts the synergistic chemotherapy and CDT mediated by DSF/DOX@ZIF-8@Cu-TA in vivo. Intratumoral DSF-Cu2+ chelating results in extremely toxic bis (N, N-diethyl dithiocarbamate) copper(II) complexes (CuL2) and reactive oxygen species (ROS), and DSF/DOX@ZIF-8@Cu-TA continuously releases Cu^{2}+, DSF, and DOX in situ in the moderately acidic TME.

hazardous chemicals. However, it is possible that transition metals, like copper ions, released into the body could cause unanticipated damage. Nanomedicines can also accumulate heavily in the liver and spleen, posing challenges for their clinical application (Dessale et al. 2022). To address these concerns, future advancements in coordination chemistry may lead to the development of safer nanomedicines with enhanced biosafety, achieved through the careful selection of transition metals and organic ligands.

We can address this challenge by the development of nanocatalytic formulations that allow for precise control over the co-delivery of drugs and transition metal ions. By using empty mesoporous silica nanoparticles as functional nanocarriers, researchers can load drugs and metal ions separately and achieve their simultaneous release in the tumor microenvironment. However, the potential toxicity of metal ions and the accumulation of nanomedicines in certain organs pose challenges for clinical application. The design of safer nanomedicines with enhanced biosafety is crucial for their successful translation into clinical practice. Future advancements in coordination chemistry may offer solutions to these challenges (Al-Zoubi and Al-Zoubi 2022). By fine-tuning the coordination bonds between the nanocarrier and the metal ions, researchers can achieve controlled release of the metal ions and minimize their toxicity. Additionally, the development of biodegradable nanocarriers can facilitate the clearance of nanomedicines from the body, reducing the risk of accumulation and potential long-term side effects.

15.9 CONCLUSION

Despite the development of certain anti-disease drugs that are now being researched and developed, chemotherapy is still a successful method for eliminating dangerous malignant growth cells. A thorough examination of the science of malignant growth has led to the successful use of a wide range of chemotherapeutic prescriptions with various mechanisms of action. This has significantly increased the variety of chemotherapy alternatives available for treating specific types of malignant growths. Nanomedicine's potential to facilitate the mixing of chemotherapy with other treatment modalities has shown promise in increasing the therapeutic efficacy of cancer treatment. Various combinations of cancer treatments have been investigated. Finding the right dosages of these nanomedicines to work in synergy can be difficult, though. This can lead to wasted medication or adverse effects. The therapeutic efficacy and biosafety of nanomedicines can be improved by strict regulation of their structure, components, and other factors. Nanomedicine-enabled chemotherapy combined with other treatment modalities could greatly improve cancer care in the clinic if these problems could be solved. Finally, the co-delivery of medicines and transition metal ions in nanocatalytic formulations for cancer treatment shows significant promise for increasing the efficacy of chemotherapy and attaining synergistic tumor therapy. However, the dosing techniques and biosafety of these nanomedicines need more work before they can be successfully applied in clinical settings.

REFERENCES

Ahmed, Asma, and Stephen W. G. Tait. 2020. "Targeting Immunogenic Cell Death in Cancer." *Molecular Oncology* 14 (12): 2994–3006. https://doi.org/10.1002/1878-0261.12851.

Al-Zoubi, Mazhar Salim, and Raed M. Al-Zoubi. 2022. "Nanomedicine Tactics in Cancer Treatment: Challenge and Hope." *Critical Reviews in Oncology/Hematology* 174: 103677. https://doi.org/10.1016/j.critrevonc.2022.103677.

Chen, Xiao-Jie, Xue-Qiong Zhang, Qi Liu, Jing Zhang, and Gang Zhou. 2018. "Nanotechnology: A Promising Method for Oral Cancer Detection and Diagnosis." *Journal of Nanobiotechnology* 16 (1). https://doi.org/10.1186/s12951-018-0378-6.

Chen, Yu, Yujie Gao, Yuce Li, Ke Wang, and Jintao Zhu. 2019. "Synergistic Chemo-Photodynamic Therapy Mediated by Light-Activated Ros-Degradable Nanocarriers." *Journal of Materials Chemistry B* 7 (3): 460–8. https://doi.org/10.1039/c8tb03030h.

Cui, Dong, Jiaguo Huang, Xu Zhen, Jingchao Li, Yuyan Jiang, and Kanyi Pu. 2019. "A Semiconducting Polymer Nano-prodrug for Hypoxia-activated Photodynamic Cancer Therapy." *Angewandte Chemie International Edition* 58 (18): 5920–4. https://doi.org/10.1002/anie.201814730.

Dessale, Mesfin, Getachew Mengistu, and Hylemariam Mihiretie Mengist. 2022. "Nanotechnology: A Promising Approach for Cancer Diagnosis, Therapeutics and Theragnosis." *International Journal of Nanomedicine* 17: 3735–49. https://doi.org/10.2147/ijn.s378074.

Entzian, Kristin, and Achim Aigner. 2021. "Drug Delivery by Ultrasound-Responsive Nanocarriers for Cancer Treatment." *Pharmaceutics* 13 (8): 1135. https://doi.org/10.3390/pharmaceutics13081135.

Feng, Qianhua, Yuanyuan Zhang, Wanxia Zhang, Yongwei Hao, Yongchao Wang, Hongling Zhang, Lin Hou, and Zhenzhong Zhang. 2017. "Programmed Near-Infrared Light-Responsive Drug Delivery System for Combined Magnetic Tumor-Targeting Magnetic Resonance Imaging and Chemo-Phototherapy." *Acta Biomaterialia* 49: 402–13. https://doi.org/10.1016/j.actbio.2016.11.035.

Filadi, Riccardo, Agnese De Mario, Matteo Audano, Patrizia Romani, Silvia Pedretti, Cesar Cardenas, Sirio Dupont, Cristina Mammucari, Nico Mitro, and Paola Pizzo. 2023. "Sustained IP3-Linked Ca2+ Signaling Promotes Progression of Triple Negative Breast Cancer Cells by Regulating Fatty Acid Metabolism." *Frontiers in Cell and Developmental Biology* 11. https://doi.org/10.3389/fcell.2023.1071037.

Galluzzi, Lorenzo, Juliette Humeau, Aitziber Buqué, Laurence Zitvogel, and Guido Kroemer. 2020. "Immunostimulation with Chemotherapy in the Era of Immune Checkpoint Inhibitors." *Nature Reviews Clinical Oncology* 17 (12): 725–41. https://doi.org/10.1038/s41571-020-0413-z.

Gu, Dihai, Peijing An, Xiuli He, Hongshuai Wu, Zhiguo Gao, Yaojia Li, Fanghui Chen, et al. 2020. "A Novel Versatile Yolk-Shell Nanosystem Based on Nir-Elevated Drug Release and GSH Depletion-Enhanced Fenton-Like Reaction for Synergistic Cancer Therapy." *Colloids and Surfaces B: Biointerfaces* 189: 110810. https://doi.org/10.1016/j.colsurfb.2020.110810.

Ha, Ji-Hui, and Young-Jin Kim. 2021. "Photodynamic and Cold Atmospheric Plasma Combination Therapy Using Polymeric Nanoparticles for the Synergistic Treatment of Cervical Cancer." *International Journal of Molecular Sciences* 22 (3): 1172. https://doi.org/10.3390/ijms22031172.

Han, Yue, Bixi Ding, Ziqiang Zhao, Huaqing Zhang, Bo Sun, Yuanpei Zhao, Lei Jiang, Jianping Zhou, and Yang Ding. 2018. "Immune Lipoprotein Nanostructures Inspired Relay Drug Delivery for Amplifying Antitumor Efficiency." *Biomaterials* 185: 205–18. https://doi.org/10.1016/j.biomaterials.2018.09.016.

Hao, Ying, Yuwen Chen, Xinlong He, Yongyang Yu, Ruxia Han, Yang Li, Chengli Yang, Danrong Hu, and Zhiyong Qian. 2020. "Polymeric Nanoparticles with Ros-responsive Prodrug and Platinum Nanozyme for Enhanced Chemophotodynamic Therapy of Colon Cancer." *Advanced Science* 7 (20). https://doi.org/10.1002/advs.202001853.

Hassan, Taimoor, Xiaojia Huang, Chao Zhou, Muhammad Sikander Khan, and Sana Saeed. 2022. "Nanoparticles in Cancer Treatment: A Narrative Review." *Proceedings of the Pakistan Academy of Sciences: B. Life and Environmental Sciences* 58 (3): 1–18. https://doi.org/10.53560/ppasb(58-3)664.

He, Yu-Chu, Zi-Ning Hao, Zhuo Li, and Da-Wei Gao. 2023. "Nanomedicine-Based Multimodal Therapies: Recent Progress and Perspectives in Colon Cancer." *World Journal of Gastroenterology* 29 (4): 670–81. https://doi.org/10.3748/wjg.v29.i4.670.

Hou, Shanshan, Muhammad Hasnat, Ziwei Chen, Yinong Liu, Mirza Muhammad Faran Ashraf Baig, Fuhe Liu, and Zelong Chen. 2022. "Application Perspectives of Nanomedicine in Cancer Treatment." *Frontiers in Pharmacology* 13. https://doi.org/10.3389/fphar.2022.909526.

Huang, Lingling, Jianqin Wan, Honghui Wu, Xiaona Chen, Qiong Bian, Linlin Shi, Xinchi Jiang, Anran Yuan, Jianqing Gao, and Hangxiang Wang. 2021. "Quantitative Self-Assembly of Photoactivatable Small Molecular Prodrug Cocktails for Safe and Potent Cancer Chemo-Photodynamic Therapy." *Nano Today* 36: 101030. https://doi.org/10.1016/j.nantod.2020.101030.

Jabalera, Ylenia, Alberto Sola-Leyva, María P. Carrasco-Jiménez, Guillermo R. Iglesias, and Concepcion Jimenez-Lopez. 2021. "Synergistic Photothermal-Chemotherapy Based on the Use of Biomimetic Magnetic Nanoparticles." *Pharmaceutics* 13 (5): 625. https://doi.org/10.3390/pharmaceutics13050625.

Jani, R. K., and K. M. Gohil. 2018. "Liposomal Formulations in Cancer Therapy: Basic Concepts to Advanced Strategies." *International Journal of Pharmaceutical Sciences and Drug Research* 10 (5). https://doi.org/10.25004/ijpsdr.2018.100505.

Kang, Tianyi, Yang Li, Yong Wang, Jiao Zhu, Ling Yang, Yulan Huang, Meimei Xiong, et al. 2019. "Modular Engineering of Targeted Dual-Drug Nanoassemblies for Cancer Chemoimmunotherapy." *ACS Applied Materials & Interfaces* 11 (40): 36371–82. https://doi.org/10.1021/acsami.9b11881.

Kemp, Jessica A., Min Suk Shim, Chan Yeong Heo, and Young Jik Kwon. 2016. "'Combo' Nanomedicine: Co-Delivery of Multi-Modal Therapeutics for Efficient, Targeted, and Safe Cancer Therapy." *Advanced Drug Delivery Reviews* 98: 3–18. https://doi.org/10.1016/j.addr.2015.10.019.

Lee, Gayoung, Jin-Yong Joung, Jung-Hyo Cho, Chang-Gue Son, and Namhun Lee. 2018. "Overcoming P-Glycoprotein-Mediated Multidrug Resistance in Colorectal Cancer: Potential Reversal Agents Among Herbal Medicines." *Evidence-Based Complementary and Alternative Medicine* 2018: 1–9. https://doi.org/10.1155/2018/3412074.

Lee, In-Hyun, Sukyung An, Mi Kyung Yu, Ho-Keun Kwon, Sin-HyeogIm, and Sangyong Jon. 2011. "Targeted Chemoimmunotherapy Using Drug-Loaded Aptamer-Dendrimer Bioconjugates." *Journal of Controlled Release* 155 (3): 435–41. https://doi.org/10.1016/j.jconrel.2011.05.025.

Lei, Guang, Yilei Zhang, Pranavi Koppula, Xiaoguang Liu, Jie Zhang, Steven H. Lin, Jaffer A. Ajani, et al. 2020. "The Role of Ferroptosis in Ionizing Radiation-Induced Cell Death and Tumor Suppression." *Cell Research* 30 (2): 146–62. https://doi.org/10.1038/s41422-019-0263-3.

Li, Honghui, Ying Zhang, Lingxia Liang, Jiaxing Song, Zixuan Wei, Shuyue Yang, Yunong Ma, Wei R. Chen, Cuixia Lu, and Liewei Wen. 2022. "Doxorubicin-Loaded Metal-Organic Framework Nanoparticles as Acid-Activatable Hydroxyl Radical Nanogenerators for Enhanced Chemo/Chemodynamic Synergistic Therapy." *Materials* 15 (3): 1096. https://doi.org/10.3390/ma15031096.

Li, Man, Yuting Yang, Chaoqun Xu, Jiaojie Wei, Yingke Liu, Xingli Cun, Qianwen Yu, et al. 2019. "Tumor-Targeted Chemoimmunotherapy with Immune-Checkpoint Blockade for Enhanced Anti-Melanoma Efficacy." *The AAPS Journal* 21 (2). https://doi.org/10.1208/s12248-018-0289-3.

Li, Xiang, Yupeng Wang, Qiankun Shi, Nuo Zhen, Jin Xue, Jingsheng Liu, Dongfang Zhou, and Hao Zhang. 2022. "Zein-Based Nanomedicines for Synergistic Chemodynamic/Photodynamic Therapy." *ACS Omega* 7 (33): 29256–65. https://doi.org/10.1021/acsomega.2c03404.

Li, Zhiyan, Xianghui Li, Shichao Ai, Song Liu, and Wenxian Guan. 2022. "Glucose Metabolism Intervention-Facilitated Nanomedicine Therapy." *International Journal of Nanomedicine* 17: 2707–31. https://doi.org/10.2147/ijn.s364840.

Liu, Dong, Fang Yang, Fei Xiong, and Ning Gu. 2016. "The Smart Drug Delivery System and Its Clinical Potential." *Theranostics* 6 (9): 1306–23. https://doi.org/10.7150/thno.14858.

Liu, Ken, Xiang Zhang, Weiqi Xu, Jinbiao Chen, Jun Yu, Jennifer R Gamble, and Geoffrey W McCaughan. 2017. "Targeting the Vasculature in Hepatocellular Carcinoma Treatment: Starving Versus Normalizing Blood Supply." *Clinical and Translational Gastroenterology* 8 (6). https://doi.org/10.1038/ctg.2017.28.

Liu, Quan, Zhongjian Xie, Meng Qiu, Inseob Shim, Yunlong Yang, Sisi Xie, Qinhe Yang, et al. 2020. "Prodrug-Loaded Zirconium Carbide Nanosheets as a Novel Biophotonic Nanoplatform for Effective Treatment of Cancer." *Advanced Science* 7 (24). https://doi.org/10.1002/advs.202001191.

Liu, Zongjun, Tuo Li, Fang Han, You Wang, Yang Gan, Junhui Shi, Tianran Wang, Muhammad Luqman Akhtar, and Yu Li. 2019. "A Cascade-Reaction Enabled Synergistic Cancer Starvation/ROS-Mediated/Chemo-Therapy with an Enzyme Modified FE-Based MOF." *Biomaterials Science* 7 (9): 3683–92. https://doi.org/10.1039/c9bm00641a.

Luo, Qiuhua, Ling Zhang, Cong Luo, and Mingyan Jiang. 2019. "Emerging Strategies in Cancer Therapy Combining Chemotherapy with Immunotherapy." *Cancer Letters* 454: 191–203. https://doi.org/10.1016/j.canlet.2019.04.017.

Man, Francis, Twan Lammers, and Rafael T. M. de Rosales. 2018. "Imaging Nanomedicine-Based Drug Delivery: A Review of Clinical Studies." *Molecular Imaging and Biology* 20 (5): 683–95. https://doi.org/10.1007/s11307-018-1255-2.

Meng, Xiangyu, Kaiying Jia, Kai Sun, Liming Zhang, and Zhifei Wang. 2021. "Smart Responsive Nanoplatform via in Situ Forming Disulfiram-Copper Ion Chelation Complex for Cancer Combination Chemotherapy." *Chemical Engineering Journal* 415: 128947. https://doi.org/10.1016/j.cej.2021.128947.

Meng, Xiangyu, Zhuoxuan Lu, QingyuLv, Yongqiang Jiang, Liming Zhang, and Zhifei Wang. 2022. "Tumor Metabolism Destruction via Metformin-Based Glycolysis Inhibition and Glucose Oxidase-Mediated Glucose Deprivation for Enhanced Cancer Therapy." *Acta Biomaterialia* 145: 222–34. https://doi.org/10.1016/j.actbio.2022.04.022.

Mishra, Alok K., Amjad Ali, Shubham Dutta, Shahid Banday, and Sunil K. Malonia. 2022. "Emerging Trends in Immunotherapy for Cancer." *Diseases* 10 (3): 60. https://doi.org/10.3390/diseases10030060.

Niza, Enrique, Alberto Ocaña, José Antonio Castro-Osma, Iván Bravo, and Carlos Alonso-Moreno. 2021. "Polyester Polymeric Nanoparticles as Platforms in the Development of Novel Nanomedicines for Cancer Treatment." *Cancers* 13 (14): 3387. https://doi.org/10.3390/cancers13143387.

Norouzi, Mohammad, and Pierre Hardy. 2021. "Clinical Applications of Nanomedicines in Lung Cancer Treatment." *Acta Biomaterialia* 121: 134–42. https://doi.org/10.1016/j.actbio.2020.12.009.

Peer, Dan, Jeffrey M. Karp, Seungpyo Hong, Omid C. Farokhzad, Rimona Margalit, and Robert Langer. 2007. "Nanocarriers as an Emerging Platform for Cancer Therapy." *Nature Nanotechnology* 2 (12): 751–60. https://doi.org/10.1038/nnano.2007.387.

Pham, Son H., Yonghyun Choi, and Jonghoon Choi. 2020. "Stimuli-Responsive Nanomaterials for Application in Antitumor Therapy and Drug Delivery." *Pharmaceutics* 12 (7): 630. https://doi.org/10.3390/pharmaceutics12070630.

Prasad, Preethy, Adam Shuhendler, Ping Cai, Andrew M. Rauth, and Xiao Yu Wu. 2013. "Doxorubicin and Mitomycin C Co-Loaded Polymer-Lipid Hybrid Nanoparticles Inhibit Growth of Sensitive and Multidrug Resistant Human Mammary Tumor Xenografts." *Cancer Letters* 334 (2): 263–73. https://doi.org/10.1016/j.canlet.2012.08.008.

Prendergast, George C., William J. Malachowski, Arpita Mondal, Peggy Scherle, and Alexander J. Muller. 2018. "Indoleamine 2,3-Dioxygenase and Its Therapeutic Inhibition in Cancer." *International Review of Cell and Molecular Biology*: 175–203. https://doi.org/10.1016/bs.ircmb.2017.07.004.

Qi, Jing, Feiyang Jin, Yuchan You, Yan Du, Di Liu, Xiaoling Xu, Jun Wang, et al. 2021. "Synergistic Effect of Tumor Chemo-Immunotherapy Induced by Leukocyte-Hitchhiking Thermal-Sensitive Micelles." *Nature Communications* 12 (1). https://doi.org/10.1038/s41467-021-24902-2.

Rasool, Mahmood, Arif Malik, Sulayman Waquar, Mahwish Arooj, Sara Zahid, Muhammad Asif, Sumaira Shaheen, Abrar Hussain, Hamid Ullah, and Siew Hua Gan. 2022. "New Challenges in the Use of

Nanomedicine in Cancer Therapy." *Bioengineered* 13 (1): 759–73. https://doi.org/10.1080/21655979.2021.2012907.

Rezvantalab, Sima, Natascha Ingrid Drude, Mostafa Keshavarz Moraveji, Nihan Güvener, Emily Kate Koons, Yang Shi, Twan Lammers, and Fabian Kiessling. 2018. "PLGA-Based Nanoparticles in Cancer Treatment." *Frontiers in Pharmacology* 9. https://doi.org/10.3389/fphar.2018.01260.

Roy, Aniruddha, Manu Smriti Singh, Pramod Upadhyay, and Sangeeta Bhaskar. 2013. "Nanoparticle Mediated Co-Delivery of Paclitaxel and a TLR-4 Agonist Results in Tumor Regression and Enhanced Immune Response in the Tumor Microenvironment of a Mouse Model." *International Journal of Pharmaceutics* 445 (1–2): 171–80. https://doi.org/10.1016/j.ijpharm.2013.01.045.

Sandesh Arun Patil, Kajal Sunil Shinde, Heena Bholaram Choudhary, Rohan Rajkumar Patekar, and Sachin Devidas Rede. 2021. "Novel Approach in Various Types of Cancer Treatments." *World Journal of Advanced Research and Reviews* 10 (3): 403–11. https://doi.org/10.30574/wjarr.2021.10.3.0291.

Seth, Anushree, Min Beom Heo, and Yong Taik Lim. 2014. "Poly (γ-Glutamic Acid) Based Combination of Water-Insoluble Paclitaxel and TLR7 Agonist for Chemo-Immunotherapy." *Biomaterials* 35 (27): 7992–8001. https://doi.org/10.1016/j.biomaterials.2014.05.076.

Shi, Jinjun, Philip W. Kantoff, Richard Wooster, and Omid C. Farokhzad. 2016. "Cancer Nanomedicine: Progress, Challenges and Opportunities." *Nature Reviews Cancer* 17 (1): 20–37. https://doi.org/10.1038/nrc.2016.108.

Spadavecchia, Jolanda, Dania Movia, Caroline Moore, Ciaran Manus Maguire, Hanane Moustaoui, Sandra Casale, Yuri Volkov, and Adriele Prina-Mello. 2016. "Targeted Polyethylene Glycol Gold Nanoparticles for the Treatment of Pancreatic Cancer: From Synthesis to Proof-of-Concept in Vitro Studies." *International Journal of Nanomedicine*: 791. https://doi.org/10.2147/ijn.s97476.

Su, Shishuai, Yanping Ding, Yiye Li, Yan Wu, and Guangjun Nie. 2016. "Integration of Photothermal Therapy and Synergistic Chemotherapy by a Porphyrin Self-Assembled Micelle Confers Chemosensitivity in Triple-Negative Breast Cancer." *Biomaterials* 80: 169–78. https://doi.org/10.1016/j.biomaterials.2015.11.058.

Taheri-Ledari, Reza, Wenjie Zhang, Maral Radmanesh, Seyedeh Shadi Mirmohammadi, Ali Maleki, Nicole Cathcart, and Vladimir Kitaev. 2020. "Multi-stimuli Nanocomposite Therapeutic: Docetaxel Targeted Delivery and Synergies in Treatment of Human Breast Cancer Tumor." *Small* 16 (41). https://doi.org/10.1002/smll.202002733.

Tian, Hailong, Mengzhu Zhang, Guoxia Jin, Yue Jiang, and Yuxia Luan. 2021. "Cu-MofChemodynamic Nanoplatform via Modulating Glutathione and H2O2 in Tumor Microenvironment for Amplified Cancer Therapy." *Journal of Colloid and Interface Science* 587: 358–66. https://doi.org/10.1016/j.jcis.2020.12.028.

Tilsed, Caitlin M., Scott A. Fisher, Anna K. Nowak, Richard A. Lake, and W. Joost Lesterhuis. 2022. "Cancer Chemotherapy: Insights into Cellular and Tumor Microenvironmental Mechanisms of Action." *Frontiers in Oncology* 12. https://doi.org/10.3389/fonc.2022.960317.

Vanneman, Matthew, and Glenn Dranoff. 2012. "Combining Immunotherapy and Targeted Therapies in Cancer Treatment." *Nature Reviews Cancer* 12 (4): 237–51. https://doi.org/10.1038/nrc3237.

Wang, Jingxue, Ju Huang, Weichen Zhou, Jiawen Zhao, Qi Peng, Liang Zhang, Zhigang Wang, Pan Li, and Rui Li. 2021. "Hypoxia Modulation by Dual-Drug Nanoparticles for Enhanced Synergistic Sonodynamic and Starvation Therapy." *Journal of Nanobiotechnology* 19 (1). https://doi.org/10.1186/s12951-021-00837-0.

Wang, Yi, Guoqing Wei, Xiaobin Zhang, Xuehui Huang, Jingya Zhao, Xing Guo, and Shaobing Zhou. 2017. "Multistage Targeting Strategy Using Magnetic Composite Nanoparticles for Synergism of Photothermal Therapy and Chemotherapy." *Small* 14 (12). https://doi.org/10.1002/smll.201702994.

Wei, Guoqing, Yu Wang, Guang Yang, Yi Wang, and Rong Ju. 2021. "Recent Progress in Nanomedicine for Enhanced Cancer Chemotherapy." *Theranostics* 11 (13): 6370–92. https://doi.org/10.7150/thno.57828.

Wu, Wencheng, Yinying Pu, and Jianlin Shi. 2022. "Nanomedicine-Enabled Chemotherapy-Based Synergetic Cancer Treatments." *Journal of Nanobiotechnology* 20 (1). https://doi.org/10.1186/s12951-021-01181-z.

Wu, Wencheng, Luodan Yu, Quzi Jiang, Minfeng Huo, Han Lin, Liying Wang, Yu Chen, and Jianlin Shi. 2019. "Enhanced Tumor-Specific Disulfiram Chemotherapy by *in Situ* Cu2+ Chelation-Initiated Nontoxicity-to-Toxicity Transition." *Journal of the American Chemical Society* 141 (29): 11531–39. https://doi.org/10.1021/jacs.9b03503.

Xie, Angel, Sumaira Hanif, Jiang Ouyang, Zhongmin Tang, Na Kong, Na Yoon Kim, Baowen Qi, Dylan Patel, Bingyang Shi, and Wei Tao. 2020. "Stimuli-Responsive Prodrug-Based Cancer Nanomedicine." *EBioMedicine* 56: 102821. https://doi.org/10.1016/j.ebiom.2020.102821.

Yu, Jie, Xidong He, Zigui Wang, Sha Liu, Dengyuan Hao, Xiaoyuan Li, and Yubin Huang. 2021. "Combination of Starvation Therapy and PT-NP Based Chemotherapy for Synergistic Cancer Treatment." *Journal of Materials Chemistry B* 9 (32): 6406–11. https://doi.org/10.1039/d1tb01222c.

Yu, Shuangjiang, Zhaowei Chen, Xuan Zeng, Xuesi Chen, and Zhen Gu. 2019. "Advances in Nanomedicine for Cancer Starvation Therapy." *Theranostics* 9 (26): 8026–47. https://doi.org/10.7150/thno.38261.

Zhang, Dan, Lin Liu, Jian Wang, Hong Zhang, Zhuo Zhang, Gang Xing, Xuan Wang, and Minghua Liu. 2022. "Drug-Loaded Peg-Plga Nanoparticles for Cancer Treatment." *Frontiers in Pharmacology* 13. https://doi.org/10.3389/fphar.2022.990505.

Zhang, Xiaojuan, Chuanchuan He, Yun Sun, Xiaoguang Liu, Yan Chen, Chen Chen, Ruicong Yan, et al. 2021. "A Smart O2-Generating Nanocarrier Optimizes Drug Transportation Comprehensively for Chemotherapy Improving." *Acta Pharmaceutica Sinica B* 11 (11): 3608–21. https://doi.org/10.1016/j.apsb.2021.04.021.

Zhang, Xinyu, Haiyan Ge, Yanling Ma, Linlin Song, Yansong Ma, Guanglong Tian, Lei Wang, Qingwei Meng, and Xiao Sun. 2023. "Engineered Anti-Cancer Nanomedicine for Synergistic Ferroptosis-Immunotherapy." *Chemical Engineering Journal* 455: 140688. https://doi.org/10.1016/j.cej.2022.140688.

Zhu, Ruirui, Fangyuan Zhang, Yudong Peng, Tian Xie, Yi Wang, and Yin Lan. 2022. "Current Progress in Cancer Treatment Using Nanomaterials." *Frontiers in Oncology* 12. https://doi.org/10.3389/fonc.2022.930125.

Zou, Lili, Hong Wang, Bin He, Lijuan Zeng, Tao Tan, Haiqiang Cao, Xinyu He, Zhiwen Zhang, Shengrong Guo, and Yaping Li. 2016. "Current Approaches of Photothermal Therapy in Treating Cancer Metastasis with Nanotherapeutics." *Theranostics* 6 (6): 762–72. https://doi.org/10.7150/thno.14988.

16 Strategies Using Nanomedicine to Manage Drug Resistance in Cancer

Divya Dhawal Bhandari, Anuradha Derashri, Nitin Kolhe, Akanksha Dwivedi, Hitesh Chopra, Akriti Sharma, and Arundhati

ABBREVIATIONS

Acronym	Full Form
FDA	Food and Drug Administration
DNA	deoxyribonucleic acid
RNA	ribonucleic acid
RFA	radiofrequency ablation
CT	computed tomography scan
MRI	magnetic resonance imaging
SCID	severe combined immunodeficiency
ADA	adenosine deaminase

16.1 INTRODUCTION

Cancer, a disease, is indicated by the changes in regulatory mechanism involved in the survival, proliferation, and differentiation of cell. Any abnormality in the genetic material of affected cell results in cancer. Genesis of tumor, or tumorigenesis, is a process including multiple steps resulting in mutations in suppressor genes and oncogenes, thus associated with dysregulation of the cell cycle (Nelson, Ferguson, and Denny 2004). Cancer is not only confined to cells but also goes to tissues, resulting in complete loss of connection between epithelial cells and their underlined stromal cells (Bissell and Radisky 2001). Cancer usually forms as a solid tumor, whereas the benign tumors is confined to only one part of the body, does not spread, and is not even threating to life, only except very rare exceptions.

The International Agency for Research on Cancer (IARC) estimated 12.4 million cancer patients by the end of the year 2012, with that number expected to almost triple by 2030 (Sudhakar 2009). Predominately, cancer is thought to be a group of diseases caused by environmental factors, but genetics also commands the risk of many cancers. The use of tobacco, improper diet, obesity, viral infections, and exposure to harmful radiations, stress, lack of physical activity, and environmental pollutants are considered to be the primary factors that contribute to cancer development. It was postulated that these aforementioned factors lead to various abnormalities in the genetic flora and fauna of the cells (Kumar, Abbas, and Aster 2021).

Carcinogenesis involves two major genes, namely, tumor-suppressor genes and oncogenes. Proto-oncogenes (normal genes), which are found in all cells and also act as the regulators of cell cycle, as well as cellular functions, give rise to oncogenes. Any alteration of the genetic material of

DOI: 10.1201/9781003463191-19

proto-oncogenes results in the activation of oncogenes. These alterations may include chromosomal rearrangement, gene amplification, and point mutations, resulting in alteration of the genetic material. The carcinogenic agents involved in altering genes include various chemical agents, radiations, and viruses. These mutations are called somatic mutations, or some mutations may be inherited, known as germ line mutations. The activation of oncogenes results in the production of either normal genes or abnormal genes in infinite number, leading to deregulation of the growth of normal cells, thus imparting growth advantage to cells and increasing probability of neoplastic transformation (Henderson, Bernstein, and Ross 2003). In comparison, tumor-suppressor genes control and inhibit inappropriate cellular growth. Gene mutation results in loss of control over normal cell growth (Abbas et al. 2018).

16.2 VARIOUS AVAILABLE THERAPIES FOR THE TREATMENT OF CANCER

The treatment options available for cancer can be categorized as conventional (traditional) therapies and advanced therapies. As given in Figure 16.1, both traditional and advance therapies are further categorized, where traditional or conventional therapies include radiotherapy, chemotherapy, and surgical removal, while advanced or modern therapies are based on stem cell therapy, targeted drug delivery, gene therapy, antioxidants, immunotherapy, etc. (DiPiro et al. 2017). In today's world, more than 50% of ongoing treatments include clinical trials focused only on cancer treatments (Charmsaz et al. 2019). The treatment option to be selected is based on the site of cancer, its type, and its severity.

16.2.1 Conventional/Traditional Cancer Therapies

The conventional or traditional treatments of cancer comprise the removal of tumor via surgery and then followed by radiations, such as X-rays, as in radiotherapy, or chemicals, as in chemotherapy (Arruebo et al. 2011).

Among the available treatments, the removal of a tumor via surgery is considered one of the most effective way to deal with cancer at an early stage. Radiation therapy can also result in the destruction of healthy cells or organs as well as tissues, whereas chemotherapy is associated with a reduced rate of mortality as well as morbidity. But all chemotherapeutic agents are also associated with damage of rapidly dividing and growing healthy cells (Moses, Brem, and Langer 2003).

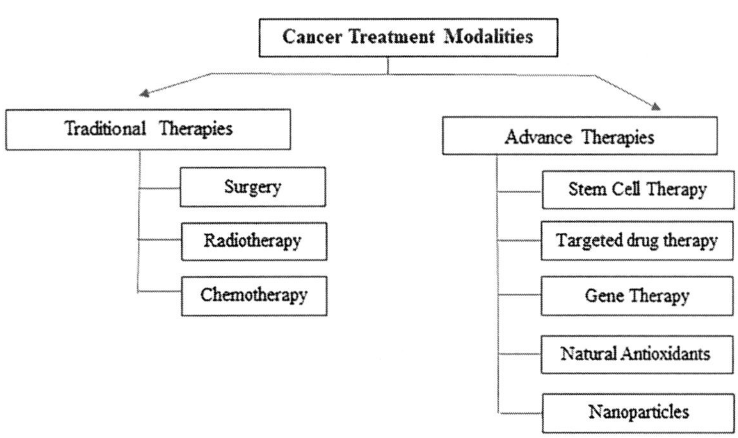

FIGURE 16.1 Modalities of cancer treatment. The flowchart illustrates the classification of cancer treatment modalities into conventional/traditional methods, such as surgery and chemotherapy, and advanced methods, such as stem cell therapy, gene therapy, natural antibodies, etc.

The major problem with chemotherapy is drug resistance, wherein cancer cells develop resistance against anticancer drugs, for which they were getting suppressed earlier due to reduced uptake of drug and increased efflux of drug (Shapira et al. 2011). Another limitation associated with conventional cancer therapies includes difficulty in dose selection, nonspecificity, and fast metabolism of drug and toxic effects (Mondal, Panigrahi, and Khuda-Bukhsh 2014)

16.2.2 Advance and Innovative Cancer Therapies

In lieu of limitations with traditional cancer treatment, some advance and novel cancer treatments, including their advantages and challenges, are stem cell therapy, RFA therapy, gene therapy, ablation cancer therapy, and targeted drug therapy (El-Readi and Althubiti 2019).

16.2.2.1 Stem Cell Therapy

A safe and effective strategy for cancer is stem cell strategy because of their application in the repair of harmed tissues. A number of clinical trials make use of mesenchymal stem cells (MSCs) (Naji et al. 2019) by HSC transplantation (Copelan 2006), infusions of MSC (Casper et al. 2010), therapeutic transporters (Sage, Thakrar, and Janes 2016), generation of immune impactor cells (Dai et al. 2016), and vaccine generation (Batlle and Clevers 2017).

The major drawbacks of stem cell therapy are (1) genesis of tumor, (2) adverse effects associated with allogeneic HSC transplantation, (3) drug toxicity as well as drug resistance, (4) elevated immune responses as well as autoimmunity, and (5) viral infection (Chu et al. 2020). Though a number of trials have been proved successful and also showed promising results, there are associated challenges of dose control, tumor site retention, safety, efficacy, and low cell targeting.

16.2.2.2 Targeted Drug Therapy

Targeted drug therapy is based on the mechanism of blocking growth and the spread of cancer by interfering with growth molecules (Bethesda n.d.). As it is difficult to select cancer cells by chemotherapy, since they look like normal cells, targeted therapy is more appropriate, which works at the cellular level, such as in the induction of apoptosis, preventing proliferation, interfering in metabolic reprogramming, and cell cycle arrest. Targeted therapy is mainly focused toward attacking only cancer cells while providing little damage to normal cells (Debela et al. 2021).

Targeted therapy has resulted in an increased rate of survival for certain conditions; for example, the survival rate increased from 17 to 24% in pancreatic cancer by adding erlotinib to chemotherapy, whereas in case of chronic myeloid leukemia, imatinib had a dramatic effect. Similarly, in case of renal and breast cancer, rituximab, sunitinib, and trastuzumab have revolutionized the treatment (Weber 2006).

Targeted therapy works by various ways, such as enzyme inhibitors, which work by inhibiting signals for the growth of cancer cells (Citri and Yarden 2006), or by inducing apoptosis, such as serine/threonine kinase, protein kinase B (PKB/Akt), which are associated with cell survival promotion (Luo, Manning, and Cantley 2003).

Additionally, they prevent the tumors from growing by preventing them from growing new blood vessels, which cut off the tumors' blood supply (Hurwitz et al. 2004). Various types of target agents include:

- Monoclonal antibodies
- Small molecule inhibitors

16.2.2.3 Ablation Cancer Therapy

Ablation, a technique associated with the destruction of tumor cell without their removal, is thus recommended only for tumors which are less than 3 cm in size. This technique is not preferred for tumors which are found near the diaphragm, bile ducts, or any other major blood vessels, as it results in the destruction of useful tissues of the body also (Salati et al. 2017). It includes thermal ablation as well as cryoablation.

16.2.2.4 RFA Therapy

RFA makes use of high-frequency electric current to destroy cancer cells, or alternatively, it can be called a minimally invasive procedure, also known as image-guided technique, and is far better than earlier available imaging techniques, such as ultrasound, CT, and MRI, because they insert needle electrodes into tumor cells. RFA is effective only in treating very little-size tumors, which are less than 3 cm in diameter, or it can be used as a combination technique with conventional cancer options (Izzo et al. 2019).

16.2.2.5 Gene Therapy

Gene therapy includes adding a copy of normal gene into a defective one to get rid of specific kinds of disorder. It was first included in 1990 with the help of a retroviral vector in patients of SCID (severe combined immunodeficiency) (Brace 2011). The vector was broken down to get ADA, that is, adenosine deaminase gene, into T cells. As of now, about 2,900 clinical trials are going on based on gene therapy, out of which 1,933 trials are related to the treatment of various types of cancer. These trials are based on strategies including expressions of tumor suppressor genes of wild type, proapoptotic genes, chemosensitizing genes, and oncogene silencing (Freeman et al. 1993; Ahrendt et al. 2003; Raty et al. 2008; Elbashir et al. 2001; Weiss, Davidkova, and Zhou 1999; Putney et al. 1999).

16.2.2.6 Natural Antioxidants

Natural antioxidants, such as vitamins, plant-derived compounds, and polyphenols, possess anti-inflammatory and antioxidant properties, which make use of them in studying drugs against cancer (Bernardini et al. 2018). The most actively screened *in vitro* and *in vivo* natural antioxidants are vitamins, alkaloids, flavonoids, curcumin, and quercetin (Chikara et al. 2018). These natural antioxidants are associated with various challenges, such as low bioavailability, and there are also chances of toxicity with their translation (Pucci, Martinelli, and Ciofani 2019); (Imran et al. 2018). Curcumin is one of the most effective natural antioxidants to date, which is under clinical trials to study tumors of the brain, lung, blood, pancreas, and hepatocellular cells. Similarly, berberine and quercetin are also under clinical trials for their chemopreventive activities, as they modulate many signaling pathways and can be used in combination with other available chemotherapeutic agents (Farooqi et al. 2019). These natural antioxidants show poor solubility, thus making path for various other strategies to facilitate their delivery through tumor cells (Liu et al. 2017). Among them, nanotechnology is one of the current methods to be focused on in oncology for the development of safe and effective anticancer drugs (Yang et al. 2015).

16.3 DEVELOPMENT OF DRUG RESISTANCE IN CANCER

Tolerance of cancer to already-available pharmaceutical treatments is well-known as drug resistance (Urruticoechea et al. 2010). Drug resistance is one of the main challenges during anticancer treatment, which arises from a number of factors, including genetic mutation, changes in various cellular and molecular mechanism, upregulation of drug efflux, or epigenetic changes (Baskar et al. 2012; Damin and Lazzaron 2014), as shown in Figure 16.2. Drug resistance in cancer also develops via inactivation of drug therapy, alterations in the target of drug, DNA mutations, inhibition of cell death, and DNA damage repair. The advance cancer treatments are surgery, chemotherapy, targeted therapy, immunotherapy, and radiation therapy, but despite advancement in all these available methods, the major problem to date is resistance of cancer cells towards chemotherapy, which act as the main cause of death in cancer (Lumachi et al. 2011; Mondal, Panigrahi, and Khuda-Bukhsh 2014). Drug resistance in cancer poses significant challenges in managing the disease. The overexpression of ATP-binding cassette (ABC) transporter proteins on cancer cell membranes leads to reduced

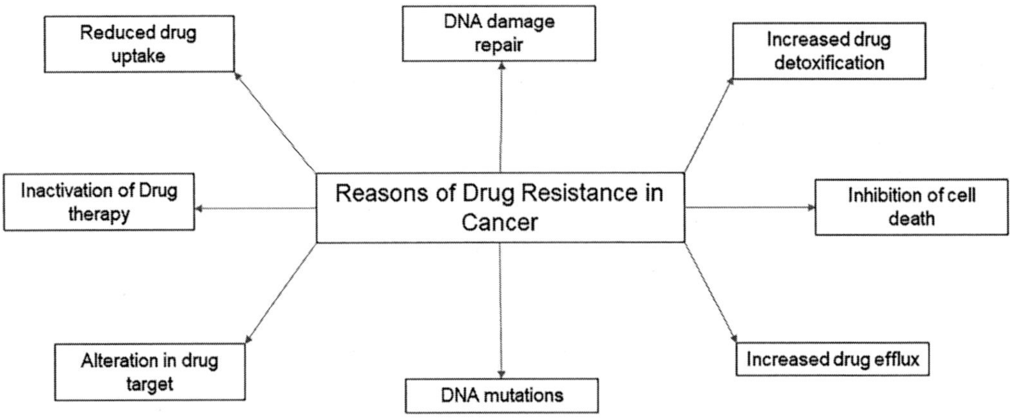

FIGURE 16.2 Various mechanisms/pathways for the development of drug resistance in cancer. The figure describes the various mechanisms involved in developing resistance against cancer treatment. There are a number of pathways involved, some of which include increased efflux of drug, reduced uptake of drug, mutations in the DNA, alterations in the drug target, inactivation of drug therapy, or an increase in drug detoxification.

drug uptake, increased drug detoxification, and improved drug efflux efficiency. This, along with other physiological abnormalities, hinders the therapeutic efficacy of drugs (Seyedi et al. 2023).

Resistance in cancer opens up various paths to screen the tumor mass and its rate of growth, physical barriers, immunological behavior, environment of the cell, irreversible genetic mutation, and side effects of available treatment approaches. To overcome drug resistance, various strategies have been explored, including co-delivery of drugs with MDR inhibitors, augmented dosage regimens, and combinatorial treatment options which can overcome intrinsic drug resistance (before treatment) associated with the changes in drug efflux and uptake (Lin-Rahardja et al. 2023). While treatment of acquired drug resistance (developed after treatment) due to certain epigenetic abnormalities is a clinical challenge (Nikolaou et al. 2018), the complexity of drug resistance in cancer suggests the use of either combination therapy or personalized therapy based on the type of resistance developed. The recent advancements in nanomedicines or nanotechnology are opening up various pathways to overcome drug resistance through a number of mechanisms, some of which include increasing pharmacokinetics, reducing toxicity associated with chemotherapy as they selectively target the cancer cells. Also, nanoformulations increase the therapeutic index of the drug to be delivered (Nikolaou et al. 2018). Further advancements are being done toward nanotechnology-based cancer treatments having less side effect as compared to conventional therapies. Industries are working more on nanotechnology these days to get them through biological barriers and to detect molecular mechanisms involved in cancer. Overall, drug resistance can be stated as:

- *Prime determinant for drug resistance.* Basically, cancer is a three-tier system which includes therapy, population of cancer cells, and a host environment.
- *Overcoming drug resistance.* Drug resistance can be overcome by early diagnosis, enhanced response surveillance of cancer therapy and adaptable strategies, and utilization of cancer dependence.
- *Nanotechnology against drug resistance.* Nanotechnology or nanomedicines are opening up novel approaches for reaching the most profound level of solid tumors with chemotherapeutic drugs delivered at the genomic level, giving new possibilities for anticancer treatment. The pharmaceutical nanomedicine-based anticancer treatments include polymeric composite vehicles and self-assembling nanoscale structures, such as micelles and dendrimers (Sharma et al. 2022).

16.4 ROLE OF NANOTECHNOLOGY FOR OVERCOMING CANCER DRUG RESISTANCE

Uncountable efforts are going on by various researchers toward the achievement of the most efficacious cancer treatment and a substitute for chemotherapy (Setyawati et al. 2017; Tay, Setyawati, and Leong 2017). Amidst the various endeavors to cure and enhance the effectiveness of anticancer medications, nanotechnologies have surfaced as a novel domain (Wang et al. 2018; Ge et al. 2020). Properties such as small size, surface charge, and mass density, give a relatively large surface area, facilitating the functionalization of nanoparticles with all the possible ligand, such as DNA, RNA, peptides, antibodies, etc. (Ganbold et al. 2019; Jia et al. 2020; Guan and Zhang 2020; Marques et al. 2020). These ligands help in delivering nanoparticles at their site of action *in vivo*, thus increasing pharmacokinetics of the nanoparticles. The role of nanomedicine as a combination therapy with radio- and chemotherapy is also getting investigated (Bakshi et al. 2019; Das et al. 2019; González-Ballesteros et al. 2019; Song et al. 2019).

16.4.1 Mechanism of Action of Nanoparticles in Overcoming Drug Resistance in Cancer

Nanoparticles-induced anticancer mechanism is based on apoptosis of cancer cells, which includes a number of mechanisms, among which the reactive oxygen species–mediated apoptosis is the most suitable one (Ferrari et al. 2018). Other mechanisms involved in the action of nanoparticles in inducing apoptosis of cancer cells include down- or upregulation of proteins, intervention in immune system, inhibition of transcription, and site-specific cytotoxicity, as mentioned in Figure 16.3. In case of drug resistance, the apoptosis pathway becomes inactive due to enhanced expression of antiapoptotic family, while on the other hand, DNA repair ability increases, followed by increased drug efflux and intoxication. Thus, cancer cells can easily survive and become unresponsive to ongoing cancer treatment. Specific drug-loaded targeted nanoparticles result in upregulation of apoptosis-associated proteins and downregulation of antiapoptotic family. Also, polymer-based nanoparticles have been proven to induce more apoptosis and also results in enhancement of pharmacokinetics of anticancer drug (Hu et al. 2022).

The increased drug efflux also results in the development of drug resistance in cancer, which, in turn, is due to overexpression of ATP-binding cassete (ABC) or reduced drug intake or DNA repair activation, etc. The associted drug resistance can be overcome by achieving a high concentration of drug in the plasma and by increasing retention time of the drug. Nanoparticles release drug through a number of delivery systems, such as dendrimers, nanoshells, nanotubes, micelles, magentic naoparticles, which can overcome or inhibit or bypass such efflux pumps, resulting in a high concentration of drug at the site of action (Xue and Liang 2012).

Multidrug resistance can also be overcome by combination therapy of chemoterapeutics with nanoparticles for a targeted and controlled drug delivery.

16.4.2 Types of Nanomedicines against Cancer

The first nanoparticle-based chemotheraputic drug, Doxil, was introduced in the market in 1995, which is almost 25 years ago, but still there are very few authorized nanomedicines for the treatment of cancer. Though a number of researchers are working on nanoparticles for cancer, only few products have reached clinical trials. Only 16 nano-based cancer drugs have been approved to date by the FDA, and 75 nanoformulations are in clinical trials for cancer. The major nanomedicines available for the management of cancer are given in Figure 16.4 (He et al. 2019).

16.4.2.1 Liposome-Based Nanoparticles

Most of the drugs or nanomedicines for cancer are formulated as liposomes-based nanodrugs because of their adaptability and feasibility toward biodegradability and biocompatibility (Pandey,

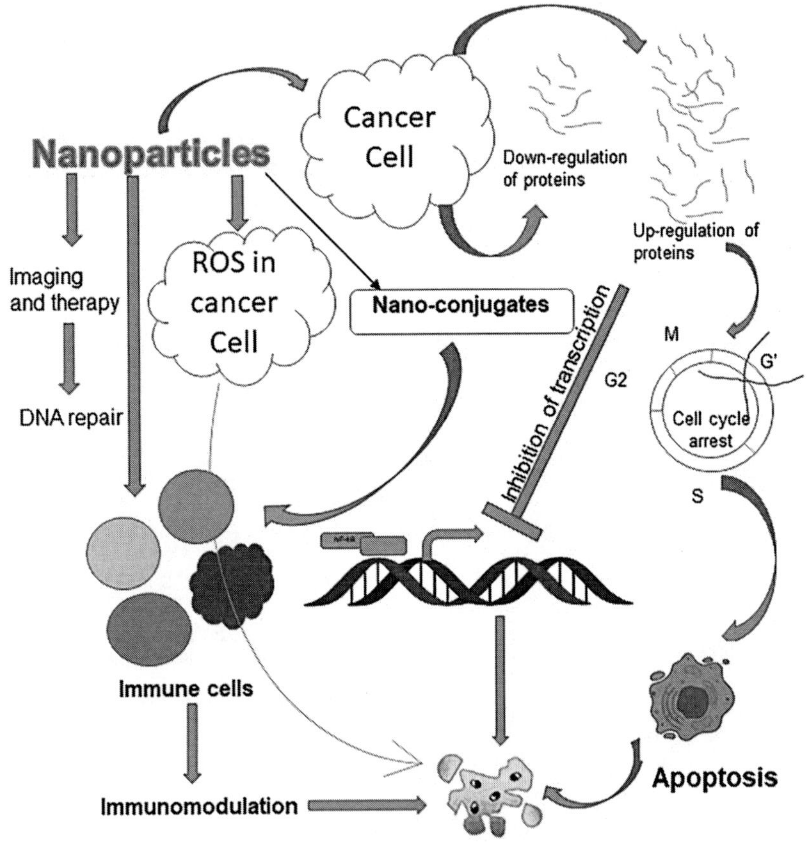

FIGURE 16.3 Nanoparticles-induced anticancer mechanism. A schematic representation illustrating anticancer action of nanoparticles through apoptosis of cancer cells via either upregulation or downregulation of cell proteins. Nanoparticles also induce their anticancer effect via ROS-mediated apoptosis of cancer cells or by inhibiting transcription process in cells.

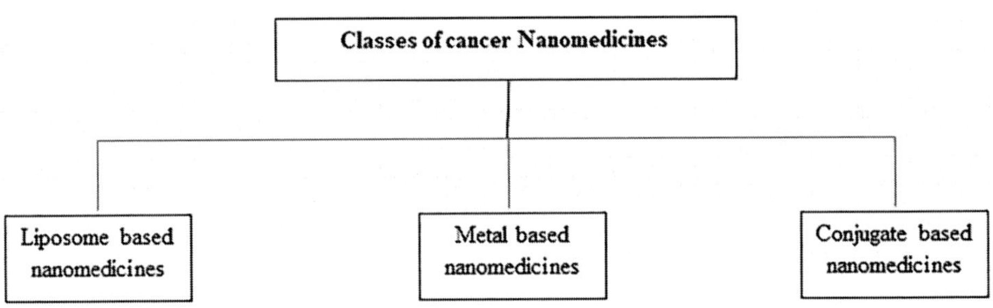

FIGURE 16.4 Various types of nanomedicines against cancer. The flowchart depicts the categories of nanomedicines available in the market for the treatment of cancer, which includes liposome-based, metal-based, and some conjugate nanomedicines.

Rani, and Agarwal 2016; Olusanya et al. 2018). Liposomes have an additional property to combine with both lipophilic as well as hydrophilic compounds; thus, they can be functionalized with numerous molecules, such as polyethylene glycol, proteins, peptides, carbohydrates, or other tiny molecules being focused on liposomes. The nature of liposome nanoparticles makes them the prime

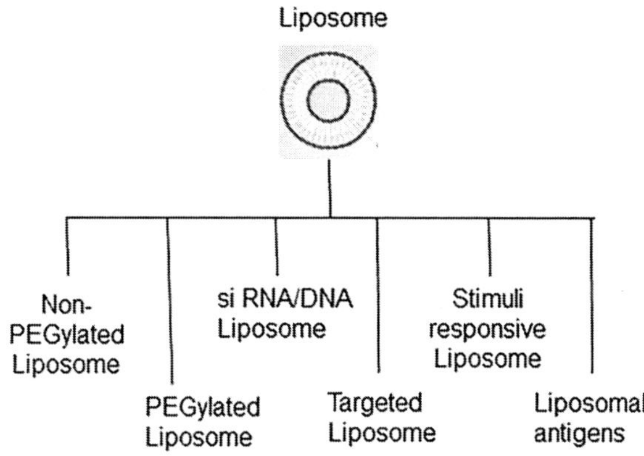

FIGURE 16.5 Various types of liposome-based nanoparticles. The flowchart depicts the category of liposome-based nanomedicines which can be further divided as PEGylated, non-PEGylated, or derived from DNA/RNA or may act as targeted, responsive to stimulus liposome, or as an antigen.

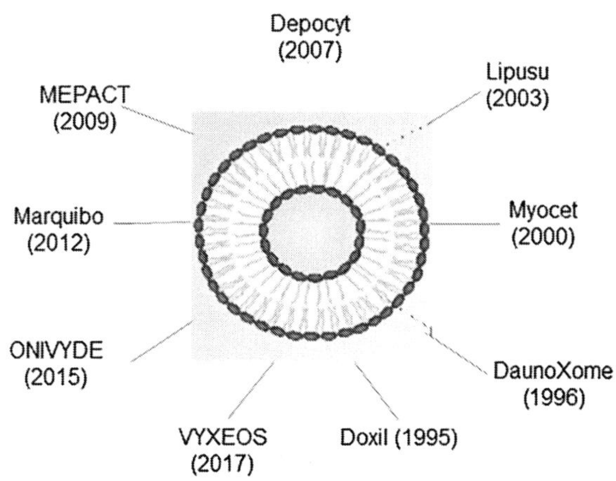

FIGURE 16.6 A liposome-based nanochemotherapeutic drug approved by the FDA. The figure describes a number of nanomedicines against cancer approved by the FDA per year, starting from 1995 to 2017, and also their approved names.

drugs in clinical trials going on cancer-based drugs. During the delivery of drug, the phospholipid bilayer, which is present in liposomes, protects the drug, which is being embedded, from the liver, from biological inactivation, and also from chemical and any immunological changes inside the body. The major advantage associated with liposomal nanoparticles is that the healthy and non-targeted cells are prevented from the vicinity of the drug. Liposome-based nanoparticles work through different pathways, including modification of liposomes for controlled and sustained drug release, or can be modified as ligand-targeted liposomes for intracellular drug delivery in resistant cancer cells and by direct interaction with glycoproteins and their inhibition through endocytosis. Various types of liposome-based nanoparticles are PEGylated, non-PEGylated, liposome antigens, siDNA/RNA-based liposomes, etc., as shown in Figure 16.5. FDA has also approved few liposome-based nanomedicines against drug resistance in cancer, as given in Figure 16.6 (Rommasi and Esfandiari 2021).

Metal/Metal Oxide based Eloxatin Aqupla Nedaplatib	**Conjugate based** Oncaspar
Polymer/Lipid Oxide based DHP107 PICN ELIGARD ABRAXANE	**Polymeric micelle based** Apealea Genoxol

FIGURE 16.7 Metal, metal oxides, polymer, and other conjugates. The illustration describes examples of metal and conjugate categories of nanomedicines. The metal-based nanomedicines include only metal or oxides of metal. They may also be polymer-based or act as conjugates with micelles or lipid oxides.

16.4.2.2 Metal-, Metal Oxide–, Polymer-, and Other Conjugates-Based Nanoparticles

Along with lipid-based nanomedicines, the drugs containing metal or the oxides of metal, polymeric micelles, polymers/lipid, or other conjugate are also in various stages of approval in clinical trials (Ndagi, Mhlongo, and Soliman 2017). Platinum is among the most exploited metals for the delivery of anticancer drugs. Another anticancer drug based on metal which was used first is cisplatin (Lakshmi et al. 2021). Another metal-based drug permitted by the FDA in combination therapy is platinol, along with carboplatin, sabriplatin, ormaplatin, oxaliplatin, etc. Platinum-based drugs are challenging to use in clinical trials, which have opened up the paths for the use of gold, silver, selenium, iron, and ruthenium (Mignani et al. 2021; Gul et al. 2021; Varlamova, Turovsky, and Blinova 2021). Future research can examine an increasing number of metal complexes due to the efficacy of metal-based nanodrugs (Figure 16.7) (Lorkowski et al. 2021).

Nanoscale self-assembled amphiphilic generated micelles have the ability to migrate across cancer cells' endothelial intersections and discharge medication in the vicinity of the tumor microenvironment; thus, these polymeric micelles are more effective than liposome and other liquid nanoparticles for the delivery of drugs, even in resistant tumor cells (Mundekkad and Cho 2022). Polymeric micelles that have core-shell structure improve the solubility of drugs, and water-insoluble drugs can also be entrapped easily by various physical and chemical conjugations (Lorkowski et al. 2021; Persano and Gigli n.d.; Jana et al. 2009). Based on properties of lipids and polymers as nanomedicines, a new system which is based on lipid-polymer nanoparticles has been discovered, which is the hybrid structure, containing polymer core surrounded by a shell of lipids (Payne et al. 2006). Metal-, metal oxide–, polymer-, and conjugate-based nanoparticles are believed to overcome drug resistance by increasing the uptake of drugs into tumor cells, accumulating more drug, inducing apoptosis of cancer cells, increasing bioavailability of drug, and suppressing glycoproteins responsible for multidrug resistance.

16.4.3 Challenges of Using Nanoparticles in Clinical Trials against Drug Resistance

Despite a number of developments being made by nanomedicines as anticancer drugs, there are a lot of challenges to bring nanodrugs from clinical trials to market against drug resistance, one of which includes the absence of proper understanding of the mechanism of action of nanoparticles with biomolecules (Ventola 2017). Some nanomedicine-based anticancer drugs, for example, DepoCyt, Clariscan, and Lumirem, have been discontinued by pharmaceutical companies due to various technical issues, even after having been approved by the FDA (Fymat 2017). Other associated challenges include:

- Predicting pattern of patient toward allergic reactions against nanomedicine
- Endotoxin quantification
- Internalization of the drug at cellular level
- Sustained release
- Breaking through biological boundaries and increasing bioavailability
- Increasing the capability of target toward tumor cells for functionalization
- Keeping control on the response of immune system toward new drug
- Lengthy drug development process
- The duration of time needed for human clinical and preclinical research
- Tedious process to obtain regulatory approval of releasing drug in the market
- Failure to load the drug effectively inside nanoparticles
- Formulation instability
- Problems associated with toxicity and biocompatibility
- Shorter time spent inside the human body
- Failure to accumulate drug formulation on target
- Incomplete biodegradation, elimination, and disappointment to translate *in vitro* results into *in vivo* studies

16.4.4 Recent Advances in Tumor Therapeutics with Nanoparticles

A number of nanodrugs against cancer have undergone a number of clinical trials in the past few years for various different types of cancers, which are given in Table 16.1.

TABLE 16.1
Nanomedicines Under Clinical Trials for Managing Cancer Drug Resistance

S. No.	Name of Nanodrug	Conventional Drug	Type of Cancer	Reference
1	Paclitaxel Nab	5-fluorouracil, epirubicin, cyclophosphamide, phenelzine sulfate, (FEC) ceritinib, cisplatin, gemcitabine hydrochloride, cetuximab, IMRT	Breast cancer, metastatic breast cancer, head and neck cancer	Wurz et al. (2014)
2	NC-6004 (NP-cisplatin)	Gemcitabine	Solid tumors	Young et al. (2011)
3	CRLX101 (cyclodextrin-based polymer)	Camptothecin	NSCLC, primary peritoneal cancer	Gargett et al. (2018)
4	CPC634 (CriPec®)	Docetaxel	Ovarian tumors	Ishikawa et al. (2021)
5	AGuIX	Polysiloxane gadolinium-chelates type nanoparticles	Brain metastases	Yardley et al. (2015)
6	Docetaxel-PNP	Taxotere	Solid tumors	Weng et al. (2020)
7	VYXEOS	Cytarabine, daunorubicin	Acute myeloid leukemia	Ogino et al. (2021)
8	ONPATTRO	Patisiran	Transthyretin amyloidosis	Gargett et al. (2018)

16.5 CONCLUSION AND FUTURE PROSPECTS

Navigating the complex realm of drug resistance within cancer treatment has been a journey illuminating diverse pathways toward effective management. It is believed that exposure to nanoparticles for a longer duration may result in damage to their penetrating power and toxicity. Use of nanomedicine in cancer diagnosis as well as therapy has opened new pathways for researchers. With the help of nanotechnology, any region of the body can be targeted easily, which is difficult for other available macromolecular drugs. For example, the original fiber-optic dosimetric device is based on nanomaterial which is used to quantify *in vivo* dose of radiations given during radiotherapy sessions (Yada et al. 2020). Also, a number of advancements have been made already in fighting with cancer; still, there are associated challenges, side effects, and toxicity issues associated with the use of other methods, along with problems related to regulation approval. The contribution of scientists, academics, regulatory authorities, and industries can result in the formation of a patient-centric nanomedicine model which may provide a new era for the development of advancements in cancer.

REFERENCES

Abbas, Zaigham, Sakina Rehman, Zaigham Abbas, and Sakina Rehman. 2018. *Neoplasm*. Intech Open. https://doi.org/10.5772/INTECHOPEN.76558.

Ahrendt, Steven A., Yingchuan Hu, Martin Buta, Michael P. McDermott, Nicole Benoit, Stephen C. Yang, Li Wu, and David Sidransky. 2003. "P53 Mutations and Survival in Stage I Non-Small-Cell Lung Cancer: Results of a Prospective Study." *Journal of the National Cancer Institute* 95 (13): 961–70. https://doi.org/10.1093/JNCI/95.13.961.

Arruebo, Manuel, Nuria Vilaboa, Berta Sáez-Gutierrez, Julio Lambea, Alejandro Tres, Mónica Valladares, and África González-Fernández. 2011. "Assessment of the Evolution of Cancer Treatment Therapies." *Cancers* 3 (3): 3279–330. https://doi.org/10.3390/CANCERS3033279.

Bakshi, Saira, Andrey Zakharchenko, Sergiy Minko, Dmitry M. Kolpashchikov, and Evgeny Katz. 2019. "Towards Nanomaterials for Cancer Theranostics: A System of DNA-Modified Magnetic Nanoparticles for Detection and Suppression of RNA Marker in Cancer Cells." *Magnetochemistry* 5 (2): 24. https://doi.org/10.3390/MAGNETOCHEMISTRY5020024.

Baskar, Rajamanickam, Kuo Ann Lee, Richard Yeo, and Kheng Wei Yeoh. 2012. "Cancer and Radiation Therapy: Current Advances and Future Directions." *International Journal of Medical Sciences* 9 (3): 193–9. https://doi.org/10.7150/IJMS.3635.

Batlle, Eduard, and Hans Clevers. 2017. "Cancer Stem Cells Revisited." *Nature Medicine* 23 (10): 1124–34. https://doi.org/10.1038/nm.4409.

Bernardini, S., A. Tiezzi, V. Laghezza Masci, and E. Ovidi. 2018. "Natural Products for Human Health: An Historical Overview of the Drug Discovery Approaches." *Natural Product Research* 32 (16): 1926–50. https://doi.org/10.1080/14786419.2017.1356838.

Bethesda, MD. n.d. "Targeted Therapy for Cancer—NCI." www.cancer.gov/about-cancer/treatment/types/targeted-therapies (accessed December 17, 2023).

Bissell, Mina J., and Derek Radisky. 2001. "Putting Tumours in Context." *Nature Reviews: Cancer* 1 (1): 46. https://doi.org/10.1038/35094059.

Brace, Chris. 2011. "Thermal Tumor Ablation in Clinical Use." *IEEE Pulse* 2 (5): 28–38. https://doi.org/10.1109/MPUL.2011.942603.

Casper, Jochen, Daniel Wolff, Wolfgang Knauf, Igor W. Blau, Tapani Ruutu, Liisa Volin, Hannes Wandt, et al. 2010. "Allogeneic Hematopoietic Stem-Cell Transplantation in Patients with Hematologic Malignancies After Dose-Escalated Treosulfan/Fludarabine Conditioning." *Journal of Clinical Oncology: Official Journal of the American Society of Clinical Oncology* 28 (20): 3344–51. https://doi.org/10.1200/JCO.2009.23.3429.

Charmsaz, Sara, Denis M. Collins, Antoinette S. Perry, and Maria Prencipe. 2019. "Novel Strategies for Cancer Treatment: Highlights from the 55th IACR Annual Conference." *Cancers* 11 (8). https://doi.org/10.3390/CANCERS11081125.

Chikara, Shireen, Lokesh Dalasanur Nagaprashantha, Jyotsana Singhal, David Horne, Sanjay Awasthi, and Sharad S. Singhal. 2018. "Oxidative Stress and Dietary Phytochemicals: Role in Cancer Chemoprevention and Treatment." *Cancer Letters* 413 (January): 122–34. https://doi.org/10.1016/J.CANLET.2017.11.002.

Chu, Dinh Toi, Tiep Tien Nguyen, Nguyen Le Bao Tien, Dang Khoa Tran, Jee Heon Jeong, Pham Gia Anh, Vo Van Thanh, Dang Tien Truong, and Thien Chu Dinh. 2020. "Recent Progress of Stem Cell Therapy in Cancer Treatment: Molecular Mechanisms and Potential Applications." *Cells* 9 (3). https://doi.org/10.3390/CELLS9030563.

Citri, Ami, and Yosef Yarden. 2006. "EGF-ERBB Signalling: Towards the Systems Level." *Nature Reviews. Molecular Cell Biology* 7 (7): 505–16. https://doi.org/10.1038/NRM1962.

Copelan, Edward A. 2006. "Hematopoietic Stem-Cell Transplantation." *The New England Journal of Medicine* 354 (17): 1813–26. https://doi.org/10.1056/NEJMRA052638.

Dai, Hanren, Yao Wang, Xuechun Lu, and Weidong Han. 2016. "Chimeric Antigen Receptors Modified T-Cells for Cancer Therapy." *Journal of the National Cancer Institute* 108 (7). https://doi.org/10.1093/JNCI/DJV439.

Damin, Daniel C., and Anderson R. Lazzaron. 2014. "Evolving Treatment Strategies for Colorectal Cancer: A Critical Review of Current Therapeutic Options." *World Journal of Gastroenterology* 20 (4): 877–87. https://doi.org/10.3748/WJG.V20.I4.877.

Das, Manisit, Limei Shen, Qi Liu, Tyler J. Goodwin, and Leaf Huang. 2019. "Nanoparticle Delivery of RIG-I Agonist Enables Effective and Safe Adjuvant Therapy in Pancreatic Cancer." *Molecular Therapy* 27 (3): 507. https://doi.org/10.1016/J.YMTHE.2018.11.012.

Debela, Dejene Tolossa, Seke G.Y. Muzazu, Kidist Digamo Heraro, Maureen Tayamika Ndalama, Betelhiem Woldemedhin Mesele, Dagimawi Chilot Haile, Sophia Khalayi Kitui, and Tsegahun Manyazewal. 2021. "New Approaches and Procedures for Cancer Treatment: Current Perspectives." *Sage Open Medicine* 9. https://doi.org/10.1177/20503121211034366.

DiPiro, Joseph T., Robert L. Talbert, Gary C. Yee, Gary R. Matzke, Barbara G. Wells, and L. M. Posey. 2017. "Pharmacotherapy: A Pathophysiologic Approach." In *Chapter 15: Hypertension*, 8th edition. The McGrawHill.

Elbashir, Sayda M., Jens Harborth, Winfried Lendeckel, Abdullah Yalcin, Klaus Weber, and Thomas Tuschl. 2001. "Duplexes of 21-Nucleotide RNAs Mediate RNA Interference in Cultured Mammalian Cells." *Nature* 411 (6836): 494–8. https://doi.org/10.1038/35078107.

El-Readi, Mahmoud Zaki, and Mohammad Ahmad Althubiti. 2019. "Cancer Nanomedicine: A New Era of Successful Targeted Therapy." *Journal of Nanomaterials* 2019: 1–15. https://doi.org/10.1155/2019/4927312.

Farooqi, Ammad Ahmad, Muhammad Zahid Qureshi, Sumbul Khalid, Rukset Attar, Chiara Martinelli, Yerzhan Sabitaliyevich Uteuliyev, Bolat Nurmurzayevich Sadykov, Simona Taverna, Palmiro Poltronieri, and Baojun Xu. 2019. "Regulation of Cell Signaling Pathways by Berberine in Different Cancers: Searching for Missing Pieces of an Incomplete Jig-Saw Puzzle for an Effective Cancer Therapy." *Cancers* 11 (4): 478. https://doi.org/10.3390/CANCERS11040478.

Ferrari, R., M. Sponchioni, M. Morbidelli, and D. Moscatelli. 2018. "Polymer Nanoparticles for the Intravenous Delivery of Anticancer Drugs: The Checkpoints on the Road from the Synthesis to Clinical Translation." *Nanoscale* 10 (48): 22701–19. https://doi.org/10.1039/C8NR05933K.

Freeman, Scott M., Camille Abboud, Scott M. Freeman, Charles H. Packman, David S. Koeplin, Frederick L. Moolten, and George N. Abraham. 1993. "The 'Bystander Effect': Tumor Regression When a Fraction of the Tumor Mass Is Genetically Modified." *Cancer Research* 53 (21): 5274–83. https://pure.johnshopkins.edu/en/publications/the-bystander-effect-tumor-regression-when-a-fraction-of-the-tumo-3.

Fymat, Alain L. 2017. "Magnetic Resonance Imaging Modalities with Contrast Enhancing Nanomaterials." *Current Trends in Clinical & Medical Imaging* 1 (1): 11–14. https://doi.org/10.19080/CTCMI.2017.01.555554.

Ganbold, Tsogzolmaa, Shuqin Han, Agula Hasi, and Huricha Baigude. 2019. "Receptor-Mediated Delivery of Therapeutic RNA by Peptide Functionalized Curdlan Nanoparticles." *International Journal of Biological Macromolecules* 126 (April): 633–40. https://doi.org/10.1016/J.IJBIOMAC.2018.12.152.

Gargett, Tessa, M. Nazim Abbas, Paul Rolan, Jason D. Price, Katharine M. Gosling, Antonio Ferrante, Andrew Ruszkiewicz, et al. 2018. "Phase I Trial of Lipovaxin-MM, a Novel Dendritic Cell-Targeted Liposomal Vaccine for Malignant Melanoma." *Cancer Immunology, Immunotherapy: CII* 67 (9): 1461–72. https://doi.org/10.1007/S00262-018-2207-Z.

Ge, Huan, Dongya Wang, Yue Pan, Yuanyuan Guo, Hongyu Li, Fan Zhang, Xinyuan Zhu, Yuehua Li, Chuan Zhang, and Ling Huang. 2020. "Sequence-Dependent DNA Functionalization of Upconversion Nanoparticles and Their Programmable Assemblies." *Angewandte Chemie International Edition* 59 (21): 8133–37. https://doi.org/10.1002/ANIE.202000831.

González-Ballesteros, N., L. Diego-González, M. Lastra-Valdor, M. C. Rodríguez-Argüelles, M. Grimaldi, A. Cavazza, F. Bigi, and R. Simón-Vázquez. 2019. "Immunostimulant and Biocompatible Gold and

Silver Nanoparticles Synthesized Using the Ulva Intestinalis L. Aqueous Extract." *Journal of Materials Chemistry B* 7 (30): 4677–91. https://doi.org/10.1039/C9TB00215D.

Guan, Baozhang, and Xingwang Zhang. 2020. "Aptamers as Versatile Ligands for Biomedical and Pharmaceutical Applications." *International Journal of Nanomedicine* 15: 1059. https://doi.org/10.2147/IJN.S237544.

Gul, Anam Rana, Farhat Shaheen, Rafia Rafique, Jyotiranjan Bal, Shahid Waseem, and Tae Jung Park. 2021. "Grass-Mediated Biogenic Synthesis of Silver Nanoparticles and Their Drug Delivery Evaluation: A Biocompatible Anti-Cancer Therapy." *Chemical Engineering Journal* 407 (March). https://doi.org/10.1016/J.CEJ.2020.127202.

He, Hongliang, Lisha Liu, Emily E. Morin, Min Liu, and Anna Schwendeman. 2019. "Survey of Clinical Translation of Cancer Nanomedicines-Lessons Learned from Successes and Failures." *Accounts of Chemical Research* 52 (9): 2673–83. https://doi.org/10.1021/ACS.ACCOUNTS.9B00228.

Henderson, Brian E., Leslie Bernstein, and Ronald K. Ross. 2003. "Hormones and the Etiology of Cancer." www.ncbi.nlm.nih.gov/books/NBK13706/.

Hu, Tingting, Hanlin Gong, Jiayue Xu, Yuan Huang, Fengbo Wu, and Zhiyao He. 2022. "Nanomedicines for Overcoming Cancer Drug Resistance." *Pharmaceutics* 14 (8). https://doi.org/10.3390/pharmaceutics14081606.

Hurwitz, Herbert, Louis Fehrenbacher, William Novotny, Thomas Cartwright, John Hainsworth, William Heim, Jordan Berlin, et al. 2004. "Bevacizumab plus Irinotecan, Fluorouracil, and Leucovorin for Metastatic Colorectal Cancer." *The New England Journal of Medicine* 350 (23): 2335–42. https://doi.org/10.1056/NEJMOA032691.

Imran, Muhammad, Azmat Ullah, Farhan Saeed, Muhammad Nadeem, Muhammad Umair Arshad, and Hafiz Ansar Rasul Suleria. 2018. "Cucurmin, Anticancer, & Antitumor Perspectives: A Comprehensive Review." *Critical Reviews in Food Science and Nutrition* 58 (8): 1271–93. https://doi.org/10.1080/10408398.2016.1252711.

Ishikawa, Takeshi, Shinichi Kageyama, Yoshihiro Miyahara, Tetsuya Okayama, Satoshi Kokura, Linan Wang, Eiichi Sato, Hideo Yagita, Yoshito Itoh, and Hiroshi Shiku. 2021. "Safety and Antibody Immune Response of CHP-NY-ESO-1 Vaccine Combined with Poly-ICLC in Advanced or Recurrent Esophageal Cancer Patients." *Cancer Immunology, Immunotherapy: CII* 70 (11): 3081–91. https://doi.org/10.1007/S00262-021-02892-W.

Izzo, Francesco, Vincenza Granata, Roberto Grassi, Roberta Fusco, Raffaele Palaia, Paolo Delrio, Gianpaolo Carrafiello, Daniel Azoulay, Antonella Petrillo, and Steven A Curley. 2019. "Radiofrequency Ablation and Microwave Ablation in Liver Tumors: An Update." *The Oncologist* 24 (10): e990–1005. https://doi.org/10.1634/THEONCOLOGIST.2018-0337.

Jana, Deblin, Shaorui Jia, Anivind Kaur Bindra, Pengyao Xing, Dan Ding, and Yanli Zhao. 2009. "Clearable Black Phosphorus Nanoconjugate for Targeted Cancer Phototheranostics." *ACS Applied Materials and Interfaces* 12 (16): 18342–51. https://doi.org/10.1021/ACSAMI.0C02718.

Jia, Xiangqian, Mingmei Guo, Qiuju Han, Yuwei Tian, Yafei Yuan, Zihua Wang, Yixia Qian, and Weizhi Wang. 2020. "Synergetic Tumor Probes for Facilitating Therapeutic Delivery by Combined-Functionalized Peptide Ligands." *Analytical Chemistry* 92 (8): 5650–5. https://doi.org/10.1021/ACS.ANALCHEM.0C00440/ASSET/IMAGES/LARGE/AC0C00440_0004.JPEG.

Kumar, Vinay, Abul Abbas, and Jon Aster. 2021. "Diseases of the Immune System—Amyloidosis." Edited by Kumar Vinay, Abul K. Abbas, and Jon C. Aster. *Robbins & Cotran Pathologic Basis of Disease*: 259–65.

Lakshmi, Buddolla Anantha, Ankireddy Seshadri Reddy, Roopkumar Sangubotla, Jong Wook Hong, and Sanghyo Kim. 2021. "Ruthenium(II)-Curcumin Liposome Nanoparticles: Synthesis, Characterization, and Their Effects against Cervical Cancer." *Colloids and Surfaces. B, Biointerfaces* 204 (August). https://doi.org/10.1016/J.COLSURFB.2021.111773.

Lin-Rahardja, Kristi, Davis T. Weaver, Jessica A. Scarborough, and Jacob G. Scott. 2023. "Evolution-Informed Strategies for Combating Drug Resistance in Cancer." *International Journal of Molecular Sciences* 24 (7): 6738. https://doi.org/10.3390/IJMS24076738.

Liu, Yue, Zhen Gang Tang, Yi Lin, Xin Guo Qu, Wei Lv, Guo Bin Wang, and Cai Li. 2017. "Effects of Quercetin on Proliferation and Migration of Human Glioblastoma U251 Cells." *Biomedicine & Pharmacotherapy = Biomedecine & Pharmacotherapie* 92 (August): 33–38. https://doi.org/10.1016/J.BIOPHA.2017.05.044.

Lorkowski, Morgan E., Prabhani U. Atukorale, Ketan B. Ghaghada, and Efstathios Karathanasis. 2021. "Stimuli-Responsive Iron Oxide Nanotheranostics: A Versatile and Powerful Approach for Cancer Therapy." *Advanced Healthcare Materials* 10 (5). https://doi.org/10.1002/ADHM.202001044.

Lumachi, Franco, Giovanni Luisetto, S. Mm Basso, U. Basso, A. Brunello, and Valentina Camozzi. 2011. "Endocrine Therapy of Breast Cancer." *Current Medicinal Chemistry* 18 (4): 469–91. https://doi.org/10.2174/092986711794480177.

Luo, Ji, Brendan D. Manning, and Lewis C. Cantley. 2003. "Targeting the PI3K-Akt Pathway in Human Cancer: Rationale and Promise." *Cancer Cell* 4 (4): 257–62. https://doi.org/10.1016/S1535-6108(03)00248-4.

Marques, A. C., P. J. Costa, S. Velho, and M. H. Amaral. 2020. "Functionalizing Nanoparticles with Cancer-Targeting Antibodies: A Comparison of Strategies." *Journal of Controlled Release: Official Journal of the Controlled Release Society* 320 (April): 180–200. https://doi.org/10.1016/J.JCONREL.2020.01.035.

Mignani, Serge, Xiangyang Shi, Valentin Ceña, João Rodrigues, Helena Tomas, and Jean Pierre Majoral. 2021. "Engineered Non-Invasive Functionalized Dendrimer/Dendron-Entrapped/Complexed Gold Nanoparticles as a Novel Class of Theranostic (Radio)Pharmaceuticals in Cancer Therapy." *Journal of Controlled Release: Official Journal of the Controlled Release Society* 332 (April): 346–66. https://doi.org/10.1016/J.JCONREL.2021.03.003.

Mondal, J., A. K. Panigrahi, and A. R. Khuda-Bukhsh. 2014. "Conventional Chemotherapy: Problems and Scope for Combined Therapies with Certain Herbal Products and Dietary Supplements." *Journal of Molecular and Cell Biology* 1 (1): 10–12. https://austinpublishinggroup.com/molecular-cellular-biology/fulltext/ajmcb-v1-id1002.php.

Moses, Marsha A., Henry Brem, and Robert Langer. 2003. "Advancing the Field of Drug Delivery: Taking Aim at Cancer." *Cancer Cell* 4 (5): 337–41. https://doi.org/10.1016/S1535-6108(03)00276-9.

Mundekkad, Deepa, and William C. Cho. 2022. "Nanoparticles in Clinical Translation for Cancer Therapy." *International Journal of Molecular Sciences* 23 (3). https://doi.org/10.3390/IJMS23031685.

Naji, Abderrahim, Masamitsu Eitoku, Benoit Favier, Frédéric Deschaseaux, Nathalie Rouas-Freiss, and Narufumi Suganuma. 2019. "Biological Functions of Mesenchymal Stem Cells and Clinical Implications." *Cellular and Molecular Life Sciences: CMLS* 76 (17): 3323–48. https://doi.org/10.1007/S00018-019-03125-1.

Ndagi, Umar, Ndumiso Mhlongo, and Mahmoud E. Soliman. 2017. "Metal Complexes in Cancer Therapy—an Update from Drug Design Perspective." *Drug Design, Development and Therapy* 11 (March): 599–616. https://doi.org/10.2147/DDDT.S119488.

Nelson, Stephanie M., Lynnette R. Ferguson, and William A. Denny. 2004. "DNA and the Chromosome—Varied Targets for Chemotherapy." *Cell & Chromosome* 3 (May): 2. https://doi.org/10.1186/1475-9268-3-2.

Nikolaou, Michail, Athanasia Pavlopoulou, Alexandros G. Georgakilas, and Efthymios Kyrodimos. 2018. "The Challenge of Drug Resistance in Cancer Treatment: A Current Overview." *Clinical & Experimental Metastasis* 35 (4): 309–18. https://doi.org/10.1007/S10585-018-9903-0.

Ogino, Misato, Takaaki Fujii, Yukio Koibuchi, Yuko Nakazawa, Daisuke Takata, and Ken Shirabe. 2021. "Phase II Study of Nab-Paclitaxel Plus Cyclophosphamide Plus Trastuzumab Neoadjuvant Chemotherapy in Early HER-2-Positive Breast Cancer." *Anticancer Research* 41 (8): 3899–904. https://doi.org/10.21873/Anticancer.15185.

Olusanya, Temidayo O. B., Rita Rushdi Haj Ahmad, Daniel M. Ibegbu, James R. Smith, and Amal Ali Elkordy. 2018. "Liposomal Drug Delivery Systems and Anticancer Drugs." *Molecules (Basel, Switzerland)* 23 (4). https://doi.org/10.3390/MOLECULES23040907.

Pandey, Himanshu, Radha Rani, and Vishnu Agarwal. 2016. "Liposome and Their Applications in Cancer Therapy." *Brazilian Archives of Biology and Technology* 59 (March): e16150477. https://doi.org/10.1590/1678-4324-2016150477.

Payne, Miranda, Paul Ellis, David Dunlop, Malcolm Ranson, Sarah Danson, Lee Schacter, and Denis Talbot. 2006. "DHA-Paclitaxel (Taxoprexin) as First-Line Treatment in Patients with Stage IIIB or IV Non-Small Cell Lung Cancer: Report of a Phase II Open-Label Multicenter Trial." *Journal of Thoracic Oncology* 1 (9): 984–90. https://doi.org/10.1016/s1556-0864(15)31631-2.

Persano, Francesca, and Giuseppe Gigli. n.d. "Lipid-Polymer Hybrid Nanoparticles in Cancer Therapy: Current Overview and Future Directions." *Nano Express* 2 (1): 2–15.

Pucci, Carlotta, Chiara Martinelli, and Gianni Ciofani. 2019. "Innovative Approaches for Cancer Treatment: Current Perspectives and New Challenges." *Ecancermedicalscience* 13 (September). https://doi.org/10.3332/ECANCER.2019.961.

Putney, Scott D., Josiah Brown, Carla Cucco, Rino Lee, Tomasz Skorski, Carlo Leonetti, Timothy Geiser, Bruno Calabretta, Gabriella Zupi, and Gerald Zon. 1999. "Enhanced Anti-Tumor Effects with Microencapsulated c-Myc Antisense Oligonucleotide." *Antisense & Nucleic Acid Drug Development* 9 (5): 451–8. https://doi.org/10.1089/OLI.1.1999.9.451.

Raty, J., J. Pikkarainen, T. Wirth, and S. Yla-Herttuala. 2008. "Gene Therapy: The First Approved Gene-Based Medicines, Molecular Mechanisms and Clinical Indications." *Current Molecular Pharmacology* 1 (1): 13–23. https://doi.org/10.2174/1874467210801010013.

Rommasi, Foad, and Neda Esfandiari. 2021. "Liposomal Nanomedicine: Applications for Drug Delivery in Cancer Therapy." *Nanoscale Research Letters* 16 (1): 95. https://doi.org/10.1186/S11671-021-03553-8.

Sage, Elizabeth K., Ricky M. Thakrar, and Sam M. Janes. 2016. "Genetically Modified Mesenchymal Stromal Cells in Cancer Therapy." *Cytotherapy* 18 (11): 1435–45. https://doi.org/10.1016/J.JCYT.2016.09.003.

Salati, Umer, Aisling Barry, Frank Y. Chou, Roy Ma, and David M. Liu. 2017. "State of the Ablation Nation: A Review of Ablative Therapies for Cure in the Treatment of Hepatocellular Carcinoma." *Future Oncology* 13 (16). https://doi.org/10.2217/FON-2017-0061.

Setyawati, Magdiel I., Chor Yong Tay, Boon Huat Bay, and David T. Leong. 2017. "Gold Nanoparticles Induced Endothelial Leakiness Depends on Particle Size and Endothelial Cell Origin." *ACS Nano* 11 (5): 5020–30. https://doi.org/10.1021/ACSNANO.7B01744/SUPPL_FILE/NN7B01744_SI_001.PDF.

Seyedi, Sareh, Valerie K. Harris, Stefania E. Kapsetaki, Shrinath Narayanan, Daniel Saha, Zachary Compton, Rezvan Yousefi, et al. 2023. "Resistance Management for Cancer: Lessons from Farmers." April. https://arxiv.org/abs/2304.00402v1.

Shapira, Alina, Yoav D. Livney, Henk J. Broxterman, and Yehuda G. Assaraf. 2011. "Nanomedicine for Targeted Cancer Therapy: Towards the Overcoming of Drug Resistance." *Drug Resistance Updates: Reviews and Commentaries in Antimicrobial and Anticancer Chemotherapy* 14 (3): 150–63. https://doi.org/10.1016/J.DRUP.2011.01.003.

Sharma, Madhu, Avijit Kumar Bakshi, Naresh Mittapelly, Shalini Gautam, Disha Marwaha, Nikhil Rai, Neha Singh, et al. 2022. "Recent Updates on Innovative Approaches to Overcome Drug Resistance for Better Outcomes in Cancer." *Journal of Controlled Release: Official Journal of the Controlled Release Society* 346 (June): 43–70. https://doi.org/10.1016/J.JCONREL.2022.04.007.

Song, Shilong, Xiaoxiao Jin, Lei Zhang, Chen Zhao, Yan Ding, Qianqian Ang, Odontuya Khaidav, and Chuanlai Shen. 2019. "PEGylated and CD47-Conjugated Nanoellipsoidal Artificial Antigen-Presenting Cells Minimize Phagocytosis and Augment Anti-Tumor T-Cell Responses." *International Journal of Nanomedicine* 14: 2465–83. https://doi.org/10.2147/IJN.S195828.

Sudhakar, Akulapalli. 2009. "History of Cancer, Ancient and Modern Treatment Methods." *Journal of Cancer Science & Therapy* 1 (2): i–iv. https://doi.org/10.4172/1948-5956.100000E2.

Tay, Chor Yong, Magdiel Inggrid Setyawati, and David Tai Leong. 2017. "Nanoparticle Density: A Critical Biophysical Regulator of Endothelial Permeability." *ACS Nano* 11 (3): 2764–72. https://doi.org/10.1021/ACSNANO.6B07806/SUPPL_FILE/NN6B07806_SI_001.PDF.

Urruticoechea, A., R. Alemany, J. Balart, A. Villanueva, F. Vinals, and G. Capella. 2010. "Recent Advances in Cancer Therapy: An Overview." *Current Pharmaceutical Design* 16 (1): 3–10. https://doi.org/10.2174/138161210789941847.

Varlamova, Elena G., Egor A. Turovsky, and Ekaterina V. Blinova. 2021. "Therapeutic Potential and Main Methods of Obtaining Selenium Nanoparticles." *International Journal of Molecular Sciences* 22 (19): 10808. https://doi.org/10.3390/IJMS221910808.

Ventola, C. Lee. 2017. "Progress in Nanomedicine: Approved and Investigational Nanodrugs." *Pharmacy and Therapeutics* 42 (12): 742. https://www.ncbi.nlm.nih.gov/pmc/articles/PMC5720487/.

Wang, Jinping, Luyao Zhang, Fei Peng, Xinghua Shi, and David Tai Leong. 2018. "Targeting Endothelial Cell Junctions with Negatively Charged Gold Nanoparticles." *Chemistry of Materials* 30 (11): 3759–67. https://doi.org/10.1021/ACS.CHEMMATER.8B00840/SUPPL_FILE/CM8B00840_SI_002.PDF.

Weber, Wolfgang A. 2006. "Positron Emission Tomography as an Imaging Biomarker." *Journal of Clinical Oncology: Official Journal of the American Society of Clinical Oncology* 24 (20): 3282–92. https://doi.org/10.1200/JCO.2006.06.6068.

Weiss, B., G. Davidkova, and L. W. Zhou. 1999. "Antisense RNA Gene Therapy for Studying and Modulating Biological Processes." *Cellular and Molecular Life Sciences: CMLS* 55 (3): 334–58. https://doi.org/10.1007/S000180050296.

Weng, Xiuhua, Xiaoting Huang, Hongchao Li, Shen Lin, Xin Rao, Xianzhong Guo, and Pinfang Huang. 2020. "First-Line Treatment with Atezolizumab Plus Nab-Paclitaxel for Advanced Triple-Negative Breast Cancer: A Cost-Effectiveness Analysis." *American Journal of Clinical Oncology* 43 (5): 340–8. https://doi.org/10.1097/COC.0000000000000671.

Wurz, Gregory T., Chiao Jung Kao, Michael Wolf, and Michael W. DeGregorio. 2014. "Tecemotide: An Antigen-Specific Cancer Immunotherapy." *Human Vaccines & Immunotherapeutics* 10 (11): 3383. https://doi.org/10.4161/HV.29836.

Xue, Xue, and Xing Jie Liang. 2012. "Overcoming Drug Efflux-Based Multidrug Resistance in Cancer with Nanotechnology." *Chinese Journal of Cancer* 31 (2): 100. https://doi.org/10.5732/CJC.011.10326.

Yada, Ryuichi, Kazusuke Maenaka, Shuji Miyamoto, Go Okada, Aki Sasakura, Motoi Ashida, Masashi Adachi, et al. 2020. "Real-Time in Vivo Dosimetry System Based on an Optical Fiber-Coupled Microsized Photostimulable Phosphor for Stereotactic Body Radiation Therapy." *Medical Physics* 47 (10): 5235–49. https://doi.org/10.1002/MP.14383.

Yang, Feiya, Liming Song, Huiping Wang, Jun Wang, Zhiqing Xu, and Nianzeng Xing. 2015. "Quercetin in Prostate Cancer: Chemotherapeutic and Chemopreventive Effects, Mechanisms and Clinical Application Potential (Review)." *Oncology Reports* 33 (6): 2659–68. https://doi.org/10.3892/OR.2015.3886.

Yardley, Denise A., Adam Brufsky, Robert E. Coleman, Pierfranco F. Conte, Javier Cortes, Stefan Glück, Jean Mark A. Nabholtz, et al. 2015. "Phase II/III Weekly Nab-Paclitaxel plus Gemcitabine or Carboplatin versus Gemcitabine/Carboplatin as First-Line Treatment of Patients with Metastatic Triple-Negative Breast Cancer (the TnAcity Study): Study Protocol for a Randomized Controlled Trial." *Trials* 16 (1). https://doi.org/10.1186/S13063-015-1101-7.

Young, Cissy, Thomas Schluep, Jungyeon Hwang, and Scott Eliasof. 2011. "CRLX101 (Formerly IT-101)–A Novel Nanopharmaceutical of Camptothecin in Clinical Development." *Current Bioactive Compounds* 7 (1): 8. https://doi.org/10.2174/157340711795163866.

Index

N

O

P